Breastfeeding and Metabolic Programming

Özlem Naciye Şahin • Despina D. Briana
Gian Carlo Di Renzo

Editors

Breastfeeding and Metabolic Programming

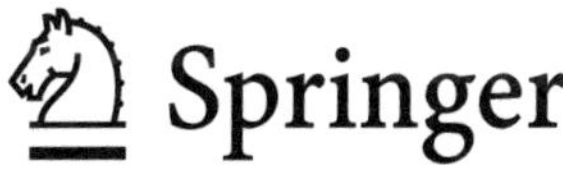 Springer

Editors
Özlem Naciye Şahin
Department of Child Health and Diseases
Arel University, Medical Faculty
Istanbul, Türkiye

Despina D. Briana
Pediatrics Department
National and Kapodistrian University of
Athens, Greece

Gian Carlo Di Renzo
Department of Obstetrics and Gynecology
University of Perugia
Perugia, Perugia, Italy

ISBN 978-3-031-33280-7   ISBN 978-3-031-33278-4   (eBook)
https://doi.org/10.1007/978-3-031-33278-4

This Springer imprint is published by the registered company Springer Nature Switzerland AG
The registered company address is: Gewerbestrasse 11, 6330 Cham, Switzerland

Preface

It is very well known that breastmilk is the healthiest option for newborns as the source of nutrients, improves immunity, and for many other known and unknown mechanisms.

Metabolic programming stands at a not well-known site. Long-term health is affected by prenatal and early postnatal environments, the developmental origins of health and illness theory suggests. Growing data from human studies show that insufficient and excessive nutrition during pregnancy can alter gene expression and have lasting effects on child phenotypes through epigenetic alterations. In light of the possibility of its application in the programming of both health and illness, epigenetics has garnered considerable interest. Little is understood, however, about the processes through which early postnatal diet can influence long-term health.

Recent research shows that several common prenatal exposures, such as intrauterine growth restriction, extremes of birth weight, maternal obesity, and maternal diabetes, are linked to increased fat mass, decreased muscle mass, and decreased bone density, with effects reported throughout infancy, childhood, and middle age. Genetic and epigenetic factors, stem cell commitment and function, mitochondrial metabolism, and maternal food are mechanisms and mediators. Changes in body composition are a typical phenotype after exposure to adverse conditions during pregnancy, and they may play a role in the prenatal programming of obesity and diabetes risk.

This book synthesizes the findings of several fields of studies into a single, accessible volume, focusing on the central idea of breastmilk and metabolic programming.

Initially, I would like to express my most heartfelt thanks to my father, Orhan Rami Atan, a well-known geology professor, who made me love science. My father told me about the importance of biological differentiation, that is, evolutionary processes, in the adaptation process of living things in the name of survival, by witnessing the changes of the same species over millennia and the fossils of geological periods he showed me in childhood. My father discovered and analyzed many fault lines, including the northern Anatolian fault line, sometimes on foot in the Taurus

Mountains, sometimes on horseback, and showed them to us by transferring them to geology education books.

I offer my sincerest appreciation to Gian Carlo Di Renzo and Despina D. Briana, who were accepted to be co-authors with me, to Cemal Cingi and Nuray Bayar Muluk, who planned and edited the "Breastfeeding: Special Conditions and Issues" section.

Last but not least, my appreciation is to Ayse Engin Arisoy, a leader or even a hero with her intelligence, wisdom, and knowledge in the newborn era of our country, and Emin Sami Arisoy, who is a hard worker but always stays calm. They guided me in planning the contents of the book.

This book will be helpful for readers and set the first step for other papers and books in this field.

Istanbul, Türkiye   Özlem Naciye Şahin
Athens, Greece   Despina D. Briana
Perugia, Perugia, Italy   Gian Carlo Di Renzo
March 2, 2023

Contents

Contributors

Nitin R. Ankle, MD Department of ENT & Head-Neck Surgery, KLE Academy of Higher Education & Research (KAHER), J. N. Medical College, Belagavi, Karnataka, India

Ayşe Engin Arısoy, MD Faculty of Medicine, Division of Neonatology, Department of Pediatrics, Kocaeli University (Emeritus), Kocaeli, Türkiye

Emin Sami Arısoy, MD Faculty of Medicine, Division of Pediatric Infectious Diseases, Department of Pediatrics, Kocaeli University (Emeritus), Kocaeli, Türkiye

İlke Özer Aslan, MD Faculty of Medicine, Department of Obstetrics and Gynecology, Tekirdag Namık Kemal University, Tekirdag, Türkiye

Mustafa Törehan Aslan, MD Division of Neonatology, Department of Pediatrics, Faculty of Medicine, Tekirdağ Namık Kemal University, Tekirdağ, Türkiye

Ali Timucin Atayoglu, MD Department of Family Medicine, Istanbul Medipol University, International School of Medicine, Istanbul, Türkiye

Ayten Guner Atayoglu, MD Department of Family Medicine, Beylikdüzü State Hospital, Istanbul, Türkiye

Elad Azizli, MD Otorhinolaryngology Specialist, Private Practice, Istanbul, Türkiye

Gabriela Kopacheva Barsova, MD, PhD Faculty of Medicine, Cyril and Methodius University of Skopje, Skopje, Republic of Macedonia

Jeffrey C. Bedrosian, MD Rhinology and Skull Base Surgery, Specialty Physician Associates, St. Luke's Medical Center, Bethlehem, PA, USA

Özlem Bekem, MD Division of Pediatric Gastroenterology, Hepatology and Nutrition, Department of Pediatrics, Health Sciences University, Dr Behcet Uz Children's Hospital, İzmir, Türkiye

Vesim Bekraki, MD Department of Pediatrics, Türkiye Hospital, İstanbul, Türkiye

Luisa Maria Bellussi, MD University of Siena- ENT Clinic, Siena, Italy

Taylan Bilici, MD Department of Otorhinolaryngology, Adana Seyhan State Hospital, Adana, Türkiye

Despina D. Briana, MD, PhD NICU, Third Department of Pediatrics, National and Kapodistrian University of Athens, University General Hospital "ATTIKON", Athens, Greece

Rezzan Budak, MD Department of Otorhinolaryngology, Şehit Sait Ertürk State Hospital, Ankara, Türkiye

Demet Can, MD Division of Allergy and Immunology, Department of Pediatrics, Izmir Dr. Behcet Uz Children's Hospital, Izmir, Türkiye

Peter Catalano, MD, FACS, FARS Department of Otolaryngology, Tufts University, School of Medicine, St. Elizabeth's Medical Center, Boston, MA, USA

İpek Dokurel Çetin, MD Faculty of Medicine, Division of Pediatric Neurology, Department of Pediatrics, Balikesir University, Balikesir, Türkiye

Aykut Ceyhan, MD Department of Otorhinolaryngology, Kutahya Evliya Çelebi Training and Research Hospital, Kutahya, Türkiye

Dennis Chua, MD Department of Otorhinolaryngology, ENT Surgeons Medical Centre, Mount Elizabeth Hospital, Singapore, Singapore

Can Cemal Cingi, PhD Faculty of Communication Sciences, Department of Communication Design and Management, Anadolu University, Eskişehir, Türkiye

Cemal Cingi, MD Medical Faculty, Department of Otorhinolaryngology, Eskisehir Osmangazi University, Eskisehir, Türkiye

Funda Çipe, MD Department of Pediatric Allergy-Immunology, Al Qassimi Women's and Children's Hospital, Sharjah, United Arab Emirates

Armando G. Correa, MD Division of Academic General Pediatrics, Department of Pediatrics, Baylor College of Medicine, and Section of International and Destination Medicine, Texas Children's Hospital, Houston, TX, USA

Tuğçe Damla Dilek, MD Cerrahpasa Medical Faculty, Division of Pediatric Neurology, Department of Pediatrics, Istanbul University, Istanbul, Türkiye

Gian Carlo Di Renzo, MD, PhD Centre of Perinatal Medicine of the University of Perugia/Sechenov University, Moscow, Russia

Keziban Doğan, MD Department of Obstetrics and Gynecology, University of Health Sciences, Bakırköy Dr. Sadi Konuk Training and Research Hospital, İstanbul, Türkiye

Riza Dundar, MD Medical Faculty, Department of Otorhinolaryngology, Bilecik Seyb Edebali University, Bilecik, Türkiye

Yusuf Dundar, MD Department of Otolaryngology-Head and Neck Surgery, Texas Tech University, Health Sciences Center, Lubbock, TX, USA

Dilek Eroğlu, PhD School of Foreign Languages, Department of Foreign Languages, Anadolu University, Eskişehir, Türkiye

Gülbin Gökçay, MD Division of Social Pediatrics, Department of Pediatrics, İstanbul Faculty of Medicine, İstanbul University, İstanbul, Türkiye

Department of Social Pediatrics, Institute of Child Health, Istanbul University, İstanbul, Türkiye

Hilal Güngör, MD Department of Internal Medicine, Eskisehir City Hospital, Eskisehir, Türkiye

Selis Gülseven Güven, MD Medical Faculty, Department of Otorhinolaryngology, Trakya University, Edirne, Türkiye

Özge Kaba, MD İstanbul Faculty of Medicine, Division of Pediatric Infectious Diseases, Department of Pediatrics, İstanbul University, İstanbul, Türkiye

İstanbul Çam and Sakura Hospital, Section of Pediatric Infectious Diseases, University of Health Science, İstanbul, Türkiye

Sheldon L. Kaplan, MD Division of Infectious Diseases, Department of Pediatrics, Baylor College of Medicine, and Infectious Disease Service, Texas Children's Hospital, Houston, TX, USA

Bülent Kara, MD Faculty of Medicine, Division of Pediatric Neurology, Department of Pediatrics, Kocaeli University, Kocaeli, Türkiye

Sait Karaman, MD Division of Allergy and Immunology, Department of Pediatrics, Manisa City Hospital, Manisa, Türkiye

Ayşe Karaoğullarindan Department of Otorhinolaryngology, Adana City Hospital, Adana, Türkiye

Sergei Karpischenko, MD Department of Otorhinolaryngology, The First Pavlov State Medical University of Saint Petersburg, St. Petersburg, Russia

Yıldız Ekemen Keleş, MD University of Health Sciences, Tepecik Training and Research Hospital, Section of Pediatric Infectious Diseases, İzmir, Türkiye

Mustafa Caner Kesimli, MD Caner Kesimli Private ENT Clinic, Istanbul, Türkiye

Gonca Keskindemirci, MD Division of Social Pediatrics, Department of Pediatrics, İstanbul Faculty of Medicine, İstanbul University, İstanbul, Türkiye

Saltuk Bugra Kilinc, MD Department of Otorhinolaryngology, Yozgat Sarıkaya State Hospital, Yozgat, Türkiye

Ahmet Köder, MD Medical Faculty, Department of Otorhinolaryngology, Trakya University, Edirne, Türkiye

Mehtap Koparal, MD Department of Otorhinolaryngology, Health Sciences University, Adıyaman Training and Research Hospital, Adıyaman, Türkiye

Nagehan Dilsad Erdogdu Küçükcan, MD Department of Otorhinolaryngology, Çukurova State Hospital, Adana, Türkiye

Nevin Cambaz Kurt, MD Department of Pediatrics, Başakşehir Çam and Sakura City Hospital, İstanbul, Türkiye

Fatma Levent, MD Division of Pediatric Infectious Diseases, Department of Pediatrics, School of Medicine, Texas Tech University, Lubbock, TX, USA

Mario Milkov, MD Faculty of Medicine, Department of Otorhinolaryngology, Varna University, Varna, Bulgaria

Nuray Bayar Muluk, MD Medical Faculty, Department of Otorhinolaryngology, Kirikkale University, Kirikkale, Türkiye

Hesham Negm, MD Faculty of Medicine, Department of Otorhinolaryngology, Cairo University, Cairo, Egypt

Derin Oygar, MD Department of Pediatric Infectious Diseases, Neurology Department, Dr. Burhan Nalbantoğlu State Hospital, Nicosia, Northern Cyprus

Seyhan Erişir Oygucu, MD Division of Neonatology, Department of Pediatrics, University of Kyrenia, Kyrenia, Cyprus

Senem Alkan Özdemir, MD Department of Neonatology, Behçet Uz Children's Hospital, Health Sciences University, İzmir, Türkiye

Samim Ozen, MD Medical Faculty, Pediatric Endocrinologiy Division, Department of Pediatrics, Ege University, Izmir, Türkiye

Aysel Özpınar, MD Medical Faculty, Department of Basic Sciences, Medical Biochemistry, Acibadem Mehmet Ali Aydinlar University, Istanbul, Türkiye

Gülten Öztürk, MD Division of Pediatric Neurology, Department of Pediatrics, Marmara University Pendik Education and Research Hospital, İstanbul, Türkiye

Fatih Palit, MD Department of Nephrology, Basaksehir Çam and Sakura City Training and Research Hospital, İstanbul, Türkiye

Muhammet Pamukcu, MD Medical Faculty, Department of Otorhinolaryngology, Istanbul Altinbas University, İstanbul, Türkiye

Desiderio Passali, MD, PhD Department of Medical, Surgical and Neuroscience Sciences, University of Siena, Siena, Italy

Department of Otorhinolaryngology, University of Siena, Siena, Italy

Özge Serçe Pehlevan, MD Faculty of Medicine, Division of Neonatology, Department of Pediatrics, Kocaeli University, Kocaeli, Türkiye

Esra Polat, MD Division of Pediatric Gastroenterology, Department of Pediatrics, Health Sciences University, Umraniye Education and Research Hospital, Istanbul, Türkiye

Özlem Naciye Şahin, MD, PhD Department of Child Health and Diseases, Arel University, Medical Faculty, Istanbul, Türkiye

Suela Sallavaci, MD, MSc, PhD Department of Otorhinolaryngology, University Hospital Centre "Mother Teresa", Tirana, Albania

Sema Saltık, MD Cerrahpasa Medical Faculty, Division of Pediatric Neurology, Department of Pediatrics, Istanbul University, Istanbul, Türkiye

Özlem Sancaklı, MD Division of Allergy and Immunology, Department of Pediatrics, Izmir Dr. Behcet Uz Children's Hospital, Izmir, Türkiye

Codrut Sarafoleanu, MD Sfanta Maria Clinical Hospital ENT&HNS Department, University of Medicine and Pharmacy "Carol Davila", Bucharest, Romania

Glenis Scadding, MD, FRCP University College Hospital London, RNENT Hospital, London, UK

Muhittin Abdülkadir Serdar, MD Medical Faculty, Department of Basic Sciences, Medical Biochemistry, Acibadem Mehmet Ali Aydinlar University, Istanbul, Türkiye

Ergun Sevil, MD Department of Otorhinolaryngology, Alaaddin Keykubat University, Alanya Training and Research Hospital, Alanya, Antalya, Türkiye

Bilal Sizer, MD Department of Otorhinolaryngology, Diyarbakir Memorial Hospital, Diyarbakir, Türkiye

Murat Sütçü, MD Division of Pediatric Infectious Diseases, Department of Pediatrics, Faculty of Medicine, Istinye University İstanbul, İstanbul, Türkiye

Soner Taşar, MD Department of Otorhinolaryngology, Afyonkarahisar State Hospital, Afyonkarahisar, Türkiye

Sinan Tüfekçi, MD Medical Faculty, Neonatology Section, Departmöent of Pediatrics, Tekirdağ Namık Kemal University, Tekirdağ, Türkiye

Dilyana Vicheva, MD, PhD Department of Otorhinolaryngology, Medical University of Plovdiv, Plovdiv, Bulgaria

Tarik Yagci, MD Medical Faculty, Department of Otorhinolaryngology, Bilecik Seyb Edebali University, Bilecik, Türkiye

Güniz Yaşöz, MD Department of Pediatrics, University of Kyrenia, Kyrenia, Northern Cyprus

Funda Yıldız, MD Faculty of Medicine, Department of Pediatrics, Istinye University İstanbul, Zeytinburnu/İstanbul, Türkiye

Fatih Yucedag, MD Faculty of Medicine, Department of Otorhinolaryngology, Karamanoglu Mehmetbey University, Karaman, Türkiye

Part I
Overview

Human Milk Composition: Nutrients and Bioactive Factors

Senem Alkan Özdemir, Özlem Naciye Şahin, and Despina D. Briana

1 Introduction

It is widely accepted that the ideal way for a human infant to be nourished up to the age of 6 months is exclusive breastfeeding. Thereafter, breastfeeding with additional sources of nutrition is suitable up to the first or second birthday, or for even more prolonged periods [1, 2]. Breast milk is the sole food which precisely addresses the developmental requirements of the infant, providing both nutritional elements and bioactive compounds to ensure survival as well as healthy growth [3]. In this chapter, the nutritional and bioactive elements of breast milk are summarised. The latter category includes cells, molecules which target infectious pathogens and dampen down inflammation, growth factors and prebiotics. Breast milk differs from artificial substitutes insofar as the latter is of essentially fixed composition, whereas breast milk varies considerably in its constituents, whether in a single nursing session, over the course of the day or over the whole period of lactation. Human milk composition differs from mother to mother, as it does between populations. There are a number of reasons for this variable composition, including factors related to both the mother and the surrounding environment, as well as to the way milk is expressed and the feeding pattern. Knowledge of the constituents of breast milk is vital, in order to best utilise the opportunities breastfeeding offers, especially for those children who are most vulnerable to adverse outcomes, and to inform

S. A. Özdemir (✉)
Department of Neonatology, Behçet Uz Children's Hospital, Health Sciences University, İzmir, Türkiye

Ö. N. Şahin
Department of Child Health and Diseases, Arel University, Medical Faculty, Istanbul, Türkiye

D. D. Briana
NICU, Third Department of Pediatrics, National and Kapodistrian University of Athens, University General Hospital "ATTIKON", Athens, Greece

© The Author(s), under exclusive license to Springer Nature Switzerland AG 2023
Ö. N. Şahin et al. (eds.), *Breastfeeding and Metabolic Programming*,
https://doi.org/10.1007/978-3-031-33278-4_1

discussion about how breast milk can potentially be stored and whether it should be pasteurised. The chapter will also discuss bioactive factors which have been identified as potential prophylactic or therapeutic agents and may be suitable to undergo pharmaceutical development and testing [3–5].

2   Stages of Lactation

The initial milk expressed by the mother postpartum is colostrum, which differs from mature milk in the amount expressed, its appearance and constituents. This early milk is expressed in low volumes over the initial days after delivery and contains abundant immune-related cells and humoral factors, notably secretory IgA, lactoferrin and white blood cells. It also contains factors that direct development, such as epidermal growth factor (EGF) [4–6]. The level of lactose in colostrum is low and it appears that this fluid is optimised for immune support and directing growth more than for supplying nutrition. The electrolyte composition of colostrum also differs from transitional or mature milk, being richer in sodium, chloride and magnesium ions, but lower in potassium and calcium [5, 6]. The rising of milk lactose concentration heralds the onset of transitional milk. Within the breast, this reflects a structural change, with the epithelium developing tight junctions between cells. The exact point at which this change occurs varies from mother to mother, however the expression of transitional milk, known as the second stage of lactogenesis, generally begins a few days after delivery. The second stage is considered delayed if it has not started by 72 h postpartum. This delay seems to be associated with neonatal prematurity and maternal obesity. It also correlates with specific metabolic biomarkers [7, 8]. The changes in biochemical composition that confirm the onset of the second stage include sodium concentration, sodium to potassium ratio, as well as citrate and lactose levels [9].

Transitional milk somewhat resembles colostrum, although it involves a considerable step up in milk production as called for by the infant's rapid development and growth, which impose greater metabolic demands. The usual period during which transitional milk is expressed is from 5 days to 2 weeks after delivery. It is followed by the stage of mature milk. Mature milk contains all the expected elements at around 4–6 weeks after birth. Thereafter, there are only relatively minor adjustments to the constituents contained in breast milk, although compositional variety is always a feature of human milk [10, 11].

3   Studies of Breast Milk Composition

Studies concerning the composition of breast milk, as indexed in Medline, have steadily increased in number over the last half-century. There are still announcements of newly discovered constituents in human milk, and an active global research effort is underway to determine the functions of each constituent. There have been multiple studies examining the composition of breast milk in different groups of mothers. These studies employed a range of methods to collect, store and analyse human milk. The ideal method of sampling is to obtain multiple samples of milk from the same mother at different points during a 24-h period [10, 11]. This sampling technique suffers from the disadvantage that it is costly and may discourage mothers from enrolling in a study. A second technique that allows for standardisation is to take all samples at a particular point during the day, such as in the morning, and to collect the entire milk content of whichever breast has not been used to feed the infant in the preceding 2–3 h. This procedure needs to be repeated several times in the same study participant on different days [12]. The majority of studies in the literature, nonetheless, are based on milk obtained in a non-standardised way from milk banks, where the milk arrives at different times and different points during nursing and is expressed from mothers at different stages of lactation. These studies on the composition of breast milk also lack standardisation in how and for how long milk was stored, how frequently was frozen and defrosted and whether it was pasteurised or not. All these factors may partly explain the heterogeneity in the results obtained.

4 Nutritional Constituents within Breast Milk

There are three sources for the nutritional components of breast milk. The lactocytes synthesise a number of compounds for secretion into milk. The maternal diet supplies other components, whilst others come from the body stores of the mother. In general, breast milk retains its nutritional value despite maternal dietary deficiencies, but there are specific vitamins and fatty acids which must be present in the maternal diet for these compounds to be present in breast milk. This issue is discussed elsewhere in this volume [12–14].

4.1 Macronutrients

The level of macronutrients in breast milk does exhibit a degree of variation between individuals and over the whole course of breastfeeding, but there is a notable consistency in macronutrient content in different groups, despite differences in maternal diets. On average, the concentration of protein in mature milk is calculated to lie between 0.9 and 1.2 g/dL, of lipids from 3.2 to 3.6 g/dL and of lactose from 6.7 to 7.8 g/dL. The calorific value of breast milk is estimated at between 65 and 70 kcal/dL and is mostly related to the lipid content. There are differences between milk expressed following a term pregnancy and that seen from mothers of preterm infants. Preterm milk generally contains a higher concentration of protein and lipids. A study undertaken in the Californian city of Davis examined mature milk expressed 4 months after delivery and related its macronutrient composition to specific characteristics of the mother. There were a number of maternal characteristics found to be of significance, in particular body mass index (BMI), dietary protein, parity, whether menses had recommenced and how often the infant was fed. Individual mothers whose milk production was greater generally produced milk that was less rich in lipids and protein but richer in lactose.

Breast milk proteins can be separated into those that aggregate in the whey and those that are in the casein fraction. Each fraction contains a surprisingly varied range of different proteins and peptides [14, 15]. The proteins present at the highest concentration are casein, α-lactalbumin, lactoferrin, secretory immunoglobulin IgA, lysozyme and serum albumin [16, 17]. Around 25% of the nitrogen contained in breast milk is not in protein form, being found as urea, urate, creatine, creatinine, amino acids or nucleotides. There is a significantly higher level of protein in breast milk from mothers of preterm infants. Whatever the stage of pregnancy when delivery occurred, protein content falls in breast milk between the first and fourth to sixth weeks. If a preterm infant is fed by donor milk, the concentration of protein and amino acids is insufficient unless artificially supplemented. This is because most donor milk is of mature type and provided by mothers who delivered a term infant. The level of protein in breast milk does not depend on what the mother eats, but it does rise if the BMI is greater and falls when the volume of milk expressed is very high [10, 18].

The typical lipid composition of breast milk involves a high volume of palmitic acid and oleic acid residues attached to triacylglycerides. Palmitic acid is generally attached mid-chain to the glycerol moiety, whereas oleic acid is attached to either of the terminal carbons. The macronutrient category subject to the most variation in breast milk is lipid. The lipid content of hindmilk, the end portion of a feed, potentially contains three-fold more lipid than the initial foremilk [19]. One study which evaluated milk sampled from 71 women over the course of a full day reported that the lipid concentration was highest during the afternoon or evening and this finding was of statistical significance [20]. A different study correlated a quarter of the variation in fat contained in breast milk with variation in maternal protein consumption [10].

The aliphatic acid content of breast milk is affected by maternal dietary consumption, especially consumption of long chain polyunsaturated fatty acids (LCPUFAs). In Western countries, most fatty acids of this type in the diet are omega-6 aliphatic acids, with less consumption of omega-3 acids than is ideal. In North American mothers, breast milk is markedly deficient in docosahexaenoic acid; therefore lactating mothers whose diet lacks this nutrient should be advised to consume supplements to remedy the defect [18, 21, 22].

The main type of sugar within breast milk is lactose, a disaccharide. Lactose varies the least amongst the macronutrients found in breast milk, although it has been noted that women with a high milk volume do secrete greater concentrations of lactose into milk [10]. Oligosaccharides are also a major carbohydrate component in breast milk. They are typically present at a concentration of around 1 g/dL, although this varies according to the stage in breastfeeding and the genetic composition of the mother [23–25]. Oligosaccharides in breast milk are not nutritive, but they perform other biological functions, as described later.

Figures representing the mean concentration of macronutrients in breast milk are helpful, but should not be allowed to give the misleading impression that individual samples of milk vary little in their composition. The opposite, in fact, applies, and this variation is especially apparent in lipid and protein concentrations. The total protein concentration in breast milk from mothers who delivered at term ranges from 0.6 to 1.4 g/dL. The range for lipids is from 1.8 to 8.9 g/dL, for lactose from 6.4 to 7.6 g/dL and the calorific value is between 50 and 115 kcal/dL [26]. There are significant differences between milk from mothers who delivered at term and those whose delivery was premature. Accordingly, when a nutritional plan for an infant at high risk is being formulated, the milk available needs to be analysed and fortified as necessary, whilst also monitoring effects on the infant's growth [27].

4.2 Micronutrients

Breast milk provides the standard to which artificial formula needs to approach to achieve optimal nutritional value. However, there is significant variation in the micronutrient content of breast milk as a result of variation in maternal diet and body stores. This especially applies to vitamins A, B_1, B_2, B_6, B_{12}, D, and iodine. Given the fact that mothers frequently consume a suboptimal diet, mothers can be advised to keep taking multivitamins whilst breastfeeding continues [28, 29]. The level of vitamin K in breast milk is always low, whatever the mother's dietary intake. This is the reasoning behind the American Academy of Paediatrics' recommendation that vitamin K should be administered intramuscularly to all neonates to prevent haemorrhagic disease of the newborn [28]. The level of vitamin D in breast milk is also low, especially if the mother has inadequate exposure to sunlight. Due to lifestyle changes, this is now frequently the case all across the globe [30]. Although benefit from supplementing the diet of breastfeeding mothers with vitamin D has not yet been proven experimentally, current guidelines advise supplying additional vitamin D to all new breastfeeding mothers and their offspring. The inability to provide a thorough, detailed review of every micronutrient contained in breast milk is a limitation of this chapter. Interested readers can find several detailed reviews available elsewhere in the literature [28, 29, 31].

5 Bioactive Constituents and Their Sources

One definition of bioactive constituents in the diet considers them as substances which 'affect biological processes or substrates which hence have an impact on body function or condition and ultimately health' [32, 33]. The bioactive molecules found in breast milk originate from several different sources. The epithelial cells of breast produce and secrete certain such compounds, whilst cellular components of milk are the source of others. Furthermore, the breast epithelium recognises and actively transports some molecules from the plasma to the milk, by means of specific receptor interactions. The epithelial cells secrete milk fat globules (MFGs), which contain within them various proteins attached to membranes as well as specific lipid components [34]. These different sources all contribute to the abundance of bioactive molecules within breast milk. In women who are breastfeeding, B-lymphocytes are drawn towards the breast, and secretory immunoglobulin produced by these cells is then transferred into the milk ducts via polymeric immunoglobulin receptors (pIgR) [35]. In contrast, vascular endothelial growth factor (VEGF) concentrations are significantly higher in breast milk than in maternal circulation, which suggests that VEGF is manufactured and secreted by the breast itself [36, 37]. A knowledge of where the constituents of breast milk that possess bioactivity originate is helpful in understanding the varying levels of secreted maternal medications in milk.

There are a number of ways in which research into the bioactive breast milk compounds can impact clinical practice. A key concept that both patients and the wider public need to grasp is that the research so far clearly shows that breast milk is more sophisticated than just another type of food. Indeed, breast milk provides infants with a number of compounds which enhance both survival and healthy growth. Accordingly, for infants at risk and where the mother cannot supply her own milk, donor breast milk is vital, provided it is safe to use. Proteomic studies reveal that the types of proteins present differ according to the stage of breastfeeding, in addition to differences associated with whether delivery occurred at term or prematurely [14, 15]. Thus, wherever the possibility exists, donor milk should be from a donor whose own infant is at the same stage of development as the patient. In actual clinical practice, this precise matching may not be achievable. Recognition of the role of bioactive compounds in breast milk has led to a rethink in how donor milk is collected, stored and pasteurised. Retaining bioactivity has become the goal. Furthermore, the mechanisms by which bioactive milk constituents enhance infant health offer new targets for future pharmaceutical or other therapeutic interventions [36, 37].

This chapter does not aim to comprehensively review the entire spectrum of bioactivity in breast milk. Instead, the objective is to examine a subset of bioactive factors in breast milk and relate their changing levels to the developmental requirements of the infant. The patterns of secretion associated with term and premature delivery are described, as well as the variations associated with the stage of lactation. In many cases, the bioactive factors function in a synergistic manner, which means that replacement or supplementation of individual bioactive molecules or sets thereof is generally less efficacious than supplying complete breast milk [38].

6 Growth Factors

Multiple different growth factors have been identified in breast milk. These molecules act on various infant organs, such as the gut, circulatory, nervous and endocrine systems [36–38].

6.1 Epidermal Growth Factor (EGF): Development and Repair of the Intestinal System

EGF plays a vital role in healthy development and repair of the gut lining. It is detectable in breast milk as well as amniotic fluid [38–40]. EGF remains intact even in the highly acidic gastric interior, and is not degraded by digestive enzymes. Within the intestines it has a stimulatory effect upon the gut lining, promoting the synthesis of DNA and cellular replication. It also increases water and glucose uptake by the gut and promotes protein manufacture [41, 42]. EGF also performs several protective roles within the infant gut, such as preventing excessive apoptosis and opposing the action of tumour necrosis factor-alpha (TNF-α). The latter promotes inflammation and alters the tight junctions between different enterocytes and between hepatocytes [43]. Heparin-binding growth factor also belongs to the same family of related proteins. This is the principal signalling molecule involved in resolving hypoxic injury, ischaemic-reperfusion damage, shock secondary to haemorrhage, resuscitation injury and necrotising enterocolitis [44]. The highest concentration of EGF occurs at the beginning of the lactation period, decreasing as lactation continues [45, 46]. The mean concentration of EGF in colostrum exceeds the mother's circulating level by 2000 times. In mature milk, EGF is 100 times more abundant than in maternal circulation [41]. Additionally, the level in breast milk of mothers who delivered prematurely is higher than in cases where delivery occurred at term [45, 46].

6.2 Neuronal Growth Factors: Normal Maturation

The intestinal system of infants is immature in several different ways, including the development of the enteric nervous system, which depends for proper maturation on the presence of brain-derived neurotrophic factor (BDNF) and glial cell-line-derived neurotrophic factor (GDNF). Peristaltic intestinal motion is often dysfunctional in premature infants. This function improves in the presence of BDNF. Rodent models exhibit severe deficiency of neurones in the gut of animals without GDNF. Ciliary neurotrophic factor (CNF) is a protein with similarities to BDNF and GDNF. All three molecules are present in breast milk for a period lasting 90 days after delivery. When neurones were exposed to GDNF isolated from human milk, cellular survival improved and the cells developed new projections [30, 31].

6.3 The Insulin-like Growth Factor (IGF) Superfamily and Its Effects on Tissues

Breast milk contains several IGF-related proteins, notably IGF-I and II, as well as IGF-binding proteins and proteases with specificity for IGF. These molecules are most abundant in colostrum, but their levels steadily fall as lactation proceeds. Preterm and term milk do not importantly differ in their level of IGF apart from IGF-binding protein-2 being more abundant in preterm samples. Rodents exposed to surgical stress and fed by total parenteral nutrition exhibited higher levels of tissue growth and lower levels of gut atrophy when administered IGF-I. This effect has not been demonstrated in human subjects so far [1, 2]. IGF-I potentially also increases cellular survival when the gut is exposed to oxidative injury. Breastfeeding increases the concentration of IGF-I in the circulation. IGF absorbed through the gut retains its bioactivity and can enter the vascular circulation. Exactly how IGF taken up by this route functions so far remains unknown, however it has been shown that IGF-I administered by an enteral route at physiological concentrations increases red cell synthesis and raises the haematocrit [32, 33].

6.4 Vascular Endothelial Growth Factor (VEGF): Regulating Vascular Development

The development of new blood vessels is mostly regulated by the balance between VEGF and molecules which antagonise its effect. Colostrum contains the greatest level of VEGF amongst different types of breast milk. Term milk has a greater concentration of VEGF than preterm milk [34, 35]. The pathogenesis of retinopathy of prematurity is believed to arise from a combination of immaturity of the lungs, therapeutic oxygen administration and down-regulation of VEGF. This then causes the retina to grow blood vessels in a disorganised fashion [36, 37]. It is possible that breast milk, which contains VEGF, may be beneficial in mitigating the severity of this condition.

6.5 Erythropoietin: Promoting Development of the Gut and Preventing Anaemia

Erythropoietin is the principal hormone which stimulates erythrocyte synthesis. Haemorrhage, disease of the gut and under-developed haematopoiesis are factors contributing to the anaemia which may affect premature infants. This condition then severely harms normal growth and development [36–41]. It has been proposed that exogenous administration of erythropoietin may be beneficial in the prevention of anaemia of prematurity, however results of this practice have produced unclear benefit [38]. Nonetheless, it has been demonstrated that where erythropoietin and iron are co-administered, a potential increase in haemoglobin and haematocrit occurs [39]. A trial involving low numbers of premature infants who were administered erythropoietin enterally found increased numbers of reticulocytes in the circulation. Furthermore, erythropoietin has significant trophic effects and leads to tighter integration of the enterocytic junctions. It appears that exogenous erythropoietin may partially prevent vertical transmission of HIV and may lower the incidence of necrotising enterocolitis [36–41].

6.6 Calcitonin and Somatostatin: Regulation of Growth

There are high concentrations of both calcitonin and the precursor molecule, procalcitonin, in breast milk [40]. The calcitonin receptor is present on cells of the intestines from the latter stages of pregnancy into the first year of life, as demonstrated by immunochemical methods. In normal circumstances, somatostatin undergoes swift degradation within the jejunum. It is not absorbed via the gut lining. When this hormone is delivered in breast milk, however, degradation does not occur and it remains bioactive in the intestines. The usual physiological role of somatostatin is inhibition of the action of growth factors. Its exact functions in breast milk is, however, still not fully elucidated [41, 42].

6.7 Adiponectin and Related Hormones: The Regulation of Metabolism and How the Body Is Composed

Adiponectin has a high molecular weight and possesses multiple endocrine functions, in particular the regulation of metabolism and inhibition of inflammatory responses. It is present at high concentration in breast milk and traverses the gut lining, after which it has an apparent regulatory function in metabolism in the infant. There is an inverse correlation between the concentration of breast milk adiponectin and both the infant body mass and BMI in exclusively breastfed infants. It has been hypothesised that adiponectin in breast milk may help to prevent individuals becoming obese or overweight at a later stage in life, but this has not yet been proven to occur. There are several other hormones with a regulatory role in metabolism that can be detected in breast milk. This group includes leptin, resistin and ghrelin, all of which significantly influence energy production and the relative proportions of fat and muscle, as well as orexigenesis [1, 42, 43].

7   Oligosaccharides: Selection of Optimal Gut Microbial Flora

Human milk oligosaccharides (HMO) are unique to humans and consist of chains of sugars between 3 and 32 residues in length [23, 24]. Despite their non-nutritional function, these sugars form a strikingly large component within breast milk, at a level similar to that of proteins overall. The synthesis of HMO depends on the action of glycosyltransferases, a group of enzymes which participate in the synthesis of other carbohydrates. HMO function as prebiotics, i.e. they assist the growth of a beneficial (probiotic) intestinal flora. Many pathogens remain in the gut by attachment to oligosaccharides attached to the enterocytic membrane. The HMO and conjugated proteins within the lumen act as alternative binding sites for pathogens, thus acting as a decoy and preventing their adhering to the intestinal lining. There is a variety in the particular HMO secreted by different mothers, the so-called lactotype, which bears comparison with blood groups [23–25]. However, there is no aspect of the lactotype corresponding to donor–recipient incompatibility, as occurs with blood transfusions. Thus, an infant may consume milk from any non-related mother. The different lactotypes have probably evolved because of varying binding affinities amongst pathogens. Certain patterns of HMO secretion are able to prevent diarrhoea secondary to infection by specific pathogens, and to inhibit HIV transmission. There is a need for more detailed research focusing on the secretion patterns for HMO and lactose in preterm milk [44, 45].

The traditional medical belief that breast milk is normally sterile has been overturned, and it now appears that breast milk has its own associated microbiota. There are various maternal factors that alter the composition of this microbiota. It also varies as breastfeeding progresses [46, 47]. The specific HMO in milk affect which microbial species colonise the gut and may partly determine which bacteria are present in breast milk.

8   Conclusion

Breast milk is a fluid which is dynamic in composition and acts in numerous different ways to promote the healthy development of the infant. It has both a nutritive and bioactive function. The constituents differ at different stages of breastfeeding and between term and preterm milk samples. Despite the numerous investigations into how breast milk is composed, research continues to identify previously unrecognised constituents. There is a pressing requirement for a study examining in a standard way breast milk samples from multiple populations. This will then allow a thorough, detailed and complete reference for the nutritive and bioactive factors in human milk to be compiled. At present, we are still at the discovery stage in understanding how breast milk contributes to the healthy development of human infants [1, 2, 48].

References

1. Ballard O, Morrow AL. Human Milk composition: nutrients and bioactive factors. Pediatr Clin N Am. 2013;60(1):49–74. https://doi.org/10.1016/j.pcl.2012.10.002.
2. Breastfeeding and the use of human milk. Pediatrics. 2012;129(3):e827–41.
3. Oftedal OT. The evolution of milk secretion and its ancient origins. Animal. 2012;6(3):355–68.
4. Castellote C, Casillas R, Ramirez-Santana C, Perez-Cano FJ, Castell M, Moretones MG, Lopez- Sabater MC, Franch A. Premature delivery influences the immunological composition of colostrum and transitional and mature human milk. J Nutr. 2011;141(6):1181–7.
5. Pang WW, Hartmann PE. Initiation of human lactation: secretory differentiation and secretory activation. J Mammary Gland Biol Neoplasia. 2007;12(4):211–21.
6. Kulski JK, Hartmann PE. Changes in human milk composition during the initiation of lactation. Aust J Exp Biol Med Sci. 1981;59(1):101–14.
7. Henderson JJ, Hartmann PE, Newnham JP, Simmer K. Effect of preterm birth and antenatal corticosteroid treatment on lactogenesis II in women. Pediatrics. 2008;121(1):e92–100.
8. Nommsen-Rivers LA, Dolan LM, Huang B. Timing of stage II lactogenesis is predicted by antenatal metabolic health in a cohort of primiparas. Breastfeed Med. 2012;7(1):43–9.
9. Cregan MD, De Mello TR, Kershaw D, McDougall K, Hartmann PE. Initiation of lactation in women after preterm delivery. Acta Obstet Gynecol Scand. 2002;81(9):870–7.
10. Nommsen LA, Lovelady CA, Heinig MJ, Lonnerdal B, Dewey KG. Determinants of energy, protein, lipid, and lactose concentrations in human milk during the first 12 mo of lactation: the DARLING study. Am J Clin Nutr. 1991;53(2):457–65.
11. Bauer J, Gerss J. Longitudinal analysis of macronutrients and minerals in human milk produced by mothers of preterm infants. Clin Nutr (Edinburgh, Scotland). 2011;30(2):215–20.
12. Geraghty SR, Davidson BS, Warner BB, Sapsford AL, Ballard JL, List BA, Akers R, Morrow AL. The development of a research human milk bank. J Hum Lact. 2005;21(1):59–66.
13. Prentice A. Regional variations in the composition of human milk. In: Jensen RG, editor. Handbook of milk composition. San Diego, CA: Academic Press, Inc.; 1995. p. 919.
14. Liao Y, Alvarado R, Phinney B, Lonnerdal B. Proteomic characterization of human milk whey proteins during a twelve-month lactation period. J Proteome Res. 2011;10(4):1746–54.
15. Gao X, McMahon RJ, Woo JG, Davidson BS, Morrow AL, Zhang Q. Temporal changes in milk proteomes reveal developing milk functions. J Proteome Res. 2012;11(7):3897–907.
16. Lonnerdal B. Human milk proteins: key components for the biological activity of human milk. Adv Exp Med Biol. 2004;554:11–25.
17. Jensen RG. Handbook of milk composition. San Diego, CA: Academic Press, Inc.; 1995. Pediatr Clin North Am. Author manuscript; available in PMC 2014 February 01.
18. Valentine CJ, Morrow G, Fernandez S, Gulati P, Bartholomew D, Long D, Welty SE, Morrow AL, Rogers LK. Docosahexaenoic acid and amino acid contents in pasteurized donor Milk are low for preterm infants. J Pediatr. 2010;157(6):906–10.
19. Saarela T, Kokkonen J, Koivisto M. Macronutrient and energy contents of human milk fractions during the first six months of lactation. Acta Paediatr. 2005;94(9):1176–81.
20. Kent JC, Mitoulas LR, Cregan MD, Ramsay DT, Doherty DA, Hartmann PE. Volume and frequency of breastfeedings and fat content of breast milk throughout the day. Pediatrics. 2006;117(3):e387–95.
21. Valentine CJ, Morrow G, Pennell M, Morrow AL, Hodge A, Haban-Bartz A, Collins K, Rogers LK. Randomized controlled trial of docosahexaenoic acid supplementation in midwestern U.S. human milk donors. Breastfeed Med. 2012; https://doi.org/10.1089/bfm.2011.0126.
22. Martin MA, Lassek WD, Gaulin SJ, Evans RW, Woo JG, Geraghty SR, Davidson BS, Morrow AL, Kaplan HS, Gurven MD. Fatty acid composition in the mature milk of Bolivian forager- horticulturalists: controlled comparisons with a US sample. Matern Child Nutr. 2012;8(3):404–18.
23. Newburg DS, Ruiz-Palacios GM, Morrow AL. Human milk glycans protect infants against enteric pathogens. Annu Rev Nutr. 2005;25:37–58.

24. Morrow AL, Ruiz-Palacios GM, Jiang X, Newburg DS. Human-milk glycans that inhibit pathogen binding protect breast-feeding infants against infectious diarrhea. J Nutr. 2005;135(5):1304–7.
25. Gabrielli O, Zampini L, Galeazzi T, Padella L, Santoro L, Peila C, Giuliani F, Bertino E, Fabris C, Coppa GV. Preterm milk oligosaccharides during the first month of lactation. Pediatrics. 2011;128(6):e1520–31.
26. Michaelsen KF, Skafte L, Badsberg JH, Jorgensen M. Variation in macronutrients in human bank milk: influencing factors and implications for human milk banking. J Pediatr Gastroenterol Nutr. 1990;11(2):229–39.
27. Arslanoglu S, Moro GE, Ziegler EE. The Wapm Working Group on nutrition. Optimization of human milk fortification for preterm infants: new concepts and recommendations. J Perinat Med. 2010;38(3):233–8.
28. Greer FR. Do breastfed infants need supplemental vitamins? Pediatr Clin N Am. 2001;48(2):415–23.
29. Allen LH. B vitamins in breast milk: relative importance of maternal status and intake, and effects on infant status and function. Adv Nutr. 2012;3(3):362–9.
30. Dawodu A, Zalla L, Woo JG, Herbers PM, Davidson BS, Heubi JE, Morrow AL. Heightened attention to supplementation is needed to improve the vitamin D status of breastfeeding mothers and infants when sunshine exposure is restricted. Matern Child Nutr. 2012;10:383.
31. Pediatrics, AAo. Pediatric nutrition handbook. 6th ed. Elk Gove Village, IL: American Academy of Pediatrics; 2009.
32. Korhonen H, Marnila P, Gill HS. Milk immunoglobulins and complement factors. Br J Nutr. 2000 Nov;84 Suppl 1:S75–80.
33. Garofalo R. Cytokines in human milk. J Pediatr. 2010;156(2 Suppl):S36–40.
34. Cavaletto M, Giuffrida MG, Conti A. The proteomic approach to analysis of human milk fat globule membrane. Clin Chim Acta. 2004;347(1–2):41–8.
35. Van de Perre P. Transfer of antibody via mother's milk. Vaccine. 2003;21(24):3374–6.
36. Kobata R, Tsukahara H, Ohshima Y, Ohta N, Tokuriki S, Tamura S, Mayumi M. High levels of growth factors in human breast milk. Early Hum Dev. 2008;84(1):67–9.
37. Patki S, Patki U, Patil R, Indumathi S, Kaingade P, Bulbule A, Nikam A, Pishte A. Comparison of the levels of the growth factors in umbilical cord serum and human milk and its clinical significance. Cytokine. 2012;59(2):305–8.
38. Hirai C, Ichiba H, Saito M, Shintaku H, Yamano T, Kusuda S. Trophic effect of multiple growth factors in amniotic fluid or human milk on cultured human fetal small intestinal cells. JPGN. 2002;34:524–8.
39. Chailler P, Menard D. Ontogeny of EGF receptors in the human gut. Front Biosci. 1999;4:87–101.
40. Wagner CL, Taylor SN, Johnson D. Host factors in amniotic fluid and breast milk that contribute to gut maturation. Clinic Rev Allerg Immunol. 2008;34:191–204.
41. Read LC, Upton FM, Francis GL, Wallace JC, Dahlenberg GW, Ballad FJ. Changes in the growth- promoting activity of human milk during lactation. Pediatr Res. 1984;18(2):133–9.
42. Chang C-Y, Chao JC-J. Effect of human milk and epidermal growth factor on growth of human intestinal caco-2 cells. JPGN. 2002;34:394–401.
43. Khailova L, Dvorak K, Arganbright KM, Williams CS, Halpern MD, Dvorak B. Changes in hepatic cell junctions structure during experimental necrotizing enterocolitis: effect of EGF treatment. Pediatr Res. 2009;66(2):140–4.
44. Radulescu A, Zhang H-Y, Chen C-L, Chen Y, Zhou Y, Yu X, Otabor I, Olson JK, Besner GE. Heparin-binding EGF-like growth factor promotes intestinal anastomotic healing. J Surg Res. 2011;171:540–50.
45. Dvorak B, Fituch CC, Williams CS, Hurst NM, Schanler RJ. Increased epidermal growth factor levels in human milk of mothers with extremely premature infants. Pediatr Res. 2003;54(1):15–9.

46. Dvorak B, Fituch CC, Williams CS, Hurst NM, Schanler RJ. Concentrations of epidermal growth factor and transforming growth factor-alpha in preterm milk. In: Pickering LK, et al., editors. Protecting infants through human milk. Kluwer Academic/Plenum Publishers; 2004. p. 407–9.

47. Rodrigues D, Li A, Nair D, Blennerhassett M. Glial cell line-derived neurotrophic factor is a key neurotrophin in the postnatal enteric nervous system. Neurogastroenterol Motil. 2011;23:e44–56.

48. Boesmans W, Gomes P, Janssens J, Tack J, Berghe PV. Brain-derived neurotrophic factor amplifies neurotransmitter responses and promotes synaptic communication in the enteric nervous system. Gut. 2008;57:314–22.

Perinatal Maternal Nutrition and Breast Milk Composition

Vesim Bekraki, Gian Carlo Di Renzo, and Ayşe Engin Arısoy

1 Introduction

The American Academy of Pediatrics (AAP) and the World Health Organization (WHO) recommend infants should be exclusively breastfed up to a minimum age of 6 months [1, 2]. The composition of breast milk is optimized for the infants to grow and develop healthily, with the appropriate balance of carbohydrates, lipids, and proteins. Breast milk contains bioactive compounds that play particularly significant roles at critical points when the central nervous, gastrointestinal, and immune systems are maturing. Infants breastfeeding are less prone to respiratory, middle ear, and gastrointestinal infections.

Breastfeeding also benefits the entire life, leading to better cognitive function and a lesser incidence of circulatory disorders, obesity, and diabetes mellitus. Furthermore, research indicates several advantages to breastfeeding mothers, notably a decreased incidence of hypertension, hyperlipidemia, and circulatory diseases. Some studies reported breastfeeding women are at lower risk of breast and ovary malignancies [3, 4].

Although breastfeeding results in undoubtedly better outcomes for infants and mothers, the actual number of breastfeeding mothers is below the ideal level.

V. Bekraki (✉)
Section of Pediatrics, Türkiye Hospital, Istanbul, Türkiye

G. C. Di Renzo
Centre of Perinatal Medicine of the University of Perugia, Perugia, Italy

Sechenov University, Moscow, Russia
e-mail: giancarlo.direnzo@unipg.it

A. E. Arısoy
Emeritus, Division of Neonatology, Department of Pediatrics, Faculty of Medicine, Kocaeli University, Kocaeli, Türkiye

Ö. N. Şahin et al. (eds.), *Breastfeeding and Metabolic Programming*,
https://doi.org/10.1007/978-3-031-33278-4_2

Healthcare professionals influence to a significant degree whether mothers will decide to breastfeed and, if so, how successful breastfeeding is. By providing that mothers know the proven benefits of breastfeeding to themselves and their infants in their early and later life stages, healthcare professionals can provide mothers make informed choices. For physicians to inform mothers of the benefits of breastfeeding and give appropriately qualified advice, they should know in detail how the mammary gland functions and how breast milk provides nutrition and protection to breastfed babies [5].

2 The Mother's Perinatal Nutritional Status

The composition of the maternal diet and the way the mother eats may influence the development of the growing fetus directly, by physiological adaptation, or indirectly, due to some stresses on the fetus altering the resulting phenotypical expression of genes. Supplementing maternal diets is no panacea, and robust evidence for the beneficial effects of most supplements is not available. Maternal diets with a low glycemic index and of Mediterranean type have an apparent benefit on subfertility linked to ovulation, render premature delivery less likely, and lower the incidence of gestational diabetes.

Overall, the female population in high-income countries is adequately nourished, but subgroups have vitamin D, folic acid, and iodine deficiencies. However, women in several low- and middle-income countries can not sufficiently be fed and may have many vitamin, trace elements, and mineral deficiencies. It is recommended that all women of childbearing age consume multivitamin supplements daily since this guarantees an adequate supply of vitamins, micronutrients, and folic acid, in case a pregnancy occurs.

Pregnant women should be carefully evaluated in terms of diet and guidelines about the degree of acceptable increase in body mass attributable to pregnancy, compared to baseline basal metabolic index. Clinicians should recommend a Mediterranean-style diet with omega-3 fatty acids sourced from oily fish or in a supplement. Some evidence exists indicating that supplementary calcium reduces the risk of pre-eclampsia. The importance of vitamin D in the strength of the bones, maintaining normoglycemia, boosting immunity, and ensuring the uterus can contract effectively during labor was demonstrated. Calcium intake should be sufficiently maintained, and vitamin D levels need to remain sufficient during pregnancy. For the latter purpose, the women's skin needs to be exposed to sunlight or supplementation provided [6].

2.1 Carbohydrates

Carbohydrates are the principal energy source in human metabolism, particularly for the central nervous system (CNS). In pregnancy, maternal consumption of carbohydrates is critical to fetal growth since glucose derived from complex carbohydrates provides most of the necessary calories [7]. Pregnant women should consume 175 g of carbohydrates each day. Carbohydrates should come from high-quality dietary sources that have a satisfactory glycemic index. Suitable sources include unprocessed foods, whole grains, vegetables without a high starch content, fruits, pulses such as beans, peas, and lentils, and reduced-fat dairy products.

Carbohydrates also occur in several food items, generally as simple sugars. Foods in this category include table sugar, honey, corn syrup, concentrated fruit juices, and treacle. The dietary intake of these simple carbohydrates must be kept at a minimum in all individuals, not just pregnant women. Added sugar is common in many processed foods, such as candies and desserts, and soft drinks, such as lemonade, fruit juice, and especially cola. Many people add table sugar to hot beverages, such as tea or coffee. A Malaysian study found that a maternal diet rich in fruit and vegetables resulted in higher weight, length, and head circumference of the infant at birth, and no association was discernible with any specific type of micronutrient [8].

2.2 Proteins

Protein from the diet supplies the amino acids used for growth, developing, and repairing bodily injury. Amino acids are utilized in the body's structural proteins and for synthesizing the enzymes needed to provide metabolism to function normally [9]. Considering how a dietary component should be supplemented, it is necessary to assess the level of other available nutrients, as this affects the fate of the supplement in the body. For example, if individuals are deficient in protein and caloric intake, supplementing protein only is hazardous, whereas average growth is aided when protein and additional calories are supplied in appropriate amounts. Likewise, iron and folic acid are generally co-administered. Thus, the overall dietary composition should not be overlooked when planning an adequate maternal diet.

Pregnant women's recommended protein intake is 1.1 g/kg, approximately 70 g daily from the second trimester onward. This amount exceeds the recommended daily protein intake in non-pregnant women by 25 g daily. Dietary items rich in protein include white and red meat, egg, seafood, nuts, seeds, dairy products such as cheese, milk, and yogurt, and pulses such as beans and lentils. Protein also exists in vegetables and grains, although at a lower concentration [9].

2.3   Lipids

Lipids are an essential dietary component for pregnancy to proceed healthily. The body mainly treats lipids as an energy source. Lipids are also involved in the absorption of lipid-soluble A, D, E, and K vitamins and provide essential fatty acids. Lipids must come from the diet because the human body cannot synthesize essential fatty acids [9].

No amount has been officially recommended as the ideal dietary intake of lipids in pregnant women. One approach for fat consumption may be to adhere to the current US guidelines that limit lipid calories to 25–35% of the total energy intake [10, 11]. The nature of the lipids consumed is another important factor since certain fatty acids are more beneficial in health. The scientific evidence supports that the diet should contain omega-3 polyunsaturated fatty acids (PUFAs), saturated acids should not supply more than 7–10% of the daily calories, and trans-fatty acids should be eliminated from the diet whenever feasible [12].

Pregnant women consuming a lipids-rich diet may demonstrate signs of insulin resistance. Diets containing higher saturated fat levels are associated with abnormal glucose metabolism and a raised likelihood of gestational diabetes mellitus in pregnant women. Gestational diabetes is more likely in women whose diet includes high levels of animal fats and cholesterol at pre-conception and those consuming diet with raised saturated fat levels during pregnancy [13–15].

The normal development of the CNS and retina in the fetus and infant depends on adequate docosahexaenoic acid (DHA) and omega-3 fatty acids. Thus dietary intake is vital in the last trimester and the first year of life. Foods rich in omega-3 fatty acids include oily fish, seafood, and walnuts. It is recommended that pregnant women eat around 350 g of oily fish weekly or take a suitable dietary supplement [9].

2.4   Iron

The serum iron level in the days around conception predicts whether iron deficiency will develop and pregnant women will become anemic. Providing an iron supplement, generally in combination with folic acid, to pregnant women in areas where anemia is endemic increases their babies' birth weight [16]. Approximately 12% of women suffer from iron deficiency and anemia in the USA, but this rate rises to around 18% in pregnant women [9]. The corresponding figures in low- and middle-income countries are 43% for non-pregnant and 75% for pregnant women. The very high levels of iron deficiency and anemia in women in low- and middle-income countries are mainly attributable to inadequate diet, especially the restricted availability of foods containing iron, and chronic blood loss due to hookworm infections of the gut [9].

The health and welfare of the mother vitally depend on the body's iron store remaining at a safe level. Fetal growth is not restricted until the maternal hemoglobin concentration falls below 6 g/dL; however, one in five or more global maternal deaths are attributable to hemorrhage in an anemic woman [17]. A mild degree of anemia, corresponding to a hemoglobin level of 8 and 10.9 g/dL, sometimes represents a normal physiological response to pregnancy. This occurs due to the rise in the circulation volume in pregnancy, which may be linked to a smoother blood flow through the placental capillary bed permitted by a lower blood viscosity; this unimpeded flow enables a more efficient gaseous exchange to take place [18].

Cantor et al. [19], in the U.S. Preventive Services Task Force literature review, concluded that no advantages exist for routinely offering iron supplementation to pregnant women living in high-income countries. However, if a woman has an iron deficiency or is at risk of significant bleeding due to placenta praevia, placental abruption, and coagulopathy, supplementing dietary iron is essential for the patient's safety [9].

2.5 Folate and Folic Acid

Folate, a water-soluble vitamin within the B vitamins group, is acquired from dietary sources or, in its acid form, folic acid, from supplemental vitamin preparations. Folate donates a methyl moiety when deoxyribonucleic acid (DNA) is synthesized and is required for cellular replication. Folate is essential for normal neural tube formation, which develops within 28 days of the zygote stage. Maternal low-folate status is associated with neural tube defects; folate prevents the occurrence of neural tube defects [20–22].

Folate is essential for normal brain and spinal cord development. The 28th day of pregnancy is when the neural tube closure occurs in normal development. Closure failure at the caudal pole of the tube results in spina bifida. A more extensive deficit in neural tube closure may cause anencephaly, where the brain structures fail to develop [9].

The U.S. Federal Drug Administration (FDA) ruling implemented in 1998 mandates cereal grains to be fortified with 0.14 mg of folic acid per 100 g. Following this ruling, the overall incidence of neural tube defects has declined by 30–40% in the USA. The incidence of spina bifida and anencephaly declined by 31% and 16%, respectively. However, incidence differences exist depending on race and ethnic origin. Moreover, the hypothesis has been proved that the essential way to reduce the incidence of neural tube defects further is by modifying women's diets to include items rich in folate [23]. As currently implemented, supplementation has provided a 20% decline in the incidence of neural tube defects. But a tenfold increase in the added daily folate intake would achieve an 82% reduction in incidence. The number of infants with neural tube defects would fall from 300,000 to 90,000–150,000 annually when other countries apply the US approach toward folate fortification of diet [9]. The folate administration in pregnant women reduces premature delivery in the 20th–32nd week [24–27]. However, some studies do not support this conclusion [28].

Women of reproductive age are advised to take a 0.4 mg folate supplement daily or consume foods with added folate alongside foods in which folate naturally occurs at a high level because the bioavailability of folate derived from the diet is low. Following conception, the folate supplement should supply 0.6 mg daily. When breastfeeding, 0.5 mg of folate daily is required. If a woman has previously had a pregnancy in which a neural tube defect in the fetus or newborn occurred, the required folate is 4 mg daily, ten times the usual amount. The folate intake at this dose should begin at least 1 month before trying for conception. Folate is abundant in beans, peas, orange juice, and green leafy vegetables. Vitamins sold for use before conception generally include 0.8–1 mg of folic acid in each tablet.

Excessively low dietary folate levels of less than 0.15 mg daily and high levels exceeding the normal recommended dietary allowance (RDA) by fourfold were associated with neoplasia in animal models [29]. The activity of the hepatic enzymes involved in folic acid metabolism may not increase sufficiently to prevent the folic acid build-up in circulation. Furthermore, high circulating folic acid levels impede the cytotoxic capabilities of natural killer (NK) cells [30].

2.6 Iodine

The need for iodine rises in pregnant women due to the 50% more synthesis of thyroxine (T4). The fetus cannot produce thyroid-stimulating hormone (TSH) before the 10th–12th week of pregnancy. The timing roughly coincides with the developing thyroid gland's ability to sequestrate iodine and synthesize iodothyronines. Despite this potential ability, the fetus's actual thyroid hormone expression rarely occurs until 18–20 weeks [1]. With an increased need for iodine in pregnancy, a greater than usual renal secretion of iodine into the urine exists.

The mother supplies fetal requirements for thyroid hormones up to the 20th week of gestation. If the mother's diet contains low iodine, her thyroid hormone synthesis will also be minimal. Unless thyroid hormones are present at sufficient levels, the migration of neurons, synthesis of myelin and transmission across the synapses, and neuronal plasticity will all be impaired. At specific points in pregnancy, abnormal fetal nervous system development secondary to iodine deficiency results in brain damage, which cannot afterward be repaired [2]. This damage may lower the child's intelligence quotient (IQ) by up to 20. Iodine deficiency is the most prevalent cause of learning disability globally, for which prevention is possible [31]. The other complications of iodine deficiency in pregnancy are goiter in the fetus, hypothyroidism, and cretinism in the child.

2.7 Vitamin D

The stores of vitamin D in pregnant women must be sufficient to allow calcium mobilization to lay down the crystallization of fetal bones. During pregnancy, 25–30 g of calcium are carried from the mother to the fetus, and the daily transfer across the placenta reaches 250 mg in the third trimester. Vitamin D-rich foods include oily fish, such as salmon, egg yolk, milk with added vitamin D, margarine, yogurt, and orange juice [1, 5]

Considerable discussion and disagreement exist about the need to screen pregnant women for vitamin D levels and how low levels should be supplemented. Some reports advocate that no evidence exists to show that screening all pregnant women for vitamin D deficiency is beneficial.

A serum concentration of at least 20 ng/mL, equal to 50 nmol/L, of 25-hydroxy vitamin D indicates healthy bone. The U.S. Institute of Medicine has advised women to intake 600 IU of vitamin D daily since 2010. Most experts concur that vitamin D deficiency in pregnancy may be corrected by administering 1000–2000 IU of vitamin D daily. Some experts even offer a maximum daily dose of 4000 IU of vitamin D for pregnant or breastfeeding women. The U.S. Department of Health and Human Services considers vitamin D a nutrient with significant consequences for public health [31].

3 Biochemical Properties of Breast Milk

Breast milk, a fluid with multiple actions, including the supply of nutrients, boosting infant immunity, and promoting healthy development, is unique to humans; as the infant grows and matures, its requirements alter, and the breast milk composition adapts accordingly [32]. The cells producing and secreting the milk into the lumen have multiple functions. The ways that nutrients are processed and packaged into breast milk vary, depending on the developmental stage reached by the infant. Colostrum, or early-stage milk, contains fewer lipids than mature milk, although protein and minerals are present in more significant amounts. The opposite pattern emerges as the infant grows and develops, with later-stage milk having a higher fat content [5].

Alongside the composition variation in the milk providing the infant's changing metabolic requirements, the milk composition varies within each session the baby feeds. The fore milk, the initial portion, has a relatively low-fat content that steadily increases. The hind milk, the last portion, provides the signals that make the infant feel satiated. Also, some differences occur in milk composition at different times of the day. These compositional differences are the consequences of the mother's diet and her changing hormone levels over the day [5].

3.1 Breast Milk Enzymes That Assist Digestion in the Neonate

Many breast milk enzymes, such as lactose synthetase, fatty acid synthetase, and thioesterase, act to generate milk components within the breast. Some other enzymes in breast milk assist the infant in digesting protein, lipids, and carbohydrates in breast milk. Furthermore, some breast milk enzymes act as packaging or for transporting minerals, notably zinc, selenium, and magnesium [5].

3.2 Structural Elements of Breast Milk

Breast milk contains structural elements that separate different components. Different compartments for specific nutrients in breast milk are separated from various bioactive molecules. Fats are the most striking example of compartmentalization in breast milk [5]. The fats are in milk-fat globules packaged within a plasma membrane derived from the epitheliocytes in the breast. The fat globule also transports specific proteins, growth factors, and vitamins in or within its membrane.

Separating membranes helps stabilize a fluid with hydrophilic and hydrophobic (fatty) elements. Lipids may be broken down before being released slowly into the aqueous phase of the milk, also termed milk serum. The membrane has amphiphilic properties, allowing the milk to remain an emulsion. Fat globules release aliphatic acids and cholesterol in the infant's small intestine, where micelles are formed to absorb the hydrophobic components [5].

3.3 Proteins, Carbohydrates, and Lipids for Development of the Nervous System

Breast milk has optimal levels of proteins, carbohydrates, and lipids for infants born at term. Proteins in breast milk mainly consist of alpha-lactalbumin and whey, while carbohydrates are primarily found as lactose. Lipids in breast milk exist in various kinds, such as cholesterol, triacyl glycerides, short-chain aliphatic acids, and long-chain polyunsaturated fatty acids (LCPFAs), with a carbon backbone of 18–22 carbon atoms essential for the formation processes of CNS and retina. Before and shortly after birth, a need for large amounts of specific LCPFAs, especially the omega-3 and -6 forms, occurs in the developing brain and retina. The main LCPFAs involved are arachidonic acid (AA) and docosahexaenoic acid (DHA), with 20 and 22 carbon atoms, respectively [1, 5, 6].

Infants, especially preterm newborns, potentially cannot produce adequate amounts of AA and DHA from linoleic and linolenic precursors. For this reason, AA and DHA are essential dietary components for infants. Accordingly, these acids are added singly or in combination with formula (artificial breast milk) preparations. The level of AA and DHA in breast milk depends on maternal dietary consumption [32–35]. A further role for aliphatic acids in breast milk is developing innate and adaptive immune systems [5].

Before AA and DHA were routinely added to formulas, advantages were detected regarding visual acuity and cognitive ability for breastfed infants compared to bottle-fed infants at 4 months [36]. However, not all studies have reached the same conclusion, and the benefit of DHA and AA supplementation remains a contentious issue. When the effects of adjusting mothers' diets to include more AA and DHA were studied, no differences were detected between groups in terms of neurodevelopmental outcomes [37]. A study of children aged 5 years compared the children of mothers who received early supplemental DHA with those whose mothers did not [38]. The supplement was continued until the infants were aged 4 months, and all the children studied were breastfed. Sustained attention was superior in the group receiving the supplemental DHA.

It is still uncertain whether adding AA and DHA to the formula is advantageous since infants can convert longer fatty acids to AA and DHA. The groups where the most significant benefit is likely to occur are sick infants born at term or premature infants, the most likely to have specific requirements for AA or DHA [5]. Breast milk, further than a single component, such as AA, DHA, or any other compound, contributes to a number of factors leading to the development of infants. It is probable that breastfed infants, further than gaining additional advantages regarding visual acuity or cognitive development, can develop these abilities since the molecular components and growth factors required to grow are present and act synergistically [5].

Dallas et al. [39] compared the breast milk of mothers who delivered preterm and term infants. The protease content, which assisted with the breakdown of proteins in preterm breast milk, was significantly above that found in the term milk. In preterm breast milk samples, plasmin, cytosol aminopeptidase, and carboxypeptidase B2 were more active than in the term milk. These findings have been concluded as evidence that breast milk contains a mechanism for assisting digestion in premature infants with an insufficiently developed digestive tract.

Preterm formula, artificial baby milk formulated for premature infants, has been found to promote better bone mineralization than the usual formula for term infants. Infants whose birth weight was exceptionally low also grow and develop better with the preterm formula [40].

4   Bioactivity in Breast Milk

Bioactive molecules, such as epidermal growth factor (EGF), granulocyte colony-stimulating factor (G-CSF), insulin-like growth factors (IGFs), interleukins (ILs), nerve growth factor (NGF), and transforming growth factors (TGFs) alpha and beta, are contained in breast milk. The growth factors in breast milk are synthesized by several cell types such as the epitheliocytes in the breast, activated macrophages, lymphocytes, particularly T-lymphocytes, and neutrophils in the milk itself.

Epidermal growth factor and TGF-alpha are at higher concentrations in the breast milk of mothers who delivered preterm newborns than in the breast milk of mothers of term babies. Epidermal growth factor plays a crucial role in how the epithelial lining of the intestines repairs itself and regenerates following injury. Fetal small intestinal cells proliferate in response to EGF and TGF-alpha of breast milk [41]. So, the presence of EGF in breast milk explains why breastfed infants have a reduced necrotizing enterocolitis (NEC) risk.

5 Conclusion

Breast milk is essential for the appropriate physical and neurological development of newborns, especially preterm infants. The ideal development and growth of newborns depend on breast milk components. The constituents of breast milk are optimized for the infants to grow and develop in a healthy way. Bioactive compounds of breast milk have significant roles in developing and maturating organ systems. The composition of the maternal diet influences the development of the growing fetus. Pregnant women may not sufficiently be fed and may have several vitamin, trace elements, and mineral deficiencies. Pregnant women should be carefully evaluated in terms of diet and needs for vitamin and mineral supplementations. Exclusive breastfeeding should be promoted and supported as a public health priority.

References

1. World Health Organization. Global strategy for infant and young child feeding. Geneva: World Health Organization; 2003. p. 1–30. https://www.who.int/publications/i/item/9241562218. Accessed 20 Feb 2023.
2. Meek JY, Noble L, Section on Breastfeeding, American Academy of Pediatrics. Policy statement: breastfeeding and the use of human milk. Pediatrics. 2022;150(1):e2022057988.
3. Zhou Y, Chen J, Li Q, Huang W, Lan H, Jiang H. Association between breastfeeding and breast cancer risk: evidence from a meta-analysis. Breastfeed Med. 2015;10:175–82.
4. Babic A, Sasamoto N, Rosner BA, et al. Association between breastfeeding and ovarian cancer risk. JAMA Oncol. 2020;6(6):e200421.
5. Tauber KA. Human milk and lactation (updated: Jun 29, 2021). In: Nimavat DJ, editor. Medscape. https://emedicine.medscape.com/article/1835675-overview#a7. Accessed 20 Feb 2023.
6. Barger MK. Maternal nutrition and perinatal outcomes. J Midwifery Womens Health. 2010;55:502–11.
7. Clapp JF 3rd. Maternal carbohydrate intake and pregnancy outcome. Proc Nutr Soc. 2002;61:45–50.
8. Loy SL, Marhazlina M, Azwany YN, Jan JMH. Higher intake of fruits and vegetables in pregnancy is associated with birth size. Southeast Asian J Trop Med Public Health. 2011;42:1214–23.

9. Lowensohn RI, Stadler DD, Naze C. Current concepts of maternal nutrition. Obstet Gynecol Surv. 2016;71:413–26.
10. National Institutes of Health. Clinical guidelines on the identification, evaluation, and treatment of overweight and obesity in adults. Obes Res. 1998;(Suppl 2):s51–209. [Erratum: Obes Res. 1998;Nov6(6):464].
11. Eckel RH, Jakicic JM, Ard JD, et al. 2013 AHA/ACC guideline on lifestyle management to reduce cardiovascular risk: a report of the American College of Cardiology/American Heart Association task force on practice guidelines. Circulation. 2014;129(25 Suppl 2):s76–99.
12. Vannice G, Rasmussen H. Position of the academy of nutrition and dietetics: dietary fatty acids for healthy adults. J Acad Nutr Diet. 2014;114:136–53.
13. Chen X, Scholl TO, Leskiw M, Savaille J, Stein TP. Differences in maternal circulating fatty acid composition and dietary fat intake in women with gestational diabetes mellitus or mild gestational hyperglycemia. Diabetes Care. 2010;33:2049–54.
14. Bowers K, Tobias DK, Yeung E, Hu FB, Zhang C. A prospective study of prepregnancy dietary fat intake and risk of gestational diabetes. Am J Clin Nutr. 2012;95:446–53.
15. Park S, Kim MY, Baik SH, et al. Gestational diabetes is associated with high energy and saturated fat intakes and with low plasma visfatin and adiponectin levels independent of prepregnancy BMI. Eur J Clin Nutr. 2013;67:196–201.
16. Mishra V, Thapa S, Retherford RD, Dai X. Effect of iron supplementation during pregnancy on birthweight: evidence from Zimbabwe. Food Nutr Bull. 2005;26:338–47.
17. Bhutta ZA, Cabral S, Chan CW, Keenan WJ. Reducing maternal, newborn, and infant mortality globally: an integrated action agenda. Int J Gynaecol Obstet. 2012;119(suppl 1):s13–7.
18. Reveiz L, Gyte MLG, Cuervo GL. Treatments for iron-deficiency anaemia in pregnancy. Cochrane Database Syst Rev. 2007;2:CD003094.
19. Cantor AG, Bougatsos C, Dana T, Blazina I, McDonagh M. Routine iron supplementation and screening for iron deficiency anemia in pregnancy: a systematic review for the US preventive services task force. Ann Intern Med. 2015;162:566–76.
20. Crider KS, Bailey LB, Berry RJ. Folic acid food fortification-its history, effect, concerns, and future directions. Nutrients. 2011;3:370–84.
21. Jagerstad M. Folic acid fortification prevents neural tube defects and may also reduce cancer risks. Acta Paediatr. 2012;101:1007–12.
22. Chang H, Zhang T, Zhang Z, et al. Tissue-specific distribution of aberrant DNA methylation associated with maternal low-folate status in human neural tube defects. J Nutr Biochem. 2011;22:1172–7.
23. Ahrens K, Yazdy MM, Mitchell AA, Werler MM. Folic acid intake and spina bifida in the era of dietary folic acid fortification. Epidemiology. 2011;22:731–7.
24. Siega-Riz AM, Savitz DA, Zeisel SH, Thorp JM, Herring A. Second trimester folate status and preterm birth. Am J Obstet Gynecol. 2004;191:1851–7.
25. Martí-Carvajal A, Peña-Martí G, Comunián-Carrasco G, et al. Prematurity and maternal folate deficiency: anemia during pregnancy study group results in Valencia, Venezuela. Arch Latinoam Nutr. 2004;54:45–9.
26. Bukowski R, Malone FD, Porter FT, et al. Preconceptional folate supplementation and the risk of spontaneous preterm birth: a cohort study. PLoS Med. 2009;6(5):e1000061.
27. Shaw GM, Carmichael SL, Yang W, Siega-Giz AM. Periconceptional intake of folic acid and food folate and risks of preterm delivery. Am J Perinatol. 2011;28:747–52.
28. Chiaffarino F, Ascone GB, Bortolus R, et al. Effects of folic acid supplementation on pregnancy outcomes: a review of randomized clinical trials. Minerva Ginecol. 2010;62:293–301. [article in Italian, abstract in English].
29. Kloosterman J, de Jong N, Rompelberg CJM, van Kranen HJ, Kampman E, Ocke EK. Folic acid fortification: prevention as well as promotion of cancer. Ned Tijdschr Geneeskd. 2006;150:1443–8. [article in Dutch, abstract in English.]

30. Troen AM, Mitchell B, Sorensen B, et al. Unmetabolized folic acid in plasma is associated with reduced natural killer cell cytotoxicity among postmenopausal women. J Nutr. 2006;136:189–94.
31. US Department of Health and Human Services and US Department of Agriculture. Dietary Guidelines for Americans 2015–2020, 8th ed.; 2015, pp. 1–122. https://health.gov/sites/default/files/2019-09/2015-2020_Dietary_Guidelines.pdf. Accessed 20 Feb 2023.
32. Crawford MA, Doyle W, Drury P, Lennon A, Costeloe K, Leighfield M. N-6 and n-3 fatty acids during early human development. J Intern Med Suppl. 1989;731:159–69.
33. Arterburn LM, Hall EB, Oken H. Distribution, interconversion, and dose-response of n-3 fatty acids in humans. Am J Clin Nutr. 2006;83(6 suppl):s1467–76.
34. Mosca F, Gianni ML. Human milk: composition and health benefits. Pediatr Med Chir. 2017;39(2):47–52.
35. Hand IL, Noble L. Premature infants and breastfeeding. In: Lawrence RA, Lawrence RM, Noble L, Rosen-Carole C, Stuebe AM, editors. Breastfeeding: a guide for the medical profession. 9th ed. Philadelphia: Elsevier; 2021. p. 502–45.
36. Birch E, Birch D, Hoffman D, Hale L, Everett M, Uauy R. Breastfeeding and optimal visual development. J Pediatr Ophthalmol Strabismus. 1993;30:33–8.
37. Crawford MA. The role of essential fatty acids in neural development: implications for perinatal nutrition. Am J Clin Nutr. 1993;57(5 suppl):s703–10.
38. Jensen CL, Voigt RG, Llorente AM, et al. Effects of early maternal docosahexaenoic acid intake on neuropsychological status and visual acuity at five years of age of breastfed term infants. J Pediatr. 2010;157:900–5.
39. Dallas DC, Smink CJ, Robinson RC, et al. Endogenous human milk peptide release is greater after preterm birth than term birth. J Nutr. 2015;145:425–33.
40. Hay WW Jr, Hendrickson KC. Preterm formula use in the preterm very low birth weight infant. Semin Fetal Neonatal Med. 2017;22:15–22.
41. Sullivan S, Schanler RJ, Kim JH, et al. An exclusively human milk-based diet is associated with a lower rate of necrotizing enterocolitis than a diet of human milk and bovine milk-based products. J Pediatr. 2010;156:562–7.

Immunological Aspects of Breast Milk

Hilal Güngör and Sinan Tüfekçi

1 Introduction

For term infants whose mothers are healthy and have a satisfactory dietary intake, breast milk is the ideal mode of nutrition. The recommendation is that infants up to the age of 6 months be solely breastfed, after which breastfeeding should continue alongside the introduction of solid food up to at least the age of 2 years. The composition of breast milk varies over the course of a single feed, and according to when in the day feeding occurs, as well as the stage of lactation. Alongside this intra-individual variation in composition, the composition varies from mother to mother and from population to population. Both the environment and the woman's genetics affect composition, as does whether the infant is a boy or girl, if an infection occurs, and any change in the mother's lifestyle, such as changes in diet [1].

Birth is a key milestone in the maturation of the immune system. The unborn child encounters a wide range of non-self-antigens, mostly of maternal origin, and the immune system must learn to tolerate these antigens for normal development to occur. Once birth occurs, the immune system must respond in a more nuanced manner. Exposure to a wide range of antigens occurs via the skin and mucosae. It must attack microbes that act as potential pathogens, whilst commensal organisms and macromolecules in the diet must not provoke a response (i.e. tolerance must occur). The newborn is able to mount an immune response comparable to that of a fully mature adult in some respects, but there are a number of components of the immune

H. Güngör (✉)
Department of Internal Medicine, Eskisehir City Hospital, Eskisehir, Türkiye

S. Tüfekçi
Neonatology Section, Department of Pediatrics, Medical Faculty, Tekirdağ Namık Kemal University, Tekirdağ, Türkiye
e-mail: stufekci@nku.edu.tr

Ö. N. Şahin et al. (eds.), *Breastfeeding and Metabolic Programming*,
https://doi.org/10.1007/978-3-031-33278-4_3

system that are not yet developed in the infant and thus, even in normal infants, it is normal for a degree of immunodeficiency to exist, which later disappears [2–4].

In this chapter we will examine the immune response in neonates, noting where the system is fully operational and where it has yet to develop its mature functionality.

2   The Immune System in General

There are two principal arms of the human immune system, providing both innate (non-specific) and acquired (specific) immunity. The innate defences involve responses that can come into play without the need for the immune system to have previously encountered a specific antigen or microbe. Included amongst the innate defences are the physical barriers presented by the skin and mucosal surfaces, provided these barriers have not been disrupted, and generalised chemical defences, such as hydrochloric acid in the stomach and the pancreatic enzymes [5]. Deep to the mucosal and cutaneous surfaces phagocytes lurk in readiness to engulf any microorganisms able to pass through the barrier. There are a number of proteins, both in the tissues themselves and within the circulation, the effect of which is to enhance the phagocytic actions of the innate defences. The acquired arm of the system is mainly made up of T-cells, acting at the cellular level, and B-cells, whose effects are humoral, i.e. through production of antibodies.

The development of complete immunocompetence depends on the maturation of both arms of the immune system, innate and acquired. These arms function in a highly integrated way and depend on each other for efficient elimination of threats. Key effectors within the innate arm are neutrophils and cells derived from monocytic precursors or differentiated macrophages, which normally act to engulf and digest microbes invading into the tissues. Both monocytes and macrophages process the antigens from ingested matter [6].

3   Haematopoiesis: Overview

The earliest haematopoieses occur within extra-embryonic mesoderm forming the yolk sac, but as the foetus keeps developing, blood begins to be produced in the liver and eventually the bone marrow. The yolk sac blood production is active between week 3 and weeks 8 or 10 of gestation. The liver becomes haematopoietically active in week 5 and remains so until weeks 20–24. The liver mainly produces red blood cells. There are numerous progenitor cells of the myeloid lineage visible in sections of foetal liver, but mature neutrophils are absent. Bone marrow blood production first becomes evident by week 11, at which point the clavicle is seen to synthesise differentiated progenitor cells of the granular series. By week 20, most blood production has already permanently shifted to the bone marrow, which continues to generate cells to keep the blood cell numbers at an adequate level.

The cells of the immune system all die within a certain amount of time, and there is a need for the pluripotent stem cells to divide constantly to supply precursors, which then differentiate into each type [6, 7]. The precise way in which pluripotent stem cells become committed to a specific lineage still awaits elucidation, but it is clear that this is the origin of the cellular immune components within the circulation. The division of progenitor cells and their maturation into different types is generally under the control of growth factors secreted into the matrix surrounding haematopoietic cells by fibroblasts, endothelial cells and macrophages. Data are also accumulating to show that the extracellular matrix itself plays a part in how progenitor cells differentiate. There are particular glycoproteins in the matrix exercising a regulatory function. [6, 7]

4 Polymorphonucleocytes (PMNs) and Neutrophils

The PMNs in infants, whether premature or term, are less adept at chemotactic pursuit, phagocytosis and killing of microbes than their mature counterparts. There is plentiful evidence to show that haematopoietic growth factors stimulate greater production of neutrophils and increase their ability to perform their physiological roles. Administration of granulocyte colony-stimulating factor (G-CSF), and Granulocyte-macrophage colony-stimulating factor (GM-CSF), raises the levels of reserve neutrophils, causes a rise in circulating neutrophil levels and renders these cells more effective in multiple ways. It has been demonstrated in a meta-analysis that administering G-CSF to newborn infants with sepsis lowered the death rate [8]. Nonetheless, when this analysis was repeated to encompass studies that lacked randomisation, the result was no longer of statistical significance. Newborn infants typically exhibit good tolerance for G-CSF injections, with the result that it is now common for G-CSF of recombinant origin to be utilised in neonatal units treating infants with severe neutropenia, i.e. a count below 500 lasting for 48 hours or maintained between 500 and 100 for at least 5 or 7 days [9]. Despite this practice being common, the evidence base currently is insufficient to justify a general recommendation to use growth factors in newborns suffering from sepsis with the aim of decreasing severity and fatal outcomes. There is a requirement for more evidence to be obtained about outcomes in particular risk subgroups amongst these patients. The initial studies appear to show greater efficacy in particular risk groups. G-CSF is now available in forms that have a more prolonged therapeutic action, and these may be suitable for treating newborns with neutropenic sepsis. The modified forms of G-CSF are obtained through conjugation with polyethylene glycol or by glycosylation.

5   Mononuclear Phagocytes

Mononuclear phagocytes in neonates home more slowly and in fewer numbers to the site of inflammation than in adults. This weaker response is probably the result of less effective chemotaxis by circulating monocytes in the newborn infant. However, mononucleocytes are equally good at engulfing and destroying microbes in both adults and neonates. The evidence base for in vivo macrophage activity at birth and in neonates is restricted at present; however, macrophages located in the pulmonary alveoli in those cases investigated up to now appear to possess normal capabilities.

6   Humoral Defences

It is currently unknown whether complement is only partially functional in newborns, but if so, this may lead to immunodeficiency. If the classical or alternative pathways are defective, this probably renders infants more prone to infection, particularly if the infant was delivered preterm. Neonates possess a certain limited number of immunoglobulins of maternal origin that cross the placenta. The immunoglobulins are mostly of IgG. IgM is not transferred. Immunoglobulins with specificity for Gram-negative organisms are notably absent. During the perinatal period, the classic pathway offers minimal protection. Since the classic pathway for complement activation depends on the presence of specific immune defences, i.e. immunoglobulins, and this branch of the immune system is immature at birth, the alternative and lectin pathways are of vital importance in early neonatal bacterial infections. In the majority of cases where a newborn is fighting a bacterial infection, the polymorphonucleocytes are relatively ineffective, and any deficiency in complement activation is likely to be of major clinical significance. In cases where neonatal sepsis has been proven by microbiological culture, there is a relative deficiency of mannose-binding lectin and the ficolins [10].

7   Cytokines and Chemokines

Neonates are at increased risk of infections due to the relative state of immunodeficiency at this stage in life. Stimulation and regulation of immune defences belonging to the acquired immune system are under the control of a number of interacting messengers (cytokines and chemokines) in the form of glycoproteins and phospholipids. These signals control how the immune defences react to perceived threats and determine the ultimate cell type into which precursor cells of both immune and non-immune lineages develop. Infants need to be able to generate a proportionate and sufficient degree of inflammation to destroy invading pathogens without leaving lasting damage to the infant's own tissues. If there is overdominance of pro- or anti-inflammatory signals, the risk of death and complications rises. An imbalanced expression of cytokines in newborns potentially contributes to necrotising enterocolitis, bronchopulmonary dysplasia and central nervous system hypoxic or ischaemic damage. Previously unknown cytokines are constantly being discovered. The following sections describe the cytokines of principal significance in pathogenic infections and other perceived threats, as well as outline how they develop in utero and during the neonatal period. The way the cytokine response is orchestrated in sepsis in newborns is also addressed [6].

8 Molecular Biological Aspects of Cytokines and Chemokines

8.1 The Interleukin-1 Superfamily

The interleukin (IL)-1 superfamily consists of 11 distinct cytokines, which produce a complicated pattern of both increasing and suppressing inflammation. IL-1α, IL-1β and the IL-1 receptor antagonist (IL-1ra) are the most heavily studied members of this family. The initial stage in the synthesis of interleukins 1α and 1β involves production of precursor molecules, i.e. pro-IL-1α and pro-IL-1β. The former already possesses bioactivity and is found within the cellular cytoplasm. It may also function in intercellular communication after being translocated to the outer cell membrane. The only situation where this cytokine is found in plasma is in severe disease states. Although the amino-acid sequence differs considerably between IL-1α and IL-1β, they both attach to the same receptor and have an identical tertiary structure. Pro-IL-1β, by contrast, is a normal constituent of plasma. It is inactive until acted upon by IL-1β converting enzyme/caspase I, a cysteine protease, after which it enters the circulation. Interleukin-1ra competes with other cytokines in the superfamily and prevents their acting. It does not itself act agonistically. Interleukins have two different types of receptor, types I and II. All the members of the superfamily are capable of binding to type I, but only IL-1β is capable of attaching to type II. The receptors are themselves members of a superfamily, in this case the IL-1 receptor/Toll-like receptor (TLR) superfamily [11].

A large number of different types of cell produce interleukin-1, such as monocytes, histiocytes, neutrophils and cells of the endothelium and epithelium. Production of interleukins begins in response to molecules of microbial origin found during an inflammatory response. The interleukins are key mediators of how inflammation occurs. Infant monocytes and macrophages express IL-1 in the same way as adults, regardless of whether the infant was born at term or prematurely. However, in acute sepsis, monocytic expression of this cytokine is frequently reduced in premature infants [6].

8.2   Interleukin-6 (IL-6)

IL-6 undergoes a number of modifications post-translationally, which means it assumes various different forms. This cytokine is manufactured in response to various stimulatory signals, in particular other cytokines (such as IL-1 and IL-6 itself), platelet-derived growth factor and epidermal growth factor. Synthesis of IL-6 also occurs in response to invading viruses or bacteria, and the presence of particular compounds, namely double-stranded RNA, endotoxins and Cyclic adenosine monophosphate (cAMP). IL-6 has an associated receptor, which is formed from two separate subunits. The first subunit (IL-6R) binds IL-6, but does not generate the response, for which the second subunit, gp130, is responsible. The receptor is also found as a soluble molecule (sIL-6Ra), to which IL-6 may attach, following which the receptor–ligand complex can attach to gp130, triggering a response. This means that even cells lacking the full receptor are capable of being stimulated by IL-6. Extraneous IL-6, when administered to human subjects, does provoke both pyrexia and chills, but produces a lesser degree of toxicity than either IL-1β or tumour necrosis factor (TNF). The known actions of IL-6 include activation of both B-lymphocytes and T-lymphocytes, enhanced maturation of megakaryocytes, elevated expression of proteins found in the acute-phase response and stimulation of action by the natural killer cells. When monocytes derived from infants delivered at term were exposed to lipopolysaccharide, they expressed normal levels of IL-6, but IL-1 production was below adult levels. There was a defective level of IL-6 secretion in monocytes taken from premature infants, regardless of the method used to stimulate a response. The plasma concentration of IL-6 in neonates is below that of their mothers, but more of the monocytes express IL-6 in neonates than in the mothers, regardless of whether they were born at term or prematurely.

8.3   The Interleukin-10 (IL-10) Superfamily

The IL-10 protein superfamily consists of IL-10 itself and a number of other related cytokines, which each regulate some aspect of immune function, such as interleukin-19, -20, -22, -24, -26, -28 and -29 [6]. IL-10 is manufactured by monocytes, macrophages and both B- and T-lymphocytes following exposure to whole bacteria, components of bacteria, and viral, fungal or parasitic organisms. It is a polypeptide that can powerfully inhibit inflammation. It acts to reduce expression of a large range of pro-inflammatory cytokines whilst simultaneously stimulating expression of cytokines that can act to inhibit other cytokines with a pro-inflammatory action, such as IL-1ra. IL-10 manufacture is upgraded following stimulation by several cytokines, notably TNF and interleukin-1, -6 and -12. However, IL-10 does also increase B-lymphocytic efficacy and stimulates maturation of cytotoxic T-lymphocytes. The interleukin-10 receptor is formed from two subcomponents. They are within the class II cytokine receptor family. Expression of IL-10 in newborns is below adult levels [6, 11].

8.4   Interleukin-12 (IL-12) and Interferon-Gamma (IFN-γ)

The IL-12 cytokine is a heterodimeric molecule. The two constituent subcomponents are referred to as p35 and p40, which are translated from separate genes [12]. It is the p40 portion of the molecule that attaches to the associated receptor (IL-12R) and the p35 portion then triggers a signal cascade. Two p40 molecules may also attach to each other forming a homodimeric molecule that can attach as strongly to IL-12R as the heterodimer, but then fails to elicit a cellular response. It is probable that the homodimeric form has a regulatory effect on IL-12 signalling. There are separate mechanisms governing expression of each of the IL-12 subunits. In certain circumstances, the concentration of homodimer exceeds that of the 'p35 + p40' form between 10- and a 100-fold. Phagocytes (especially monocytes and macrophages) synthesise IL-12 when exposed to whole bacteria or components thereof, microbes of intracellular type or viruses. The IL-12R falls within the gp130 cytokine receptor superfamily and is formed of two subcomponents. The receptor only triggers a signal cascade if both subcomponents are activated. The main cells regulated by IL-12 are T-lymphocytes and natural killer cells. In response to IL-12, IFN-γ expression is stepped up and cellular division occurs. Cell-killing activity increases. Mononucleocytes taken from cord samples and stimulated by bacterial endotoxin express lower than normal levels of IL-12, except when presented with *Staphylococcus aureus* components in the form of heat-killed organisms.

A number of different cells express IFN-γ in response to stimulation by interleukin-1, -12, -15 and -18, as well as TNF. These cells include the natural killer cells, T-helper 1 cells and cytotoxic T-lymphocytes. The IFN-γ receptor is made up of two subunits, to one of which the ligand attaches, whilst the other triggers an intracellular signalling cascade. The actions of IFN-γ involve stimulating antigen presentation by the major histocompatibility complex class II and activation of macrophages. This molecule strengthens the immune response to intracellular pathogenic agents and performs a number of other roles. Its level of manufacture is very low in newborns compared to adults [12, 13].

9   The Tumour Necrosis Factor (TNF) Superfamily

There are 18 molecules within the TNF superfamily grouping, with varied roles, such as assisting development, provoking inflammation and stimulating cytotoxic killing [14]. The two molecules in the superfamily that have attracted most interest are TNF (which may also be referred to as TNF-α or cachectin) and lymphotoxin-alpha (also referred to as TNF-β). TNF can exist in two forms, i.e. as a membrane-bound pro-hormone or as a truncated trimeric molecule, which is soluble. This latter is produced by enzymatic cleavage of the pro-hormone by disintegrin, a matrix metalloproteinase. Both the pro-hormone and soluble form possess potential bioactivity. As is the case with IL-1, molecules released by microbes under inflammatory attack can stimulate expression of TNF. It is also synthesised in response to IL-1, and TNF itself. Whilst multiple cell types have the capacity to express TNF, it is mainly secreted in soluble form by monocytes and macrophages.

TNF-α and lymphotoxin-α have their own receptors, TNF-RI and RII. Agonists acting on TNF-RI reproduce multiple actions attributed to TNF, such as encouraging cytotoxic killing and increased expression of molecules of adhesion. A section of the TNF-RI receptor within the cytoplasm consisting of 80 amino-acid residues controls apoptosis. It seems probable that TNF-RII mainly assists the attachment of TNF to the type I receptor.

10 Platelet-Activating Factor (PAF)

PAF is a phospholipid molecule with a potent mode of action and a short half-life. It is enzymatically degraded by acetylhydrolase. Multiple cell populations may synthesise PAF, but regulation of secretion has only been demonstrated in macrophages and eosinophils. The main location for the molecule is facing the extracellular space and it functions in intercellular signalling. If extraneous PAF is given intravenously to laboratory animals, it causes a fall in systemic tension, the capillaries become leaky, there is a rise in the pulmonary arterial tension, a reduction in neutrophils and platelets and the intestines undergo ischaemic necrosis. PAF has a powerful stimulatory effect on neutrophils. Its expression is upgraded in response to exposure to bacterial lipopolysaccharides, low oxygen tension, haematopoietic growth factors, TNF, IL-1, thrombin, bradykinin and leukotriene C4. There is also a stimulatory effect from PAF on several other immune processes, reflected in raised levels of TNF, complement activity, oxygen-derived reactive species, prostaglandin synthesis, thromboxane expression and leukotriene signalling. Raised levels of PAF in newborns are strongly associated with necrotising enterocolitis, although this does not necessarily imply causality [13].

11 Conclusion

The T-lymphocytes in neonates are less capable than adult T-cells of mounting a T-helper 1 response. Their expression of IFN-γ and TNF is muted in response to stimulatory signals, even when the cluster of differentiation (CD)3 T-cell receptor is activated. In the neonatal period, T-lymphocytes are relatively immature and thus less efficacious than in adults. However, the T-lymphocytes in neonates are capable of synthesising cytokines at the level found in adults if there is sufficient co-stimulation of a T-helper 1 response. Furthermore, cytotoxic T-cells in newborns can differentiate into long-lived memory cells capable of responding to a number of different viruses, notably cytomegalovirus and Rous sarcoma virus. Thus there is potential for a vaccination strategy in neonates aiming to treat viral infections.

The lower effectiveness of T-lymphocytes and other antigen-presenting cells than their fully mature counterparts may be partially attributable to their being qualitatively dissimilar. T-lymphocytes obtained from neonates appear to need a greater level of co-stimulation to mount an effective T-helper 1 response, both in their normal body environment and in the test tube. The weaker T-helper 1 response in newborns may be a consequence of less effective antigen presentation by cells other than lymphocytes. This conclusion appears supported by noting that boosts to antigen presentation in newborns may permit a more vigorous, adult-level T-helper 1 response to occur.

References

1. Bravi F, Wiens F, Decarli A, Dal Pont A, Agostoni C, Ferraroni M. Impact of maternal nutrition on breast-milk composition: a systematic review. Am J Clin Nutr. 2016;104(3):646–62. https://doi.org/10.3945/ajcn.115.120881. Epub 2016 Aug 17.
2. Amulic B, Cazalet C, Hayes GL, et al. Neutrophil function: from mechanisms to disease. Annu Rev Immunol. 2012;30:459–89.
3. Artis D, Spits H. The biology of innate lymphoid cells. Nature. 2015;517:293–301.
4. Barnie PA, Lin X, Liu Y, et al. IL-17 producing innate lymphoid cells 3 (ILC3) but not Th17 cells might be the potential danger factor for preeclampsia and other pregnancy associated diseases. Int J Clin Exp Pathol. 2015;8:11,100–7.
5. Bharat A, Bhorade SM, Morales-Nebreda L, et al. Flow cytometry reveals similarities between lung macrophages in humans and mice. Am J Respir Cell Mol Biol. 2016;54:147–9.
6. Benjamin JT, Maheshwari A. Chapter 47 developmental immunology. In: Fanaroff and Martin's neonatal-perinatal medicine, diseases of the fetus and infant. 11th ed. Elsevier; 2000. ISBN: 978-0-323-56711-4.
7. Yoder MC. Aortic tissue as a niche for hematopoiesis. Circulation. 2012;125:565–7.
8. Christensen RD, Jensen J, Maheshwari A, Henry E. Reference ranges for blood concentrations of eosinophils and monocytes during the neonatal period defined from over 63 000 records in a multihospital health-care system. J Perinatol. 2010;30:540–5.
9. Bernstein HM, Pollock BH, Calhoun DA, Christensen RD. Administration of recombinant granulocyte colony-stimulating factor to neonates with septicemia: a meta-analysis. J Pediatr. 2001;138:917–20.
10. Schlapbach LJ, Mattmann M, Thiel S, et al. Differential role of the lectin pathway of complement activation in susceptibility to neonatal sepsis. Clin Infect Dis. 2010;51:153–62.
11. Vignali DA, Kuchroo VK. IL-12 family cytokines: immunological playmakers. Nat Immunol. 2012;13:722–8.
12. Walker JC, Smolders MA, Gemen EF, et al. Development of lymphocyte subpopulations in preterm infants. Scand J Immunol. 2011;73:53–8.
13. O'Neill LA, Golenbock D, Bowie AG. The history of toll-like. Receptors—redefining innate immunity. Nat Rev Immunol. 2013;13:453–60.
14. Del Vecchio A, Christensen RD. Neonatal neutropenia: what diagnostic evaluation is needed and when is treatment recommended? Early Hum Dev. 2012;88(suppl 2):S19–24.

Immunological and Anti-Infectious Benefits of Breastfeeding

Mustafa Törehan Aslan, Ayşe Engin Arısoy, and Armando G. Correa

1 Introduction

Breast milk, with its nutritional, immunological, and anti-infectious properties, is always an indispensable food for infants due to the many diseases it can protect against in infancy, childhood, and even adulthood. Therefore, exclusive breastfeeding for about the first 6 months and continued breastfeeding along with appropriate complementary foods for up to 2 years of age or older is advised [1–3]. This chapter summarizes the immunological and anti-infectious benefits of breastfeeding.

2 Immunological Aspects of Breast Milk

Breast milk contains abundant molecules, such as immunoglobulins (Igs), lactoferrin, lysozymes, and cytokines, which provide immunological functions, directly or indirectly conferring active or passive immunity in breastfed infants [3, 4].

M. T. Aslan (✉)
Division of Neonatology, Department of Pediatrics, Faculty of Medicine, Tekirdağ Namık Kemal University, Tekirdağ, Türkiye

A. E. Arısoy
Division of Neonatology, Department of Pediatrics, Faculty of Medicine, Kocaeli University (Emeritus), Kocaeli, Türkiye

A. G. Correa
Division of Academic General Pediatrics, Department of Pediatrics, Baylor College of Medicine, and Section of International and Destination Medicine, Texas Children's Hospital, Houston, TX, USA
e-mail: acorrea@bcm.edu

Ö. N. Şahin et al. (eds.), *Breastfeeding and Metabolic Programming*, https://doi.org/10.1007/978-3-031-33278-4_4

2.1 Immunoglobulins

Immunoglobulins (Igs) of all classes (A, D, E, G, and M) are found in breast milk; however, secretory IgA (sIgA) is the type present at the highest level. After birth, until the onset of the endogenous neonatal sIgA synthesis, breast milk sIgA is a significant contributor to passive immunity. Humans are relatively defenseless against pathogens that invade the gut; hence the protection provided by breast milk sIgA is critical. In premature infants, the time period until endogenous sIgA synthesis begins is even longer. Thus, the protection provided by sIgA depends to an even greater degree on maternal sIgA delivered via breast milk [5].

The mother and her baby coexist in close proximity and come to carry the same microbial flora. Thus, the organisms targeted by the mother's immunoglobulins are the same ones threatening the infant. The mother's immune system surveys the flora of the gastrointestinal and respiratory tracts and synthesizes IgA according to the potential pathogens detected. These immunoglobulins pass via the blood and lymph to the breast and then are secreted into breast milk. Immunoglobulin A is packaged in a particular way before being released into breast milk, such that it is protected from being denatured in the acidic environment of the infant's gastric cavity and allowing it to pass undamaged into the small intestine [4].

2.2 Other Molecules with Immunological Functions

Breast milk also contains multiple other molecules possessing immunological functions, acting on the gastrointestinal tract's flora and shaping it in healthy ways. The most significant protein in the whey proteins portion of breast milk is lactoferrin, which possesses a range of antimicrobial and anti-inflammatory actions. Lactoferrin assists in establishing a healthy bacterial flora, promoting beneficial species, and inhibiting the growth of pathogens [6]. One of its actions is the sequestration of iron, an element that numerous pathogenic species rely on to multiply. Lactoferrin can stop bacteria from attaching themselves to the walls of the gut. Lactoferricin, formed from lactoferrin, is a positively charged peptide that can destroy bacteria.

Lactose and fats are the constituents of breast milk at the highest concentrations. Human milk oligosaccharides (HMOs) are the third most abundant constituent. These oligosaccharides directly affect the infant's gastrointestinal flora as they act as food for some microorganisms, promoting healthy flora and preventing harmful species' attachment to the gastrointestinal lining [7]. Maternal and genetic factors influence the expression pattern of the HMOs secreted into the milk. Considerable variability in breast milk HMOs exists between women and in the same person at different stages of breastfeeding [4, 8].

Human milk glycoproteins (HMGPs), also immunologically active breast milk constituents, can inhibit the multiplication of many pathogenic microorganisms.

The mucins play highly significant extracellular roles within this group of molecules by preventing pathogens from invading the gut lining, modulating cellular signaling, and influencing gene expression [9].

The science behind how all these bioactive molecules interact with the microbes in the gastrointestinal tract and how this affects healthy development is still at an early stage. However, the bioactive components of breast milk have a significant and lasting effect on the health of breastfed individuals, beginning in infancy and continuing at every stage of life [5, 10–12].

2.3 Leukocytes

Leukocytes in breast milk assist the infant in gaining immunity to infection in several ways, including phagocytic engulfment of pathogens, synthesis of biologically active immune system molecules, aiding the maturation of the neonatal immune system, and altering the composition of the infant gut flora favorably [13]. Significant alterations exist in the leukocyte population of breast milk at different stages of breastfeeding. Trend et al. [14] noted that the total white blood cell count and the proportions of the cell types changed according to the lactation stage. The leukocytic concentration was around 146,000 cells per mL in colostrum, lower in transitional milk at 27,500 cells per mL from 8 to 12 days after delivery, and even lower in mature milk at 23,650 cells per mL from 26 to 30 days.

2.4 Passive Immunity Conferred by Breastfeeding

Before the infant has gained a mature immune system, passive immunity is provided by several different immunologically active components in breast milk. These components act in concert to provide passive protection from birth up to a few months [15]. Passive immunity provided by breast milk results in a lowered incidence of infections of the gastrointestinal and respiratory tracts, particularly in the first year of life [3, 16, 17].

Growing data support the hypothesis that immunologically active components of breast milk "train" the gut and immune system of the newborn to recognize and react appropriately to specific antigens, including the signals to release. Breast milk training function may be the reason why breastfed infants are less likely to develop allergic hypersensitivity to ingested or inhaled antigens and have a lowered incidence of autoimmune disorders. Since allergic and autoimmune disorders involve multiple factors, establishing a mechanism for such effects is highly complex and challenging [4].

3   Beneficial Effects of Breastfeeding

3.1   *Respiratory Tract and Middle Ear Infections*

The likelihood of being admitted to the hospital following a lower respiratory tract infection falls by 72% in children exclusively breastfed for at least 4 months [18, 19]. The risk of pneumonia is four times higher in infants exclusively breastfed for 4–6 months than in infants exclusively breastfed for more than 6 months [20]. Bronchiolitis due to the respiratory syncytial virus (RSV) is 74% less severe in exclusively breastfed infants than those who never breastfed or where breastfeeding was not exclusive [21]. This lesser severity is reflected in a lower hospital admission rate and decreased need for supplementary oxygen.

Furthermore, when infants breastfed at any point are compared with those who only received formula, a 23% lower rate of middle ear infections is seen in those breastfed [18]. Infants exclusively breastfed over a minimum of 3 months have half the risk of otitis media. Moreover, a 63% reduction exists in severe coryza or ear, nose, and throat (ENT) infections in infants where the duration of exclusive breastfeeding is 6 months [1, 22].

3.2   *Gastrointestinal Tract Infections*

Breastfeeding, regardless of duration, results in a 64% lower risk of gastrointestinal infections [18, 19, 22, 23]. This risk reduction persists for 2 months after cessation of breastfeeding.

3.3   *Necrotizing Enterocolitis*

Meta-analysis of four randomized clinical trials between 1983 and 2005 revealed an association between the feeding of premature neonates with breast milk and a 58% decrease in the rate of necrotizing enterocolitis (NEC) [18, 24]. Another study reported a lower NEC rate in premature infants exclusively breastfed compared with those fed breast milk and supplementary formula based on bovine milk [25]. It has been estimated that one NEC case is prevented for every ten infants exclusively breastfed. Similarly, for every eight infants solely breastfed, one case of severe NEC (defined as leading to mortality or surgery) is averted [1, 24].

3.4 Sudden Infant Death Syndrome

A meta-analysis of studies where the breastfeeding amount was explicitly defined and adjustment for potential confounders was made, including the known associations with sudden infant death syndrome (SIDS), found that being breastfed lowered infants' risk of SIDS by 36% [18]. The recent data comparing exclusive breastfeeding with breastfeeding of any degree show that breastfeeding is protective against SIDS; this effect is more substantial for exclusive breastfeeding [25]. Some 21% of infant deaths in the United States of America (USA) probably result from, among other factors, the lack of breastfeeding, which increases SIDS [26]. A case-control study involving large numbers of infants who slept in a supine position confirmed that the reduction in SIDS associated with breastfeeding was separate from any effect due to infants' sleeping position [27, 28].

If the rate of exclusive breastfeeding up to the age of 6 months in the USA rose to 90%, it has been estimated that some 900 infant fatalities would be prevented annually [29]. Ninety percent of global infant deaths occur in 42 low- and middle-income countries. In these countries, approximately 13% of such demises (around 1,000,000 cases) could be prevented if children were exclusively breastfed for up to 6 months and weaned after 1 year [1, 30].

3.5 Allergic Disorders

Exclusive breastfeeding for 3–4 months is accompanied by a reduction in the rates of symptomatic asthma, atopic dermatitis, and eczema; the level of decline depends on the background risk [31]. For infants at low overall risk, the reduction is 27%, but this increases to 42% in families with a family history of atopy [18]. Studies assessing the optimal time to introduce solid food into the infant diet after 4 months to lower the risk of allergic complications, such as food allergy, atopic dermatitis, and asthma, produced inconsistent findings for both infants at high and low risks [31]. Likewise, suggesting that potentially allergy-triggering foods should not be introduced before 6 months seems to lack evidence [32–35]. The fact that exclusive breastfeeding in six-month-old infants is relatively unusual makes analysis of the data challenging. The conclusions of studies investigating the allergic disorder risk in infants given breast milk and solid food are potentially not valid for infants exclusively breastfed [21].

3.6 Celiac Disease

The risk of developing celiac disease is reduced by 52% if breastfeeding is ongoing when the infant first encounters gluten [36]. In general, the further that breastfeeding is extended, the lower the risk of developing the celiac disease as defined by the detection of characteristic celiac antibodies. This protective effect seems crucially dependent on the continuation of breastfeeding, not the age at which the infant first encounters gluten. Accordingly, infants should be tried with gluten-containing food when exclusive breastfeeding occurs, not after introducing formula or other forms of cow's milk [1].

3.7 Inflammatory Bowel Disorders

Breastfed infants also have a 31% lower risk of developing inflammatory bowel disorders during childhood [37]. One hypothesis to explain this risk reduction suggests that breast milk has immunomodulatory effects that interact with the disease phenotype expression in those with genetic risk factors. Furthermore, breast milk also influences the gut microbiome, and changes in flora may exert protective effects on the gastrointestinal tract [38].

3.8 Obesity

Campaigns aiming to lower obesity generally include advocating breastfeeding since breastfed infants have a significantly decreased chance of later becoming obese [39, 40]. Despite the multifactorial nature of obesity and the difficulty in separating various factors in studies, it is clear that any duration of breastfeeding lowers the likelihood of being obese during adolescence or adulthood by between 15% and 30% compared to no breastfeeding [18, 41]. Breastfeeding during infancy has been associated with a lower body mass index (BMI) and a greater level of high-density lipoprotein in adulthood [42]. A study examining siblings where one sibling was breastfed and the other formula-fed found that the breastfed siblings had a body mass 6.35 kg below the formula-fed sibling and a lower likelihood of attaining a BMI consistent with obesity [43].

One of the weaknesses of these studies was the failure to distinguish between infants fed directly from the breast and those provided breast milk via a bottle. Such difference plays a significant role later in life since infants breastfed directly learn to control how much they ingest, regardless of how much milk volume is available from the breast; this learned ability to self-regulate the ingested food amount has a significant effect on the propensity to gain weight in adulthood [44]. This difference is also reflected in the fact that bottle-fed infants, whether fed with breast milk or formula, tend to empty the bottle, have less ability to decide when they are full, and thus gain more body mass above the age of 6 months than infants exclusively breastfed [45, 46].

3.9 Diabetes Mellitus

Infants exclusively breastfed for a minimum of 3 months have a lower risk of type 1 diabetes mellitus by approximately 30% [47]. A proposed explanation for this risk reduction is that bovine milk-fed children are exposed to bovine beta-lactoglobulin, which is antigenic and causes a cross-reaction with the infants' pancreatic beta-cells. Breastfeeding is also associated with a 40% lower risk of type 2 diabetes [48]. Such a decrease may reflect the beneficial effects of exclusive breastfeeding on the ability to regulate the amount of food consumed and the resultant body mass.

3.10 Childhood Leukemia and Lymphoma

An inverse correlation was reported between breastfeeding duration and leukemia risk [19, 49]. If infants are breastfed for a minimum of 6 months, acute lymphocytic leukemia (ALL) risk decreases by 20%, and acute myeloid leukemia (AML) risk by 15% [50, 51]. If breastfeeding is shorter than 6 months, some decline in risk still occurs, but of a smaller proportion, namely 12% for AML and 10% for ALL. However, it is unclear how breastfeeding confers this lower risk.

3.11 Neurodevelopmental Outcomes

Some studies reported that breastfed and formula-fed infants differ in neurodevelopmental levels. However, the direct comparison is complicated by numerous confounding variables, such as parents' education level, intelligence quotient (IQ), domestic circumstances, and socioeconomic level [18, 52]. The findings of the Promotion of Breastfeeding Intervention Trial (PROBIT), which enrolled high numbers of infants and randomized the intervention, showed that, even after adjustment for confounders, the IQ level and teachers' ratings of breastfed infants were superior to those of formula-fed peers [53–55]. Furthermore, being exclusively breastfed for a minimum of 3 months led to higher intelligence and more significant academic potential, as rated by teachers. The incidence of neurodevelopmental abnormalities is higher than usual in premature infants; however, substantial advantages exist in the neurodevelopmental outcomes of breastfed babies [56–59].

3.12   Prematurity and Donor Breast Milk

Breastfeeding infants results in several significant health benefits that last over a lifetime. Moreover, these benefits appear to depend on the breastfeeding duration: the longer the infant is breastfed, the greater the benefit. Thus, prompting and supporting breastfeeding should be considered a public health priority. However, beginning and continuing breastfeeding in premature neonates is more challenging than in term infants [60, 61]. In addition, the breast milk composition of mothers who delivered prematurely significantly differs from that of mothers of near-term infants [4].

Several studies examined donor breast milk where the mother can not feed the infant with her milk. Donor milk requires pasteurization to be safe and is also usually fortified. Despite this mandatory processing, donor milk may remain superior to standard formulas when the mother does not provide breast milk for her baby [1]. However, processing donor milk alters the composition and reduces its vitamin, active enzyme, and nutrient constituents, meaning that its bioactivity is inferior to that of unprocessed breast milk [62]. The extent to which compositional alterations are caused by processing donor milk and some innovative breast milk processing methods, such as high-pressure sterilization, are currently being investigated [63, 64].

Necrotizing enterocolitis in extremely premature infants is less common if fed with processed donor milk [65]. Nonetheless, formula milk promotes superior gains in body mass, growth in length, and head circumference to those gained using donor milk. Despite these benefits, formula milk is not preferable to donor milk [66]. When the mother can not provide breast milk to a premature infant, donor breast milk remains the best option [4].

Several studies have reported that premature infants fed either with breast milk from their mothers or donated samples have a lower risk of infections or NEC during the neonatal period [24, 65]. In addition, since these feeding methods lower infection rates and are more nutritionally valuable than formula feeding, premature infants fed with breast milk are anticipated to show superior cognitive outcomes as they grow up, as determined by higher verbal IQ, for example [67].

4   Conclusion

Breast milk has many invaluable components, including some with immunological and anti-infectious properties. Breast milk is essential for the appropriate physical and neurological development of all newborns, particularly preterm infants. Breastfeeding protects against NEC, the most common acquired gastrointestinal disease in preterm infants. Breast milk also protects against infectious diseases, SIDS, allergic conditions, autoimmune diseases such as celiac disease, inflammatory bowel diseases, endocrine-metabolic afflictions, diabetes mellitus, and obesity.

Childhood leukemia and lymphoma incidence are lower in breastfed than in formula-fed children. Prompting and supporting exclusive breastfeeding should be advocated as a public health priority.

References

1. Meek JY, Noble L, Section on Breastfeeding, American Academy of Pediatrics. Policy statement: breastfeeding and the use of human milk. Pediatrics. 2022;150(1):e2022057988.
2. World Health Organization. Breastfeeding. https://www.who.int/health-topics/breastfeeding#tab=tab_1. Accessed 10 Feb 2023.
3. Goldman AS. The immune system in human milk and the developing infant. Breastfeed Med. 2007;4:195–204.
4. Tauber KA. Human milk and lactation (updated: Jun 29, 2021). In: Nimavat DJ, editor. Medscape. https://emedicine.medscape.com/article/1835675-overview#a7. Accessed 10 Feb 2023.
5. Young L, McGuire W. Immunologic properties of human milk and clinical implications in the neonatal population. NeoReviews. 2020;12:809–16.
6. Embleton ND, Berrington JE, McGuire W, Stewart CJ, Cummings SP. Lactoferrin: antimicrobial activity and therapeutic potential. Semin Fetal Neonatal Med. 2013;18:143–9.
7. Thai JD, Gregory KE. Bioactive factors in human breast milk attenuate intestinal inflammation during early life. Nutrients. 2020;12(2):581.
8. Borewicz K, Gu F, Saccenti E, et al. The association between breastmilk oligosaccharides and faecal microbiota in healthy breastfed infants at two, six, and twelve weeks of age. Sci Rep. 2020;10(1):4270.
9. Liu B, Newburg DS. Human milk glycoproteins protect infants against human pathogens. Breastfeed Med. 2013;8:354–62.
10. Mshvildadze M, Neu J, Mai V. Intestinal microbiota development in the premature neonate: establishment of a lasting commensal relationship? Nutr Rev. 2008;66:658–63.
11. Walker AW, Duncan SH, Harmsen HJ, Holtrop G, Welling GW, Flint HJ. The species composition of the human intestinal microbiota differs between particle-associated and liquid-phase communities. Environ Microbiol. 2008;10:3275–83.
12. Bardanzellu F, Peroni DG, Fanos V. Human breast milk: bioactive components, from stem cells to health outcomes. Curr Nutr Rep. 2020;9:1–13.
13. Witkowska-Zimny M, Kaminska-El-Hassan E. Cells of human breast milk. Cell Mol Biol Lett. 2017;22:11.
14. Trend S, de Jong E, Lloyd ML, et al. Leukocyte populations in human preterm and term breast milk identified by multicolour flow cytometry. PLoS One. 2015;10(8):e0135580.
15. Elwakiel M, Boeren S, Hageman JA, Szeto IM, Schols HA, Hettinga KA. Variability of serum proteins in Chinese and Dutch human milk during lactation. Nutrients. 2019;11(3):499.
16. Mosca F, Gianni ML. Human milk: composition and health benefits. Pediatr Med Chir. 2017;39:47–52.
17. Beaudry M, Dufour R, Marcoux S. Relation between infant feeding and infections during the first six months of life. J Pediatr. 1995;126:191–7.
18. Ip S, Chung M, Raman G, et al. Breastfeeding and maternal and infant health outcomes in developed countries. Evid Rep Technol Assess (Full Rep). 2007;153:1–186.
19. Ip S, Chung M, Raman G, Trikalinos TA, Lau J. A summary of the Agency for Healthcare Research and Quality's evidence report on breastfeeding in developed countries. Breastfeed Med. 2009;4(suppl 1):17–30.
20. Chantry CJ, Howard CR, Auinger P. Full breastfeeding duration and associated decrease in respiratory tract infection in US children. Pediatrics. 2006;117:425–32.

21. Nishimura T, Suzue J, Kaji H. Breastfeeding reduces the severity of respiratory syncytial virus infection among young infants: a multi-center prospective study. Pediatr Int. 2009;51:812–6.
22. Duijts L, Jaddoe VW, Hofman A, Moll HA. Prolonged and exclusive breastfeeding reduces the risk of infectious diseases in infancy. Pediatrics. 2010;126(1):e18–25.
23. Quigley MA, Kelly YJ, Sacker A. Breastfeeding and hospitalization for diarrheal and respiratory infection in the United Kingdom millennium cohort study. Pediatrics. 2007;119:e837–42.
24. Sullivan S, Schanler RJ, Kim JH, et al. An exclusively human milk-based diet is associated with a lower rate of necrotizing enterocolitis than a diet of human milk and bovine milk-based products. J Pediatr. 2010;156:562–7.
25. Hauck FR, Thompson JMD, Tanabe KO, Moon RY, Vennemann MM. Breastfeeding and reduced risk of sudden infant death syndrome: a metaanalysis. Pediatrics. 2011;128:1–8.
26. Chen A, Rogan WJ. Breastfeeding and the risk of postneonatal death in the United States. Pediatrics. 2004;113:e435–9.
27. Vennemann MM, Bajanowski T, Brinkmann B, et al. Does breastfeeding reduce the risk of sudden infant death syndrome? Pediatrics. 2009;123(3):e406–10.
28. Moon RY. Task force on sudden infant death syndrome. SIDS and other sleep-related infant deaths: expansion of recommendations for a safe infant sleeping environment. Pediatrics. 2011;128:1030–9.
29. Bartick M, Reinhold A. The burden of suboptimal breastfeeding in the United States: a pediatric cost analysis. Pediatrics. 2010;125:1048–56.
30. Jones G, Steketee RW, Black RE, Bhutta ZA, Morris SS, Bellagio Child Survival Study Group. How many child deaths can we prevent this year? Lancet. 2003;362(9377):65–71.
31. Greer FR, Sicherer SH, Burks AW, American Academy of Pediatrics Committee on Nutrition, American Academy of Pediatrics Section on Allergy and Immunology. Effects of early nutritional interventions on the development of atopic disease in infants and children: the role of maternal dietary restriction, breastfeeding, timing of introduction of complementary foods, and hydrolyzed formulas. Pediatrics. 2008;121:183–91.
32. Zutavern A, Brockow I, Schaaf B, et al. Timing of solid food introduction in relation to atopic dermatitis and atopic sensitization: results from a prospective birth cohort study. Pediatrics. 2006;117:401–11.
33. Poole JA, Barriga K, Leung DYM, et al. Timing of initial exposure to cereal grains and the risk of wheat allergy. Pediatrics. 2006;117:2175–82.
34. Zutavern A, Brockow I, Schaaf B, et al. Timing of solid food introduction in relation to eczema, asthma, allergic rhinitis, and food and inhalant sensitization at the age of 6 years: results from the prospective birth cohort study LISA. Pediatrics. 2008;121(1):e44–52.
35. Nwaru BI, Erkkola M, Ahonen S, et al. Age at the introduction of solid foods during the first year and allergic sensitization at age 5 years. Pediatrics. 2010;125:50–9.
36. Akobeng AK, Ramanan AV, Buchan I, Heller RF. Effect of breast feeding on risk of coeliac disease: a systematic review and metaanalysis of observational studies. Arch Dis Child. 2006;91:39–43.
37. Barclay AR, Russell RK, Wilson ML, Gilmour WH, Satsangi J, Wilson DC. Systematic review: the role of breastfeeding in the development of pediatric inflammatory bowel disease. J Pediatr. 2009;155:421–6.
38. Penders J, Thijs C, Vink C, et al. Factors influencing the composition of the intestinal microbiota in early infancy. Pediatrics. 2006;118:511–21.
39. Perrine CG, Shealy KM, Scanlon KS, et al. Centers for Disease Control and Prevention (CDC). Vital signs: hospital practices to support breastfeeding-United States, 2007 and 2009. MMWR Morb Mortal Wkly Rep. 2011;60(30):1020–5.
40. US Department of Health and Human Services, The Surgeon General's call to action to support breastfeeding (last reviewed: May 14, 2019). www.surgeongeneral.gov/topics/breastfeeding/. Accessed 9 Feb 2023.

41. Owen CG, Martin RM, Whincup PH, Smith GD, Cook DG. Effect of infant feeding on the risk of obesity across the life course: a quantitative review of published evidence. Pediatrics. 2005;115:1367–77.
42. Parikh NI, Hwang SJ, Ingelsson E, et al. Breastfeeding in infancy and adult cardiovascular disease risk factors. Am J Med. 2009;122:656–63.
43. Metzger MW, McDade TW. Breastfeeding as obesity prevention in the United States: a sibling difference model. Am J Hum Biol. 2010;22:291–6.
44. Dewey KG, Lönnerdal B. Infant self-regulation of breast milk intake. Acta Paediatr Scand. 1986;75:893–8.
45. Li R, Fein SB, Grummer-Strawn LM. Association of breastfeeding intensity and bottle-emptying behaviors at early infancy with infants' risk for excess weight at late infancy. Pediatrics. 2008;122(suppl 2):77–84.
46. Li R, Fein SB, Grummer-Strawn LM. Do infants fed from bottles lack self-regulation of milk intake compared with directly breastfed infants? Pediatrics. 2010;125(6):e1386–93.
47. Rosenbauer J, Herzig P, Giani G. Early infant feeding and risk of type 1 diabetes mellitus—a nationwide population-based case-control study in pre-school children. Diabetes Metab Res Rev. 2008;24:211–22.
48. Das UN. Breastfeeding prevents type 2 diabetes mellitus: but, how and why? Am J Clin Nutr. 2007;85:1436–7.
49. Bener A, Hoffmann GF, Afify Z, Rasul K, Tewfik I. Does prolonged breastfeeding reduce the risk for childhood leukemia and lymphomas? Minerva Pediatr. 2008;60:155–61.
50. Rudant J, Orsi L, Menegaux F, et al. Childhood acute leukemia, early common infections, and allergy: the ESCALE study. Am J Epidemiol. 2010;172:1015–27.
51. Kwan ML, Buffler PA, Abrams B, Kiley VA. Breastfeeding and the risk of childhood leukemia: a metaanalysis. Public Health Rep. 2004;119:521–35.
52. Der G, Batty GD, Deary IJ. Effect of breast feeding on intelligence in children: prospective study, sibling pairs analysis, and metaanalysis. BMJ. 2006;333(7575):945.
53. Kramer MS, Fombonne E, Igumnov S, et al. Promotion of Breastfeeding Intervention Trial (PROBIT) Study Group. Effects of prolonged and exclusive breastfeeding on child behavior and maternal adjustment: evidence from a large, randomized trial. Pediatrics. 2008;121(3):e435–40.
54. Kramer MS, Aboud F, Mironova E, et al. Promotion of Breastfeeding Intervention Trial (PROBIT) Study Group. Breastfeeding and child cognitive development: new evidence from a large randomized trial. Arch Gen Psychiatry. 2008;65:578–84.
55. Kramer MS, Chalmers B, Hodnett ED, et al. Promotion of Breastfeeding Intervention Trial (PROBIT): a randomized trial in the Republic of Belarus. JAMA. 2001;285:413–20.
56. Vohr BR, Poindexter BB, Dusick AM, et al. NICHD Neonatal Research Network. Beneficial effects of breast milk in the neonatal intensive care unit on the developmental outcome of extremely low birth weight infants at 18 months of age. Pediatrics. 2006;118(1):e115–223.
57. Vohr BR, Poindexter BB, Dusick AM, et al. National Institute of Child Health and Human Development National Research Network. Persistent beneficial effects of breast milk ingested in the neonatal intensive care unit on outcomes of extremely low birth weight infants at 30 months of age. Pediatrics. 2007;120(4):e953–9.
58. Lucas A, Morley R, Cole TJ. Randomised trial of early diet in preterm babies and later intelligence quotient. BMJ. 1998;317(7171):1481–7.
59. Isaacs EB, Fischl BR, Quinn BT, Chong WK, Gadian DG, Lucas A. Impact of breast milk on intelligence quotient, brain size, and white matter development. Pediatr Res. 2010;67:357–62.
60. Goldman AS. Evolution of immune functions of the mammary gland and protection of the infant. Breastfeed Med. 2012;7:132–42.
61. Crippa BL, Colombo L, Morniroli D, et al. Do a few weeks matter? Late preterm infants and breastfeeding issues. Nutrients. 2019;11(2):312.

62. Peila C, Emmerik NE, Giribaldi M, et al. Human milk processing: a systematic review of innovative techniques to ensure the safety and quality of donor milk. J Pediatr Gastroenterol Nutr. 2017;64:353–61.
63. Moukarzel S, Wiedeman AM, Soberanes LS, Dyer RA, Innis SM, Lamers Y. Variability of water-soluble forms of choline concentrations in human milk during storage, after pasteurization, and among women. Nutrients. 2019;11(12):3024.
64. Wesolowska A, Brys J, Barbarska O, et al. Lipid profile, lipase bioactivity, and lipophilic antioxidant content in high pressure processed donor human milk. Nutrients. 2019;11(9):1972.
65. Lapidaire W, Lucas A, Clayden JD, Clark C, Fewtrell MS. Human milk feeding and cognitive outcome in preterm infants: the role of infection and NEC reduction. Pediatr Res. 2022;91(5):12.
66. Embleton N, Cleminson J. Randomized trial of exclusive human milk versus preterm formula diets in extremely premature infants. Acta Paediatr. 2017;106:1538.
67. Quigley M, Embleton ND, McGuire W. Formula versus donor breast milk for feeding preterm or low birth weight infants. Cochrane Database Syst Rev. 2018;6(6):CD002971.

Physiological Aspects of Lactation

Nevin Cambaz Kurt and Gian Carlo Di Renzo

1 Introduction

Milk production by the human breast is the end result of a long series of physiological changes. The breast alters in form, size and overall shape as the girl grows and develops into an adult woman. The key developmental stages include puberty, pregnancy and lactation. For breastfeeding to be fully possible, there must have been a series of physiological adaptations well before the neonate latches onto the breast for the first time. In this chapter, the way the breast develops its adult form (mammogenesis), the way the mammary gland develops the ability to produce milk (lactogenesis) and the way the milk is then delivered to the infant (lactation) are all discussed [1–4].

Any illness or injury that affects the development of the breast or hinders lactogenesis may prevent successful breastfeeding. For example, a woman who has undergone surgery to alter the breast size may find breastfeeding difficult or impossible, although this depends on where the surgical incision was made. Procedures where the incision is transaxillary are less disruptive of the ability to breastfeed than the 'smile' type periareolar incision [1].

After delivery, some mothers struggle to succeed at breastfeeding if their mammary glands produce too little milk, the milk does not easily leave the breast or if the diet includes too few calories to allow the body to commit to producing milk. At present, guidelines suggest that women who are lactating should consume at least

N. C. Kurt (✉)
Department of Pediatrics, Başakşehir Çam and Sakura City Hospital, İstanbul, Türkiye

G. C. Di Renzo
Centre of Perinatal Medicine of the University of Perugia, Perugia, Italy

Sechenov University, Moscow, Russia
e-mail: giancarlo.direnzo@unipg.it

Ö. N. Şahin et al. (eds.), *Breastfeeding and Metabolic Programming*,
https://doi.org/10.1007/978-3-031-33278-4_5

500 calories a day above the usual metabolic requirement to allow milk to be produced in sufficient quantity. It is also recommended that lactating mothers empty the breast as frequently as they can, usually every 2–3 h, as this ensures that milk production continues to occur [5–8].

In order to understand the physiological aspects of lactation, it is necessary to be familiar with the normal gross and microscopic anatomy of the breast first. In the healthy breast, there are two major anatomical components, i.e. the ducts and lobules. Histology reveals two populations of epithelial cells, namely luminal and myoepithelial, and two types within the stroma, namely interlobular and intralobular. There are between six and ten major duct orifices that converge at the nipple. The terminal portion of the ducts is lined by a keratinised squamous epithelium, with an abrupt transition to an epithelial surface consisting of two layers, one containing luminal cells, the other myoepithelial cells. This latter lining continues into the smaller calibre ducts within the lobules. Multiple small acini are clustered together, resembling a bunch of grapes, forming the lobules. The terminal portion of the duct connects the acini to the rest of the duct. Lobules are classified into three types, numbered 1–3. At different stages of female development, different types of lobules form. When pregnancy occurs, the stroma is progressively replaced by lobular tissue, such that, by the time of delivery, the majority of the mammary gland consists of lobular tissue, with minimal stromal tissue. Pregnancy is the necessary trigger for the breast to assume its final form, in which it is capable of lactation [1–9].

2   Breast Development

Puberty is the trigger for formation of type 1 lobules. The fluctuating endocrine profile during the menstrual cycle (affecting the level of oestrogen and progesterone) stimulates proliferation of new alveolar buds. The breast then passes through further developmental stages, as first type 2 and then type 3 lobular structures are formed. The end of puberty arrests further development of the mammary gland until the woman becomes pregnant, when further changes occur [1].

In the pregnant female, stage II of mammogenesis occurs, during which the alveoli develop more and the epithelium takes on a mature form. These changes are mainly stimulated by the rise in progesterone. The larger than usual size of the breasts in pregnant women occurs due to formation of greater amounts of secretory tissue. At the beginning of pregnancy, chorionic gonadotrophin stimulates type 3 lobular development. Type 3 lobules are larger and contain a greater volume of epithelial cells within the acini. Towards the end of pregnancy, new acini cease to be formed, and the lumen fills with colostrum and other secretions [1].

The lobular tissue of the breast grows and differentiates even further as labour proceeds and when breastfeeding commences. The mammary gland begins to secrete milk. During the whole lactation phase, the vast majority of the breast tissue is of glandular type, with stromal tissue only constituting a minor element [1].

When the phase of lactation comes to an end, the breast shows involutionary change in response to the absence of endocrine signals needed to promote lactogenesis. Glandular tissue undergoes apoptosis triggered by autocrine signalling and the breast tissue architecture becomes remodelled. The mammary gland never returns fully to its pre-pregnant state, however, and there are always more lobules and their magnitude is greater following a pregnancy. Once lactation has occurred, the breast retains the ability to secrete milk if the gland is regularly stimulated [1].

3 Functional Aspects

All mothers need to decide whether they intend to nurse their infants or to express milk to a container for later feeding. It is the duty of healthcare professionals to ensure mothers are aware of the entire range of advantages that being breastfed provides to neonates. The nutritional composition of human milk is optimal in terms of protein, lipid, carbohydrates, minerals and vitamins and neonates can more easily digest human than bovine (formula) milk. Furthermore, the immunoglobulins within breast milk are important sources of infant immunity to bacterial and viral pathogens. Immunoglobulins, especially of the IgA type, are key, but breast milk also provides other immunologically active components in the form of maternal leucocytes, whey (which contains lysozyme and lactoferrin) and human milk oligosaccharides. This immune function of breast milk means that breastfed infants have a lower average incidence of asthma, allergic disorders, otitis, respiratory tract infections, diarrhoeal illness, diabetes mellitus and obesity [1].

4 Breast Physiology

The process by which the breast becomes capable of releasing milk is known as lactogenesis. It depends on alveolar cell maturation. There are two main phases, namely secretory initiation and secretory activation [1], as follows:

- Secretory initiation (also termed stage I lactogenesis) occurs in the latter half of pregnancy. The elevated concentration of progesterone synthesised by the placenta effectively halts complete maturation of the milk-producing alveolar units. By the 16th week of pregnancy, a low volume of milk may be secreted by the breast and towards the end of the pregnancy, some mothers find they can already secrete colostrum.
- Secretory activation (i.e. the second stage of lactogenesis) is indicated by the availability of large volumes of milk from the breast following delivery of the infant. Delivery of the placenta causes the circulating progesterone level to fall precipitously, and the levels of prolactin, cortisol and insulin at this point are high. These endocrine signals initiate stage II lactogenesis. On the second or

third day after delivery, the majority of mothers find their breasts swell and milk begins to be available in large quantities. For women giving birth for the first time, there is a short delay in the onset of copious milk production, and the volume of milk at the start is lower than in multiparous women. Caesarean delivery also results in less milk production than vaginal delivery. Delays in secretory activation are also noted in mothers where the entire placenta has not been delivered, those who have diabetes mellitus, or where vaginal delivery has been unusually traumatic for the woman. If portions of the placenta are retained, the maternal progesterone level will remain elevated and stage II lactogenesis will not fully occur until these fragments are removed from the uterus.

The maintenance of lactation depends on the breast being regularly emptied of milk and the nipple being stimulated. This stimulation of the breast sends signals to the adenohypophysis to secrete prolactin and to the neurohypophysis to release oxytocin. Unless the mammary gland continues to receive endocrine stimulation, it will cease to produce milk. There are different receptors on the mammary gland cells for the two hormones, but both receptors must be stimulated if the breast is to continue to generate and release milk [1].

The structure of the prolactin hormone has similarities to other polypeptides, specifically growth hormone and lactogen produced by the placenta. It is manufactured by the lactotrophic cells of the adenohypohysis. There is regulation of prolactin that can both increase and suppress its release; however, the principal factor affecting its release is inhibition of the lactotrophs by dopamine acting on D2-receptors. This dopamine is manufactured in the hypothalamus. Prolactin itself stimulates ducts to grow within the breast and epithelial cells to divide. It also stimulates manufacture of proteins found in breast milk. The key factor in the release of prolactin is the release of milk in response to the infant suckling on the nipple. This action causes stimulation of nerve fibres within the nipple, which then relay the signal to higher centres [1].

The letdown or ejection of milk falls under the control of oxytocin. When the nipple and areola are stimulated by the suckling infant, nervous signals pass up to the hypothalamus, which responds by releasing oxytocin. Oxytocin then induces the myoepithelial cells to contract. This action squeezes milk out of the lumen of each alveolus and into the duct, which empties to the exterior at the nipple. In addition to this action, oxytocin also alters the mother's emotional state, causing her to feel calmer and less anxious. The bonding between infant and mother is increased by breastfeeding, partly through the action of this hormone [1].

After lactation has begun and is continuing, there are a number of physical and biochemical factors that act to ensure that breastfeeding is possible. When the breast ceases to be emptied regularly, the pressure within the breast rises and a substance accumulates that prevents further secretion of milk and triggers involutional change in the breast. Provided the breast milk continues to be taken away, this inhibitory feedback mechanism cannot operate and the breast continues to generate fresh milk. The build-up of an inhibitory factor allows the demand for milk by the infant to be supplied in the right amount by the mammary gland. If the infant feeds more, the breast works harder, but a reduction in demand by the infant leads to a reduction in milk production by the mother [1].

5 Formation of the Mammary Gland (Mammogenesis)

An understanding of mammogenesis is key to appreciating how breast physiology adapts so as to permit lactation. The mammary gland begins to be formed during foetal life, when the initial differentiation steps occur on the path leading eventually to fully functioning lactation. In the 18th or 19th week of foetal development, the primordial breast bud can be noted, with a characteristic bulbar outline. Within this bud a simple system of ducts is formed and this is how the breast appears at the time of birth. Until the girl reaches puberty, the gland simply grows in size to match the overall size of the child [10, 11].

The healthy human mammary gland contains between 15 and 20 lobes consisting of glandular tissue. The lobes themselves consist of multiple lobules, the sites for the eventual synthesis of milk when the woman becomes pregnant. The usual number of lobules in each lobe is between 20 and 40. Each lobule is connected to a lobar lactiferous duct. These lactiferous ducts join together such that at the nipple there are between five and ten main lactiferous ducts converging. The milk passes along this network of ducts and exits at the nipple. If the infant is latched onto the nipple, milk flows directly out of the breast into the infant's mouth [10].

6 Lobule Types 1–4

The lobules can be of four distinct types. Type 1 is the type present from week 18 or 19 of foetal life until puberty begins. The onset of puberty sees an alteration in the oestrogen and progesterone levels, as menstruation commences. These hormones fluctuate and the breast responds to the fluctuation by forming type 2 lobules, which contain newly formed alveolar buds. The breast undergoes no further change after puberty has finished unless pregnancy subsequently occurs [10].

In pregnant women, the breast undergoes remodelling, leading to an increase in the dimensions and number of lobules. During pregnancy the mammary gland composition alters, such that type 3 lobules are by far the most common type. Once the lobules are synthesising and releasing milk, they are classified as type 4 lobules. The ending of breastfeeding causes these milk-producing type 4 lobules to revert to type 3. This occurs since the lactogenic hormones cease to circulate and the breast itself produces autocrine signals that prompt programmed cell death and remodelling of the microarchitecture of the breast [10].

7   Lactogenesis

Lactogenesis is the process by which the breast becomes capable of producing and releasing milk. Thus it refers to the multiple steps by which the breast is transformed from a relatively undifferentiated organ at the beginning of pregnancy to a specialised milk-producing organ shortly after the birth of the infant. Lactogenesis is divided into two principal stages, as follows [10]:

Stage 1 is complete by the time the first 20 weeks of pregnancy are ending. At this point the breast can already produce and release milk. The level of lactose, antibodies and protein overall rises and the concentration of the electrolytes sodium and potassium falls in the fluid produced by the glands. The breast at the end of stage 1 can potentially secrete milk, and some women do experience a small volume of nipple discharge in the middle and final semester, this discharge consisting of colostrum. Because maternal progesterone and oestrogen levels are high, however, at this point milk is not actively secreted [10].

The second stage of lactogenesis takes place at the end of pregnancy. The breast begins secreting a high volume of milk once the maternal progesterone level falls due to the absence of placental hormones. Prolactin, cortisol and insulin levels are high, too, which also encourages milk production. The fact that the mammary epithelium loses its receptors for progesterone, which further decreases the braking effect of this hormone, has been shown by Haslam and Shyamala [12, 13]. In the second stage of lactogenesis, the concentrate of citrate rises, to the extent that it acts as a biomarker indicating that lactogenesis stage II has started.

The many steps by which lactation is possible are outlined below, following the scheme outlined by Riordan and Auerbach in their seminal 1998 work [14].

7.1 *Mammogenesis*

Mammogenesis involves an increase in the mass and dimensions of the mammary gland [10].

7.2 *Lactogenesis*

- Stage 1 (complete by around week 20). The cells of the alveoli develop a specialised secretory ability.
- Stage 2 (begins around the second or third day post-partum and is complete by the eighth day). The tight junctions between alveolar cells increase. The breast starts to secrete milk in large quantities. The mammary glands are full. Milk production is predominantly under local (autocrine) control, which matches milk supply with the demand from the infant [10].

7.3 *Galactopoiesis*

This stage is the point at which the breast is regularly and reliably secreting copious amounts of milk. Control of the process still depends on mainly autocrine factors.

7.4 *Involutionary Stage*

The mean point at which involution starts is 40 days after the last time the infant is breastfed. The trigger for involution is accumulation of peptides with an anti-lactogenic action [10].

8 Lactation

The second stage of lactogenesis occurs when the mammary gland can produce milk as required. Milk production can only continue if the appropriate endocrine signals are present. The stimulation of the nipple and areolar tissue triggers a nervous signal to the central nervous system, in response to which oxytocin and prolactin are released by the pituitary. These two hormones act independently, but unless both signals are present, breastfeeding will not be able to succeed [10].

8.1 *Prolactin*

- Lactotrophic cells within the adenohypophysis are responsible for the synthesis of prolactin. This molecule is a polypeptide endocrine signalling molecule. When the hormone attaches to receptors of the epithelial cells within the breast, it triggers production of milk. Expression of the prolactin receptor is suppressed by a high level of circulating progesterone, which occurs during pregnancy. However, once the infant (and the placenta) has been delivered, there is a fall in the circulating progesterone level, which results in upregulation of the prolactin receptor, so that the epithelial cells of the mammary gland begin to respond to prolactin by synthesising milk.
- Over the last few decades, there has been an accumulation of knowledge about how prolactin functions. Animals with deleted genes for prolactin and related molecules show that the hormone plays an essential part in both lactation and reproduction. The majority of the tissues on which prolactin acts do not depend on prolactin but are regulated by its changing levels [15].

8.2 *Oxytocin*

- Alongside prolactin, another hormone plays a vital part in lactation, by stimulating the myoepithelial cells of the mammary gland to contract, forcing milk along the ducts. This milk letdown reflex is under the control of oxytocin. Oxytocin release is caused by the stimulation of the nipple by a suckling infant. This reflex passes from the nipple and surrounding areolar tissues to the central nervous system via the intercostal nerves and the dorsal root ganglia [14, 16, 17]. The signals pass along an ascending afferent path within the spinal cord to the hypothalamic paraventricular nuclei. Here oxytocin is generated and released by the neurohypophysis. The paraventricular nuclei secrete oxytocin, which descends the infundibulum towards the posterior portion of the hypophysis. Here oxytocin is accumulated awaiting release [10].
- The afferent signals that begin when the infant suckles cause the neurohypophysis to release pulses of oxytocin into the pituitary portal system, after which these molecules travel to the breast, where they act on the myoepithelial cells and induce contraction. The myoepithelial cells are located within the ductal lining. The effect of their contraction causes it to propel milk out of the alveoli and into the ducts, which converge at the nipple. Thus the breast milk passes directly out of the breast into the waiting mouth of the infant [10].

The amount of milk released to the infant's mouth closely corresponds to the volume of milk generated. The system of milk production demonstrates high efficiency. There is a surprisingly constant rate of milk production, with the usual daily total equal to around 800 mL. The amount of milk actually released is dependent on the level of feedback inhibitor of lactation within the milk in the breast. If the breast is full, synthesis slows, whereas the emptying of the milk creates a situation where milk synthesis proceeds rapidly [10].

The extent to which milk is synthesised depends on the mother's general health and well-being. Mothers who are under high stress or are overly fatigued produce less milk. This inhibition of milk production is under the control of dopamine ± noradrenaline. Raised dopamine and/or noradrenaline slow the generation of milk. Thus, for a woman to be able to breastfeed effectively, she needs to feel relaxed and unstressed [10].

References

1. Pillay J, Davis TJ. Physiology, lactation. [Updated 2022 Jul 18]. In: StatPearls [Internet]. Treasure Island (FL): StatPearls Publishing; 2022 Jan. https://www.ncbi.nlm.nih.gov/books/NBK499981/
2. Ventrella D, Forni M, Bacci ML, Annaert P. Non-clinical models to determine drug passage into human breast Milk. Curr Pharm Des. 2019;25(5):534–48.
3. Levine S, Muneyyirci-Delale O. Stress-induced hyperprolactinemia: pathophysiology and clinical approach. Obstet Gynecol Int. 2018;2018:9253083.

4. Hård AL, Nilsson AK, Lund AM, Hansen-Pupp I, Smith LEH, Hellström A. Review shows that donor milk does not promote the growth and development of preterm infants as well as maternal milk. Acta Paediatr. 2019;108(6):998–1007.
5. Bernard V, Young J, Binart N. Prolactin—a pleiotropic factor in health and disease. Nat Rev Endocrinol. 2019;15(6):356–65.
6. Weaver G, Bertino E, Gebauer C, Grovslien A, Mileusnic-Milenovic R, Arslanoglu S, Barnett D, Boquien CY, Buffin R, Gaya A, Moro GE, Wesolowska A, Picaud JC. Recommendations for the establishment and operation of human milk banks in Europe: a consensus statement from the European Milk Bank Association (EMBA). Front Pediatr. 2019;7:53.
7. Hahn-Holbrook J, Saxbe D, Bixby C, Steele C, Glynn L. Human milk as "chrononutrition": implications for child health and development. Pediatr Res. 2019;85(7):936–42.
8. Wallace TC, Blusztajn JK, Caudill MA, Klatt KC, Natker E, Zeisel SH, Zelman KM. Choline: the underconsumed and underappreciated essential nutrient. Nutr Today. 2018;53(6):240–53.
9. Sampieri CL, Montero H. Breastfeeding in the time of Zika: a systematic literature review. PeerJ. 2019;7:e6452.
10. Tauber KA. Human milk and lactation. In: Nimavat DJ, editor. Medscape. Updated: Jun 29, 2021. https://emedicine.medscape.com/article/1835675-overview#a7. Accessed 2 Dec 2022.
11. Hassiotou F, Geddes D. Anatomy of the human mammary gland: current status of knowledge. Clin Anat. 2013;26(1):29–48.
12. Haslam SZ, Shyamala G. Effect of oestradiol on progesterone receptors in normal mammary glands and its relationship with lactation. Biochem J. 1979;182(1):127–31.
13. Haslam SZ, Shyamala G. Progesterone receptors in normal mammary glands of mice: characterization and relationship to development. Endocrinology. 1979;105(3):786–95.
14. Auerbach KG, Riordan J. Breastfeeding and human lactation. Boston: Jones and Bartlett Publishers; 1993.
15. Bernard V, Young J, Chanson P, Binart N. New insights in prolactin: pathological implications. Nat Rev Endocrinol. 2015;11(5):265–75.
16. Neville MC. Physiology of lactation. Clin Perinatol. 1999;26(2):251–79. v
17. Black RF, Jarman L, Simpson JB. The process of breastfeeding. Lactation specialist self-study series. Sudbury, MA: Jones and Bartlett Publishers; 1998.

Breast Milk Oligosaccharides

Özlem Naciye Şahin, Aysel Özpınar, and Despina D. Briana

1 Introduction

Oligosaccharides are polymeric molecules typically consisting of between three and around ten monosaccharide subunits. Human breast milk differs from that found in the majority of mammalian species by virtue of the rich mixture of oligosaccharides (at least 150 different types) that it contains at high levels. Human milk oligosaccharides (HMOs) in mature human milk are even more abundant than milk proteins. They are usually present at a concentration of 5–15 g/L, which means that, if the water content is disregarded, they are exceeded in amount only by disaccharide lactose and milk fats [1, 2].

The monosaccharide subunits out of which HMOs are constructed consist of five types: glucose (Glc), galactose (Gal), *N*-acetylglucosamine (GlcNAc), fucose, and sialic acid. The variety of HMOs comes about through different combinations of these monosaccharide subunits and the type of linkages present in the oligosaccharide [1]. The scheme by which the different HMOs are assembled is illustrated. The common feature of the HMOs is the presence of a lactose at the reducing end of the polymeric chain. The lactose contains the Galβ1–4Glc linkage. To this growing chain either the disaccharide lacto-*N*-biose or *N*-acetyllactosamine can be added. In

Ö. N. Şahin (✉)
Department of Child Health and Diseases, Arel University, Medical Faculty, Istanbul, Türkiye

A. Özpınar
Medical Faculty, Department of Basic Sciences, Medical Biochemistry, Acibadem Mehmet
Ali Aydinlar University, Istanbul, Türkiye
e-mail: aysel.ozpinar@acibadem.edu.tr

D. D. Briana
NICU, Third Department of Pediatrics, National and Kapodistrian University of Athens,
University General Hospital "ATTIKON", Athens, Greece

© The Author(s), under exclusive license to Springer Nature
Switzerland AG 2023
Ö. N. Şahin et al. (eds.), *Breastfeeding and Metabolic Programming*,
https://doi.org/10.1007/978-3-031-33278-4_6

the former disaccharide there is a Galβ1–3GlcNAc linkage, whereas in the latter the linkage occurs as Galβ1–4GlcNAc. Sialic acid can be conjugated either to the initial lactose or to the tetramer through an α2–3 or α2–6 linkage. Likewise, fucose can also link to the dimer or tetramer by forming α1–2, α1–3 or α1–4 bonds. In this way a vast range of different polymers can be generated. The different monomeric subunits may confer different properties on the polymer as a whole. Sialic acid, for example, makes the polymer negatively charged overall, since it carries a carboxyl moiety. This charge affects the conformation of the polymer. The structure of the HMO frequently determines its physiological role [1, 2].

The basis of HMO variety is the same in every woman and up to now at least 150 different oligosaccharides have been discovered in breast milk. A key point is that there are wide differences in the HMO content of different women's milk. Nonetheless, each individual woman secretes milk with a fairly consistent HMO content whilst lactating [3, 4]. To date, the HMO content of milk from over 10,000 different human mothers has been analysed in various studies, with samples taken from multiple different countries. The principal components are plotted graphically. A heterogeneity of HMO content in different samples of human milk can be observed, yet the clustering of data also shows that specific lactotypes exist.

HMOs represent a group of polysaccharides not joined to other molecules that form a family of related polymers with a wide degree of heterogeneity. They are all found only in human milk in significant quantities. Scientific discovery of HMOs occurred in studies looking at milk components that promote the growth of *Bifidobacteria* in the infantile gut. Currently they are considered to play a greater role than merely nourishing beneficial microbiota. There is growing evidence to show that HMOs also prevent pathogens from attaching to the infant mucosae, thus making it harder for viruses, pathogenic bacteria or protozoa to cause infections. They are molecules found floating freely within the gut to which the pathogen attaches, rather than attaching itself to a similar molecule on the mucosal surface. Furthermore, they may regulate how the epithelium and immune system reacts, preventing white cells from entering the mucosa in massive numbers to fight infection, reducing the incidence of necrotising enterocolitis and supplying sialic acid, which is probably necessary for the central nervous system to develop normally. This evidence, however, has mostly been gathered from in vitro or ex vitro research or work on non-human animals, with a few studies of cohort design looking at mothers and their offspring. More robust evidence in the form of randomised, controlled studies of sufficient statistical power is called for to state with certainty that these mechanisms apply in human babies. This chapter will examine the history of research into HMOs, describe the structural differences between the types and outline the current state of knowledge regarding HMO production in the human breast and how they are metabolised in infants fed breast milk. The later part of the chapter looks at what benefits HMOs confer on infants, looks at the situation in related species and in artificial baby milk, and states what barriers and goals affect research into HMOs at present and in the future.

2 Why Is there Such Variety in the HMOs Contained in Milk?

Some of the many factors that add to the variety in HMOs are illustrated. One of the most crucial factors driving variety appears to be genetic. The separation into right and left seen on the principal component 1 axis is mainly attributable to a single nucleotide polymorphism (SNP). Indeed, a single base pair substitution in a genome containing 3 giga base pairs in total accounts for one of the main lactotype pairs: secretory and non-secretory phenotypes. These two phenotypes result in major differences in the HMO content of breast milk. The SNP is found in the region coding for the FUT2 gene (fucosyltransferase 2). This enzyme links fucose by an α1–2 bond either to the invariable disaccharide HMO precursor or to a longer precursor polysaccharide chain [5]. Certain nucleotide substitutions result in coding for ending protein assembly, meaning that the fucosyltransferase 2 product is truncated and non-functional. In the secretory phenotype this enzyme is functional and the HMO composition includes abundant oligosaccharides that contain α1–2-linked fucose subunits, notably 2′-fucosyllactose (2′FL) or lacto-*N*-fucopentaose (LNFP) I. Women with the non-secretory phenotype have virtually none of these HMOs in their breast milk [4]. Furthermore, the non-functioning FUT2 creates many other changes in HMO composition beyond the ones attributable to defective α1–2 fucosylation. There are analogous, although less profound, changes attributable to polymorphism in the genetic region containing the FUT3 gene (fucosyltransferase 3). This gene is linked to expression of the Lewis blood group glycoproteins. FUT3 links fucose to the disaccharide or lengthier precursor of the HMO via an α1–3 or α1–4 bond [6]. Whether the FUT3 gene codes for a functional or non-functional enzyme explains the formation of the lactotype pair – Lewis positive and negative.

Fucosyltransferases 2 and 3 only catalyse a small number of the steps within the HMO synthetic pathways. There is at present only a limited understanding of these pathways, meaning that a substantial portion of the biosynthetic machinery in humans still awaits characterisation. This area of biosynthesis has unusual characteristics: it is only active in a single species (*Homo sapiens*), is confined to a single organ (i.e. the breast) and only in lactating or pregnant females. Because of these characteristics, mapping out the steps involved is highly challenging. However, a greater knowledge of this area of biosynthesis may help to find features unique to our species. Methods that may be employed to investigate HMO biosynthesis include genome-wide association techniques, RNA characterisation in milk, milk metabolomics, computed pathway simulations and target validation in vitro.

The genetic composition of the mother is not the sole factor influencing which HMOs are present in milk. Maternal dietary intake, her level of exercise, consumption of dietary supplements, health in general and drug history when pregnant and whilst lactating, all potentially influence HMO levels in milk [3]. Research using a murine model indicates that a lipid-rich diet results in reducing HMO levels, whereas being physically active increases the HMO content of milk. A trial in which pregnant women were assigned to receive a combined probiotic or none noted differences in HMO levels and type between the two groups [7]. At present, it has not been fully established what effects on HMO arise from maternal obesity, gestational diabetes or maternal chronic inflammatory conditions. Studies to answer these questions are being undertaken.

3   The Fate of HMOs Following Ingestion

HMOs are mostly unaltered by the highly acidic infantile gastric environment. The enzymes excreted by the pancreas and found on the small intestinal brush border do not dismantle the oligosaccharide chain apart from possibly type 2 polysaccharide chains. In this type of polysaccharide, lactase can separate the last galactose subunit off the chain by cleaving the $\beta1$–4 linkage. Around 1% of the HMOs entering the gut undergo absorption and are detectable in the systemic circulation and within the infant's urine [8, 9]. This suggests that HMOs have effects that are not solely exerted within the gut itself. The majority of HMOs travel unaltered to the terminal small bowel and large intestine. Here they are consumed by the microbiota or pass out in the faeces.

4   Possible Roles for HMOs

HMOs have frequently been considered as simply prebiotics within milk that can provide nutritional support for healthy microbiota within the infant's digestive system [10]. There is, nonetheless, evidence suggesting that this is not the only role they play. There are grounds for supposing that the original evolutionary advantage from HMOs came not from a prebiotic, but an antibiotic effect. In other words, they may have evolved to stop bacterial growth rather than shape the microbial flora [11]. The origins of milk appear to lie in the creation of a substance capable of maintaining the moisture content of eggs. Since moist eggs were at risk of hosting bacteria or fungi, there would have been an evolutionary advantage if this substance had an antimicrobial function. It appears that such naturally occurring microbicides probably included oligosaccharides. Despite lactose being an invariable component of all current HMOs, this sugar is believed to have originated later than this egg-moistening stage, possibly through its role in energy production. If this is so, then HMOs were originally antimicrobial substances, with the prebiotic effect only evolving afterwards. Some studies have found that particular HMOs can arrest the multiplication of certain bacterial species, such as *Streptococci* belonging to Group B [12]. HMOs also resemble components of the cell surface receptors that many viral, bacterial and protozoal pathogens utilise for attachment, proliferation and, sometimes, invasion and infection [1]. They represent a kind of decoy that remain within the gut lumen. Pathogens attach to these decoys rather than to the gut wall, thus preventing attachment, proliferation and infection [1]. That HMOs can prevent attachment of strains of *Campylobacter jejuni* has been demonstrated both in vivo and in other species [13]. A study following a cohort of infants and their mothers found that these same oligosaccharides were present in cases of diarrhoea originating lower down in the gut and associated with *Campylobacter* spp. [14]. Subsequently, HMOs that possess the ability to prevent enteropathogenic *Escherichia coli* strains (EPEC) from adhering to the gut and causing disease have been discovered. For these studies tissue culture or a murine model was used [15].

5 Do HMOs Have a Pre- or Antibiotic Function?

Most probably, not all HMOs perform the same role. Commensal bacterial species like the *Bifidobacteria* have an apparent preference for the shorter, less complex HMOs [16]. The longer, more complex oligosaccharides appear better suited to an antibiotic role. Indeed, the fact that the shorter HMOs, such as fucosyllactose, sialyl lactose and lacto-*N*-tetraose or lacto-*N*-neotetraose, serve as ready nutrition for microbes means the microbes preferentially metabolise these compounds, rather than breaking down the longer HMOs, which have antibiotic abilities.

Nonetheless, evolutionary pressure is unrelenting, and it is expected that some microorganisms would find ways to exploit HMOs. A recent study [16] demonstrated that a certain variant of the rotavirus possessing a G10P spike protein was more capable of infecting cells when particular HMOs were present in tissue culture [17]. It was noted that for infants who showed the symptoms of a rotavirus infection, their mothers produced milk containing high levels of the same specific HMOs. In this case, the virus seems to have taken the evolutionary advantage. It has been suggested, however, that the same mechanism may be used to render vaccination more effective, conferring benefit to the host. The Rotavac vaccination consists of a live, attenuated virus. This strain also infects tissue cultures more effectively when specific HMOs are present. Administering the vaccine together with these HMOs may be a way to make vaccination more effective.

Beyond their role in modulating the interaction of the infant with microbes, there are also specific associations between particular HMOs and infant body composition. A study involving 25 infants and their mothers in the USA found associations between particular HMOs and the infant's body mass, lean mass and fat mass [18]. A further study, which employed the same analytical equipment, looked at 30 infant and mother pairs living in Denmark and established associations between excessive infant body mass and particular HMOs [19]. In both these studies, there was a negative association between body mass and adipose deposition and lacto-*N*-neotetraose, whilst 2′-fucosyllactose had a positive association with increased infant body mass. The two studies referenced have low numbers of participants, but a larger study involving 802 infants and their mothers has been undertaken in Finland, although the results are yet to be published. However, pre-publication results indicate that the same associations were established, but with the additional information that the association with increased infant body mass persisted up to the age of 5 years, at which point breastfeeding had long ceased. Thus, a longer lasting effect on the child's growth and body structure seems to exist. However, these results should be interpreted with caution, as statistical association does not establish causality.

6 The Role of HMOs in Immunomodulation

The direct and indirect effects of HMOs on the infant gut lining and immune system that have so far been proven. For innate immunity to occur, the initial defence consists of a healthy gut lining, which acts as a physical barrier. In the intestinal epithelium, the cells at the base of the crypts undergo division, moving up along the crypts as they mature into fully functional epithelial cells. The Paneth cells present an exception, as their migration is in the opposite direction. HMOs decrease the division of cells in the crypt bases [20–24], accelerate the development of the lining cells [24] and strengthen the integrity of the barrier [24]. The goblet cells secrete a lubricating and protective mucinous substance formed of glycoproteins, which separates the epithelium from the material within the gut lumen. It is possible that HMOs modulate the behaviour of mucin-secreting cells. This effect has been observed with galactose-containing oligosaccharides [25]. HMOs can influence the synthesis of immune molecules by the mucosa, an effect that may be direct [23–25] or indirect [26], via an effect on the gut flora [26]. As previously discussed, HMOs have a probiotic effect on beneficial microbial flora, especially *Bifidobacteria* spp. and *Bacteroides* spp. [27]. This is shown by 7. HMOs also reduce the infective potential of viral and bacterial pathogens through acting as decoys or interfering with pathogen attachment to the epithelial glycoprotein receptors [12, 13, 28]. This is shown by 8. Furthermore, oligosaccharides in the diet are found along the walls of the gut, which increase the variety of glycoproteins found at that site [29]. HMOs are metabolised by *Bifidobacterium infantis* within the intestines of the infant [8, 16]. This organism secretes peptides that cause the intestine to assume a healthy state of permeability via increased synthesis of proteins forming tight junctions. This was shown in a murine colitis model [30]. HMOs have a probable role in promoting the survival of other beneficial bacteria within the intestine. The way the intestine performs its barrier role then also influences the function of the immune system, both locally and systemically [31]. HMOs have effects on both the numbers of each type of immunocytes and the release of cytokines [28, 32]. There is also absorption of HMOs into the systemic circulation [33–35]. Here they may cause monocytes, lymphocytes or neutrophils to attach to the vascular lining [36] and stimulate neutrophilic attachment to thrombocytes [37].

7 HMOs May Modulate the Immune Response through Binding of Carbohydrates

A significant mechanism by which the immune system exerts its responses is through the use of carbohydrate signals and the proteins that bind to them. Individual cells carry distinctive glycoproteins on their surface composed of particular molecular motifs. These signals are transferred to other cells and the surrounding environment [38, 39]. The glycoproteins located on the plasma membrane are similar to those located on the surface of microbes or in food, such as breast milk. This circumstance means that there are many ways in which the infant, the microorganism and the HMOs can interact.

The lectins are a class of proteins located on the plasma membrane, which have the ability to recognise certain molecular signatures and the way these are laid out, and to translate recognition into a cellular response. Lectins are classified according to the carbohydrate recognition domain (CRD) they carry. More than 12 CRDs are recognised in mammalian species. However, the three categories of lectins of a special significance in immunomodulation by the HMOs are the C-type lectins, siglecs (sialic acid-binding Ig-like lectins) and galectins.

Calcium must be present for the C-type lectins to perform their role. This group encompasses the selectins, mannan-binding protein and dendritic cell-specific intercellular adhesion molecule 3-grabbing non-integrin (DC-SIGN). This class of lectins is bound to the outer plasma membrane of dendritic cells, where they may either activate a lymphocytic response to an antigen or ignore it (i.e. immunotolerance) [40]. The DC-SIGN molecule is especially relevant to understanding how HMOs modulate the immune response, since its carbohydrate-binding domain can recognise fucosyl groups and it is present on the plasma membrane of certain gut cells in infants [41]. The cells expressing DC-SIGN have a probable antigen presentation role, since this molecule is typically found on other cells specialised to present antigen, such as dendritic cells [39]. Whilst the attachment of DC-SIGN to fucose-containing carbohydrates is a part of the development of immunotolerance, further recognition events must happen at the same time for a cellular response to be stimulated [39].

Siglecs can recognise sialic acid residues and are generally expressed on particular types of immune cells [42]. A minimum of 16 different siglecs exist, such as sialoadhesin (siglec-1), CD22 (siglec-2), myelin-associated glycoprotein (MAG, siglec-4), siglec-15, and CD33-related siglecs. These are found on various white cells. The particular recognition abilities of individual siglecs depend on variety in their secondary binding sites [39]. Siglecs bind to recognised antigens and then trigger endocytosis to engulf the antigen and bring it into the cytoplasm for further processing. The majority of cells bearing siglecs are specialised to process and present antigens [39]. Molecules that carry a sialic acid group can be endocytosed by macrophages following recognition by siglecs on the outer plasma membrane [42].

In mammalian species there are certain carbohydrates that include sialic acid, the purpose of which is to induce tolerance to innocuous antigens by classifying them as 'self'. After specific siglecs recognise an antigen, interleukin-10 (IL-10) release is triggered [43].

The galectins play a key role in cellular proliferation and immunomodulation. Galectins specifically recognise the beta-galactosides. Removal of sialic acid residues results in a greater concentration of galactosyl units on the outer plasma membrane. CD45, for example, is a molecule containing sialic acid in an alpha configuration bound from the second carbon atom of one unit to the sixth carbon on the second. This molecule is expressed on unactivated T-lymphocytes. When this bond is cleaved in the activated cell, the lymphocyte may undergo apoptosis after being bound to galectin-1 [44]. If HMOs containing sialic acid bind to cells, this prevents galectins from triggering programmed cell death.

8 The Immunomodulatory Role of HMOs on Mucosae

Cell culture methods have been used to study how HMOs affect the degree to which genes related to immunity are expressed and their products are synthesised in cells of the gut. To simulate the effect of infection by a bacterium [24], various experiments have been undertaken, including incubating cells with oligosaccharides [23], bacterial organisms [44] or lipopolysaccharides. In Caco-2 gut cell cultures incubated with *Bifidobacterium* organisms, where HMOs were added there was decreased expression of chemokine-related genes when compared with cultures using glucose or lactose in place of HMOs [24]. In contrast, HT-29 cell cultures, to which HMOs were added but without simultaneous presence of any bacterium, reacted by upregulating expression of a number of chemokine-related genes [23]. Further studies utilising cell cultures of T84 and HCT8 lineages have demonstrated that inflammatory responses by these cells are downgraded in the presence of a mixture of HMOs or 2′-fucosyllactose alone [24].

It has also been shown that HMOs can alter the progression of a gastrointestinal infection caused by a virus. One study modelled infection with rotavirus using a technique that isolated the ileum in a 21-day piglet without removing it from the animal. The section of intestine inoculated with rotavirus and simultaneous application of HMOs expressed fewer mRNA transcripts for the viral protein NSP-4 (non-structural protein 4). This result demonstrates that HMOs limit viral replication in intestinal cells [45]. Nonetheless, the application of HMOs had no effect on production of cytokines or chemokines. In the piglet model, expression of the viral protein was reduced in the presence of both neutral and acidic HMOs. This contrasts with the result from in vitro studies, where virus-limiting effects were only seen with acidic HMOs [45].

9 Systemic Immunomodulatory and Protective Role of HMOs

Since HMOs are present in the peripheral circulation of breastfed infants at a level between 1 and 133 mg/L [33, 35], it seems probable that HMOs in breast milk may directly modulate the infant immune cell systemic responses. As stated earlier, many of the immunoreceptors are bound by proteoglycans and the oligosaccharide portion of the molecule is key to recognition [12, 13]. Furthermore, the structural similarities between HMOs and selectin ligands [12] suggest the possibility that HMOs may cause direct activation of circulating immunocytes and provoke the release of immune signals that alter the balance and behaviour of various immune cells. To take an example, P- and E-selectins can bind to CD15s, a carbohydrate sequence found on multiple HMOs [9]. A further point to consider is that selectin binding is frequently affected by the addition of fucose or sialic acid to a glycan and HMOs frequently exhibit such modifications [46]. HMOs have been shown to be capable of preventing pavementing [36] and recruitment [37] of neutrophils by disrupting the binding of immune proteins and glycans. When peripheral mononucleocytes (PMNs) taken from newborn pigs were examined ex vivo, it was noted that HMOs influenced their propensity to divide and to express cytokines [32]. When HMOs only were supplied to PMNs, they responded by synthesising IL-10, a cytokine involved in immune regulation [32]. Separate studies have noted that IL-10 synthesis increases in response to acidic HMOs. Ex vivo studies with mononucleocytes derived from human umbilical cord samples have shown that interferon gamma increases in the presence of acidic HMOs [41]. PMNs divided more rapidly when HMOs were administered to PMNs that had been primed with phytohaemagglutinin, which stimulates T-cell proliferation. Meanwhile, PMNs primed to divide by being presented with lipopolysaccharide increased their rate of division when HMOs containing sialic acid residues were present [32]. If PMNs were not stimulated and remained in culture for 3 days, the presence of 2′-fucosyllactose prevented their division. Accordingly, we can expect HMOs to have different effects on infant immune systems depending on their state of activation. If there is no stimulus present to encourage immune proliferation, HMOs keep proliferation levels low, whereas they increase division when immunocytes are already proliferating.

Currently, limited research has examined the immunological response to feeding infants HMOs [24, 25, 47–49, 52]. Although one study did supply dietary 2′-fucosyllactose to piglets [53], the reports only concern growth and toxicity. A recent trial compared the immunological effects of artificial baby milk containing varying amounts of HMOs with normal breast milk [49]. The artificial milk contained 2.4 g/L oligogalactose, 2.2 g/L oligogalactose plus 0.2 g/L 2′-fucosyllactose or 1.4 g oligogalactose plus 1.0 g 2′-fucosyllactose. The human infants in the trial received artificial milk between the ages of 5 days and 4 months, with blood sampling at the age of 6 weeks to quantify cytokine levels, phenotype the immunocytes present and observe the effects of stimulating ex vivo PMNs separated from the blood samples. There were similarities between the control group and the infants who received either type of artificial milk containing 2′-fucosyllactose. These subjects expressed decreased levels of inflammatory cytokines than those taking formula milk containing no HMOs. Furthermore, looking at the results of cytokine secretion by the isolated PMNs, when respiratory syncytial virus was inoculated into these samples, investigators could observe similarities between the breastfed infants and those receiving supplemental 2′-fucosyllactose in the formula preparations. These infants had lower levels of tumour necrosis factor (TNF)-alpha and interferon gamma, with a tendency to decrease levels of IL-1Ra, IL-6, and IL-1β, as compared with the babies receiving standard artificial milk [49].

References

1. Bode L. Human milk oligosaccharides: structure and functions. Nestle Nutr Inst Workshop Ser. 2020;94:115–23. https://doi.org/10.1159/000505339. Epub 2020 Mar 11.
2. Bode L, Contractor N, Barile D, et al. Overcoming the limited availability of human milk oligosaccharides: challenges and opportunities for research and application. Nutr Rev. 2016;74:635–44.
3. Bode L. Human milk oligosaccharides: every baby needs a sugar mama. Glycobiology. 2012;22:1147–62.
4. Azad MB, Robertson B, Atakora F, et al. Human milk oligosaccharide concentrations are associated with multiple fixed and modifiable maternal characteristics, environmental factors and feeding practices. J Nutr. 2018;148:1733–42.
5. Jantscher-Krenn E, Bode L. Structure-function relationships of human milk oligosaccharides. Adv Nutr. 2012;3:383S–91S.
6. Kumazaki T, Yoshida A. Biochemical evidence that secretor gene, Se, is a structural gene encoding a specific fucosyltransferase. Proc Natl Acad Sci U S A. 1984;81:4193–7.
7. Stahl B, Thurl S, Henker J, et al. Detection of four human milk groups with respect to Lewis-bloodgroup-dependent oligosaccharides by serologic and chromatographic analysis. Adv Exp Med Biol. 2001;501:299–306.
8. Ruhaak LR, Stroble C, Underwood MA, et al. Detection of milk oligosaccharides in plasma of infants. Anal Bioanal Chem. 2014;406:5775–84.
9. Rudloff S, Obermeier S, Borsch C, et al. Incorporation of orally applied (13)C-galactose into milk lactose and oligosaccharides. Glycobiology. 2006;16:477–87.
10. German JB, Freeman SL, Lebrilla CB, et al. Human milk oligosaccharides: evolution, structures and bioselectivity as substrates for intestinal bacteria. Nestlé Nutr Workshop Ser Pediatr Program. 2008;62:205–18; discussion 218–222.
11. Oftedahl OT. The evolution of milk secretion and its ancient origins. Animal. 2012;6:355–68.
12. Lin AE, Autran CA, Szyszka A, et al. Human milk oligosaccharides inhibit growth of group B streptococcus. J Biol Chem. 2017;292:11,243–9.
13. Ruiz-Palacios GM, Cervantes LE, Ramos P, et al. Campylobacter jejuni binds intestinal H (O) antigen (Fucα1,2Galβ1, 4GlcNAc), and fucosyloligosaccharides of human milk inhibit its binding and infection. J Biol Chem. 2003;278:1411214120.
14. Morrow AL, Ruiz-Palacios GM, Altaye M, et al. Human milk oligosaccharides are associated with protection against diarrhea in breast-fed infants. J Pediatr. 2004;145:297–303.
15. Manthey CF, Autran CA, Eckmann L, Bode L. Human milk oligosaccharides protect against enteropathogenic E. coli attachment in vitro and colonization in suckling mice. J Pediatr Gastroenterol Nutr. 2014;58:167–70.

16. LoCascio RG, Ninonuevo MR, Freeman SL, et al. Glycoprofiling of bifidobacterial consumption of human milk oligosaccharides demonstrates strain specific, preferential consumption of small chain glycans secreted in early human lactation. J Agric Food Chem. 2007;55:8914–9.
17. Ramani S, Stewart CJ, Laucirica DR, et al. Complex interplay between human milk oligosaccharides, milk microbiome and infant gut microbiome modulates neonatal rotavirus infection. Nat Commun. 2018;9:5010.
18. Alderete TL, Autran CA, Brekke BE, et al. Associations between human milk oligosaccharides and infant body composition in the first six months of life. Am J Clin Nutr. 2015;102:13811388.
19. Larsson MW, Lind MV, Laursen RP, et al. Human milk oligosaccharide composition is associated with excessive weight gain during exclusive breastfeeding—an explorative study. Front Pediatr. 2019;7:297.
20. Jantscher-Krenn E, Aigner J, Reiter B, et al. Evidence of human milk oligosaccharides in maternal circulation already during pregnancy—a pilot study. Am J Physiol Endocrinol Metab. 2019;316:E347–57.
21. Donovan SM, Comstock SS. Human milk oligosaccharides influence neonatal mucosal and systemic immunity. Ann Nutr Metab. 2016;69(Suppl 2):42–51. https://doi.org/10.1159/000452818. Epub 2017 Jan 20.
22. Hester SN, Donovan SM. Individual and combined effects of nucleotides and human milk oligosaccharides on proliferation, apoptosisandnecrosis in a humanfetalintestinalcellline. Food Nutr Sci. 2012;3:1567–76.
23. Lane JA, O'Callaghan J, Carrington SD, Hickey RM. Transcriptional response of HT-29 intestinal epithelial cells to human and bovine milk oligosaccharides. Br J Nutr. 2013;110:2127–37.
24. Holscher HD, Davis SR, Tappenden KA. Human milk oligosaccharides influence maturation of human intestinal Caco-2Bbe and HT-29 cell lines. J Nutr. 2014;144:586–91.
25. Bhatia S, Prabhu PN, Benefiel AC, Miller MJ, Chow J, Davis SR, Gaskins HR. Galacto-oligosaccharides may directly enhance intestinal barrier function through the modulation of goblet cells. Mol Nutr Food Res. 2015;59:566–73.
26. He Y, Liu S, Kling DE, Leone S, Lawlor NT, Huang Y, Feinberg SB, Hill DR, Newburg DS. The human milk oligosaccharide 2′-fucosyllactose modulates CD14 expression in human enterocytes, thereby attenuating LPS-induced inflammation. Gut. 2016;65:33–46.
27. Mezoff EA, Hawkins JA, Ollberding NJ, Karns R, Morrow AL, Helmrath MA. The human milk oligosaccharide 2′-fucosyllactose augments the adaptive response to extensive intestinal resection. Am J Physiol Gastrointest Liver Physiol. 2016;310:G427–38.
28. Wise A, Robertson B, Choudhury B, et al. Infants are exposed to human milk oligosaccharides already in utero. Front Pediatr. 2018;6:270.
29. Wickramasinghe S, Pacheco AR, Lemay DG, Mills DA. Bifidobacteria grown on human milk oligosaccharides downregulate the expression of inflammation-related genes in Caco-2 cells. BMC Microbiol. 2015;15:172.
30. Marcobal A, Sonnenburg JL. Human milk oligosaccharide consumption by intestinal microbiota. Clin Microbiol Infect. 2012;18(suppl 4):12–5.
31. Kavanaugh D, O'Callaghan J, Kilcoyne M, Kane M, Joshi L, Hickey RM. The intestinal glycome and its modulation by diet and nutrition. Nutr Rev. 2015;73:359–75.
32. Ewaschuk JB, Diaz H, Meddings L, Diederichs B, Dmytrash A, Backer J, Looijer-vanLangen M, Madsen KL. Secreted bioactive factors from *Bifidobacterium infantis* enhance epithelial cell barrier function. Am J Physiol Gastrointest Liver Physiol. 2008;295:1025–34.
33. Macpherson AJ, Geuking MB, McCoy KD. Immune responses that adapt the intestinal mucosa to commensal intestinal bacteria. Immunology. 2005;115:153–62.
34. Comstock SS, Wang M, Hester SN, Li M, Donovan SM. Select human milk oligosaccharides directly modulate peripheral blood mononuclear cells isolated from 10-d-old pigs. Br J Nutr. 2014;111:819–28.
35. Goehring KC, Kennedy AD, Prieto PA, Buck RH. Direct evidence for the presence of human milk oligosaccharides in the circulation of breastfed infants. PLoS One. 2014;9:e101692.

36. Marriage BJ, Buck RH, Goehring KC, Oliver JS, Williams JA. Infants fed a lower calorie formula with 2′-fucosyllactose (2′FL) show growth and 2′FL uptake like breast-fed infants. J Pediatr Gastroenterol Nutr. 2015;61:649–58.
37. Ruhaak LR, Stroble C, Underwood MA, Le-brilla CB. Detection of milk oligosaccharides in plasma of infants. Anal Bioanal Chem. 2014;406:5775–84.
38. Bode L, Kunz C, Muhly-Reinholz M, Mayer K, Seeger W, Rudloff S. Inhibition of monocyte, lymphocyte, and neutrophil adhesion to endothelial cells by human milk oligosaccharides. Thromb Haemost. 2004;92:1402–10.
39. Bode L, Rudloff S, Kunz C, Strobel S, Klein N. Human milk oligosaccharides reduce platelet-neutrophil complex formation leading to a decrease in neutrophil beta 2 integrin expression. J Leukoc Biol. 2004;76:820–6.
40. Rabinovich GA, Croci DO. Regulatory circuits mediated by lectin-glycan interactions in auto-immunity and cancer. Immunity. 2012;36:322–35.
41. Schnaar RL. Glycans and glycan-binding proteins in immune regulation: a concise introduction to glycobiology for the allergist. J Allergy Clin Immunol. 2015;135:609–15.
42. Geijtenbeek TB, vanVliet SJ, Engering A, 'tHart BA, van Kooyk Y. Self-and nonself-recognition by C-typel ectins on dendritic cells. Annu Rev Immunol. 2004;22:33–54.
43. Koning N, Kessen SF, Van Der Voorn JP, Appelmelk BJ, Jeurink PV, Knippels LM, Garssen J, Van Kooyk Y. Human milk blocks DC-SIGN-pathogen interaction via MUC1. Front Immunol. 2015;6:112.
44. Macauley MS, Crocker PR, Paulson JC. Si-glec-mediated regulation of immune cell function in disease. Nat Rev Immunol. 2014;14:653–66.
45. Stephenson HN, Mills DC, Jones H, Milioris E, Copland A, Dorrell N, Wren BW, Crocker PR, Escors D, Bajaj-Elliott M. Pseudaminic acid on *Campylo bacterjejuni* flagella modulates dendritic cell IL-10 expression via Si-glec-10 receptor: a novel flagellin-host interaction. J Infect Dis. 2014;210:1487–98.
46. Earl LA, Bi S, Baum LG. N-and O-glycans modulate galectin-1 binding, CD45 signaling, and T cell death. J BiolChem. 2010;285:2232–44.
47. Hester SN, Chen X, Li M, Monaco MH, Comstock SS, Kuhlenschmidt TB, Kuhlen-schmidt MS, Donovan SM. Human milk oligosaccharides inhibit rotavirus infectivity in vitro and in acutely infected piglets. Br J Nutr. 2013;110:1233–42.
48. Luhn K, Wild MK. Human deficiencies of fucosylation and sialylation affecting selectin ligands. Semin Immunopathol. 2012;34:383–99.
49. Castillo-Courtade L, Han S, Lee S, Mian FM, Buck R, Forsythe P. Attenuation of food allergy symptoms following treatment with human milk oligosaccharides in a mouse model. Allergy. 2015;70:1091–102.
50. Johnson PH, Watkins WM. Purification of the Lewis blood-group gene associated α-3/4fucosyltransferase from human milk: an enzyme transferring fucose primarily to type 1 and lactose-based oligosaccharide chains. Glycoconj J. 1992;9:241–9.
51. Seppo AE, Kukkonen AK, Kuitunen M, et al. Association of maternal probiotic supplementation with human milk oligosaccharide composition. JAMA Pediatr. 2019;173:286–8.

Breast Milk as a Biological System

Ayten Guner Atayoglu

1 Introduction

According to official recommendations, mothers should exclusively breastfeed their infants up to the age of 6 months [1], since the data show this reduces the infant's chances of developing various illnesses and of dying [2]. Globally, there are many large public-health campaigns devoted to encouraging women to breastfeed their infants. Human milk (i.e. breast milk) may be considered a system possessing various active roles and capable of delivering benefit to neonates in terms of nutrition, immunological support at the point when neonates have the least effective immune defences of their own, and support for healthy growth and development, including that of the gastrointestinal tract. Furthermore, breastfeeding is also beneficial for maternal health [3]. The more that human milk is investigated, the more apparent it becomes that milk cannot be adequately understood as simply a source of infant nutrition. Instead, milk both affects the infant and mother and is affected by them, working in a complex way to deliver its benefits. In this chapter the terms 'milk', 'breast milk' or 'human milk' will be used interchangeably to refer to the milk generated by the human mammary gland and consumed by another human being. Milk may be from the mother of the infant herself (mother's own milk, MOM), in which case it is provided to the infant directly from the breast or after being expressed into a container, or it may be a donated sample from another woman, in which case it is referred to as donated or banked milk. Although banked milk is broadly similar to MOM, it is not exactly the same. The use of banked milk is generally recommended for where MOM is unavailable or is of insufficient quantity to supply the infant's needs [4].

A. G. Atayoglu (✉)
Department of Family Medicine, Beylikdüzü State Hospital, Istanbul, Türkiye
e-mail: ayten.atayoglu@saglik.gov.tr

© The Author(s), under exclusive license to Springer Nature Switzerland AG 2023
Ö. N. Şahin et al. (eds.), *Breastfeeding and Metabolic Programming*,
https://doi.org/10.1007/978-3-031-33278-4_7

Infants who breastfeed soon after delivery (less than an hour after completion) and consume colostrum have a greater rate of survival than those who do not [5]. Breastfeeding that continues beyond the age of 6 months is beneficial to the infant, both in terms of immunity and for consuming an adequate diet, particularly if the foods for supplementing breastfeeding are unsatisfactory or consist of a very limited range of items. Although it is generally held that the amount of breast milk and several of its key constituents are independent of inadequacies in the mother's diet (provided the dietary inadequacy is not severe) [6], scientific understanding of several micronutrients and molecules possessing bioactivity in milk is still at an early stage. The health status and diet consumed by the mother are potentially key factors impinging upon the success and benefits of breastfeeding, even if further research is still needed to clarify exactly why this is so [4, 7].

2   How Breast Milk Functions as a Biological System

Breast milk is the factor of most importance in how infants grow and develop in a healthy way. It is clear that breast milk contains many essential nutrients and molecules possessing bioactivity necessary for infant health, but there remain questions about how it comes to be produced, the mutual interactions between milk, mother and child and the way that the many components of this fluid function. In many respects, milk may be best considered another physiological system of the body [4].

Breast milk is a biofluid with a unique composition. Its sophistication reflects millions of years of evolution in mammals, where the composition of each species' milk reflects the needs of the offspring. In humans, some of the key functions performed by this biofluid are rectifying the deficits caused by the immaturity of the gastrointestinal and immune systems at birth [8, 9].

2.1   Development of the Human Breast

The breast, or mammary gland, is an organ with a highly specialised exocrine function. It is under a complex set of endocrine and other physiological signals, the details of which are increasingly better understood [9]. Development of the fully functional mammary gland can be divided into three separate phases, starting during foetal life and extending over the lifetime of the human female, so that an embryonic, pubertal and adult reproductive phase can be identified. At the time of birth, the rudimentary breast organ is already present, and this organ continues to grow during childhood up until puberty occurs, when the breast tissues differentiate further, with an increase in ductal branching. At this stage the breast becomes capable of exocrine function and is responsive to growth hormone, oestrogen and insulin-like growth factor (IGF-1). The combined signals of a raised progesterone and prolactin level during pregnancy cause the alveolar lobules to differentiate into milk-producing cells. As the phase of lactation draws to an end and the infant begins weaning, the breast undergoes an involutionary change, reverting to a tissue architecture resembling that existing before pregnancy occurred. It is already known that diet (both in terms of macro- and micronutrient content) affects endocrine activity, therefore diet is likely to affect the anatomy and physiology of the breast. It has been hypothesised, for example, that vitamin A and retinoic acid play a role in the development of the breast in utero [10]. Furthermore, there are potential environmental effects on breast physiology. It has been demonstrated that molecules that interfere with endocrine signalling, as well as being exposed to heavy metals, have negative effects on in utero development [11]. The way the breast develops and its functionality are both impacted by how women respond to psychosocial and environmental stress when pregnant [12].

2.2   Constituents of Milk

Knowledge concerning the individual constituents in breast milk and how their associated bioactivity affects the healthy development of infants is increasing currently. The macronutrients in breast milk (namely lipids, proteins and carbohydrates) have been intensively researched for several decades now, and micronutrients (in particular vitamins, minerals, aliphatic acids and individual amino acids) have also been quantified in breast milk samples. Studies addressing the specific role of micronutrients in infant metabolism have only rarely, however, been published [4].

2.3   The Chronobiology of Breast Milk

The composition of breast milk varies widely between different women, but there are also differences within the breast milk of any particular woman at different stages of lactation. Colostrum, for example, which is produced for around 4–5 days after delivery, contains abundant carotenoids, high electrolyte levels (especially sodium and calcium ions) and a high concentration of protein, including antibodies. Its lactose and lipid concentration is low. Transitional milk is the type produced from around the fifth to tenth day post-partum. Finally, at around day 10 post-partum, mature milk begins to be secreted, and lactation is considered fully under way at that point. There is a variable lipid content in breast milk of different kinds, mature milk containing a higher level (3.6% on average) than either transitional milk or colostrum. The lipid content is also affected by the time of day the milk is secreted, the mother's dietary intake and how long feeding continues. The extent of the interval between feeds also influences the lipid level [13]. The vitamin content of breast milk is known to be influenced by the duration of feeding and circadian rhythm [14]. Women taking vitamin supplements secrete a higher vitamin content into the milk, not only the lipid-soluble vitamins A and D, but also those that are hydrophilic, such as B vitamins (1, 2, 5, 12 and 6) and vitamin C. Comparison of the rates of vitamins detected in breast milk from different countries reveals a wide range of values. There is only a slender evidence base on which the daily allowances recommended for infants and during breastfeeding by, for example, the Institute for Medicine or the World Health Organisation (WHO) are based. Indeed, the recommendations for vitamin A were based on data from 3 patients, whilst that for niacin was based on 23 patients [7]. A recently published review on the subject of vitamin A in breast milk found that colostrum held the highest amount of retinol:fat and retinol, but this was markedly lower within days and reached a baseline value around weeks 2–4 of breastfeeding [15]. It appears likely that the levels of other micronutrients also rise or fall depending on the stage of breastfeeding [16]. How the volume of milk produced affects the level of nutrients in breast milk is not fully known. It is clear, however, that the energy content of milk mainly depends on lipid levels, and lipid levels in milk are likely to be related to the mother's dietary intake of fats, especially as free fatty acids.

3 How Extracellular Vesicles in Breast Milk Behave as a Biological System

All types of cells in mammals appear to possess the ability to secrete extracellular vesicles or exosomes. These exosomes are particles less than a micron in diameter that are wrapped in plasma membrane derived from the cell and are secreted into extracellular compartments. The main way exosomes act is in transportation of specific cellular machinery (which may consist of protein, lipids or nucleic acids) from one cell to another. Exosomes can initiate major, complicated alterations in the cells with which they combine, with effects on normal physiology and pathological processes [17, 18]. The discovery of the exosomic transportation mechanism and its ability to trigger changes in the cells to which exosomes fuse was rewarded by a Nobel Prize in 2013 for the co-discoverers, Rothman, Schekman and Südhof, in the category of Physiology or Medicine [19, 20].

Breast milk is a sophisticated biologically active liquid that may act in a dynamic way to support the growing infant through the delivery of nutrients as well as boosting the infant's immunity to various conditions [21–24]. It has been demonstrated in clinical trials as well as through epidemiological methods that breast milk offers greater benefit to the child than artificial baby milk in terms of susceptibility to necrotising enterocolitis, sepsis in the newborn period, infections of the gut and respiratory tract, atopic conditions, obesity, diabetes mellitus and neoplasia [21–24]. Scientific understanding of the ways in which specific parts of this biological system contribute to healthy development in childhood and early adulthood is increasing. There are several constituents of breast milk, the biological activity of which has been clearly demonstrated, namely various proteins (antibodies, lactoferrin), growth factors, cytokines, adipokines, non-digestible oligosaccharides

(20-fucosyllactose [20FL], lacto-*N*-tetraose [LNT], lacto-*N*-neotetraose [LNnT], sialyllactoses [3SL, 6SL]), white blood cells and stem cells [25–28]. Exosomes containing major histocompatibility proteins of class I and II were identified by Admyr et al. in 2007 [29]. These exosomes potentially suppress immune responses. The current understanding of milk exosomes is that they play functional roles in breast milk. More research is now needed to clarify how molecular signalling between the mother and infant occurs and the long-term effects this has on the child's future health [20].

4 Biogenesis and Subpopulations

Three distinct types of vesicle are recognised as extracellular vesicles, namely exosomes, microvesicles and apoptotic bodies. All three types of vesicle consist of components of the cytosol and outer cell membrane derived from an ordinary human cell, but they originate in different ways from cells and fulfil different purposes, hence their magnitude and precise constituents differ [30, 31]. Exosomes have a diameter of around 40–150 nm. They are formed when endosomes created by invagination of cell membrane into the cytosol join together to form multivesicular bodies (MVBs). These MVBs move towards the outer cell membrane, with which they fuse, afterwards releasing exosomes out into the extracellular environment [32, 33]. There are a minimum of two separate pathways that lead to the formation of MVBs. These pathways include apportioning specific molecules to intraluminal vesicles. One of the pathways involves ESCRT—Endosomal Sorting Complex Required for Transport – an array of as many as 30 distinct proteins. The proteins that make up ESCRT can be classified into four main groups, namely ESCRT-0, -I, -II and -III. In addition there is the ATPase Vps4 complex [34–37]. The actions of ESCRT-0 include recognition and sorting of ubiquitin-tagged cargo proteins, so that they can be apportioned to the lipid-rich area of the vesicle [38, 39]. ESCRT-I and II cause invagination of the membrane of late-stage endosomes, which allows budding with specific sorted proteins intended to be transported [40, 41]. ESCRT-III removes ubiquitin from the proteins carried in the vesicle [42, 43]. It joins with the Vps4 complex to be able to perform molecular scission. The ESCRT-III-Vps4 complex can shape intraluminal vesicles, which are then put together as MVBs [44–46]. Vps4 is also involved in disassembling ESCRT and gathering molecular subunits that can be used again in generating further vesicles [47, 48]. There is also a second pathway leading to generation of MVBs, which does not depend on ESCRT [32, 33, 49]. This pathway forms MVBs from the raft-based microdomains of the endosome. Ceramide is synthesised from sphingolipids by the action of the neutral sphingomyelinase 2 (nSMase2) enzyme [50]. When the sphingolipid is converted into ceramide, the microdomains coalesce, forming larger units. The generation of intraluminal vesicles and MVBs is then initiated by these domains, and involves budding [32, 49]. Whilst blocking the action of nSMase 2 does downgrade the production of exosomes by several cell populations, this reduction in exosomal formation is not seen in all cell types. It seems, therefore, that ceramide may play different roles in the formation of exosomes in different cell types [20, 33, 49–54].

At present, the evidence points to human milk extracellular vesicles (hMEVs) originating within the breast itself, as well as from elsewhere in the body [29, 55, 56]. The majority of hMEVs are generated and released by epithelial cells of the breast in the course of lactation [29, 55]. A portion of the hMEVs is bound to the external surface of the milk fat globules. Some of the extracellular vesicles present in breast milk are likely generated by cells in the milk. Such cells include lymphocytes, macrophages and stem cells. However, some extracellular vesicles also arrive from more distant parts of the body, travelling to the breast via the blood stream [26, 27, 29, 56]. The ratio of the extracellular vesicles of mammary gland origin to those from elsewhere in the body has not yet been ascertained, due to the limits of the current techniques. It would be a useful figure to know, as it would help clarify the wider understanding of how extracellular vesicles in breast milk function overall. One possibility is that techniques where a single extracellular vesicle is isolated and its characteristics investigated [57–60] may be employed to categorise the extracellular vesicles in breast milk and thus provide an insight into their originating organ system and its relative contribution to the biological activity of milk [20].

5 Molecular Constituents

The formation of exosomes is vitally dependent on the tetraspanin proteins (such as CD9, CD63 and CD81), as well as Tsg101 and Alix. In experiments involving separation of hMEVs from milk, these proteins are measured to indicate how successful enrichment has been. Some other proteins may also be used in this way, namely lactadherin (also termed Milk Fat Globule-EGF factor VIII [MFGE8]), butyrophilin and xanthine dehydrogenase/oxidase. These are important constituents of the breast milk fat globules [61, 62]. Butyrophilin, major histocompatibility complex (MHC) proteins and transforming growth factor-β (TGF-β) probably act synergistically to regulate the immune system of the infant, a process known to involve hMEVs [20, 29, 63, 64].

References

1. Department of Nutrition for Health and Development, Department of Child and Adolescent Health and Development. The optimal duration of exclusive breastfeeding: report of an Expert Consultation. Geneva, Switzerland: World Health Organization; 2001.
2. Black RE, Victora CG, Walker SP, Bhutta ZA, Christian P, de Onis M, Ezzati M, Grantham-Mcgregor S, Katz J, Martorell Ret al.. Maternal and child undernutrition and overweight in low-income and middle-income countries. Lancet North Am Ed 2013;382:427–451.

3. Chowdhury R, Sinha B, Sankar MJ, Taneja S, Bhandari N, Rollins N, Bahl R, Martines J. Breastfeeding and maternal health outcomes: a systematic review and meta-analysis. Acta Paediatr. 2015;104:96–113.

4. Christian P, Smith ER, Lee SE, Vargas AJ, Bremer AA, Raiten DJ. The need to study human milk as a biological system. Am J Clin Nutr. 2021;113(5):1063–72. https://doi.org/10.1093/ajcn/nqab075.

5. Smith ER, Hurt L, Chowdhury R, Sinha B, Fawzi W, Edmond KM, Neovita Study Group. Delayed breastfeeding initiation and infant survival: a systematic review and meta-analysis. PLoS One. 2017;26(12):e0180722. https://journals.plos.org/plosone/article/file?id=10.1371/journal.pone.0180722&type=printable. Accessed 2 Oct 2020.

6. Pérez-Escamilla R, Buccini GS, Segura-Pérez S, Piwoz E. Perspective: should exclusive breastfeeding still be recommended for 6 months? Adv Nutr. 2019;10:931–43.

7. Allen LH, Donohue JA, Dror DK. Limitations of the evidence base used to set recommended nutrient intakes for infants and lactating women. Adv Nutr. 2018;9:295S–312S.

8. Garofalo RP, Goldman AS. Cytokines, chemokines, and colony-stimulating factors in human milk: the 1997 update. Neonatology. 1998;74:134–42.

9. Macias H, Hinck L. Mammary gland development. WIREs Dev Biol. 2012;1:533–7.

10. Cabezuelo MT, Zaragozá R, Barber T, Viña JR. Role of vitamin A in mammary gland development and lactation. Nutrients. 2019;12:80.

11. Lee S, Kelleher SL. Biological underpinnings of breastfeeding challenges: the role of genetics, diet, and environment on lactation physiology. Am J Physiol Endocrinol Metab. 2016;311:E405–22.

12. Avivar-Valderas A, Wen HC, Aguirre-Ghiso JA. Stress signaling and the shaping of the mammary tissue in development and cancer. Oncogene. 2014;33:5483–90.

13. Andreas NJ, Kampmann B, Le-Doare KM. Human breast milk: a review on its composition and bioactivity. Early Hum Dev. 2015;91:629–35.

14. Hampel D, Shahab-Ferdows S, Islam MM, Peerson JM, Allen LH. Vitamin concentrations in human milk vary with time within feed, circadian rhythm, and single-dose supplementation. J Nutr. 2017;147:603–11.

15. Dror DK, Allen LH. Overview of nutrients in human milk. Adv Nutr. 2018;9:278S–94S.

16. Dror DK, Allen LH. Retinol-to-fat ratio and retinol concentration in human milk show similar time trends and associations with maternal factors at the population level: a systematic review and meta-analysis. Adv Nutr. 2018;9:332S–46S.

17. Couch Y, Buzàs EI, Di Vizio D, Gho YS, Harrison P, Hill AF, Lötvall J, Raposo G, Stahl PD, Théry C, et al. A brief history of nearly EV-erything—the rise and rise of extracellular vesicles. J Extracell Vesicles. 2021;10:e12144.

18. Raposo G, Stahl PD. Extracellular vesicles: a new communication paradigm? Nat Rev Mol Cell Biol. 2019;20:509–10.

19. Bonifacino JS. Vesicular transport earns a Nobel. Trends Cell Biol. 2014;24:3–5.

20. Chutipongtanate S, Morrow AL, Newburg DS. Human milk extracellular vesicles: a biological system with clinical implications. Cell. 2022;11(15):2345. https://doi.org/10.3390/cells11152345.

21. AAP. Section on breastfeeding breastfeeding and the use of human milk. Pediatrics. 2012;129:e827–41.

22. Horta BL. Breastfeeding: investing in the future. Breastfeed Med Off J Acad Breastfeed Med. 2019;14:S11–2.

23. Kanaprach P, Pongsakul N, Apiwattanakul N, Muanprasat C, Supapannachart S, Nuntnarumit P, Chutipongtanate S. Evaluation of fetal intestinal cell growth and antimicrobial biofunctionalities of donor human milk after preparative processes. Breastfeed Med. 2018;13:215–20.

24. Chiangjong W, Panachan J, Vanichapol T, Pongsakul N, Pongphitcha P, Siriboonpiputtana T, Lerksuthirat T, Nuntnarumit P, Supapannachart S, Srisomsap C, et al. HMP-S7 is a novel anti-leukemic peptide discovered from human Milk. Biomedicine. 2021;9:981.

25. Ballard O, Morrow AL. Human milk composition: nutrients and bioactive factors. Pediatr Clin N Am. 2013;60:49–74.
26. Hassiotou F, Hartmann PE. At the dawn of a new discovery: the potential of breast milk stem cells. Adv Nutr. 2014;5:770–8.
27. Vizzari G, Morniroli D, Ceroni F, Verduci E, Consales A, Colombo L, Cerasani J, Mosca F, Giannì ML. Human milk, more than simple nourishment. Children. 2021;8:63.
28. Chutipongtanate S, Morrow AL, Newburg DS. Human milk oligosaccharides: potential applications in COVID-19. Biomedicine. 2022;10:346.
29. Admyre C, Johansson SM, Qazi KR, Filén J-J, Lahesmaa R, Norman M, Neve EPA, Scheynius A, Gabrielsson S. Exosomes with immune modulatory features are present in human breast milk. J Immunol. 2007;179:1969–78.
30. Lötvall J, Hill AF, Hochberg F, Buzás EI, Di Vizio D, Gardiner C, Gho YS, Kurochkin IV, Mathivanan S, Quesenberry P, et al. Minimal experimental requirements for definition of extracellular vesicles and their functions: a position statement from the International Society for Extracellular Vesicles. J Extracell Vesicles. 2014;3:26,913.
31. Théry C, Witwer KW, Aikawa E, Alcaraz MJ, Anderson JD, Andriantsitohaina R, Antoniou A, Arab T, Archer F, Atkin-Smith GK, et al. Minimal information for studies of extracellular vesicles 2018 (MISEV2018): a position statement of the International Society for Extracellular Vesicles and update of the MISEV2014 guidelines. J Extracell Vesicles. 2018;7:1535750.
32. Dreyer F, Baur A. Biogenesis and functions of exosomes and extracellular vesicles. Methods Mol Biol. 2016;1448:201–16.
33. Hessvik NP, Llorente A. Current knowledge on exosome biogenesis and release. Cell Mol Life Sci. 2018;75:193–208.
34. Henne WM, Stenmark H, Emr SD. Molecular mechanisms of the membrane sculpting ESCRT pathway. Cold Spring Harb Perspect Biol. 2013;5:a016766.
35. Vietri M, Radulovic M, Stenmark H. The many functions of ESCRTs. Nat Rev Mol Cell Biol. 2020;21:25–42.
36. Calistri A, Reale A, Palù G, Parolin C. Why cells and viruses cannot survive without an ESCRT. Cell. 2021;10:483.
37. Olmos Y. The ESCRT machinery: remodeling, repairing, and sealing membranes. Membranes. 2022;12:633.
38. Raiborg C, Bache KG, Gillooly DJ, Madshus IH, Stang E, Stenmark H. Hrs sorts ubiquitinated proteins into clathrin-coated microdomains of early endosomes. Nat Cell Biol. 2002;4:394–8.
39. Mayers JR, Fyfe I, Schuh AL, Chapman ER, Edwardson JM, Audhya A. ESCRT-0 assembles as a heterotetrameric complex on membranes and binds multiple ubiquitinylated cargoes simultaneously. J Biol Chem. 2011;286:9636–45.
40. Katzmann DJ, Babst M, Emr SD. Ubiquitin-dependent sorting into the multivesicular body pathway requires the function of a conserved endosomal protein sorting complex, ESCRT-I. Cell. 2001;106:145–55.
41. Babst M, Katzmann DJ, Snyder WB, Wendland B, Emr SD. Endosome-associated complex, ESCRT-II, recruits transport machinery for protein sorting at the multivesicular body. Dev Cell. 2002;3:283–9.
42. Agromayor M, Martin-Serrano J. Interaction of AMSH with ESCRT-III and deubiquitination of endosomal cargo. J Biol Chem. 2006;281:23083–91.
43. Kyuuma M, Kikuchi K, Kojima K, Sugawara Y, Sato M, Mano N, Goto J, Takeshita T, Yamamoto A, Sugamura K, et al. AMSH, an ESCRT-III associated enzyme, deubiquitinates cargo on MVB/late endosomes. Cell Struct Funct. 2007;31:159–72.
44. Wollert T, Wunder C, Lippincott-Schwartz J, Hurley JH. Membrane scission by the ESCRT-III complex. Nature. 2009;458:172–7.
45. Adell MAY, Vogel GF, Pakdel M, Müller M, Lindner H, Hess MW, Teis D. Coordinated binding of Vps4 to ESCRT-III drives membrane neck constriction during MVB vesicle formation. J Cell Biol. 2014;205:33–49.

46. Schöneberg J, Pavlin MR, Yan S, Righini M, Lee I-H, Carlson L-A, Bahrami AH, Goldman DH, Ren X, Hummer G, et al. ATP-dependent force generation and membrane scission by ESCRT-III and Vps4. Science. 2018;362:1423–8.
47. Davies BA, Azmi IF, Payne J, Shestakova A, Horazdovsky BF, Babst M, Katzmann DJ. Coordination of substrate binding and ATP hydrolysis in Vps4-mediated ESCRT-III disassembly. Mol Biol Cell. 2010;21:3396–408.
48. Caillat C, Macheboeuf P, Wu Y, McCarthy AA, Boeri-Erba E, Effantin G, Göttlinger HG, Weissenhorn W, Renesto P. Asymmetric ring structure of Vps4 required for ESCRT-III disassembly. Nat Commun. 2015;6:8781.
49. Trajkovic K, Hsu C, Chiantia S, Rajendran L, Wenzel D, Wieland F, Schwille P, Brügger B, Simons M. Ceramide triggers budding of exosome vesicles into multivesicular endosomes. Science. 2008;319:1244–7.
50. Menck K, Sönmezer C, Worst TS, Schulz M, Dihazi GH, Streit F, Erdmann G, Kling S, Boutros M, Binder C, et al. Neutral sphingomyelinases control extracellular vesicles budding from the plasma membrane. J Extracell Vesicles. 2017;6:1378056.
51. Kosaka N, Iguchi H, Yoshioka Y, Takeshita F, Matsuki Y, Ochiya T. Secretory mechanisms and intercellular transfer of microRNAs in living cells. J Biol Chem. 2010;285:17442–52.
52. Lang JK, Young RF, Ashraf H, Canty JMJ. Inhibiting extracellular vesicle release from human cardiosphere derived cells with lentiviral knockdown of nSMase2 differentially effects proliferation and apoptosis in cardiomyocytes, fibroblasts and endothelial cells in vitro. PLoS One. 2016;11:e0165926.
53. van Niel G, Charrin S, Simoes S, Romao M, Rochin L, Saftig P, Marks MS, Rubinstein E, Raposo G. The tetraspanin CD63 regulates ESCRT-independent and -dependent endosomal sorting during melanogenesis. Dev Cell. 2011;21:708–21.
54. Phuyal S, Hessvik NP, Skotland T, Sandvig K, Llorente A. Regulation of exosome release by glycosphingolipids and flotillins. FEBS J. 2014;281:2214–27.
55. Gallier S, Vocking K, Post JA, Van De Heijning B, Acton D, Van Der Beek EM, Van Baalen T. A novel infant milk formula concept: mimicking the human milk fat globule structure. Colloids Surf B Biointerfaces. 2015;136:329–39.
56. Alsaweed M, Lai CT, Hartmann PE, Geddes DT, Kakulas F. Human milk miRNAs primarily originate from the mammary gland resulting in unique miRNA profiles of fractionated milk. Sci Rep. 2016;6:20680.
57. Smith ZJ, Lee C, Rojalin T, Carney RP, Hazari S, Knudson A, Lam K, Saari H, Ibañez EL, Viitala T, et al. Single exosome study reveals subpopulations distributed among cell lines with variability related to membrane content. J Extracell Vesicles. 2015;4:28533.
58. Sharma P, Ludwig S, Muller L, Hong CS, Kirkwood JM, Ferrone S, Whiteside TL. Immunoaffinity-based isolation of melanoma cell-derived exosomes from plasma of patients with melanoma. J Extracell Vesicles. 2018;7:1435138.
59. Chiang C-Y, Chen C. Toward characterizing extracellular vesicles at a single-particle level. J Biomed Sci. 2019;26:9.
60. Hilton SH, White IM. Advances in the analysis of single extracellular vesicles: a critical review. Sens Actuators Rep. 2021;3:100052.
61. Vaswani KM, Peiris H, Qin Koh Y, Hill RJ, Harb T, Arachchige BJ, Logan J, Reed S, Davies PSW, Mitchell MD. A complete proteomic profile of human and bovine milk exosomes by liquid chromatography mass spectrometry. Expert Rev Proteom. 2021;18:719–35.
62. Sedykh S, Kuleshova A, Nevinsky G. Milk exosomes: perspective agents for anticancer drug delivery. Int J Mol Sci. 2020;21:6646.
63. Zeng F, Morelli AE. Extracellular vesicle-mediated MHC cross-dressing in immune homeostasis, transplantation, infectious diseases, and cancer. Semin Immunopathol. 2018;40:477–90.
64. Arnett HA, Viney JL. Immune modulation by butyrophilins. Nat Rev Immunol. 2014;14:559–69.

Microbiota Composition of Breast Milk

Seyhan Erişir Oygucu and Özlem Bekem

1 Introduction

The community of microorganisms, including bacteria, viruses, fungi, and protozoa residing within the human intestinal tract, which is defined as gut microbiota, plays a significant role in metabolic, neurobehavioral, endocrine, and immune pathways influencing child growth and development [1–3].

Early microbiota colonization, which starts with birth, is affected by maternal obesity and diet, birth mode, antibiotic exposure, and feeding type [4]. Breast milk modifies gut microbial composition by prebiotic properties of human milk oligosaccharides and anti-infective properties of lactoferrin, lysozyme, and immunoglobulins [5]. In addition, breast milk itself is a significant source of microbes for the infant's gut [6–8]. An infant consuming about 800 mL breast milk daily has been reported to ingest about 8×10^4–8×10^6 commensal bacteria by suckling [9]. It provides vertical microbiota transmission from mothers to their infants, which formats infant gut microbiota [10].

Scientists have been interested in microbiological components of human milk since the 1890s, mostly focusing on pathogenic effects on infant's health [11]. Until the 2000s, human milk has been traditionally considered sterile. Based on the studies reporting the presence of lactic acid bacteria in breast milk, it was suggested that human breast milk might be a source of potentially probiotic bacteria and may be

S. Erişir Oygucu (✉)
Department of Pediatrics, Division of Neonatology, Faculty of Medicine,
University of Kyrenia, Kyrenia, Cyprus

Ö. Bekem
Department of Pediatrics, Division of Pediatric Gastroenterology, Hepatology and Nutrition,
Health Sciences University, Dr Behcet Uz Children's Hospital, İzmir, Türkiye

Ö. N. Şahin et al. (eds.), *Breastfeeding and Metabolic Programming*,
https://doi.org/10.1007/978-3-031-33278-4_8

considered a symbiotic food [9, 12]. Today, it is recognized that the dynamics of human milk microbiota in the mammary gland ecosystem are essential for infant and mother health together [13].

2   Origins of Human Milk Microbiota

Although the mechanism of action of human milk microbiota formation is not entirely understood, two main hypotheses are suggested as sources of human milk microbiota: retrograde flow and the entero-mammary pathway [14].

Retrograde flow is the transmission of areolar bacteria and the infant's oral inhabitants back into the mammary ducts during nursing, which has been shown by infrared photography [15]. This could be an explanation for the presence of bacteria derived from maternal areolar microbial flora and infant oral cavity in breast milk [16, 17].

The second hypothesis suggests that the source of breast milk microbiota is the entero-mammary pathway that links the milk-gut bacteria [18]. Dendritic cells that cross the intestinal epithelium of the mother take the bacteria from the intestinal lumen and through lymphoid circulation transfers to mammary glands, including precolostrum and milk anaerobes [19–24]. This theory was also supported by the detection of a single strain of Bifidobacterium breve in the maternal intestine, breast milk, and infant stool in an infant delivered via the caesarian section [17].

3   Human Milk Microbiota Composition

Human milk contains a complex community of microorganisms with bacterial, viral, fungal, and archaeal components [25, 26]. Culture-dependent methods reported the presence of Streptococcus, Enterococcus, and Staphylococcus in addition to lactic acid bacteria such as Lactobacillus, Lactococcus, and Bifidobacterium [9, 12, 27]. The implementation of culture-independent techniques made it possible to determine higher microbial diversity in breast milk [26, 28, 29]. Methods including polymerase chain reaction (PCR) [30–34], PCR-denaturing gradient gel electrophoresis (DGGE) [35], 16S rRNA gene sequencing [36–40], matrix-assisted laser desorption ionization-time of flight mass spectrometry (MALDI-TOF-MS) [24, 41, 42],and metagenomic shotgun sequencing [41, 43, 44] were used for identification of microbiota composition. Diversity of microbiota in human milk was reported to be higher than in maternal or infant feces [20, 45–47].

3.1 Bacterial Component

In a recent review, 820 species of bacteria have been identified in human milk, mainly composed of Gram-negative Proteobacteria and Gram-positive Firmicutes [48]. Proteobacteria phyla include Escherichia, Pseudomonas, Serratia, Enterobacter, Ralstonia, Sphingomonas, and Bradyrhizobium whereas Firmicutes phyla include Streptococcus, Staphylococcus, Lactobacillus, Bifidobacterium, Enterococcus, Veilonella, Gemella, and Clostridium. Human milk also contains Propionibacterium, Actinomyces, Corynebacterium from Actinobacteria and Prevotella from Bacteroidetes phyla [49]. The "core" bacterium representing about half of the milk microbial content in human milk consists of nine genera: Streptococcus, Staphylococcus, Pseudomonas, Serratia, Sphingomonas, Ralstonia, Bradyrhizobium, Propionibacterium, and Corynebacterium [50]. Results of the studies varying in geographic locations, collection and storage of samples, and analytic methods showed that the predominant species are Staphylococcus and Streptococcus followed by Bifidobacterium, Lactobacillus, Propionibacterium, and Enterococcus [51].

3.2 Viral Component and Phages

Recent studies have demonstrated that human milk also contains eukaryotic viruses (Herpesviridae, Poxviridae, Mimiviridae, and Iridoviridae) and bacterium-infecting viruses named bacteriophages (Myoviridae, Siphoviridae, and Podoviridae) [52]. The majority of the human milk virome is consisted of bacteriophages and they are transmitted to the infant from the mother by breastfeeding, to colonize and shape the infant's gut microbiome [53, 54].

3.3 Fungal and Other Microbial Components

Fungal component of the human milk microbiome, also named as "mycobiome," is suggested to have a potential beneficial role in infant's gut mycobiome development. The first study investigating the presence of fungi in human milk detected DNA of fungi in 85% of the milk samples, which were belonging to two phyla (Ascomycota and Basidiomycota) and ten species (Malassezia globosa, Calocera cornea, Guepiniopsis buccina, Podospora anserine, Sordaria macrospora, Candida dubliniensis, Malassezia restricta, Talaromyces stipitatus, and Yarrowia lipolytica) [41]. The fungal load of human milk has been estimated as 3.5×10^5 cells/mL with a composition dominated by Malassezia, Candida, and Saccharomyces [7]. Although a core mycobiome was formed by Malassezia, Davidiella, Penicillium, and Sistotrema, changes in mycobiome composition were detected, associated with geographic location and delivery mode [55].

Other than bacteria, viruses, and fungi, archaea and eukaryotes also contribute to the breast milk microbiota. Researchers have been focusing on human archaeome, with recognition of the importance of human-archaeal-bacterial mutualism for human health and metabolism through methanogenesis. Methanobrevibacter smithii, which is the main human methanogenic archaea, has been shown to improve energy harvest by consuming end products of microbial fermentation [56, 57]. The correlation between decreased frequency of Methanobrevibacter smithii in human feces and obesity supports the critical commensal role of archaea on weight regulation [58, 59]. The study investigating the presence of archaea in human milk has detected Methanobrevibacter smithii and Methanobrevibacter oralis in human colostrum and milk by using culture and real-time PCR. Interestingly, compared with lean mothers, Methanobrevibacter smithii count was higher in milk samples of overweight mothers. Additionally, differences in the distribution of maternal body mass index (BMI) correlated with the presence of Methanobrevibacter smithii supported the association of this neglected element of breast milk microbiota with maternal metabolic phenotype [60]. Furthermore, in the study comparing milk samples of mothers with or without mastitis, the metagenomic analysis demonstrated the presence of archaeal DNA in 80% of milk samples only collected from healthy mothers, thus proposing a protective effect for maternal health [41].

4 Factors That Influence the Composition of Human Milk Microbiota

Breast milk harbors a unique, complex, and dynamic ecosystem that plays a critical role in seeding the infant gut microbiota [12, 13, 24, 38, 42, 47, 61, 62]. Multiple factors influence the composition, including mode of delivery, lactation stage, gestational age, antibiotic usage, genetics, mode of breastfeeding, method of milk expression, parity, ethnicity, maternal BMI, and infant gender [29, 38, 63].

4.1 Mode of Delivery

The effect of mode of delivery on breast milk microbiota composition is still a topic of interest among scientists since studies report contradictory and debatable findings. Three studies reported no difference in microbial profiles based on the mode of delivery [64–66], while others demonstrated that colostrum and milk following vaginal delivery have been shown to display higher microbial diversity and abundance of Bifidobacterium and Lactobacillus spp. compared to cesarean delivery [30, 67–70]. A recent study reported a remarkable difference in the microbial composition of breast milk between cesarean section and vaginal deliveries [16]. Compared with vaginal delivery, mothers who gave birth by elective cesarean section showed a different microbial composition with low amounts of Leuconostocaceae and high amounts of Carnobacteriaceae. Interestingly microbiota composition of mothers who gave birth by nonelective cesarean section was more similar to mothers who gave vaginal delivery than the elective cesarean group. This result was interpreted as the results of changes in the microbial transmission process affected by physiological stress and hormonal signals [16]. In a similar study, colostrum obtained from mothers who underwent vaginal delivery had higher biodiversity with a higher abundance of Haemophilus and Streptococcus genera and a lower abundance of Finegoldia, Halomonas, Prevotella, Pseudomonas, and Staphylococcus genera compared to cesarean delivery group [71]. Colostrum bacterial networks were also identified by using Auto contractive maps in both groups and bacteria having three or more connections with others were accepted as main bacterial hubs. Haemophilus genera, which was more abundant in the colostrum of the vaginal delivery group, acted as a main bacterial hub only in the cesarean colostrum group, which had interactions with Peptostreptococcus, Achromobacter, and Kluyvera spp. This result was interpreted as a supportive finding for the idea that the pathogenicity of a microorganism does not only depend on its abundance but also on other factors, including the relationship with other microorganisms [71]. In addition, a study investigating the impact of perinatal factors on bifidobacteria and lactobacilli species in human milk of healthy mothers demonstrated that isolation of Lactobacillus fermentum and Lactobacillus salivarius were higher in the breast milk of women who gave birth by vaginal delivery compared to cesarean section. A similar effect was seen in women who received anesthesia during delivery as the same species were more frequent in the breast milk samples of women who did not receive anesthesia [68].

Differences in virome and mycobiota compositions of human milk have also been documented in relation to the delivery mode. In the study comparing the virome compositions of transient and mature human milk, the bacteriophage counts of both groups were found to be higher in the spontaneous vaginal delivery group than in cesarean section deliveries [72]. Mycobiota compositions of breast milk samples of mothers from different geographic origins who delivered vaginally showed statistically significant higher counts of Cryptococcus than breast milk samples of mothers who gave birth by cesarean delivery [55]. In another study, Malassezia globosa was reported as the most abundant species in the normal spontaneous vaginally delivery group, whereas Saccharomyces cerevisiae and Penicillium Rubens were the most abundant species in transient and mature milk samples of mothers who underwent cesarean delivery, respectively [73].

4.2 Gestational Age

Differences in microbial composition are reported between breast milk of mothers of preterm and term babies. The quantity of Enterococcus spp. was significantly lower in colostrum, while the quantity of Bifidobacterium spp. was significantly higher at all lactation stages of mothers of term babies. Furthermore, a direct correlation was present between Bifidobacterium content and gestational age in all stages, while there was no correlation with Staphylococcus, Streptococcus, and Lactobacillus counts [30]. Breast milk samples collected from mothers of very preterm babies (27.6 ± 2.6 weeks gestation) showed individualized microbial profiles, which changed over time with an increase in abundance of Stenotrophomonas, Acinetobacter, and Lactobacillus and a decrease in Staphylococcus and Corynebacterium. Additionally, changes in microbial composition were found to be related to maternal BMI, antibiotic usage, and mode of delivery [74].

4.3 Lactation Stage

Breast milk is classified into three stages according to the time of production: colostrum (first 5 days postpartum), transitional (5 days to 2 weeks postpartum), and mature milk (2 weeks and onwards) [75]. Colostrum is produced in low quantities with relatively low lactose concentrations but rich in proteins, triacylglycerol, immune active substances, and growth factors [76–78]. Levels of macronutrient, micronutrient, immunological, and bioactive components change throughout the lactation period accompanied by changes in microbial composition [30, 77, 79–82]. Colostrum, containing Weisella, Leuconoctoc, Streptococcus, Staphylococcus, and Lactococcus as the most common genera, has been reported to have higher bacterial diversity than transition and mature milk. Typical oral cavity inhabitants like Leptotrichia, Veillonella, and Prevotella have been shown to progressively increase in addition to lactic acid bacteria genera at later stages of lactation [16]. In addition, total bacteria count, Bifidobacterium and Enterococcus spp. were shown to be significantly lower in colostrum than in transitional and mature milk [30]. In one study, mature milk was shown to contain a greater quantity of anaerobic bacteria compared with colostrum [83]. Conversely, other researchers reported consistent composition in some breast milk samples over time and significant variation in others [84]. Results of other studies showed relatively constant milk microbiome composition with minor changes in less abundant genera like Veillonella, Propionibacterium, Granulicatella, and Prevotella [65] or no effect of the stage of lactation at all [85]. The subsequent studies supported the findings of previous ones showing the effect of the lactation stage on human milk microbiota. A recent longitudinal study reported the highest microbial diversity in colostrum, which decreased gradually over lactation. Staphylococcus, Streptococcus, Acinetobacter, Pseudomonas, and Lactobacillus were predominant in colostrum samples. The abundance of

Proteobacteria was shown to increase while Firmicutes decreased across lactation [86]. Additionally, the study observing the lactation period from birth to postnatal 24 weeks reported a significant decrease in the diversity of human milk microbiota throughout lactation. Nine predominating genera including Streptococcus, Staphylococcus, Acinetobacter, Pseudomonas, Bifidobacterium, Brevundimonas, Mesorhizobium, Rhodococcus, and Flavobacterium showed apparent changes over time. Streptococcus was shown to predominate at weeks 1 and 24, whereas Pseudomonas had the highest mean relative abundance at weeks 4 and 8. Bifidobacterium and Lactobacillus predominated in week 4 [66].

In the study investigating the virome composition of transient and mature milk, it was reported that bacteriophages were predominant in both groups (79.5%), mainly composed of Siphoviridae, Podoviridae, and Myoviridae families and eukaryotic viruses accounted for 20.5% of the total count with Herpesviridae as the most abundant order. When the two groups were compared, bacteriophages were found to be predominant at 87.6% in transient human milk and decreased to 67% in mature milk. While Podoviridae and Myoviridae were predominant in transient human milk, a decrease in the abundance of Podoviridae and an increase in the abundance of Siphoviridae family were observed in mature human milk [72].

Regarding fungal composition, Saccharomyces cerevisiae (33.3%) and Aspergillus glaucus (27.4%) were reported to be the most abundant species in transient human milk whereas Penicillium Rubens (35.5%), followed by Aspergillus glaucus (33.7%) were predominant in mature human milk [73].

5 Maternal Health Status

Maternal pathologies including obesity, hypertension, perinatal antibiotherapy, celiac disease, and human immunodeficiency virus (HIV) status, also have been linked to differences in microbial diversity and composition of human milk [16, 34, 87, 88]. Deviations in gut microbiota, which is a transmissible trait, are linked to obesity by the abundance of specific microbes with increased capacity to harvest energy [89]. Prepregnancy weight and BMI of women were shown to be correlated with the abundance of Bacteroides, Clostridium, Staphylococcus, and excessive weight gain over pregnancy was associated with high Bacteroides concentrations in gut microbiota [90]. Maternal BMI has been shown to influence milk microbiota composition as well. Studies investigating the impact of obesity on the composition of human milk microbiota report different compositions. Breast milk microbiota from obese mothers showed less diversity compared with normal-weight mothers. Higher maternal BMI was correlated with a higher proportion of Lactobacillus in colostrum and a higher proportion of Staphylococcus accompanied with lower numbers of Bifidobacterium in mature milk. Immoderate weight gain during pregnancy was also found to be related with higher counts of Staphylococcus in breast milk samples obtained at postnatal 1 month with higher Lactobacillus and lower Bifidobacterium counts in breast milk samples obtained at 6 months [16]. In another study, postpartum BMI had a negative correlation with Lactobacillus and a positive correlation with Staphylococcus counts [37].

No association was found between pre-pregnancy BMI with the most prevalent bacterial taxa, but breast milk of obese and overweight mothers had higher relative counts of Granulicatella than milk produced by normal-weight mothers. In addition, relative abundance of some bacteria was found to be associated with the maternal diet. Relative abundance of Gemella was positively correlated with protein intake whereas relative abundance of Corynebacterium was negatively associated with saturated fatty acid and monounsaturated fatty acid intakes. Total disaccharides, carbohydrates, and lactose consumption were inversely associated with Firmicutes. Consumption of diet with highly insoluble fiber had a positive effect on the abundance of Rothia [65]. Breastfeeding habits have been shown to have an additional effect on milk microbiota profile modulated with mother BMI, as a higher abundance of Bifidobacterium genus and significantly higher richness and diversity were observed in milk samples obtained from exclusively breastfeeding mothers with pre-gestational normal weight compared to overweight mothers [91].

Breast milk samples from mothers with celiac disease under a gluten-free diet have been reported to contain significantly lower levels of interleukin-12, transforming growth factor-β1, secretory immunoglobulin A with a significant reduction in Bifidobacterium spp. and Bacteroides spp. in comparison with healthy mothers' milk [88]. Acinetobacter ursingii, Rothia mucilaginosa, and Bacillus cereus were found in increased abundance in transient milk samples from mothers with celiac disease. At the same time, Bacteroides, Faecalibacterium prausnitzii, Clostridiales, and Gemella were abundant in milk samples from healthy mothers [92]. Interestingly increased abundance of Rothia mucilaginosa and decreased abundance of Faecalibacterium prausnitzii have been previously linked to autoimmune inflammatory conditions [93, 94]. Regarding viral composition, Dill cryptic virus 2, and Rosellinia necatrix partitivirus 2 were found in increased abundance in the breast milk of healthy women compared with milk samples from mothers with celiac disease [92].

A recent study compared the microbiota profiles of mature milk samples from mothers with celiac disease to investigate the role of breast milk microbiota profiles in the development of the disease in the offspring. Milk of mothers whose children also developed celiac disease later on contained a high proportion of Verrucomicrobia and Beijerinckiaceae species in addition to increased abundance of operational taxonomic units of Methylobacterium komagatae, Methylocapsa palsarum, Parabacteroides distasonis, and Bacteroides vulgatus [95].

Gestational hypertensive status is another maternal factor that affects human milk bacterial composition. Reduction of microbial diversity and richness were observed in colostrum, transition milk, and mature milk of mothers with gestational prehypertension compared with those from normotensive mothers [86].

The presence of HIV infection also has an impact on the microbiological composition of human milk. Although total bacterial counts showed no difference between HIV RNA positive and negative milk samples, the frequency of Lactobacillus is reported to be higher while the frequencies of Staphylococcus hominis and Staphylococcus aureus were statistically significantly lower in samples with HIV RNA positive samples [34].

Perinatal antibiotic consumption may alter breast milk microbiota by decreasing Lactobacillus and Bifidobacterium counts [68]. In the study analyzing the effect of delivery mode and intrapartum antibiotic administration on human milk microbiota one month after delivery, although no statistically significant differences were detected in the most abundant families which were Streptococcaceae and Staphylococcaceae, Bifidobacterium spp. was only detected in milk samples of mothers who did not use antibiotics [70].

High maternal psychosocial distress has been shown to decrease the bacterial diversity of breast milk. Increased human milk bacterial diversity among women with low maternal psychosocial distress has been related to a decrease in the relative abundance of Staphylococcus as the leading bacterial genera, accompanied with increased abundance of Lactobacillus, Acinetobacter, and Flavobacterium [96].

6 Geographic Location

The geographic location and lifestyle factors are known to affect milk microbiota diversity and taxonomic composition [97]. Breast milk samples originating from developing countries or rural sites have been reported to have a higher diversity of bacteria compared to samples from developed or urban sites [98]. It has been reported that the microbiota profile of Spanish and South African milk samples were more diverse than Finnish and Chinese milk samples. Breast milk of Spanish women had the highest levels of Bacteroidetes, while South African women's milk samples had a high abundance of Proteobacteria. Conversely, milk samples from Finland contained lower levels of Proteobacteria and higher levels of Firmicutes. As well Chinese women had the highest level of Actinobacteria in their milk samples [97]. The study, which explored the microbiota network of mature milk and colostrum samples from Burundian and Italian mothers using an auto-contractive map, documented different bacterial hubs and central nodes in two groups, which were attributed to different lifestyles and dietary habits [83]. The systematic review of human milk microbiota, including 12 studies from Finland, Spain, Türkiye, Switzerland, Canada, and the United States, demonstrated the predominance of Staphylococcus and Streptococcus in human milk microbiota [51]. In addition, even though every sample revealed a unique microbial profile, Staphylococcus and Streptococcus have been reported as the most prevalent genera, while Lactobacillus and Bifidobacterium were detected in very small counts in milk samples from Taiwan [99]. The suggestion of universal predominance of these two genera [51] was supported by the study analyzing milk samples of 11 populations from Africa, Europe, North and South America by demonstration of Staphylococcus and Streptococcus as the core microbiota in all human milk samples [98].

7 Mode of Breastfeeding, Method of Milk Expression

Variations in feeding methods have been reported to alter the composition of human milk microbiota. Exclusively breastfeeding mothers contained a higher proportion of Staphylococcus parasanguinis in their milk samples compared to women who reported mixed infant feeding [34]. Breast milk obtained by pump versus manual expression was associated with lower bacterial richness. In addition, Nocardioides, Gemellaceae, and Vogesella showed higher relative abundances with direct breastfeeding, whereas Pseudomonas and Enterobacteriaceae were relatively more abundant with indirect breastfeeding [38].

8 Infant Gender

The biological sex of the infant is described as a factor influencing the composition of human milk microbiota. Several studies have reported lower diversity and richness in addition to higher counts of Streptococcus and lower counts of Staphylococcus in milk samples of mothers of male infants compared to mothers of female infants [38, 65], while others showed no statistically significant association [6, 64, 66].

9 Future Perspectives

Metabolic programming, which starts at the prenatal period and continues throughout infancy with nutrition, may result with increased risk for cardiovascular diseases, type 2 diabetes, and obesity [100, 101]. In addition to dietary factors, intestinal microbiome composition also has an impact on metabolic programming. Even though gut microbiota profile has been shown to be related to childhood obesity [102, 103], studies report discordant results. While the relative abundance ratio of Firmicutes and Bacteroidetes has been reported to be significantly higher in the gut microbiota of obese children [104], another study has reported the opposite, with decreased counts of Lactobacillus and Bifidobacterium [105]. In addition to modulating the effects of breastfeeding on gut microbial colonization, interventions to use breast milk as a source of microbes remains to be determined. Even though maternal oral Lactobacillus reuteri supplementation for the last 4 weeks of pregnancy was associated with a higher abundance of the organism in colostrum [106], maternal probiotic supplementation with Lactobacillus rhamnosus GG, Lactobacillus acidophilus La-5, and Bifidobacterium animalis ssp. lactis Bb-12 during 1 month prenatal and 3 months postnatal periods, has been shown not to have a significant effect on the composition of breast milk [39]. Further studies are needed, including mothers from different geographic locations with varying health status, and nutritional and environmental conditions, to increase our knowledge about breast milk microbiota and modulation of its composition, in order to reduce the risk of diseases related to imbalanced microbiota profiles.

References

1. Bull MJ, Plummer NT. Part 1: the human gut microbiome in health and disease. Integr Med (Encinitas). 2014;13:17–22.
2. Robertson RC, Manges AR, Finlay BB, Prendergast AJ. The human microbiome and child growth – first 1000 days and beyond. Trends Microbiol. 2019;27:131–47. https://doi.org/10.1016/j.tim.2018.09.008.
3. Valdes AM, Walter J, Segal E, Spector TD. Role of the gut microbiota in nutrition and health. BMJ (Online). 2018;361:36–44. https://doi.org/10.1136/bmj.k2179.
4. Jian C, Carpén N, Helve O, et al. Early-life gut microbiota and its connection to metabolic health in children: perspective on ecological drivers and need for quantitative approach. EBioMedicine. 2021;69:103475.
5. O'Sullivan A, Farver M, Smilowitz JT. The influence of early infant-feeding practices on the intestinal microbiome and body composition in infants. Nutr Metab Insights. 2015;8:1–9. https://doi.org/10.4137/NMI.S29530.
6. Pannaraj PS, Li F, Cerini C, et al. Association between breast Milk bacterial communities and establishment and development of the infant gut microbiome. JAMA Pediatr. 2017;171:647–54. https://doi.org/10.1001/jamapediatrics.2017.0378.
7. Boix-Amorós A, Martinez-Costa C, Querol A, et al. Multiple approaches detect the presence of fungi in human breastmilk samples from healthy mothers. Sci Rep. 2017;7:13016. https://doi.org/10.1038/s41598-017-13270-x.
8. Duranti S, Lugli GA, Mancabelli L, et al. Maternal inheritance of bifidobacterial communities and bifidophages in infants through vertical transmission. Microbiome. 2017;5:66. https://doi.org/10.1186/s40168-017-0282-6.
9. Heikkilä MP, Saris PEJ. Inhibition of Staphylococcus aureus by the commensal bacteria of human milk. J Appl Microbiol. 2003;95:471–8. https://doi.org/10.1046/j.1365-2672.2003.02002.x.
10. Asnicar F, Manara S, Zolfo M, et al. Studying vertical microbiome transmission from mothers to infants by strain-level metagenomic profiling. mSystems. 2017:2. https://doi.org/10.1128/msystems.00164-16.
11. Dudgeon LS, Jewesbury RC. The bacteriology of human milk. J Hyg (Lond). 1924;23:54–76.
12. Martín R, Langa S, Reviriego C, et al. Human milk is a source of lactic acid bacteria for the infant gut. J Pediatr. 2003;143:754–8. https://doi.org/10.1016/j.jpeds.2003.09.028.
13. Fernández L, Pannaraj PS, Rautava S, Rodríguez JM. The microbiota of the human mammary ecosystem. Front cell Infect Microbiol. 2020;10:10.
14. McGuire MK, McGuire MA. Got bacteria? The astounding, yet not-so-surprising, microbiome of human milk. Curr Opin Biotechnol. 2017;44:63–8.
15. Ramsay DT, Kent JC, Owens RA, Hartmann PE. Ultrasound imaging of milk ejection in the breast of lactating women. Pediatrics. 2004;113:361–7. https://doi.org/10.1542/peds.113.2.361.
16. Cabrera-Rubio R, Collado MC, Laitinen K, et al. The human milk microbiome changes over lactation and is shaped by maternal weight and mode of delivery. Am J Clin Nutr. 2012;96:544–51. https://doi.org/10.3945/ajcn.112.037382.
17. Kordy K, Gaufin T, Mwangi M, et al. Contributions to human breast milk microbiome and enteromammary transfer of Bifidobacterium breve. PLoS One. 2020;15:e0219633. https://doi.org/10.1371/journal.pone.0219633.
18. Civardi E, Garofoli F, Tzialla C, et al. Microorganisms in human milk: lights and shadows. J Matern Fetal Neonatal Med. 2013;26:30–4.
19. Martín R, Langa S, Reviriego C, et al. The commensal microflora of human milk: new perspectives for food bacteriotherapy and probiotics. Trends Food Sci Technol. 2004;15:121–7.
20. Perez PF, Doré J, Leclerc M, et al. Bacterial imprinting of the neonatal immune system: lessons from maternal cells? Pediatrics. 2007;119:e724–32. https://doi.org/10.1542/peds.2006-1649.
21. Rescigno M, Urbano M, Valzasina B, et al. Dendritic cells express tight junction proteins and penetrate gut epithelial monolayers to sample bacteria. Nat Immunol. 2001;2:361–7. https://doi.org/10.1038/86373.

22. Thum C, Cookson AL, Otter DE, et al. Can nutritional modulation of maternal intestinal microbiota influence the development of the infant gastrointestinal tract? J Nutr. 2012;142:1921–8. https://doi.org/10.3945/jn.112.166231.

23. Rodríguez JM. The origin of human milk bacteria: is there a bacterial entero-mammary pathway during late pregnancy and lactation? Adv Nutr. 2014;5:779–84. https://doi.org/10.3945/an.114.007229.

24. Damaceno QS, Souza JP, Nicoli JR, et al. Evaluation of potential probiotics isolated from human milk and colostrum. Probiotics Antimicrob Proteins. 2017;9:371–9. https://doi.org/10.1007/s12602-017-9270-1.

25. Consales A, Cerasani J, Sorrentino G, et al. The hidden universe of human milk microbiome: origin, composition, determinants, role, and future perspectives. Eur J Pediatr. 2022;181:1811–20.

26. Notarbartolo V, Giuffre M, Montante C, et al. Composition of human breast Milk microbiota and its role in children's health. Pediatr Gastroenterol Hepatol Nutr. 2022;25:194–210. https://doi.org/10.5223/pghn.2022.25.3.194.

27. Martín R, Jiménez E, Heilig H, et al. Isolation of bifidobacteria from breast milk and assessment of the bifidobacterial population by PCR-denaturing gradient gel electrophoresis and quantitative real-time PCR. Appl Environ Microbiol. 2009;75:965–9. https://doi.org/10.1128/AEM.02063-08.

28. Selma-Royo M, Calvo Lerma J, Cortés-Macías E, Collado MC. Human milk microbiome: from actual knowledge to future perspective. Semin Perinatol. 2021;45:151450. https://doi.org/10.1016/j.semperi.2021.151450.

29. Zimmermann P, Curtis N. Breast milk microbiota: a review of the factors that influence composition. J Infect. 2020;81:17–47.

30. Khodayar-Pardo P, Mira-Pascual L, Collado MC, Martínez-Costa C. Impact of lactation stage, gestational age and mode of delivery on breast milk microbiota. J Perinatol. 2014;34:599–605. https://doi.org/10.1038/jp.2014.47.

31. Huang MS, Cheng CC, Tseng SY, et al. Most commensally bacterial strains in human milk of healthy mothers display multiple antibiotic resistance. Microbiology. 2019;8:e00618. https://doi.org/10.1002/mbo3.618.

32. Aakko J, Kumar H, Rautava S, et al. Human milk oligosaccharide categories define the microbiota composition in human colostrum. Benef Microbes. 2017;8:563–7. https://doi.org/10.3920/BM2016.0185.

33. Collado MC, Delgado S, Maldonado A, Rodríguez JM. Assessment of the bacterial diversity of breast milk of healthy women by quantitative real-time PCR. Lett Appl Microbiol. 2009;48:523–8. https://doi.org/10.1111/j.1472-765X.2009.02567.x.

34. González R, Mandomando I, Fumadó V, et al. Breast milk and gut microbiota in African mothers and infants from an area of high HIV prevalence. PLoS One. 2013;8:e80299. https://doi.org/10.1371/journal.pone.0080299.

35. Obermajer T, Lipoglavšek L, Tompa G, et al. Colostrum of healthy Slovenian mothers: microbiota composition and bacteriocin gene prevalence. PLoS One. 2015;10 https://doi.org/10.1371/journal.pone.0123324.

36. Ojo-Okunola A, Nicol M, du Toit E. Human breast milk bacteriome in health and disease. Nutrients. 2018;10

37. Ding M, Qi C, Yang Z, et al. Geographical location specific composition of cultured microbiota and: lactobacillus occurrence in human breast milk in China. Food Funct. 2019;10:554–64. https://doi.org/10.1039/c8fo02182a.

38. Moossavi S, Sepehri S, Robertson B, et al. Composition and variation of the human milk microbiota are influenced by maternal and early-life factors. Cell Host Microbe. 2019;25:324–335.e4. https://doi.org/10.1016/j.chom.2019.01.011.

39. Simpson MR, Avershina E, Storrø O, et al. Breastfeeding-associated microbiota in human milk following supplementation with lactobacillus rhamnosus GG, lactobacillus acidophilus La-5, and Bifidobacterium animalis ssp. lactis bb-12. J Dairy Sci. 2018;101:889–99. https://doi.org/10.3168/jds.2017-13411.

40. Li SW, Watanabe K, Hsu CC, et al. Bacterial composition and diversity in breast milk samples from mothers living in Taiwan and mainland China. Front Microbiol. 2017;8 https://doi.org/10.3389/fmicb.2017.00965.
41. Jiménez E, de Andrés J, Manrique M, et al. Metagenomic analysis of milk of healthy and mastitis-suffering women. J Hum Lact. 2015;31:406–15. https://doi.org/10.1177/0890334415585078.
42. Albesharat R, Ehrmann MA, Korakli M, et al. Phenotypic and genotypic analyses of lactic acid bacteria in local fermented food, breast milk and faeces of mothers and their babies. Syst Appl Microbiol. 2011;34:148–55. https://doi.org/10.1016/j.syapm.2010.12.001.
43. Pärnänen K, Karkman A, Hultman J, et al. Maternal gut and breast milk microbiota affect infant gut antibiotic resistome and mobile genetic elements. Nat Commun. 2018;9:3891. https://doi.org/10.1038/s41467-018-06393-w.
44. Ward TL, Hosid S, Ioshikhes I, Altosaar I. Human milk metagenome: a functional capacity analysis. BMC Microbiol. 2013;13
45. Murphy K, Curley D, O'callaghan TF, et al. The composition of human milk and infant faecal microbiota over the first three months of life: a pilot study. Sci Rep. 2017;7 https://doi.org/10.1038/srep40597.
46. Biagi E, Quercia S, Aceti A, et al. The bacterial ecosystem of mother's milk and infant's mouth and gut. Front Microbiol. 2017;8 https://doi.org/10.3389/fmicb.2017.01214.
47. Jost T, Lacroix C, Braegger CP, et al. Vertical mother-neonate transfer of maternal gut bacteria via breastfeeding. Environ Microbiol. 2014;16:2891–904. https://doi.org/10.1111/1462-2920.12238.
48. Togo A, Dufour J-C, Lagier J-C, et al. Repertoire of human breast and milk microbiota: a systematic review. Future Microbiol. 2019;14:623–41. https://doi.org/10.2217/fmb-2018-0317.
49. LaTuga MS, Stuebe A, Seed PC. A review of the source and function of microbiota in breast milk. Semin Reprod Med. 2014;32:68–73.
50. Moubareck CA. Human milk microbiota and oligosaccharides: a glimpse into benefits, diversity and correlations. Nutrients. 2021;13 https://doi.org/10.3390/nu13041123.
51. Fitzstevens JL, Smith KC, Hagadorn JI, et al. Systematic review of the human milk microbiota. Nutr Clin Pract. 2017;32:354–64.
52. Mohandas S, Pannaraj PS (2020) Beyond the bacterial microbiome: virome of human milk and effects on the developing infant, pp. 86–93.
53. Pannaraj PS, Ly M, Cerini C, et al. Shared and distinct features of human milk and infant stool viromes. Front Microbiol. 2018;9 https://doi.org/10.3389/fmicb.2018.01162.
54. Stinson LF, Sindi ASM, Cheema AS, et al. The human milk microbiome: who, what, when, where, why, and how? Nutr Rev. 2021;79:529–43. https://doi.org/10.1093/nutrit/nuaa029.
55. Boix-Amorós A, Puente-Sánchez F, du Toit E, et al. Mycobiome profiles in breast Milk from healthy women depend on mode of delivery, geographic location, and interaction with bacteria. Appl Environ Microbiol. 2019;85:e02994.
56. Thauer RK, Kaster AK, Seedorf H, et al. Methanogenic archaea: ecologically relevant differences in energy conservation. Nat Rev Microbiol. 2008;6:579–91.
57. Samuel BS, Gordon JI. A humanized gnotobiotic mouse model of host-archaeal-bacterial mutualism. Proc Natl Acad Sci USA. 2006;103:10,011–6.
58. Million M, Angelakis E, Maraninchi M, et al. Correlation between body mass index and gut concentrations of lactobacillus reuteri, Bifidobacterium animalis, Methanobrevibacter smithii and Escherichia coli. Int J Obes. 2013;37:1460–6. https://doi.org/10.1038/ijo.2013.20.
59. Ignacio A, Fernandes MR, Rodrigues VAA, et al. Correlation between body mass index and faecal microbiota from children. Clin Microbiol Infect. 2016;22:258.e1–8. https://doi.org/10.1016/j.cmi.2015.10.031.
60. Togo AH, Grine G, Khelaifia S, et al. Culture of methanogenic archaea from human colostrum and Milk. Sci Rep. 2019;9:18653. https://doi.org/10.1038/s41598-019-54759-x.
61. Fernández L, Langa S, Martín V, et al. The human milk microbiota: origin and potential roles in health and disease. Pharmacol Res. 2013;69:1–10.

62. Jeurink P, van Bergenhenegouwen J, Jiménez E, et al. Human milk: a source of more life than we imagine. Benef Microbes. 2013;4:17–30. https://doi.org/10.3920/BM2012.0040.
63. Gomez-Gallego C, Garcia-Mantrana I, Salminen S, Collado MC. The human milk microbiome and factors influencing its composition and activity. Semin Fetal Neonatal Med. 2016;21:400–5.
64. Urbaniak C, Angelini M, Gloor GB, Reid G. Human milk microbiota profiles in relation to birthing method, gestation and infant gender. Microbiome. 2016;4:1. https://doi.org/10.1186/s40168-015-0145-y.
65. Williams JE, Carrothers JM, Lackey KA, et al. Human Milk microbial community structure is relatively stable and related to variations in macronutrient and micronutrient intakes in healthy lactating women. J Nutr. 2017;147:1739–48. https://doi.org/10.3945/jn.117.248864.
66. Lyons KE, O'Shea C-A, Grimaud G, et al. The human milk microbiome aligns with lactation stage and not birth mode. Sci Rep. 2022;12:5598. https://doi.org/10.1038/s41598-022-09009-y.
67. Cabrera-Rubio R, Mira-Pascual L, Mira A, Collado MC. Impact of mode of delivery on the milk microbiota composition of healthy women. J Dev Orig Health Dis. 2016;7:54–60. https://doi.org/10.1017/S2040174415001397.
68. Soto A, Martín V, Jiménez E, et al. Lactobacilli and bifidobacteria in human breast milk: influence of antibiotherapy and other host and clinical factors. J Pediatr Gastroenterol Nutr. 2014;59:78–88. https://doi.org/10.1097/MPG.0000000000000347.
69. Hoashi M, Meche L, Mahal LK, et al. Human milk bacterial and glycosylation patterns differ by delivery mode. Reprod Sci. 2016;23:902–7. https://doi.org/10.1177/1933719115623645.
70. Hermansson H, Kumar H, Collado MC, et al. Breast milk microbiota is shaped by mode of delivery and intrapartum antibiotic exposure. Front Nutr. 2019;6 https://doi.org/10.3389/fnut.2019.00004.
71. Toscano M, de Grandi R, Peroni DG, et al. Impact of delivery mode on the colostrum microbiota composition. BMC Microbiol. 2017;17:205. https://doi.org/10.1186/s12866-017-1109-0.
72. Dinleyici M, Pérez-Brocal V, Arslanoglu S, et al. Article human milk virome analysis: changing pattern regarding mode of delivery, birth weight, and lactational stage. Nutrients. 2021;13 https://doi.org/10.3390/nu13061779.
73. Dinleyici M, Pérez-Brocal V, Arslanoglu S, et al. Human milk mycobiota composition: relationship with gestational age, delivery mode, and birth weight. Benef Microbes. 2020;11:151–62. https://doi.org/10.3920/BM2019.0158.
74. Asbury MR, Butcher J, Copeland JK, et al. Mothers of preterm infants have individualized breast Milk microbiota that changes temporally based on maternal characteristics. Cell Host Microbe. 2020;28:669–682.e4. https://doi.org/10.1016/j.chom.2020.08.001.
75. Ballard O, Morrow AL. Human milk composition. Nutrients and bioactive factors. Pediatr Clin N Am. 2013;60:49–74.
76. Munblit D, Treneva M, Peroni DG, et al. Colostrum and mature human milk of women from London, Moscow, and Verona: determinants of immune composition. Nutrients. 2016;8 https://doi.org/10.3390/nu8110695.
77. Akhter H, Aziz F, Ullah FR, et al. Immunoglobulins content in colostrum, transitional and mature milk of Bangladeshi mothers: influence of parity and sociodemographic characteristics. J Mother Child. 2021;24:8–15. https://doi.org/10.34763/jmotherandchild.20202403.2032.d-20-00001.
78. Morera Pons S, Castellote Bargalló A, Campoy Folgoso C, López Sabater M. Triacylglycerol composition in colostrum, transitional and mature human milk. Eur J Clin Nutr. 2000;54:878–82. https://doi.org/10.1038/sj.ejcn.1601096.
79. Samuel TM, Zhou Q, Giuffrida F, et al. Nutritional and non-nutritional composition of human milk is modulated by maternal, infant, and methodological factors. Front Nutr. 2020;7 https://doi.org/10.3389/fnut.2020.576133.
80. Gila-Diaz A, Arribas SM, Algara A, et al. A review of bioactive factors in human breastmilk: a focus on prematurity. Nutrients. 2019;11:1307. https://doi.org/10.3390/nu11061307.

81. Vass RA, Kemeny A, Dergez T, et al. Distribution of bioactive factors in human milk samples. Int Breastfeed J. 2019;14:9. https://doi.org/10.1186/s13006-019-0203-3.

82. Sinkiewicz-Darol E, Martysiak-Żurowska D, Puta M, et al. Nutrients and bioactive components of human milk after one year of lactation: implication for human milk banks. J Pediatr Gastroenterol Nutr. 2022;74:284–91. https://doi.org/10.1097/MPG.0000000000003298.

83. Drago L, Toscano M, de Grandi R, et al. Microbiota network and mathematic microbe mutualism in colostrum and mature milk collected in two different geographic areas: Italy versus Burundi. ISME J. 2017;11:875–84. https://doi.org/10.1038/ismej.2016.183.

84. Hunt KM, Foster JA, Forney LJ, et al. Characterization of the diversity and temporal stability of bacterial communities in human milk. PLoS One. 2011;6:e21313. https://doi.org/10.1371/journal.pone.0021313.

85. Sakwinska O, Moine D, Delley M, et al. Microbiota in breast milk of Chinese lactating mothers. PLoS One. 2016;11:e0160856. https://doi.org/10.1371/journal.pone.0160856.

86. Wan Y, Jiang J, Lu M, et al. Human milk microbiota development during lactation and its relation to maternal geographic location and gestational hypertensive status. Gut Microbes. 2020;11:1438–49. https://doi.org/10.1080/19490976.2020.1760711.

87. Collado MC, Cernada M, Baüerl C, et al. Microbial ecology and host-microbiota interactions during early life stages. Gut Microbes. 2012;3:352.

88. Olivares M, Albrecht S, de Palma G, et al. Human milk composition differs in healthy mothers and mothers with celiac disease. Eur J Nutr. 2015;54:119–28. https://doi.org/10.1007/s00394-014-0692-1.

89. Turnbaugh PJ, Ley RE, Mahowald MA, et al. An obesity-associated gut microbiome with increased capacity for energy harvest. Nature. 2006;444:1027–31. https://doi.org/10.1038/nature05414.

90. Collado MC, Isolauri E, Laitinen K, Salminen S. Distinct composition of gut microbiota during pregnancy in overweight and normal-weight women. Am J Clin Nutr. 2008;88:894–9. https://doi.org/10.1093/ajcn/88.4.894.

91. Cortés-Macías E, Selma-Royo M, Martínez-Costa C, Collado MC. Breastfeeding practices influence the breast milk microbiota depending on pre-gestational maternal bmi and weight gain over pregnancy. Nutrients. 2021;13 https://doi.org/10.3390/nu13051518.

92. Olshan KL, Zomorrodi AR, Pujolassos M, et al. Microbiota and metabolomic patterns in the breast milk of subjects with celiac disease on a gluten-free diet. Nutrients. 2021;13 https://doi.org/10.3390/nu13072243.

93. Bajer L, Kverka M, Kostovcik M, et al. Distinct gut microbiota profiles in patients with primary sclerosing cholangitis and ulcerative colitis. World J Gastroenterol. 2017;23:4548–58. https://doi.org/10.3748/wjg.v23.i25.4548.

94. Sokol H, Seksik P, Furet JP, et al. Low counts of Faecalibacterium prausnitzii in colitis microbiota. Inflamm Bowel Dis. 2009;15:1183–9. https://doi.org/10.1002/ibd.20903.

95. Benítez-Páez A, Olivares M, Szajewska H, et al. Breast-milk microbiota linked to celiac disease development in children: a pilot study from the PreventCD cohort. Front Microbiol. 2020;11 https://doi.org/10.3389/fmicb.2020.01335.

96. Browne PD, Aparicio M, Alba C, et al. Human milk microbiome and maternal postnatal psychosocial distress. Front Microbiol. 2019;10 https://doi.org/10.3389/fmicb.2019.02333.

97. Kumar H, du Toit E, Kulkarni A, et al. Distinct patterns in human milk microbiota and fatty acid profiles across specific geographic locations. Front Microbiol. 2016;7 https://doi.org/10.3389/fmicb.2016.01619.

98. Lackey KA, Williams JE, Meehan CL, et al. What's normal? Microbiomes in human milk and infant feces are related to each other but vary geographically: the inspire study. Front Nutr. 2019;6 https://doi.org/10.3389/fnut.2019.00045.

99. Chen PW, Lin YL, Huang MS. Profiles of commensal and opportunistic bacteria in human milk from healthy donors in Taiwan. J Food Drug Anal. 2018;26:1235–44. https://doi.org/10.1016/j.jfda.2018.03.004.

100. Barker DJP. Fetal origins of coronary heart disease. BMJ. 1995;311:171–4. https://doi.org/10.1136/bmj.311.6998.171.
101. Franks PW, Hanson RL, Knowler WC, et al. Childhood obesity, other cardiovascular risk factors, and premature death. N Engl J Med. 2010;362:485–93. https://doi.org/10.1056/NEJMoa0904130.
102. Kalliomäki M, Carmen Collado M, Salminen S, Isolauri E. Early differences in fecal microbiota composition in children may predict overweight. Am J Clin Nutr. 2008;87:534–8. https://doi.org/10.1093/ajcn/87.3.534.
103. Luoto R, Kalliomäki M, Laitinen K, Isolauri E. The impact of perinatal probiotic intervention on the development of overweight and obesity: follow-up study from birth to 10 years. Int J Obes. 2010;34:1531–7. https://doi.org/10.1038/ijo.2010.50.
104. Hou YP, He QQ, Ouyang HM, et al. Human gut microbiota associated with obesity in Chinese children and adolescents. Biomed Res Int. 2017;2017:1. https://doi.org/10.1155/2017/7585989.
105. Liang C, Guo M, Liu T, et al. Profiles of gut microbiota in children with obesity from Harbin, China and screening of strains with anti-obesity ability *in vitro* and *in vivo*. J Appl Microbiol. 2020;129:728–37. https://doi.org/10.1111/jam.14639.
106. Abrahamsson TR, Sinkiewicz G, Jakobsson T, et al. Probiotic lactobacilli in breast milk and infant stool in relation to Oral intake during the first year of life. J Pediatr Gastroenterol Nutr. 2009;49:349–54.

Renal Physiology of Pregnancy

Fatih Palit

1 Introduction

The term "physiologic" does not adequately describe the state of a woman during pregnancy. There are several shifts in biochemistry, psychology, and physiology. Every component of kidney physiology is modified by pregnancy. It is a physiological marvel that these alterations can be orchestrated. Significant volume expansion and vasodilation characterize kidney and systemic hemodynamics. Renal plasma flow (RPF) and glomerular filtration rate (GFR) rise by as much as 80% relative to pre-pregnancy values. Healthcare providers, to best serve their pregnant patients, need a thorough understanding of all how pregnancy changes their bodies [1–3].

Changes in glomerular filtration rate, tubular function, electrolyte and acid/base management, and other processes are all driven by the kidneys to ensure the health of both mother and child throughout pregnancy (Table 1).

Increased renal blood flow and glomerular filtration rate occur early in pregnancy due to systemic vasodilation, which is mediated by a change in the quantity of and a reaction to numerous hormones. Alterations in total body storage of electrolytes are brought on by the activation of the renin-angiotensin-aldosterone axis, which occurs in response to vasodilation, and by changes in renal tubular processing [4].

Hemodynamic shifts and fluid and electrolyte balance must be precisely orchestrated to develop and maintain a healthy pregnancy for both mother and child.

F. Palit (✉)

Department of Nephrology, Basaksehir Çam and Sakura City Training and Research Hospital, İstanbul, Türkiye

Ö. N. Şahin et al. (eds.), *Breastfeeding and Metabolic Programming*, https://doi.org/10.1007/978-3-031-33278-4_9

Table 1 Physiologic changes in pregnancy

Increased
• Blood volume
• Cardiac output
• Levels of nitric oxide and relaxin
• Relative resistance to vasoconstrictors
• GFR by 50%
• Urine protein excretion
Decreased
• Systemic vascular resistance
• Systemic blood pressure
• Serum creatinine

Abbreviations: *GFR* Glomerular filtration rate

2 Basic Physiology of the Kidney

Kidney function is based on the nephron, which has three different subunits: Blood vessels, including the afferent arteriole (before the glomerulus) and the efferent arteriole(after the glomerulus), and the tubules (from the proximal tubule to the more distal collecting tubule), are responsible for the selective reabsorption and secretion of several molecules (electrolytes, proteins, and glucose) (after the glomerulus). Some molecules, like glucose and amino acids, are actively exchanged for others via the sodium/potassium pump. In contrast, others, like urea and hydrogen ions, are secreted by other portions of the tubules to maintain homeostasis and ultimately contribute to the generation of urine. In a typical pregnancy, the nephron's filtration, reabsorption, and secretion mechanisms all change [1–5].

3 Hemodynamic Alterations in the Kidneys

Vasodilation and increased volume are two hallmarks of pregnancy, both resulting from a complex interplay between several hormones (Table 2). By the end of the second trimester, the average blood pressure of a pregnant woman has dropped by around 10 mmHg to 105/60 mmHg. Several factors contribute to this, such as shifts in hormone levels and modifications to the renin-angiotensin-aldosterone system (RAAS). Maternal hormones may influence pregnancy-related alterations in maternal hemodynamics. During the mid-luteal phase of menstruation, there is a decrease in vascular resistance and an increase in cardiac output, which leads to a drop in mean arterial pressure compared to the mid-follicular phase [6, 7]. Although progesterone can raise RPF and GFR, it cannot explain the dramatic rise observed during pregnancy. The corpus luteum, decidua, and placenta secrete relaxin, a vasodilating hormone. Increasing vascular gelatinase activity via the endothelium endothelin B receptor-nitric oxide pathway plays a role in mouse kidney physiology during pregnancy. As measured by Ogueh and coworkers, the levels of relaxin

Table 2 Typical laboratory values during pregnancy (Adopted from reference [6])

Variable	Average values in pregnancy
Plasma osmolality	270 mOsm/kg
Serum sodium	135 mEq/L
Serum potassium	3.8 mEq/L
Serum bicarbonate	18–20 mEq/L
Serum creatinine	0.5 mg/dL
Blood urea nitrogen	9.0 mg/dL
Uric acid	2–3 mg/dL

increased steadily during pregnancy and then declined after delivery. At least in late pregnancy and the postpartum period, clinical connections between relaxin levels and hemodynamic measures have not been shown [5–7].

RAAS is upregulated during a healthy pregnancy. The ovaries and the decidua are two extrarenal sources that secrete renin. When a pregnant woman's body generates estrogen, it stimulates the liver to make more angiotensinogen, increasing the production of angiotensin II (ANG II). Despite this, it is well documented that systolic blood pressure often drops during pregnancy. The refractoriness could explain the vasodilated condition during pregnancy to ANG II that develops at this time. The presence of additional chemicals, such as progesterone and vascular endothelial growth factor-mediated prostacyclins, and/or the monomeric form of angiotensin 1 (AT1) receptors might account for this insensitivity [2, 3]. Return of ANG II sensitivity, decreased aldosterone production, heterodimeric AT1 receptors, and the presence of autoantibodies to AT1 all indicate that the RAAS is dysregulated in pregnancy (AT1-AA). At week 8 of a healthy pregnancy, aldosterone levels begin to climb, and by the end of the third trimester, they have increased by a factor of three to six over the upper range of normal (80 to 100 ng/dL). Overall, blood volume increases by 30%–50%, or 1.1–1.6 L, compared to women who are not pregnant [6, 8, 9].

4 Changes in GFR

Renal vascular dilatation results from systemic vasodilation that occurs during pregnancy. This causes a rise in the GFR and the ERPF (RPF). By the third month of pregnancy, the glomerular filtration rate (GFR) has increased by 40–50%, reaching a maximum of 180 mL/min. This plateau lasts until around week 36 of pregnancy. Changes in blood levels of analytes and changes in the clearance of drugs eliminated by the kidneys can result from even a modest increase in GFR. Four weeks into pregnancy, creatinine clearance has increased by 25%, and by 9 weeks, it has increased by 45%. While GFR rises and glomerular membrane charge selectivity shifts, protein and albumin are excreted more significantly in the urine [10–13].

5　Measurement of GFR

Estimating GFR is essential for the management of pregnant patients. In pregnancy, like in nephrology, there is still much room for improvement regarding GFR estimates. Like its known propensity to underestimate when GFR is more than 60 mL/min, the Modification of Diet in Renal Disease (MDRD) equation overestimates GFR in pregnant women with and without preeclampsia. In research comparing both equations to 24-h urine collections in preeclamptic patients, the CKD Epidemiology Collaboration equation was shown to underestimate GFR to a comparable degree as the MDRD equation. Comparing MDRD and cystatin-C-based equations, both produce mean GFR values greater than 120 mL/min. However, cystatin C produced higher first and second-trimester GFRs, followed by a fall in GFR in the third trimester. This contradicts evidence from early studies showing that GFR increases steadily until the term. Postpartum, GFR was shown to decrease using the MDRD equation but increase using the cystatin C equation. Recent prospective research comparing cystatin-C-based GFR estimations with inulin clearances at three time points in 12 pregnant individuals revealed no association. The best method for determining GFR in expectant mothers is still a 24-h urine collection to calculate creatinine clearance. [6, 8–15].

6　Mechanism of Increased GFR

The GFR rises by around 50% from its pre-pregnancy value during pregnancy. It needs to be better understood what processes are responsible for this growth. Keep in mind that GFR is expressed in several different ways and that different parts of it change at different stages of pregnancy.

$$\text{GFR} = \left(\Delta P - \pi_{\text{GC}}\right) \times K_{\text{f}}$$

where (ΔP) is the oncotic pressure at the glomerulus and (π_{GC}) is the net hydraulic pressure in the glomerulus. Although direct measurement of transcapillary hydraulic pressure in humans is impossible, this parameter can be studied in animal models utilizing micropuncture. The π_{GC} value is calculated by averaging the afferent (π_{A}) and efferent (π_{E}) oncotic pressures. Oncotic pressure (P) at the entrance to the afferent arteriole (A) is expressed as a fraction 1 minus FF, where FF is the percent of plasma filtered by the glomerulus.

$$\pi_{\text{E}} = \pi_{\text{A}} / \left(1 - \text{FF}\right)$$

The FF value is calculated by dividing the GFR by the RPF.

$$\text{FF} = \text{GFR} / \text{RPF}$$

The capacity to ultrafiltrate through the three layers of the glomerulus is measured by the glomerular ultrafiltration coefficient, Kf, which is the product of the surface area accessible for filtration and the hydraulic permeability (k). The permeability estimate is calculated using the data obtained from the autopsy and the computer simulation.

During pregnancy, there is a significant reduction in oncotic pressure due to the increase in plasma volume, which helps to increase GFR [6]. Modifications to the filter surface area and the hydraulic permeability may also cause slight shifts in Kf. WhetherpP rises during human pregnancy is still a matter of debate. Baylis found no difference in hydrostatic or oncotic pressure in his early tests of the 12-day pregnant rat, and he credited the increase in GFR to higher RPF [16]. Pregnant women's glomerular size selectivity appeared to change, and oncotic pressure was lower, although increased P was not [17]. They reasoned that the elevated RPF was the primary cause of the improved GFR. Since RPF constantly decreases approaching the term, this explanation cannot account for the fact that GFR continues to rise later in pregnancy. An evaluation of the dynamics of glomerular filtration in postpartum humans revealed that the persistent increase in GFR after delivery was caused by either an increase in P of up to 16%, an increase in Kf of around 50%, or a combination of these two factors [18]. It is impossible to rule out the likelihood that P does vary, according to Odutayo and Hlaudunewich, because both estimated and observed changes in Kf and GC are relatively small [18].

7 Alterations in Tubular Function

Changes in tubular waste and nutrition processing occur during pregnancy. Increases in GFR and reductions in proximal tubular reabsorption contribute to increased uric acid excretion. At around 22–24 weeks of pregnancy, serum uric acid levels drop to their lowest point, between 2.0 and 3.0 mg/dL, and then gradually return to normal levels by term. It is believed that higher clearance is required to deal with the extra output from the placenta and baby during pregnancy.

After being freely filtered at the glomerulus, glucose is reabsorbed almost entirely in the proximal tubule and just a little in the collecting tubule. When glucose is excreted in the urine, it is usually because the amount filtered out is more than what the kidneys can absorb. The reabsorption of glucose is less efficient, and glucose excretion is more variable during pregnancy. Earlier research hypothesized that glucosuria with normoglycemia or physiologic glucosuria resulted when an elevated GFR and the resulting elevated filtered load of glucose exceeded the ability of the proximal tubule to reabsorb glucose. Research involving glucose infusion and simultaneous assessments of glucose excretion and inulin clearance in 29 pregnant women showed that this effect was independent of glucosuria. Those without glucosuria regained their average reabsorption ability 8–12 weeks after giving birth, but those who had had glucosuria to varied degrees during pregnancy retained a residual impairment in reabsorption capacity. Pregnancy may also reduce reabsorption efficiency at the distal end of the nephron. The fractional reabsorption of amino acids and b-microglobulin is diminished, leading to higher excretion, similar to what happens with uric acid and glucose [5–20].

Total urine protein and albumin excretion rise throughout a healthy pregnancy, peaking around week 20. Most of the protein in urine is of the Tamm-Horsfall type, with some albumin and other circulating proteins present in trace amounts. Although the time of the increase in proteinuria during pregnancy falls outside the window of the peak increase in GFR, this is generally explained as a result of the increase in GFR. In late pregnancy, there is an increase in albuminuria, although not at abnormally high levels [20]. Increases in circulating soluble antiangiogenic factors, which are present in abnormally high amounts in preeclampsia and disturb the slit diaphragm, are also observed late in normal pregnancy and may account for late-term increases in proteinuria [21]. Third-trimester selective changes in glomerular charge or the presence of additional protein substances are another possible explanation [21, 22].

Protein levels in urine, more significant than 300 mg every 24 h, are considered abnormal in pregnant women [23]. This estimate was based on a limited sample size, and subsequent research has demonstrated that average protein excretion is far lower than 200 mg/24 h [24, 25]. The 24-h urine collection remains the gold standard for quantifying proteinuria in pregnant patients, despite the widespread adoption of urine protein/creatinine for quantification of proteinuria in nonpregnant patients and its usefulness as a screening tool for the presence or absence of proteinuria. Since pregnant women's dilated urinary tracts may hold more pee than usual, a high proportion of scheduled urine samples are lost due to timing and retention issues [25].

Control of fluid and electrolyte balance by the kidneys.

During pregnancy, the body has a decreased threshold for triggering osmoreceptors associated with antidiuretic hormone (ADH) and thirst. Serum sodium levels typically drop by around 5 mEq/L, and plasma osmolality approaches 270 mOsm/kg. The hormone b-human chorionic gonadotropin may have a role in this shift, as it is elevated during the luteal phase of the menstrual cycle [26]. Vasodilation, arterial underfilling, and ADH release have all been linked to decreased serum sodium. Relaxin levels are elevated in pregnant women, and in animals, relaxin has been found to promote ADH secretion and water consumption [27]. An increase in aldosterone and its antinatriuretic effects coincides with mild hyponatremia.

Additionally, deoxycorticosterone increases the activity of sodium pumps across several membranes, which aids in salt retention. The natriuretic effects of elevated GFR, atrial natriuretic peptide, and progesterone levels counteract these effects. However, the net balance between these effects is the preferred retention of water over salt and decreased osmolality, even though the total sodium increase during pregnancy is predicted to be 900–1000 mEq. By the time pregnancy is through, the body's total supply of potassium has increased by around 320 mEq. This happens because progesterone has anti-kaliuretic actions, which counteract the effects of aldosterone's salt retention. During pregnancy, the amount of potassium excreted remains constant, whereas the amount reabsorbed by the tubules adjusts to the changing filtered load. Progesterone was not discovered to play a role in the acute control of potassium or sodium excretion in the pioneering investigation by Brown and colleagues [28].

Notably, a placental enzyme called vasopressin causes a rise in the metabolic clearance of ADH beginning about week ten and continuing through the middle of pregnancy. Enzyme activity reaches its highest point in the third trimester, remains elevated during labor and delivery, and then drops to undetectable levels within the first 2–4 weeks after giving birth. However, increased production in pregnancy often maintains average plasma ADH concentrations. Polydipsia, polyuria, high-normal blood sodium, and abnormally low urine osmolality are all symptoms of transitory diabetes insipidus (DI), which affects a small percentage of women. Compared to women without DI, these ladies can have higher vasopressinase activity. Desmopressin (DDAVP), resistant to degradation by vasopressinase, can be used to treat this condition. While many pregnant women report urinating often, genuine polyuria (0.3 L/day) is unusual [29].

8 Conclusion

During pregnancy, the kidneys are subjected to extreme stress. Hence a nephrologist needs to be familiar with the kidneys' typical responses to this situation. Numerous physiological changes occur throughout pregnancy. The kidneys play crucial roles in various pregnancy-related processes, including salt, potassium, water retention, blood pressure regulation, and many more. These shifts are governed by mechanisms that are complex and only partially understood. Our current knowledge of kidney development in the mother is mainly based on studies conducted in the 1970s and 1980s. As women live longer, they have more children later in life, and as a result, more women are experiencing complications during pregnancy. To better recognize pathology in our ever-changing patient population, it is crucial to have a firm grasp of typical physiologic changes [29].

References

1. Ökten SB, Fıçıcıoğlu C. Maternal physiology during pregnancy. In: Cingi C, Özel HE, Bayar Muluk N, editors. ENT diseases: diagnosis and treatment during pregnancy and lactation. Cham: Springer; 2022. https://doi.org/10.1007/978-3-031-05303-0_1.
2. Beers K, Patel N. Kidney physiology in pregnancy. Adv Chronic Kidney Dis. 2020;27(6):449–54.
3. Davison JM. Overview: kidney function in pregnant women. Am J Kidney Dis. 1987;9(4):248–52.
4. Dunlop W. Serial changes in renal hemodynamics during normal human pregnancy. Br J Obstet Gynaecol. 1981;88(1):1–9.

5. Ogueh O, Clough A, Hancock M, Johnson MR. A longitudinal study of the control of renal and uterine hemodynamic changes of pregnancy. Hypertens Pregnancy. 2011;30(3):243–59.
6. Cheung KL, Lafayette RA. Renal physiology of pregnancy. Adv Chronic Kidney Dis. 2013;20(3):209–14.
7. Lafayette RA, Hladunewich MA, Derby G, Blouch K, Druzin ML, Myers BD. Serum relaxin levels and kidney function in late pregnancy with or without preeclampsia. Clin Nephrol. 2011;75(3):226–32.
8. Schrier RW, Briner VA. Peripheral arterial vasodilation hypothesis of sodium and water retention in pregnancy: implications for pathogenesis of preeclampsia-eclampsia. Obstet Gynecol. 1991;77(4):632–9.
9. Abdul-Karim R, Assali NS. Pressor response to angiotonin in pregnant and nonpregnant women. Am J Obstetr Gynecol. 1961;82(2):246–51.
10. Davison JM, Noble MCB. Serial changes in 24 hour creatinine clearance during normal menstrual cycles and the first trimester of pregnancy. BJOG Int J Obstet Gynaecol. 1981;88(1):10–7.
11. Lindheimer MD, Davison JM, Katz AI. The kidney and hypertension in pregnancy: twenty exciting years. Semin Nephrol. 2001;21(2):173–89. Elsevier.
12. Tan EK, Tan EL. Alterations in physiology and anatomy during pregnancy. Best Pract Res Clin Obstet Gynaecol. 2013;27(6):791–802.
13. Suarez MLG, Kattah A, Grande JP, Garovic V. Renal disorders in pregnancy: core curriculum 2019. Am J Kidney Dis. 2019;73(1):119–30.
14. Alper AB, Yi Y, Webber LS, Pridjian G, Mumuney AA, Saade G, et al. Estimation of glomerular filtration rate in preeclamptic patients. Am J Perinatol. 2007;24(10):569–74.
15. Larsson A, Palm M, Hansson LO, Axelsson O. Cystatin C and modification of diet in renal disease (MDRD) estimated glomerular filtration rate differ during normal pregnancy. Acta Obstet Gynecol Scand. 2010;89(7):939–44.
16. Baylis C. The mechanism of the increase in glomerular filtration rate in the twelve-day pregnant rat. J Physiol. 1980;305(1):405–14.
17. Roberts MARK, Lindheimer MD, Davison JM. Altered glomerular permselectivity to neutral dextrans and heteroporous membrane modeling in human pregnancy. Am J Physiol Renal Physiol. 1996;270(2):F338–43.
18. Odutayo A, Hladunewich M. Obstetric nephrology: renal hemodynamic and metabolic physiology in normal pregnancy. Clin J Am Soc Nephrol. 2012;7(12):2073–80.
19. Davison JM, Hytten FE. The effect of pregnancy on the renal handling of glucose. BJOG Int J Obstet Gynaecol. 1975;82(5):374–81.
20. Erman A, Neri A, Sharoni R, Rabinov M, Kaplan B, Rosenfeld JB, Boner G. Enhanced urinary albumin excretion after 35 weeks of gestation and during labour in normal pregnancy. Scand J Clin Lab Invest. 1992;52(5):409–13.
21. Yoshimatsu J, Matsumoto H, Goto K, Shimano M, Narahara H, Miyakawa I. Relationship between urinary albumin and serum soluble fms-like tyrosine kinase 1 (sFlt-1) in normal pregnancy. Eur J Obstetr Gynecol Reprod Biol. 2006;128(1–2):204–8.
22. Cornelis T, Odutayo A, Keunen J, Hladunewich M. The kidney in normal pregnancy and preeclampsia. Semin Nephrol. 2011;31(1):4–14. WB Saunders.
23. Brown MA, Lindheimer MD, de Swiet M, Assche AV, Moutquin JM. The classification and diagnosis of the hypertensive disorders of pregnancy: statement from the International Society for the Study of hypertension in pregnancy (ISSHP). Hypertens Pregnancy. 2001;20(1):ix–xiv.
24. Kuo VS, Koumantakis G, Gallery ED. Proteinuria and its assessment in normal and hypertensive pregnancy. Am J Obstet Gynecol. 1992;167(3):723–8.
25. Lindheimer MD, Kanter D. Interpreting abnormal proteinuria in pregnancy: the need for a more pathophysiological approach. Obstet Gynecol. 2010;115(2 Part 1):365–75.
26. Davison JM, Shiells EA, Philips PR, Lindheimer MD. Serial evaluation of vasopressin release and thirst in human pregnancy. Role of human chorionic gonadotrophin in the osmoregulatory changes of gestation. J Clin Invest. 1988;81(3):798–806.

27. Thornton SN, Fitzsimons JT. The effects of centrally administered porcine relaxin on drinking behaviour in male and female rats. J Neuroendocrinol. 1995;7(3):165–9.
28. Brown MA, Sinosich MJ, Saunders DM, Gallery ED. Potassium regulation and progesterone-aldosterone interrelationships in human pregnancy: a prospective study. Am J Obstet Gynecol. 1986;155(2):349–53.
29. Schrier RW. Systemic arterial vasodilation, vasopressin, and vasopressinase in pregnancy. J Am Soc Nephrol. 2010;21(4):570–2.

Part II
Metabolic Programming

The Evolution and Genomic Aspects of Milk

Özlem Naciye Şahin and Gian Carlo Di Renzo

1 Introduction

Lactation can be defined as a process by which milk is secreted in large amounts by mammary glands in order to nourish the organism's offspring. It plays a key role in the reproductive strategy of mammals, so much so that the Linnaean classification that created the class Mammalia in 1758 did so on the basis of the ability to lactate, rather than on other features of anatomy shared by the group. Choosing lactation as the basis to categorize the group is reflective of the great significance lactation plays in nourishing the young of all mammalian species, including humans. Indeed, lactation is said to have created a unique nutritional environment in this group of organisms [1].

According to the fossil record and molecular evolutionary studies, the earliest mammals evolved during the Triassic era (252–201 million years ago (Mya)), from Synapsid animals which had diverged from Sauropsids within the Permian era (299–252 Mya). A comparison of genomes undertaken recently has proven that the molecules which make lactation possible have existed for a very long time. The beginnings of lactation are seen in the therapsids, developing over the course of the Triassic era. Lactation is likely to have been present in the earliest common ancestor of all current mammalian species, as well as in the mammaliaformes, by the late Triassic. Lactation appears to have evolved in cynodonts at the same times as the other features associated with the mammals as a group, such as the integumentary system, ability to generate their own body heat and growth of hair/fur [1, 2].

Ö. N. Şahin (✉)
Department of Child Health and Diseases, Arel University, Medical Faculty, Istanbul, Türkiye

G. C. Di Renzo
Centre of Perinatal Medicine of the University of Perugia/Sechenov University, Moscow, Russia
e-mail: giancarlo.direnzo@unipg.it

Ö. N. Şahin et al. (eds.), *Breastfeeding and Metabolic Programming*, https://doi.org/10.1007/978-3-031-33278-4_10

111

Thus, mammalian lactation has been evolving for over 200 million years, which has helped to generate the radical differences in reproductive strategy seen within the group. Nowhere is this more apparent than in the lactational differences, which may affect either an entire lineage or a single species. Within mammals, there are three subgroups, which diverged around 220 Mya: the Prototheria (known nowadays as the monotremes), the Metatheria (containing the marsupials), and the Eutheria (the placental mammals). There are only two families extant from the monotremes, both in Australasia, namely the platypus (*Ornithorhynchus anatinus*) and the echidnas (belonging to the genus *Tachyglossus or Zaglosus*). The monotremes lay eggs and possess a more primitive system for lactation than that found in the other two groups of mammals. Molecular-based research using genomic and transcriptomic techniques has permitted comparison between the prototherian, metatherian, and eutherian lactational systems [2–5].

There is a great deal of complexity in the way lactation occurs within different mammalian species and the process involves more than simply meeting the nutritional requirements of the offspring. Milk itself exerts a regulatory role on the mammary gland and the growth of the offspring. The complexity of the processes involved is emerging through studies of highly specialized lactational systems, such as those possessed by fur seals or marsupials [6].

2   The Evolution of Mammals and how Lactation Originated

The exact evolutionary mechanism which must have operated on the mammary gland and lactation over the course of time in the synapsid branch is much debated since direct evidence in the form of extant species showing intermediate stages or fossils indicating parental care and the changing morphology of the mammary gland are not found. In current mammalian species, lactation is a sophisticated process that exhibits many different features in terms of morphology, physiology, biochemistry, ecology, and ethology. It is improbable that such diversity could appear all at once, and a more primitive system must clearly have once existed, from which the adaptations arose. There is almost no evidence for such a primitive system in any living species. So, striking is this absence that it has even been cited as a reason why evolutionary theory may be flawed. After all, what evolutionary advantage would accrue from a system providing small quantities of low-quality secretion? This argument even goes back to the time of Charles Darwin, whose 1872 second edition of "On the Origin of Species" put forward the hypothesis that the evolutionary precursor of the mammary gland was the intrauterine brood patch identified in certain sea-dwelling animals, such as sharks and certain fish. This structure guards the eggs and provides nutrition after hatching. Darwin's hypothesis arose from the conviction that the pouch possessed by metatherian and prototherian species had evolved from the uterus. Currently, however, the consensus is that the mammary glands are specialized adaptations of the glands within the integument, and had already evolved within the therapsids [1, 7].

3 Genomic Factors Affecting Milk

Breast milk varies in its composition. There are a number of causes for this variety, such as the lactational stage, how many previous pregnancies the mother has had, the stage of gestation, mother's nutritional intake, the time feeding starts, and how long it has been continuing for [8–12]. Much of the variability in milk composition arises for normal physiological reasons and is tailored to the nutritional requirements of the child, such as the variation within a feeding session. However, there may be other, harmful causes for variation, such as when the mother's diet is unbalanced. This type of variability impairs the nutritional benefits of breast milk, and may cause malnutrition in the infant, either an insufficiency or a surfeit of calories [8].

It is overly simplistic to see breast milk as supplying only the energy requirements of the child or as providing a supply of raw materials to fuel growth. Some breast milk constituents also influence gene activity [5]. For example, aliphatic acids in breast milk not only serve as energetic metabolic substrates but also may be incorporated into plasma membranes, be modified to become immunoregulatory signaling molecules or control the expression of specific gene products [6–13]. There are now two new branches of nutritional science that attempt to understand this complexity. Nutrigenomics examines the direct or indirect mechanisms through which genetic expression is regulated by specific nutrients, while nutrigenetics examines how the genes individuals inherit determine the response to a particular nutrient [9].These new disciplines may eventually explain why the nutritional requirements differ so greatly between individuals and explain how specific individuals are likely to respond to nutritional interventions [5].

This chapter accordingly focuses on the way a lactating mother's consumption of fatty acids in the diet affects the amount of milk lipids she expresses, both through the nutrigenomic effects of the fatty acids on maternal genetic expression and the nutrigenetic effects of the mother's genetic composition on the resulting breast milk she excretes. The initial discussion covers what role fatty acids in milk play and where they originate, before discussing how the breast milk composition is influenced by maternal nutrigenomic and nutrigenetic factors.

4 Anatomy of the Breast and Fatty Acids Contained in Breast Milk

Production of milk occurs within the breast itself. The breast is made up of a variety of tissue types, namely glandular (containing the lactocytes), connective, adipose, and a stroma with its own blood supply. Within the glands, the epithelium contains two layers of different cell types, i.e., secretory cells facing the lumen and myoepithelial cells constituting the base layer. The myoepithelial cells form a branched network enveloping the alveoli and small-caliber ducts. Myoepithelial cells possess longitudinal striations [10]. When the myoepithelium contracts, milk is ejected out of the alveoli, through the smaller ducts and into the principal lactiferous duct, which terminates at the nipple [11].

The mammary glands begin to assume their adult form at puberty. When a woman becomes pregnant, the breast keeps on developing up to the point when lactation commences. The breast goes through four phases of development, i.e., mammogenesis, lactogenesis, galactopoiesis, and involution [12]. There are steady alterations in the composition of breast milk as the period of breast feeding continues, both in terms of macro- and micronutrient levels. Three specific types of breast milk have been identified, namely colostrum, transitional, and mature types. These types are different in several ways from each other [8, 14].

5 Roles Played by Aliphatic Acids in Milk

Lipids comprise the second most abundant constituent of human breast milk. They are key to the development of the infant, both as a metabolic substrate to generate energy and to supply essential fats [13, 15]. The principal lipids within milk are aliphatic acids bound to glycerol as triglycerides. Some 98% of the milk lipids are in this form [16]. These fatty acids can be categorized as saturated (containing only single bonds) or unsaturated (with one or more double bonds). The role milk lipids play as a substrate for energy generation and to dissolve lipophilic vitamins, as well as to support the child's development has been well-described elsewhere [7, 14, 17]. The aliphatic acids in milk also play a role in regulating the hepatic synthesis of lipoproteins at the transcription level [18], which ensures that infants are competent to synthesize the lipoproteins they need. Furthermore, n-3 long-chain PUFAs are essential for the development of the central nervous system (CNS) and retina [19–21]. If they are lacking, the plasticity of the CNS is impaired and neurological function is affected when the child grows into an adult [22]. The results from a number of studies support the hypothesis that mothers who consume omega-3 long-chain PUFAs while pregnant produce infants with improved cognitive function and focus than the infants of those who do not [23, 24].

6 Nutrigenomic Aspects of Aliphatic Acids in Milk

Lipids have recently been shown, in research involving rodents, cattle, and humans, to possess the ability to regulate hepatic and mammary gland expression of particular genes, so as to ensure sufficient local levels of saturated fatty acids and mono- and poly-unsaturated fatty acids [22, 23]. Fats in the diet potentially regulate the synthesis of lipids through interactions with certain transcription factors, notably the peroxisome proliferator-activated receptor (PPAR) and sterol regulatory element binding protein (SREBP), both found in the cell nucleus [23, 24]. These two receptors regulate the expression of the gene FADS1, which encodes delta-5 desaturase and FADS2, the product of which is delta-6 desaturase. They also regulate the genes which encode the elongase enzymes, i.e., ELOV-2 and 5. The PPAR superfamily of proteins includes alpha, gamma, and beta/delta variants. When the gamma and beta/delta variants are activated, the genetic expression of molecules involved in de novo manufacture of fatty acids increases. The activated alpha variant, by contrast, increases the genetic expression of molecules involved in oxidizing fatty acids [25]. SREBP denotes a group of related transcription factors, three of which have been discovered, namely SREBP1a, 1c, and 2. They have a proven role in maintaining cholesterol levels within cells and also help to control the manufacture of fatty acids and their uptake. Despite the fact that SREBP-1c and 2 share similarities in their structure, there are many differences in their hepatic function in response to endocrine signals, nutrient levels, and according to the stage in infant development [25, 26]. SREBP2 increases the manufacture of cholesterol, whereas SREBP-1a and -1c upregulate the production of fatty acids through their control of specific genes, in particular lipoprotein lipase, acetyl-CoA carboxylase α, FAS, SCD, and FADS1 and 2, as well as FA ELOVL-2 and ELOVL-5 [26, 27]. The synthesis of SREBP-1c involves an initially larger gene product that adheres to the endoplasmic reticulum. This protein is then truncated, the N-terminal region moving into the nucleoplasm, where it becomes bound to the sterol regulatory element. In this position, it can regulate its target genes [25].

7 Nutrigenetic Factors Related to Aliphatic Acids in Milk

The extent to which genetics affects the fatty acids present in milk is an ongoing research topic in cattle and other ruminants. Candidate genes for more detailed research have been identified through quantitative trait locus analysis, which linked particular patterns of fatty acids with specific regions within the genome [28, 29]. The existence of single nucleotide polymorphisms has established that genetic variability in these regions is indeed related to which fatty acids are present in milk [30–36]. These studies were driven by the commercial need to breed cattle or other ruminants that produce milk with the desired fatty acid content. Such milk offers better health benefits to human consumers or fits with the need for particular dairy products, such as butter that can be spread more easily. Once the genes were identified, the animals could be selectively bred and given a tailored diet to produce the maximum yield of milk. Currently, the dairy industry wants to produce milk that contains more C18 monounsaturated fatty acids and polyunsaturated fatty acids, especially eicosapentaenoic acid, docosahexaenoic acid, and conjugated linoleic acid [37, 38].

By contrast, there has been relatively little research on nutrigenetic factors affecting the fatty acid composition of human breast milk. This topic appears to have become of interest once it became known that specific SNPs correlated with the amounts of some fatty acids (especially LC-PUFAs) in the circulation and within the tissues. Frequently noted SNPs occurring in the region where FADS is encoded were shown by Schaeffer et al. [39] to be related to the level of LC-PUFA seen in phospholipids within the cell membrane. This finding has since been replicated [40–43]. Simultaneously, it was shown by the work of Rodriguez-Cruz *et al.* that rats express fatty acid desaturases in their mammary glands [26]. This prompted researchers to investigate whether the same enzymes might be present in human mammary glands and involved in manufacturing LC-PUFA for packaging in breast milk. Other researchers, notably Xie and Innis [44] and Moltó-Puigmartí and colleagues [45], taking this as the basis for their inquiry, found that SNPs in the FADS region had effects beyond the one shown by Schaeffer et al., viz regulation of LC-PUFA content [39].

Dietary PUFA actually serves to regulate the level in breast milk through its effects on the SREBP, which regulates the genetic expression of FADS1 and 2 and ELOVL-2 and 5. Unfortunately, maternal dietary intake of artificially produced trans-fatty acids (TFAs) has a detrimental effect on the fatty acid composition of breast milk. This is because these TFAs alter lipid metabolism.

However, the way the mother responds to dietary intake of fatty acids may alter depending on her genetics, as the association of variability within the FADS and ELOVL coding regions has been established. Specifically, mothers with two copies of the minor allele secreted breast milk with lower levels of arachidonic acid and docosahexaenoic acid (DHA) than women with at least one copy of the major allele. The levels in the maternal circulation were also lower. Furthermore, SNP mutations in the FADS encoding region were also noted by Moltó-Puigmartí et al. [45] to have an association with the level of DHA in breast milk. Mothers with the major allele secreted milk richer in DHA in response to increased dietary consumption in the form of fish, but increasing dietary consumption of DHA did not produce the same effect in women with two copies of the minor allele, within the limits of the observations. This result may have important consequences for public health since LC-PUFAs are essential for the normal development of the nervous system. Breastfed infants of mothers with two copies of the minor allele potentially face a risk of abnormal neurodevelopment. Since this initial research was published, findings connecting SNPs in the FADS encoding region with the fatty acid content of breast milk have been replicated on three occasions [45, 46]. Furthermore, the PUFA content of breast milk has now also been connected to SNPs in the regions containing the ELOVL-2 and -5 genes, which encode elongases [46]. It is reasonable to suppose that, as understanding of the metabolism of aliphatic acids moves forward and more genetic analyses are undertaken, there will emerge new associations between genetic variants and the fatty acid content of human milk. It does not appear currently that any group has studied the effect of dietary manipulation on breast milk composition in groups with different genetics, other than the study previously mentioned [45]. A knowledge of the effect that genetics plays in concert with dietary modifications to alter the composition of breast milk lays open the exciting possibility that breast milk quality can be improved as needed by nutrigenetic techniques [45].

8 Conclusion

The ideal way to feed an infant is by breastfeeding since breast milk delivers the full range of nutritional requirements and other molecules with beneficial biological activity needed for the infant to develop normally, including the nervous system. It has been shown several times that dietary modification in the mother while pregnant and lactating influences the quality of breast milk and hence affects how the child grows. This chapter has touched on both the nutrigenomics and nutrigenetic aspects of this problem, in other words, both how the mother's diet influences her expression of genes and how her genes affect the processing of nutrients.

References

1. Lefèvre CM, Sharp JA, Nicholas KR. Evolution of lactation: ancient origin and extreme adaptations of the lactation system. Annu Rev Genomics Hum Genet. 2010;11:219–38. https://doi.org/10.1146/annurev-genom-082509-141806.
2. Lemay DG, Lynn DJ, Martin WF, Neville MC, Casey TM, et al. The bovine lactation genome: insights into the evolution of mammalian milk. Genome Biol. 2009;10:R43.
3. Lefèvre CM, Sharp JA, Nicholas KR. Characterization of monotreme caseins reveals lineage-specific expansion of an ancestral casein locus in mammals. Reprod Fertil Dev. 2009;21:1015–27.
4. Andrechek ER, Mori S, Rempel RE, Chang JT, Nevins JR. Patterns of cell signaling pathway activation that characterize mammary development. Development. 2008;135:2403–13.
5. Lefèvre CM, Digby MR, Whitley JC, Strahm Y, Nicholas KR. Lactation transcriptomics in the Australian marsupial, Macropus eugenii: transcript sequencing and quantification. BMC Genomics. 2007;8:417.
6. Bird PH, Hendry KA, Shaw DC, Wilde CJ, Nicholas KR. Progressive changes in milk protein gene expression and prolactin binding during lactation in the tammar wallaby (Macropus eugenii). J Mol Endocrinol. 1994;13:117–25.
7. Oftedal OT. The origin of lactation as a water source for parchment-shelled eggs. J Mammary Gland Biol Neoplasia. 2002;7:253–66.
8. Sosa-Castillo E, Rodríguez-Cruz M, Moltó-Puigmartí C. Genomics of lactation: role of nutrigenomics and nutrigenetics in the fatty acid composition of human milk. Br J Nutr. 2017;118(3):161–8. https://doi.org/10.1017/S0007114517001854.
9. World Health Organization. Exclusive breastfeeding; 2011. http://www.who.int/nutrition/topics/exclusivebreastfeeding/en/. Accessed Jan 2022.
10. Hill DR, Newburg DS. Clinical applications of bio-active milk components. Nutr Rev. 2015;73:463–76.
11. Ballard O, Morrow AL. Human milk composition: nutrients and bioactive factors. Pediatr Clin N Am. 2013;60:49–74.
12. Bachour P, Yafawi R, Jaber F, et al. Effects of smoking, mother's age, body mass index, and parity number on lipid, protein, and secretory immunoglobulin A concentrations of human milk. Breastfeed Med. 2012;7:179–88.
13. Verduci E, Banderali G, Barberi S, et al. Epigenetic effects of human breast milk. Nutrients. 2014;24:1711–24.
14. Madsen O. Mammals (Mammalia). In: Kumar SB, editor. The Timetree of life. New York: Oxford Univ. Press; 2009. p. 459–61.

15. Richard C, Lewis ED, Field CJ. Evidence for the essentiality of arachidonic and docosahexaenoic acid in thepostnatal maternal and infant diet for the development of the infant's immune system early in life. Appl Physiol Nutr Metab. 2016;41:461–75.
16. Andreas NJ, Kampmann B, Mehring Le-Doare K. Human breast milk: a review on its composition and bio- activity. Early Hum Dev. 2015;91:629–35.
17. Mennitti LV, Oliveira JL, Morais CA, et al. Type of fatty acids in maternal diets during pregnancy and/or lactation and metabolic consequences of the offspring. J Nutr Biochem. 2015;26:99–111.
18. Fenech M, El-Sohemy A, Cahill L, et al. Nutrigenetics and nutrigenomics: viewpoints on the current status and applications in nutrition research and practice. J Nutrigenet Nutrigenomics. 2011;4:69–89.
19. Arendt LM, Kuperwasser C. Form and function: how estrogen and progesterone regulate the mammary epithelial hierarchy. J Mammary Gland Biol Neoplasia. 2015;20:9–25.
20. Riordan J. Anatomy and physiology of lactation. In: Wambach K, Riordan J, editors. Breastfeeding and human lactation. 4th ed. Boston, MA: Jones & Bartlett Learning; 2010. p. 79–86.
21. Golinelli LP, Del Aguila EM, Flosi Paschoalin VM, et al. Functional aspect of colostrum and whey proteins in human milk. J Hum Nutr Food Sci. 2014;2:1035.
22. Ibeagha-Awemu EM, Li R, Ammah AA, et al. Transcriptome adaptation of the bovine mammary gland to diets rich in unsaturated fatty acids shows greater impact of linseed oil over safflower oil on gene expression and metabolic pathways. BMC Genomics. 2016;17:104.
23. Capel F, Rolland-Valognes G, Dacquet C, et al. Analysis of sterol-regulatory element-binding protein 1c target genes in mouse liver during aging and high-fat diet. J Nutrigenet Nutrigenomics. 2013;6:107–22.
24. Neschen S, Morino K, Dong J, et al. N-3 fatty acids preserve insulin sensitivity in vivo in a peroxisome proliferator–activated receptor-alpha–dependent manner. Diabetes. 2007;56:1034–41.
25. Jump DB, Tripathy S, Depner CM. Fatty acid-regulated transcription factors in the liver. Annu Rev Nutr. 2013;33:249–69.
26. Rodriguez-Cruz M, Tovar AR, Palacios-Gonzalez B, et al. Synthesis of long-chain polyunsaturated fatty acids in lactating mammary gland: role of Delta5 and Delta6 desaturases, SREBP-1, PPAR alpha, and PGC-1. J Lipid Res. 2006;47:553–60.
27. Schennink A, Stoop WM, Visker MHPW, et al. Short communication: genome-wide scan for bovine milk-fat composition. II. Quantitative trait loci for long-chain fatty acids. J Dairy Sci. 2009;92:4676–82.
28. Stoop WM, Schennink A, Visker MH, et al. Genome-wide scan for bovine milk-fat composition. I. Quantitative trait loci for short- and medium-chain fatty acids. J Dairy Sci. 2009;92:4664–75.
29. Mele M, Conte G, Castiglioni B, et al. Stearoyl-coenzyme a desaturase gene polymorphism and milk fatty acid composition in Italian Holsteins. J Dairy Sci. 2007;90:4458–65.
30. Schennink A, Heck JM, Bovenhuis H, et al. Milk fatty acid unsaturation: genetic parameters and effects of stearoyl-CoA desaturase (SCD1) and acyl CoA: diacylglycerol acyltransferase 1 (DGAT1). J Dairy Sci. 2008;91:2135–43.
31. Conte G, Mele M, Chessa S, et al. Diacylglycerol acyl-transferase 1, stearoyl-CoA desaturase 1, and sterol regulatory element binding protein 1 gene polymorphisms and milk fatty acid composition in Italian Brown cattle. J Dairy Sci. 2010;93:753–63.
32. Nafikov RA, Schoonmaker JP, Korn KT, et al. Sterol regulatory element binding transcription factor 1 (SREBF1) polymorphism and milk fatty acid composition. J Dairy Sci. 2013;96:2605–16.
33. Marchitelli C, Contarini G, De Matteis G, et al. Milk fatty acid variability: effect of some candidate genes involved in lipid synthesis. J Dairy Res. 2013;80:165–73.
34. Nafikov RA, Schoonmaker JP, Korn KT, et al. Poly-morphisms in lipogenic genes and milk fatty acid composition in Holstein dairy cattle. Genomics. 2014;104:572–81.

35. Tăbăran A, Balteanu VA, Gal E, et al. Influence of DGAT1 K232A polymorphism on milk fat percentage and fatty acid profiles in Romanian Holstein cattle. Anim Biotechnol. 2015;26:105–11.
36. Ashes JR, Gulati SK, Scott TW. Potential to alter the content and composition of milk fat through nutrition. J Dairy Sci. 1997;80:2204–12.
37. Lock AL, Bauman DE. Modifying milk fat composition of dairy cows to enhance fatty acids beneficial to human health. Lipids. 2004;39:1197–206.
38. Lanier JS, Corl BA. Challenges in enriching milk fat with polyunsaturated fatty acids. J Anim Sci Biotechnol. 2015;6:26.
39. Schaeffer L, Gohlke H, Müller M, et al. Common genetic variants of the FADS1 FADS2 gene cluster and their reconstructed haplotypes are associated with the fatty acid composition in phospholipids. Hum Mol Genet. 2006;15:1745–56.
40. Malerba G, Schaeffer L, Xumerle L, et al. SNPs of the FADS gene cluster are associated with polyunsaturated fatty acids in a cohort of patients with cardiovascular disease. Lipids. 2008;43:289–99.
41. Martinelli N, Girelli D, Malerba G, et al. FADS geno- types and desaturase activity estimated by the ratio of arachidonic acid to linoleic acid are associated with inflammation and coronary artery disease. Am J Clin Nutr. 2008;88:941–9.
42. Rzehak P, Heinrich J, Klopp N, et al. Evidence for an association between genetic variants of the fatty acid desaturase 1 fatty acid desaturase 2 (FADS1 FADS2) gene cluster and the fatty acid composition of erythrocyte membranes. Br J Nutr. 2009;101:20–6.
43. Baylin A, Ruiz-Narvaez E, Kraft P, et al. Alpha-linolenic acid, Delta6-desaturase gene polymorphism, and the risk of nonfatal myocardial infarction. Am J Clin Nutr. 2007;85:554–60.
44. Xie L, Innis SM. Genetic variants of the FADS1 FADS2 gene cluster are associated with altered (n-6) and (n-3) essential fatty acids in plasma and erythrocyte phospholipids in women during pregnancy and in breast milk during lactation. J Nutr. 2008;138:2222–8.
45. Moltó-Puigmartí C, Plat J, Mensink RP, et al. FADS1 FADS2 gene variants modify the association between fish intake and the docosahexaenoic acid proportions in human milk. Am J Clin Nutr. 2010;91:1368–76.
46. Morales E, Bustamante M, González JR, et al. Genetic variants of the FADS gene cluster and ELOVL gene family colostrums LC-PUFA levels, breastfeeding, and child cognition. PLoS One. 2011;6:e17181.

Programming Molecules in Early Life

Özlem Naciye Şahin and Despina D. Briana

1 Introduction

Children whose mothers suffered from obesity, diabetes mellitus, or who had feeding difficulties face an increased risk of metabolic disorders, research has shown [1, 2]. Furthermore, being bottle fed or starting supplementary formula milk at an early stage may result in obesity as a child and adult [3, 4]. This research also indicates that the mother's diet plays a role in how metabolism is programmed in her offspring. Children who consume a diet with excessive amounts of lipids and proteins from an early age may lay down more fat and have an increased body mass index (BMI). A diet very rich in protein may result in raised insulin levels, which can cause insulin insensitivity. Since blood glucose also increases as a consequence of raised insulin, lipogenesis is stimulated. Infant birth weight and a maternal diet with high macronutrient levels were found to be significantly correlated [5–8].

Within developed countries, the incidence of obesity has undergone a dramatic rise, such that obesity now represents a major public health concern, since there is expected to be a greatly increased demand for healthcare as a result. It has recently been calculated that over one in three individuals within the USA qualify as obese in adulthood, whilst in the UK, more than 50% of adults are over the recommended BMI. Obesity acts to increase the risk of developing related problems with metabolism, namely diabetes mellitus type 2, circulatory disorders, high blood pressure, and osteoarthritis. The aetiology of these metabolic complications involves multiple factors related to both genetics and the environment [1].

Ö. N. Şahin (✉)
Department of Child Health and Diseases, Arel University, Medical Faculty, Istanbul, Türkiye

D. D. Briana
NICU, Third Department of Pediatrics, National and Kapodistrian University of Athens, University General Hospital "ATTIKON", Athens, Greece

121

Ö. N. Şahin et al. (eds.), *Breastfeeding and Metabolic Programming*, https://doi.org/10.1007/978-3-031-33278-4_11

Research employing an observational methodological design indicates that individuals whose diet contains elevated levels of protein are prone to obesity in adulthood. When breast milk is compared with typical artificial baby milk (formula), it can be seen that breast milk contains between 60 and 70% lower levels of protein, with a calorific value 10–18% less than formula. Intervening at an early stage in life to correct dietary problems appears necessary if the metabolic disease in later life is to be prevented. Two studies both found that disorders affecting the circulation, such as diabetes mellitus type 2, advanced hypertension and hypercholesterolaemia were less common in individuals who had been breast fed [8, 9]. Research on both humans and other mammalian species leads to the conclusion that there are biologically active molecules in human milk which ensure the infant develops optimally, with a robust immune system and a balanced metabolism. Because of these findings, both the WHO (World Health Organization) and UNICEF offer the recommendation that, up to the age of 6 months, all infants should be exclusively breast fed, that other food may begin from 6 months onward, but that breast feeding should continue up to the second birthday or beyond [9–11].

2 Programming the Growth of Infants and Their Appetite During the Perinatal Period

Prior to birth, the foetus grows in response to the supply of nutrients from the mother and according to maternal hormonal levels. The initial stage in embryological development involves cellular differentiation and organogenesis. Although the first stage is the most dramatic, the third trimester is when the maximum increase in size occurs. During the last 3 months of foetal development, insulin and IGF-1 are vital to regulating growth and the maintenance of stable glucose levels. The factors controlling appetite in the final trimester also include changes within the immediate environment surrounding the foetus. Following birth, the circulating level of molecules which sense the presence of nutrients, such as L-citrulline, rises following feeding. The offspring of mothers whose diet was rich in lipids whilst pregnant and lactating demonstrate raised levels of Agouti-related peptide and AMP-activated protein kinase, the effect of which is to stimulate appetite in the presence of L-citrulline. It has also been proven that the type of diet followed by the mother also influences the activity of the hypothalamic-pituitary axis, resulting in an increase in neuropeptide Y and Agouti-related peptide levels, which influences the way the infant manages the input of nutrients. In fact, these increases stimulate appetite to the level where obesity becomes a risk and hypothalamic dysregulation occurs, with low levels of proopiomelanocortins. Experiments on mice have demonstrated that an excess of nutrients in early life produces leptin resistance and a change in response to insulin. The individual tends to eat excessive levels of fat. Raised leptin in the period following birth has effects on orexigenesis through an effect on hypothalamic connectivity. Gupta was able to show that maternal intake which was rich in fats prior to conception and during pregnancy resulted in elevated levels of both leptin and insulin, which altered the foetal hypothalamic propensity to stimulate the release of peptide signals for appetite and satiety. The net result is believed to be that, following birth, the child overeats and becomes obese. The breastfed offspring of mothers with obesity grow rapidly and gain weight quickly following birth. This swift increase in body mass appears to be a risk factor for becoming obese later in life [12–16].

The association between the pattern of child growth and the development of disease was established by Wells, who noted the difference between the concepts of 'metabolic capacity' occurring in homeostasis and 'metabolic load', the latter influenced by an overly calorific diet and sedentary lifestyle. In the mother, the physiological processes needed to ensure the growth of the foetus may be affected where the metabolic capacity is exceeded by the metabolic load. In considering where this is likely to occur, it is important to consider the maternal body characteristics, since the same mismatch will also affect her phenotypical appearance [17].

Barker et al. [18] were the first to suggest that somehow the metabolic circumstances pertaining before birth played a role in programming metabolic problems later in life. The observation that a low weight at birth was strongly associated with the subsequent development of circulatory disease and diabetes mellitus type 2 as an adult prompted this suggestion [19, 20]. Since then, a number of studies with a retrospective methodology have confirmed that the risk of metabolic disorders in adulthood is tied to early life events [21, 22]. From such studies, there has arisen the 'thrifty phenotype' hypothesis, according to which foetal metabolic programming and the establishment of a metabolic type in early life set the stage for metabolic disorders in adulthood. According to this way of thinking, any foetal adversity resulting from an inadequate nutritional environment in utero (such as occurs with an undernourished mother) results in metabolic reprogramming. When, at a later stage in life, nutrients become available in surplus, there is a risk that this reprogrammed metabolism will result in a metabolic syndrome [20]. It is now increasingly clear, however, that if the mother eats too much whilst pregnant, this also predisposes to faulty metabolism, in this case, high birth weight and obesity. When the risk of becoming an obese adult and suffering from a metabolic syndrome is plotted against the weight at birth, a U-shaped curve result, indicating that risk arises at both extremes of the birth weight range [23].

Control of orexigenesis occurs within the hypothalamus, a system that develops early in foetal life. Whether the mother's diet is hypo- or hypercaloric, the consequence is an alteration in the orexigenic mechanism. The hypothalamus is a key area where maternal nutritional imbalance exerts long-term effects that can result in metabolic dysequilibrium. Within the hypothalamus, epigenetic modifications occur to several genes of importance in metabolic regulation. The rest of this chapter will review the latest evidence confirming the role of the hypothalamus in resetting the metabolism to produce an obese individual, plus consider what effect epigenetic modifications have in producing an abnormal phenotype in the children of mothers whose own nutritional balance was disturbed [24, 25].

2.1 Neuronal Circuitry Within the Hypothalamus Responsible for Regulating Energy Balance

There is a central mechanism controlling energy balance within the body, mostly under hypothalamic control. The key region in which the neuronal circuitry is located in the arcuate nucleus (ARC), although some of the control is exercised in the hypothalamic paraventricular nucleus (PVN) and the dorsomedial hypothalamus (DMH). The ARC is located in proximity to the median eminence and the third ventricle. It may be referred to as the 'feeding centre'. Within this part of the central nervous system, the blood-brain barrier is more permeable than elsewhere, which permits circulating endocrine messenger molecules to enter. There are neurones with a proappetite action (orexigenic) and an antiappetite action (anorexigenic). Both categories of neurone release peptide signalling molecules, and it is the overall balance between these signals that largely controls how many calories the individual consumes or expends and thus what the eventual body mass is [1].

There are projections formed by neurones within the ARC expressing proopiomelanocortin (POMC) and either Agouti-related peptide (AGP) or neuropeptide Y (NPY) toward the hypothalamic paraventricular nucleus (PVN). This circuitry regulates dietary intake and manages energy balance. The activity of these neurones is modulated by glucocorticoids, leptin, and insulin.

Key to abbreviations used in figure: *ARC* Arcuate nucleus, *AgRP* Agouti-related peptide, *GCs* Glucocorticoids, *GR* Glucocorticoid receptor, *IR* Insulin receptor, *LepR* Leptin receptor, *MC4R* melanocortin 4 receptor, *α-MSH* α melanocyte stimulating hormone, *NPY* Neuropeptide Y, *POMC* Pro-opiomelanocortin, *PVN* Paraventricular nucleus, *Y1/Y5* Y1 and Y5 receptors, *3V* Third Ventricle.

3 Anorexigenic Neurones of the Arcuate Nucleus

Within the arcuate nucleus, those expressing proopiomelanocortin (POMC) have been the subject of most scientific scrutiny, since these neurones, besides producing POMC, also express the cocaine and amphetamine-regulated transcript (CART). The latter plays a role in reducing the consumption of calories. Virtually all the POMC neurones are found within the ARC, whence they send out projections to the paraventricular and lateral hypothalamic regions plus the brainstem. All these regions play a role in regulating the balance of energy [1] (see Fig. 1).

The POMC molecule undergoes cleavage at various points, resulting in the formation of a number of important signalling peptides, especially adrenocorticotrophic hormone (ACTH), beta-endorphin, and alpha-melanocyte-stimulating hormone (α-MSH). The majority of studies of anorexigenic signals in the ARC have focused on the role played by α-MSH. This neuropeptide has agonistic action on the hypothalamic melanocortin 3 and melanocortin 4 receptors (MC3R and MC4R). The MC3R and MC4R are abundant on second-order neurones located within the

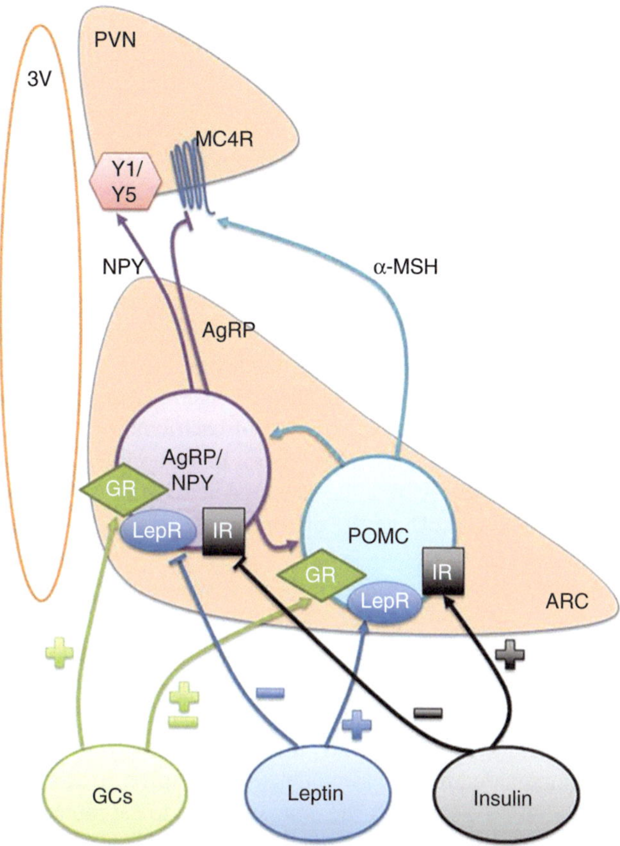

Fig. 1 Neuroendocrine circuitry responsible for energy balance. (Adopted from reference [1])

PVN. Stimulation of these receptors results in decreased appetite and higher utilisation of energy. Genetic knock-out studies have been helpful in elucidating the role played by POMC. In a murine model, complete removal of the POMC gene results in an animal that eats to excess and attains an abnormally high BMI. Moreover, loss of either type of melanocortin receptor results in obesity and increased adiposity. It has also been demonstrated in humans that mutated POMC alleles result in obesity. It is thus clear that POMC and the products derived from it play a part in decreasing appetite and lowering BMI [1, 26].

There is one more signalling molecule within the ARC which has an important role in decreasing appetite, namely, CART. It is not fully understood yet which receptors the molecule acts on, which has meant fewer studies have so far been undertaken [27]. The same neurones which express POMC also express CART, and the effects of appetite and greater energy utilisation are comparable. However, CART, unlike POMC, is expressed in multiple locations both within the CNS and elsewhere in the body. In a murine model where the CART gene was knocked out, the animals ate excessively and gained abnormal weight, as predicted. It appears that CART also regulates energy balance in the body [1, 28].

4   Neurones of Orexigenic Type within the ARC

There are also neurones located in the ARC which increase appetite (orexigenesis). The main signals they express are neuropeptide Y, Agouti-related peptide, and gamma-aminobutyric acid (GABA). Projections from the orexigenic neurones go to the PVN, the dorsomedial hypothalamic nucleus, the perifornical region, the lateral hypothalamus, and the medial preoptic region [1, 29].

A study which has recently been published revealed that all of these regions play a role. The method consisted of the deletion of each component separately. This then showed that NPY, AgRP, and GABA work in synergy to regulate appetite. If the entire orexigenic neurone within the ARC is deleted after the mouse is born, the animal fails to eat and dies. Thus, the orexigenic neurones appear to be vital for orexgenesis to occur [1, 30].

AgRP exerts an antagonistic effect on the melanocortin 4 receptor, where it can prevent stimulation of the receptor by α-MSH. This then results in greater expression of appetite. If AgRP is deleted at the neuronal level in a murine model, there are only very minor changes in the appearance of the animal and any effects only appear as the mouse ages. From the age of 6 months onward, mice lacking neuronal AgRP show decreased BMI in association with greater use of energy. Interestingly, despite the relatively undramatic effect of gene deletion of AgRP, if extraneous AgRP is injected directly into the ventricles, the animal begins to eat more and this change lasts up to 7 days. The latest studies using genetic modification techniques point to the fact that AgRP has a long term, rather than short term, effect on the tendency to eat more [1, 31, 32].

The mechanism through which neuropeptide Y affects appetite and energy balance is through acting on the hypothalamic receptors Y1 and Y5 [30]. This mechanism was elucidated by a rodent animal model involving the injection of NPY into the ventricles, after which the animals began steadily eating for several hours. When this procedure was repeated over the course of subsequent days, the animals continued to feed more than usual, to gain body mass and to lay down fat. When an antisense oligonucleotide to NPY was injected, feeding decreased and the rodents lost body mass. It is unclear exactly why animals in whom the NPY gene has been deleted still eat normally and attain a usual body mass, in addition to responding to 48 hours of fasting normally, although it suggests that there exist other signalling mechanisms operating when NPY fails.

In addition to NPY and AgRP, the neurones promoting appetite also release GABA. Research which made use of modified receptors that were activated only by a specially altered molecule produced evidence that GABA and NPY act in comparable ways. GABA can affect the beginning of the feeding and replace NPY. Thus,

GABA, NPY, and AgRP secreted by orexigenic neurones in the ARC all act to promote extra feeding [33, 34].

5 Glucocorticoids as a Regulator of Appetite

Glucocorticoids are a class of steroid hormones released by the adrenals in response to stimulation by the hypothalamo-pituitary-adrenal axis. Their function includes regulating orexigenesis in addition to conserving energy balance. These hormones bind to the glucocorticoid receptor, leading to a series of events beginning with the steroid-receptor complex binding to the glucocorticoid response elements (GREs) within the genomic DNA. The GREs are located in the promoter segments leading to the genes encoding AgRP and NPY [1, 35].

Murine models of weight gain indicate that glucocorticoids result in raised appetite and higher body mass index. This result occurs whether corticosterone (metabolically active) or 17-deoxy cortisone is administered. Metabolic syndrome and Cushing's syndrome could both be artificially induced in this manner. Both clinical conditions involve elevated glucocorticoid levels and excessive eating. Furthermore, in clinical practice, where synthetic glucocorticoids are administered long term, the side effects also resemble these conditions. If the adrenals are excised from rodents who have a genetic predisposition to obesity, resulting in a state where no glucocorticoids are naturally present, the animals lose body mass and eat less [1, 27].

6 Conclusion

There is an overwhelming volume of evidence to show that adverse metabolic conditions in early life can cause metabolism to be reprogrammed in the long term, predisposing some individuals to obesity and metabolic syndromes. The reason for this may relate to epigenetic modifications. If the mother has an unbalanced diet (excess or insufficiency of macronutrients), there occur epigenetic modifications to the genes responsible for appetite and energy use. These genes are located in neurones that form the hypothalamic circuitry controlling metabolism. A corollary of this is that the rising number of obese patients may be partially due to malnutrition in early life. When these imbalances occur and how severe they are also affect the pathophysiology. In other words, not only what we ourselves eat, but also what our mothers ate influences our current metabolism. There is still a great deal to be learned about the role of external factors, such as nutrient levels, on epigenetic modifications and more research is needed. Nonetheless, since it appears that epigenetic changes can be reset, targeted interventions to achieve this goal may play a key role in future in overcoming the obesity epidemic.

References

1. Gali Ramamoorthy T, Begum G, Harno E, White A. Developmental programming of hypothalamic neuronal circuits: impact on energy balance control. Front Neurosci. 2015;21(9):126. https://doi.org/10.3389/fnins.2015.00126.
2. Fields DA, George B, Williams M, Whitaker K, Allison D, Teague A, Demerath EW. Associations between human breast milk hormones and adipocytokines and infant growth and body composition in the first six months of life. Pediatr Obes. 2017;12(Suppl 1):S78–85.
3. Alfaradhi MZ, Ozanne SE. Developmental programming in response to maternal overnutrition. Front Genet. 2011;3(2):27.
4. Ley S, O'Connor D, Retnakaran R, Hamilton J, Sermer M, Zinman B. Impact of maternal metabolic abnormalities in pregnancy on human milk and subsequent infant metabolic development: methodolgy and design. BioMed Central Public Health. 2010;10(1):590.
5. Wen X, Triche EW, Hogan JW, et al. Prenatal factors for childhood blood pressure mediated by intrauterine and/or childhood growth. Pediatrics. 2011;127(1):713–21.
6. McCurdy CE, Bishop JM, Williams SM, Grayson BE, Smith MS, Friedman JE. Maternal high fat diet triggers lipotoxicity in the fetal livers of nonhuman pirmates. J Clin Investig. 2009;119(2):323–35.
7. Rolland-Cachera M, Deeeger M, Akrout M, Bellisle F. Influence of macronutrients on adiposity development. A follow up study of nutrition and growth from 10 months to 8 years of age. J Int Assoc Study Obes. 1995;19(8):573–8.
8. Dewey KG. Is breastfeeding protective against child obesity? J Hum Lact. 2003;19(1):9–18.
9. Haschke F, Steenhout P, Grathwohl D, Haschke-Becher E. Evaluation of growth and early infant feeding: a challenge for scientists, industry and regulatory bodies. World Rev Nutr Diet. 2013;6:33–8.
10. Harding J. The nutritional basis of the fetal origins of adult disease. Int J Epidemiol. 2001;30(1):15–23.
11. World Health organisation (WHO). 2015 http://www.who.int/nutrition.
12. Coupe B, Amarger V, Grit I, Benani A, Parnet P. Nutritional programming affects hypothalamic organization and early response to leptin. Endocrinology. 2010;151(2):702–13.
13. Stark R, Ashley SE, Andrews ZB. AMPK and the neuroendocrine regulation of apetite and energy expenditure. Mol Cell Endocrinol. 2013;366(2):215–23.
14. Glavas MM, Kirigiti MA, Xiao XQ, Enriori PJ, Fisher SK, Evans AE. Early overnutrition results in early onset arcuate leptin resistance and increased sensitivity to high fat diet. Endocrinology. 2010;151(4):1598–610.
15. Gupta A, Srinivasan M, Thamadilok E, et al. Hypathalamic alterations in fetuses of high fat dşet-fed obese female rats. J Endcorinol. 2009;200:293–300.
16. Johnstone L, Higuchi T. Food intake and leptin during pregnancy and lactation. Prog Brain Res. 2001;133:215–27.
17. Wells J. Maternal capital and the metabolic ghetto: an evolutionary perspective on transgenerational basis of health inequalities. Am J Hum Biol. 2010;22:1–17.
18. Barker DJ. The developmental origins of insulin resistance. Horm Res. 2005;64(Suppl. 3):2–7. https://doi.org/10.1159/000089311.
19. Barker DJ, Gluckman PD, Godfrey KM, Harding JE, Owens JA, Robinson JS. Fetal nutrition and cardiovascular disease in adult life. Lancet. 1993;341:938–41. https://doi.org/10.1016/0140-6736(93)91224-A.
20. Hales CN, Barker DJ, Clark PM, Cox LJ, Fall C, Osmond C, et al. Fetal and infant growth and impaired glucose tolerance at age 64. BMJ. 1991;303:1019–22. https://doi.org/10.1136/bmj.303.6809.1019.
21. Ravelli AC, van Der Meulen JH, Osmond C, Barker DJ, Bleker OP. Obesity at the age of 50 y in men and women exposed to famine prenatally. Am J Clin Nutr. 1999;70:811–6.
22. Ravelli GP, Stein ZA, Susser MW. Obesity in young men after famine exposure *in utero* and early infancy. N Engl J Med. 1976;295:349–53. https://doi.org/10.1056/NEJM197608122950701.

23. Pettitt DJ, Jovanovic L. Birth weight as a predictor of type 2 diabetes mellitus: the U-shaped curve. Curr Diab Rep. 2001;1:78–81. https://doi.org/10.1007/s11892-001-0014-x.
24. Ross MG, Desai M. Developmental programming of appetite/satiety. Ann Nutr Metab. 2014;64(Suppl. 1):36–44. https://doi.org/10.1159/000360508.
25. Stevens A, Begum G, White A. Epigenetic changes in the hypothalamic pro-opiomelanocortin gene: a mechanism linking maternal undernutrition to obesity in the offspring? Eur J Pharmacol. 2011;660:194–201. https://doi.org/10.1016/j.ejphar.2010.10.111.
26. Challis BG, Pritchard LE, Creemers JW, Delplanque J, Keogh JM, Luan J, et al. A missense mutation disrupting a dibasic prohormone processing site in pro-opiomelanocortin (POMC) increases susceptibility to early-onset obesity through a novel molecular mechanism. Hum Mol Genet. 2002;11:1997–2004. https://doi.org/10.1093/hmg/11.17.1997.
27. Morgan SA, McCabe EL, Gathercole LL, Hassan-Smith ZK, Larner DP, Bujalska IJ, et al. 11beta-HSD1 is the major regulator of the tissue-specific effects of circulating glucocorticoid excess. Proc Natl Acad Sci U S A. 2014;111:E2482–91. https://doi.org/10.1073/pnas.1323681111.
28. Kasacka I, Janiuk I, Lewandowska A, Bekisz A, Lebkowski W. Distribution pattern of CART-containing neurons and cells in the human pancreas. Acta Histochem. 2012;114:695–9.
29. Karatsoreos IN, Bhagat SM, Bowles NP, Weil ZM, Pfaff DW, McEwen BS. Endocrine and physiological changes in response to chronic corticosterone: a potential model of the metabolic syndrome in mouse. Endocrinology. 2010;151:2117–27. https://doi.org/10.1210/en.2009-1436.
30. Luquet S, Perez FA, Hnasko TS, Palmiter RD. NPY/AgRP neurons are essential for feeding in adult mice but can be ablated in neonates. Science. 2005;310:683–5. https://doi.org/10.1126/science.1115524.
31. Mahmood S, Smiraglia DJ, Srinivasan M, Patel MS. Epigenetic changes in hypothalamic appetite regulatory genes may underlie the developmental programming for obesity in rat neonates subjected to a high-carbohydrate dietary modification. J Dev Orig Health Dis. 2013;4:479–90. https://doi.org/10.1056/NEJM199602013340503.
32. Corander MP, Rimmington D, Challis BG, O'Rahilly S, Coll AP. Loss of agouti-related peptide does not significantly impact the phenotype of murine POMC deficiency. Endocrinology. 2011;152:1819–28. https://doi.org/10.1210/en.2010-1450.
33. Erickson JC, Hollopeter G, Palmiter RD. Attenuation of the obesity syndrome of Ob/Ob mice by the loss of neuropeptide Y. Science. 1996;274:1704–7. https://doi.org/10.1126/science.274.5293.1704.
34. Farooqi IS, Drop S, Clements A, Keogh JM, Biernacka J, Lowenbein S, et al. Heterozygosity for a POMC-null mutation and increased obesity risk in humans. Diabetes. 2006;55:2549–53. https://doi.org/10.2337/db06-0214.
35. Lee B, Kim SG, Kim J, Choi KY, Lee S, Lee SK, et al. Brain- specific homeobox factor as a target selector for glucocorticoid receptor in energy balance. Mol Cell Biol. 2013;33:2650–8. https://doi.org/10.1128/MCB.00094-13.

The Part Breast Milk Plays in Epigenetic Programming

Özlem Naciye Şahin

1 Introduction

For mammals, following birth, the source of their entire nutrition is milk. Milk provides a transition between placental nutrition and an adult diet. Weaning is the stage of moving onto an adult diet. Evolutionary pressures in mammals have led to milk which performs many complex functions, displays dynamic characteristics and enables molecular signalling to occur. Thus, breast milk can optimally support the infant's growth needs [1]. The nutritional environment at this early stage creates epigenetic modifications which may programme metabolism in a way that predisposes individuals in the longer term to metabolic disorders [2]. Detailed research in recent years has shown that micro-RNA (miRNA) transcripts may function in cell-to-cell molecular signalling [3–5]. These transcripts consist of RNA sequences with a typical length of around 20 nucleotides. They are highly conserved within phyla. A miRNA sequence binds to a matching messenger RNA (mRNA) sequence, preventing the mRNA being translated into the protein for which it encodes [6]. A new approach makes use of miRNA as a diagnostic probe, allowing identification of targets and visualisation [7]. Milk is secreted by lactocytes in the mammary gland as a fluid containing an unusually large volume of both RNA and miRNA [8]. The miRNAs are encased within an exosomic protective vesicle encased by a lipid bilayer and measuring around 100 nm in diameter. This extracellular vesicle is excreted by the lactocyte [9]. miRNA is thus transported and may be taken up into the infant's cells by the process of endocytosis [10–12]. The exosomes within both breast milk and milk from other mammals, such as cows, act therefore to permit genetic material to enter the body of the infant or whoever else consumes the milk.

Ö. N. Şahin (✉)
Department of Child Health and Diseases, Arel University, Medical Faculty, Istanbul, Türkiye

Ö. N. Şahin et al. (eds.), *Breastfeeding and Metabolic Programming*,
https://doi.org/10.1007/978-3-031-33278-4_12

131

It is regrettable that the epigenetic modification that can be achieved by breast milk through transfer of miRNA is not possible for infants fed using artificial baby milk. However, there is some contamination of the food chain caused by human consumption of cows' milk, and it seems that the efforts to increase the amount of milk cows can produce for human consumption is also exposing consumers to greater amounts of bovine miRNA [13, 14]. This ongoing exposure of human consumers to bovine genetic signals may risk inducing epigenetic modifications that predispose to severe chronic metabolic problems including obesity and diabetes mellitus type 2.

2 Milk Exosomes

Exosomes contained in breast milk are amongst the most essential ways for the mother–infant dyad to communicate during breastfeeding [15]. The initial isolation and characterisation of exosomes in human colostrum and breast milk was undertaken by Admyre et al. [16]. Following this study, milk exosomes have been noted to occur in the colostrum and mature milk of a number of mammals apart from humans, in particular the cow, buffalo, goat, pig, *Macropus eugenii* (a wallaby, i.e. marsupial mammal) and rodents [17–19]. Exosomes in milk either enter milk directly from lactocytes or enter via the cytoplasmic crescents within the fat globules, which appear to contain exosomes [20]. The miRNA that occurs at the highest level, miRNA-148a, is a significant ingredient in skimmed milk, both as globules and within exosomes [21–23].

3 How Well Do Milk Exosomes Survive Passage Through the Gut?

There is increasing evidence to show that milk exosomes are not degraded within the gut. The exosome performs an important function in protecting miRNA and ensuring it can be delivered in a stable form to the infant. Exogenous, artificially produced miRNA is broken down by the unfavourable conditions within the gut, but miRNAs performing immune functions and protected within exosomes survive much better [21]. When commercially produced cows' milk was examined, the milk miRNA remains stable when subjected to acid exposure, RNAse degradation or freezing, but did break down when detergents were applied or bacteria were permitted to ferment the milk [22, 24].

4   Biological Availability of miRNA Derived from Milk

The bioavailability of miRNAs derived from cows' milk was at the level of biological significance when consumed at a level typical of a normal diet by human volunteers, as evidenced by the altered genetic expression within circulating polymorphonucleocytes [25]. In another study, piglets were fed either colostrum or mature sow milk. Colostrum contained higher levels of miRNAs of immunological significance and piglets receiving this type of milk had higher circulating levels of the miRNAs in question. Thus, bioavailability depends on dose [20]. In newly born wallabies (*M. eugenii*) the circulating levels of particular miRNAs known to be secreted in milk are significantly higher than in adult animals, which supports the idea the miRNAs in the circulation have been absorbed from ingested milk [26]. A study which combined genomics with a computerised analysis concluded that transfer of miRNAs from milk to the plasma probably occurred [27]. When mice were force-fed each day with cows' milk containing exosomes labelled by a fluorescent probe, the label was detectable both in the ileal epithelium and in the cells of the spleen [28]. In a recent paper, Manca et al. demonstrated the bioavailability of bovine milk exosomes tagged with a fluorescent probe, using a murine model [29, 30]. A significant finding was that some of the exosomes were absorbed without any change in their packaging. There was hepatic and splenic accumulation of the milk-derived exosomes. In research investigating the fate of exosomes in the diet using a murine model, exosomes in bovine milk containing RNA to which a red-coloured GLOW label was attached were noted in central nervous, renal, pulmonary and hepatic tissues, leading the authors to the conclusion that RNA in the diet can ultimately reach tissues at distant sites in the body [29, 30].

5   Artificial Baby Milk Is Low in miRNAs

Cows' milk which had undergone sterilisation and evaporation to render it suitable for feeding infants first entered the market in 1929. Doctors in the 1920s saw breast milk as a food just like any other, and many mothers soon took up the option to feed their infants formula rather than rely on breastfeeding [31, 32]. Until more recently, it was unknown that breast milk could function to pass miRNAs from the mother to the neonate. At present, artificial milk lacks the majority of miRNAs found in breast milk. Thus, formula milk does not offer the protective benefits that breast milk does in terms of immunity and programming of the metabolism [12]. When Chen et al. compared artificial baby milk with untreated bovine milk, they noted the formula milk contained only a tenth as many miRNA-148a sequences as the unpasteurised milk [33]. This finding of depleted miRNAs in powder-form artificial baby milk was also noted by Golan-Gerstl et al. [34].

6 Homologous Features of miRNA Shared by Different Species

There is considerable preservation of miRNA sequences and seed sequences between different mammalian species, which is especially clear in the case of miRNA-148a-3p, as has been demonstrated in recent research [35]. Thus, the miRNA signals in mammals appear to go back far into the evolutionary past. The seed sequences for miRNA-148a-3p are the same in both cows and humans. The base pairing between the heptameric seed sequence and the complementary mRNA sequence on the DNMT1 messenger RNA transcript is very strong. If a miRNA sequence binds weakly to an mRNA sequence, inhibition of mRNA translation occurs, but if the base pairs match up exactly, the mRNA is disassembled by the cellular machinery [4]. It seems likely that consumption of miRNA-148a-3p leads to downregulation of DNMT1 mRNA expression and thus its gene product.

The p53 transcription factor performs such an important role that it is sometimes referred to as a genomic guardian [36]. There is close control on how the p53 gene (TP53) is expressed both at the level of transcription and after the mRNA has been translated [28, 37, 38]. A number of miRNAs present in large quantities in milk [20, 21, 24] act to downgrade mRNA transcribed from the TP53 gene, namely miRNA-125b, miRNA-30d and miRNA-25 [28, 37, 38]. The function of miRNA-125b in regulating p53 exhibits preservation of molecular interactions for all members of the subphylum Vertebrata [24]. Rather surprisingly, there are no differences between humans and cows in the seed sequence of this particular miRNA.

7 How Genes Involved in Development Are Activated Through CpG Demethylation of DNA

7.1 FTO

Since milk provides the entire nutritional requirements of the developing infant, it is to be expected that it will contain some mechanism capable of directing the transcribing and translating of appropriate genes. There is indirect evidence suggesting that breast milk can activate the FTO enzyme (fat mass and obesity-associated protein), which controls transcription. It can also activate translation under the control of mTORC1 (mechanistic target of rapamycin complex 1). FTO is an enzyme which catalyses the demethylation of N^6-methyladenosine (m^6A) contained in messenger RNA sequences. Messenger RNA bearing m^6A is found in many cellular processes and greatly influences the composition of the transcriptome in eukaryotic cells. It regulates the splicing, export, addressing, translation and stabilisation of mRNA. M^6A methylation/demethylation has a role in many processes under the control of RNA, such as development, circadian cycles and resetting of the programmed cellular function. Typically, RNA bearing m^6A is thought to inhibit the expression of particular genes and thus formation of the gene product. The m⁶A modification is most common on stop codons as well as on the three prime untranslated regions. These sequences are targeted by members of the human YTH domain family 2 (YTHDF2) in the course of selecting which mRNAs should be degraded. The modification also prevents mRNA from attaching to human antigen R (HuR) which increases the stability of mRNA [27, 39–47].

A mutated allele for m⁶A demethylase FTO resulting in a non-functional protein causes humans with the mutation to have delayed growth following birth. Similarly, when the FTO gene was silenced in a murine model, the animals put on less weight, exhibited metabolic changes and had delayed growth. On the other hand, when the FTO gene was overexpressed, also in a murine model, the mice gained weight and laid down more fat in proportion to the degree of overexpression. These changes were related to the animals overfeeding and eventually becoming obese. Thus, it seems clear that growth following birth and energy balance fall under the vital control of FTO. In mice with the overexpressed FTO gene, the numbers of RNA sequences with an m⁶A modification were reduced overall. There are already associations known between SNPs within the initial intron of the FTO gene and raised BMI, fat deposition and development of diabetes mellitus type 2. The FTO protein is overactive both in individuals with specific SNPs and in cases where there has occurred an epigenetic modification of the gene as a result of CpG demethylation at certain points within the initial intron. Certain miRNAs found within exosomes in milk, specifically miRNA-148a, miRNA-152, miRNA-21 and miRNA-29 s, potentially fulfil a key function in epigenetic modification of the FTO gene by blocking CpG demethylation at key points on the gene. This then means FTO expression goes up and more of the mRNA can be transcribed [48–60].

7.2 Nuclear Factor Erythroid 2-Related Factor 2 (NRF2)

The actions of FTO occur in close conjunction with those of mTORC1, a kinase whose function alters depending on nutrient levels. mTORC1 increases translation and anabolism in response to milk. It becomes activated in the presence of leucine, in particular, through the action of another enzyme, leucyl-tRNA synthase. FTO participates in the activation. In particular, the activity of mTORC1 in response to high levels of amino acids can only occur due to FTO-related demethylation events. Thus, the fact that components of milk modify how the FTO gene is expressed through epigenetic modifications means that this mechanism also has downstream effects on the activity of mTORC1.

Furthermore, there are other epigenetically mediated ways in which milk affects the activity of mTORC1, including translation of mRNA. Another transcription factor, the behaviour of which is controlled epigenetically, is nuclear factor erythroid 2-related factor 2 (NRF2). When the DNA methyltransferase enzyme is inhibited, NRF2 activity rose, both in terms of mRNA transcripts produced and gene products synthesised. This effect was mediated through NRF2 demethylating DNA. NRF2 can directly activate transcription of the MTOR gene. This gene encodes the core protein contained within the mTORC1 and 2 molecular complexes. NRF2 also stimulates RagD, a low molecular weight G-protein that makes mTORC1 more active. Furthermore, miRNA-29 production goes up under the influence of NRF2, resulting in a downgraded level of DNMT3B. This last event acts as positive feed forward for epigenetic modifications enhancing the expression of NRF2 [36, 61–70].

7.3 The Insulin Gene (INS)

Insulin plays a major role in stimulating anabolic metabolism through signals regulated by PI3K-mTORC1. Following consumption of milk, the circulating insulin level rises. Transcription of the INS (insulin) gene is controlled by methylation of the DNA sequence encoding for the gene. According to Kuroda et al., the demethylated INS is expressed in pancreatic beta cells, whilst methylated copies of the gene remain unexpressed [66, 68]. In cells synthesising insulin, the INS promoter region in particular is demethylated. Indeed the CpG demethylation of this region of the gene appears essential for the beta cell to fully differentiate and for insulin to be expressed only within a certain tissue. Accordingly, miRNAs which downregulate the activity of DNMT, namely miRNA-148a, miRNA-21 and miRNA-29s and which originate in milk may exert control over the activity of mTORC1 on translation and anabolism (see Fig. 2). This suggestion is supported by recent evidence showing that, in mice, miRNA-29a positively regulates the release of insulin in vivo [69].

7.4 Insulin-like Growth Factor-1 (IGF1)

Insulin-like growth factor-1 (IGF1) acts in a similar manner to insulin. It is the most potent factor controlling growth and acts by stimulating the mTORC1 signalling pathway [65–73]. A diet containing milk results in a significant rise in the circulating IGF1 level. Children who drink bovine milk attain a greater height. Ouni et al. [72] undertook a study investigating the effect of CpG methylation on the promoter regions for IGF1 (i.e. P1 and P2), since they already knew that this gene is responsible for growth following birth. They wondered if demethylation could account for the different levels of IGF1 seen in the plasma of children as they grow. Results showed that, where six particular CpGs, which occur proximally in the P2 region, were methylated, the circulating IGF1 level and the child's growth were both lower. The level of transcription occurring at the P2 region in the circulating polymorphonucleocytes of patients who are administered growth hormone has a negative association with the degree of CpG methylation in that region of the gene [65–73].

The cumulative evidence from transcriptomic studies points to the conclusion that miRNAs in milk play a normal role in increasing the activity of signals which themselves activate mTORC1, namely mTOR, FTO, insulin and IGF1. The miR-NAs achieve this through influencing epigenetic modification by (de)methylation.

7.5 *Caveolin 1 (CAV1)*

This molecule is a protein embedded in a microdomain of the plasma membrane. It can modify signals depending on the context in which they occur. CAV1 has inter-actions with the insulin and IGF1 receptors (IR and IGF1R), which encourages these signals to be transduced. When CAV1 is bound to low density lipoprotein receptor-related protein 6 (LRP6), the complex takes on a signalling function and can activate both the IGF1 receptor and IR, leading to strengthening of signals by Akt-mTORC1. CAV1 is, surprisingly, strongly expressed following demethylation of the initial exon and intron of the gene. This change is noted to occur when adipo-cytes are maturing. One possibility is that miRNAs derived from milk and targeting DNMTs actually strengthen signalling by insulin, IGF1 and mTORC through their epigenetic modificatory effects on the CAV1 gene, which mean CAV1 synthesis increases. The consequence of this is then that exosomes in milk are absorbed in higher quantities [74–77].

7.6 *FOXP3*

FOXP3 exerts overall control over transcriptional events in regulatory T-lymphocytes (Tregs). These lymphocytes play a key role in ensuring the immune system does not target self-antigens (i.e. does not cause autoimmunity to occur). They also prevent immunoreactivity against innocuous allergens in the environment, including in the diet. Thus, they are anti-allergenic. It has been demonstrated that when milk-derived exosomes are presented to circulating polymorphonucleocytes, the levels of Tregs expressing FOXP3 rose. The presence of this protein is sufficient to indicate that the T lymphocytes expressing it possess a unique role in immunosuppression. FOXP3 is expressed at a fixed rate when certain epigenetic switches are set on Tregs in the Treg-specific demethylated region (TSDR) of the FOXP3 gene. This region is rich in CpG sequences. Indeed, FOXP3 is only steadily expressed where this section of the DNA is demethylated. In recent studies, it has even been noted that the extent of demethylation within the TSDR region correlates directly with the level of FOXP3 in the cell. Accordingly, the TSDR is considered a key location for epigenetic control of FOXP3. If the epigenetic modifications do not occur here, Treg numbers may fluctuate widely. On the other hand, if the FOXP3 gene region contains an excessive level of methylation, Tregs fail to prevent allergic responses from developing. It is noteworthy that patients with a tendency to allergic disorders have fewer Tregs in which the FOXP3 region is demethylated [78–88].

DNMT1 and DNMT3b both act on the FOXP3 gene in CD4+ T lymphocytes. When DNA methyltransferase action was prevented by the enzyme inhibitory agent decitabine, the TSDR region remained relatively demethylated and FOXP3 was expressed steadily and at high levels. This result suggests that expression of FOXP3 can be reliably regulated at the epigenetic level by preventing DNA methyltransferase activity. This then results in adequate numbers of well-functioning Tregs. MiRNAs capable of downgrading DNMT1 and DNMT3b (i.e. miRNA-148a and miRNA-21, and miRNA-148a and miRNA-29b, respectively) and entering the body via milk exosomes are accordingly believed to participate in the epigenetic regulation of FOXP3 and thus are of major importance in stabilising the generation of competent Tregs. The evidence is growing that miRNAs found in milk exosomes play a key part in epigenetic modulation and thus influence the immunological behaviour of the gut and the body as a whole [92–96].

A study that was recently undertaken in the Netherlands examined the relationship between hypermethylated DNA generally and allergic sensitivity to bovine milk. Children with and without an allergy to milk were compared. The TSDR of FOXP3 was more highly methylated in those cases where an allergic response to milk mediated through IgE was known to occur than in children who no longer exhibited an active allergic response or in whom allergy to milk had never occurred. In a rodent model involving atopic very young rats, the rat pups were given either rat milk or artificial formula. The rat milk contained the normal level of miRNAs, unlike the formula milk. When the mesenteric lymph nodes were examined for FOXP3 expression, the pups fed rat milk had higher levels. The circulating IgE specific for beta-lactoglobulin was also lower in the rats fed rat milk. Seemingly, miRNAs have the effect of inhibiting DNA methylation and thus ensuring FOXP3 is expressed at higher levels. In such a situation, Tregs can efficiently induce immunotolerance. Thus, all evidence points to miRNAs in milk exosomes functioning to regulate FOXP3 expression at the epigenetic level, which then has a key role in halting the development of autoimmune and allergic reactions. It also seems reasonable to suppose that breast milk, through its effects on Tregs, lays the ground for appropriate immunotolerance of non-self-innocuous food antigens when the child is eventually weaned [89–95].

7.7 NRA4

There are a number of receptors within the NR4A (nuclear receptor subfamily 4a) grouping where the endogenous ligand is unknown. This subfamily is contained within the nuclear receptor superfamily. These receptors all function as transcription factors and can switch gene expression on and off, thereby regulating an intricate system of interacting pathways by which signals are transduced within the cell. A number of members of the NR4A subfamily, notably NR4A1, NR4A2 and

NR4A3 have all been implicated in modulating the growth of Tregs via an effect upon FOXP3. These receptors have a direct action on the promoter region of FOXP3. When NR4A members are stimulated artificially, Tregs begin to be produced, hence they may be considered 'nursing factors' in the growth of this cellular population [96–101].

Milk has a potential role in regulating immunological development in the infant through an epigenetic mechanism and may also regulate how the NR4A subfamily is expressed. When the promoter region underwent CpG demethylation and the surrounding histones where hyperacetylated, the result was a rise in the synthesis of the luteinising hormone receptor (LHR). When the promoter region of NR4A3 was methylated, the gene stopped being expressed, but demethylation of the same region leads to upgraded synthesis. Moreover, the effect of deactivating the HDAC1 and 3 histone deacetylases is to increase the transcription of the NR4A3 gene. DNMT1 has been frequently associated with the histone deacetylases and there are interactions between these enzymes. An important way in which methylated regions of DNA are silenced is by the interaction of methyl CpG binding protein 2 (MeCP2) with sections of methylated CpGs. In part this restriction of transcription by MeCP2 relies on the synergistic activity of histone deacetylases. To take an example, the H19 imprinting control region is not transcribed when MeCP2 and a histone deacetylase act jointly on it. If miRNA-148a from milk exosomes can downgrade the activity of DNMT1, neither MeCP2 nor the histone deacetylase can function and the histone will be hyperacetylated. This hyperacetylated state upgrades transcription of genes involved in development, in particular the NR4A orphan receptors [102–108].

7.8 Nuclear Factor Kappa B (NF-κB)

Milk importantly influences the health of the gastrointestinal system in newborns. Breastfed premature babies are at lower risk of necrotising enterocolitis (NEC) than bottle-fed infants. There is an association between NEC and a raised level of certain pro-inflammatory cytokines (especially interleukin 1 (IL1) and tumour necrosis factor alpha (TNFα)) in the peripheral circulation. These effects occur through the action of Nuclear Factor Kappa B (NF-κB). In a study involving a tissue culture model of NEC, the supernatant from breast milk was applied to plates cultured with Caco-2 gut epitheliocytes. The effect of doing so was to prevent interleukin-1β, IL-6 TNFα from being expressed. Expression of these cytokines is stimulated by NF-κB and promotes an inflammatory response. One of the key molecules with the ability to deactivate NF-κB is IκBα. It achieves this inhibition by blocking signals that precede migration of NF-κB into the nucleus. Instead, the proteins remain within the cytoplasm and lack activity. Additionally, NF-κB is prevented from attaching to DNA, a vital step in its function. IκBα is expressed more strongly by epithelial cells of the gut which lack DNA methyltransferase activity than in those where these enzymes are highly active. The extent to which the promoter region of NfκBI is CpG methylated strongly affects how the NfκB functions in gut lining cells. A high degree of demethylation results in IκBα being highly expressed, whilst extensive methylation has the opposite effect. Epithelial cells without DNMTs exhibit less activity by NFκB. Since miRNAs derived from milk decrease the level of DNMT synthesis, the anti-inflammatory effect of breast milk may occur because a lower level of demethylation occurs. This then means IκBα is relatively more active and NF-κB less active as a result. The actions of miRNAs in breast milk thus resembles that of glucocorticoids, which exert their effects through enhancing IκBα activity [109, 110].

7.9   *The Lactase Gene (LCT)*

For virtually all other mammals than humans, lactase is no longer synthesised within the gut once the young have been weaned onto adult food. Humans are unusual in this regard, namely by virtue of showing lactase persistence. The mechanism by which the expression of LCT declines so massively with age in certain humans, but not all, is not understood currently. However, the latest evidence suggests that the varying levels of mRNA transcripts of LCT expressed in different people, different cell populations or different species are accounted for by an epigenetic mechanism. It appears highly probable that the reason some adults continue to transcribe mRNA from LCT as adults is thanks to epigenetic regulation of the LCT gene. The ongoing expression of LCT in European adults has a strong association with a particular SNP in MCM6, a gene located next to the LCT region. The SNP consists of 13910C>T within intron 13. The effect of the substitution is to promote expression of the LCT gene. There are 7 different sites where epigenetic control of LCT occurs, including that at the 13910 location. Individuals who do not exhibit lactase persistence are found to have a greater extent of methylation within intron 13, the opposite being the case for those individuals demonstrating lactase persistence and therefore continuing to express a significant amount of lactase [110–115].

One possible explanation of how lactase remains available for the duration of breastfeeding is that miRNAs regulating expression of DNMTs thereby ensure intron 13 remains relatively demethylated and thus actively transcribed while breastfeeding occurs. Once breastfeeding ceases, lactase levels then would fall since miRNAs no longer prevent the silencing of the LCT gene, and it is no longer needed. In the Neolithic period, humans may have continued milk consumption after weaning and this then meant a selective pressure favouring those individuals with the 13910C>T mutation. This mutation might ensure that intron 13 remains demethylated and thus the LCT gene continues to be translated into lactase.

8 Conclusion

The earlier medical view of breast milk as a straightforward source of nutrition has altered to one in which milk is seen as a complex medium carrying both nutrients and key communicative signals between mother and child. These signals are the way the youngest children's metabolism is programmed. A major part of the signalling occurs through transfer of miRNAs via exosomes and fat globules in milk. These miRNAs are secreted by the lactocytes of the breast. Exosomes are capable of avoiding degradation in the gut and are endocytosed by the gut lining, eventually reaching the systemic circulation of the child. The miRNA expressed in the highest amount is miRNA-148a, noted in both human and bovine milk exosomes and fat globules, and known to downgrade the activity of DNMT. This enzyme plays a pivotal role in epigenetic control. miRNA-125b is a further miRNA with major effects and it regulates p53, a protein responsible for the integrity of genomic DNA. P53 has multiple effects on different processes. The fact that exosomes containing miRNAs are largely lacking in artificial baby milk but present in bovine milk, which may continue to be consumed long after infancy, raises some concerns about potential ill-effects on the health of people over the longer term [116, 117].

The current era, in which genomic studies are becoming prevalent, offers the chance that individuals at risk of specific disorders can be identified before the condition itself manifests. Genetics alone does not explain predisposition, however, since there are epigenetic modifications and environmental causes to consider. The influence of the environment is especially strong during in utero life and in the neonatal period. It is hypothesised that changes to the metabolism at this early stage in life produce effects at much older ages. One key environmental effect to consider is diet. An essential component of avoiding diseases linked to lifestyle at later ages is for neonates and infants to be breastfed. There is a steadily accumulating evidence base showing that being breastfed at this stage reduces the likelihood of the individuals becoming obese, hypertensive, dyslipidaemic or exhibiting insulin insensitivity as they grow older. Nonetheless, for a complete understanding to emerge, there need to be well-controlled studies for long periods, so that the benefits of breast milk can be properly appreciated [116, 117].

References

1. Alsaweed M, Hartmann PE, Geddes DT, Kakulas F. MicroRNAs in breastmilk and the lactating breast: potential immunoprotectors and developmental regulators for the infant and the mother. Int J Environ Res Public Health. 2015;12:13,981–4,020.
2. Godfrey KM, Costello PM, Lillycrop KA. Development, epigenetics and metabolic programming. Nestle Nutr Inst Workshop Ser. 2016;85:71–80.
3. Chen X, Liang H, Zhang J, et al. Secreted microRNAs: a new form of intercellular communication. Trends Cell Biol. 2012;22:125–32.
4. Xu L, Yang BF, Ai J. MicroRNA transport: a new way in cell communication. J Cell Physiol. 2013;228:1713–9.

5. de Candia P, De Rosa V, Casiraghi M, Matarese G. Extracellular RNAs: a secret arm of immune system regulation. J Biol Chem. 2016;291:7221–8.
6. Ambros V. The functions of animal microRNAs. Nature. 2004;431:350–5.
7. Gustafson D, Tyryshkin K, Renwick N. microRNA-guided diagnostics in clinical samples. Best Pract Res Clin Endocrinol Metab. 2016;30:563–75.
8. Weber JA, Baxter DH, Zhang S, et al. The mircoRNA spectrum in 12 body fluids. Clin Chem. 2010;56:1733–41.
9. Alsaweed M, Lai CT, Hartmann PE, et al. Human milk miRNAs primarily originate from the mammary gland resulting in unique miRNA profiles of fractionated milk. Sci Rep. 2016;6:20680.
10. Ludwig AK, Giebel B. Exosomes: small vesicles participating in intercellular communication. Int J Biochem Cell Biol. 2012;44:11–5.
11. Yáñez-Mó M, Siljander PR, Abdreu Z, et al. Biological properties of extracellular vesicles and their physiological functions. J Extracell Vesicles. 2015;4:27,066.
12. Zempleni J, Aguilar-Lozano A, Sadri M, et al. Biological activities of extracellular vesicles and their cargos from bovine and human milk in humans and implications for infants. J Nutr. 2017;147:3–10.
13. Admyre C, Johansson SM, Qazi KR, et al. Exosomes with immune modulatory features are present in human breast milk. J Immunol. 2007;179:1969–78.
14. Kosaka N, Izumi H, Sekine K, Ochiya T. microRNA as a new immune-regulatory agent on breast milk. Silence. 2010;1:7.
15. Hata T, Murakami K, Nakatani H, et al. Isolation of bovine milk-derived microvesicles carrying mRNA and microRNAs. Biochem Biophys Res Commun. 2010;396:528–33.
16. Reinhardt TA, Lippolis JD, Nonnecke BJ, Sacco RE. Bovine milk exosome proteome. J Proteome. 2012;75:1486–92.
17. Gu Y, Li M, Wang T, et al. Lactation-related microRNA expression profiles of porcine breast milk exosomes. PLoS One. 2012;7:e43691.
18. Zhou Q, Li M, Wang X, et al. Immune-related microRNAs are abundant in breast milk exosomes. Int J Biol Sci. 2012;8:118–23.
19. Izumi H, Kosaka N, Shimizu T, et al. Bovine milk contains microRNA and messenger RNA that are stable under degradative conditions. J Dairy Sci. 2012;95:4831–41.
20. Sun Q, Chen X, Yu J, et al. Immune modulatory function of abundant immune-related microRNAs in microvesicles from bovine colostrum. Protein Cell. 2013;4:197–210.
21. Modepalli V, Kumar A, Hinds LA, et al. Differential temporal expression of milk miRNA during the lactation cycle of the marsupial tammar wallaby (Macropus eugenii). BMC Genomics. 2014;15:1012.
22. Chen T, Xi QY, Ye RS, et al. Exploration of microRNAs in porcine milk exosomes. BMC Genomics. 2014;15:100.
23. Baier SR, Nguyen C, Xie F, et al. MicroRNAs are absorbed in biologically meaningful amounts from nutritionally relevant doses of cow milk and affect gene expression in peripheral blood mononuclear cells, HEK-293 kidney cell cultures, and mouse livers. J Nutr. 2014;144:1495–500.
24. Manca S, Giraud D, Zempleni J. The bioavailability and distribution of bovine milk exosomes is distinct from that of their cargos in mice. FASEB J. 2017;31:148.2.
25. Marriott M, Schoenthal L. An experimental study of the use of unsweetened evaporated milk for the preparation of infant feeding formulas. Arch Pediatr. 1929;46:135–48.
26. Manca S, Giraud D, Zempleni J. Bioavailability and biodistribution of fluorophore-labeled exosomes from cow's milk after intravenous and oral administration in C57BI/6J mice. FASEB J. 2016;30:690.8.
27. Peters T, Ausmeier K, Rüther U. Cloning of Fatso (Fto), a novel gene deleted by the Fused toes (Ft) mouse mutation. Mamm Genome. 1999;10:983–6.
28. Melnik BC, Schmitz G. Milk's role as an epigenetic regulator in health and disease. Diseases. 2017;5(1):12. https://doi.org/10.3390/diseases5010012.

29. Bryder L. From breast to bottle: a history of modern infant feeding. Endeavour. 2009;33:54–9.
30. Chen X, Gao C, Li H, et al. Identification and characterization of microRNAs in raw milk during different periods of lactation, commercial fluid, and powdered milk products. Cell Res. 2010;20:1128–37.
31. Golan-Gerstl R, Elbaum Shiff Y, Moshayoff V, et al. Characterization and biological function of milk-derived miRNAs. Mol Nutr Food Res. 2017;61 https://doi.org/10.1002/mnfr.201700009.
32. Pieters BC, Arntz OJ, Bennink MB, et al. Commercial cow milk contains physically stable extracellular vesicles expressing immunoregulatory TGF-β. PLoS One. 2015;10:e0121123.
33. Le MT, Teh C, Shyh-Chang N, et al. MicroRNA-125b is a novel negative regulator of p53. Genes Dev. 2009;23:862–76.
34. Kumar M, Lu Z, Takwi AA, et al. Negative regulation of the tumor suppressor p53 gene by microRNAs. Oncogene. 2011;30:843–53.
35. Le MT, Shyh-Chang N, Khaw SL, et al. Conserved regulation of p53 network dosage by microRNA-125b occurs through evolving miRNA-target gene pairs. PLoS Genet. 2011;7:e1002242.
36. Sasaki H, Shitara M, Yokota K, Hikosaka Y, Moriyama S, Yano M, Fujii Y. RagD gene expression and NRF2 mutations in lung squamous cell carcinomas. Oncol Lett. 2012;4:1167–70.
37. Maity A, Das B. N6methyl adenosine modification in mRNA: machinery, function and implications for health and diseases. FEBS J. 2016;283:1607–30.
38. Wu R, Jiang D, Wang Y, Wang X. N(6)-methyladenosine (m(6)A) methylationinm RNA with adynamic and reversible epigenetic modification. Mol Biotechnol. 2016;58:450–9.
39. Chhabra R. miRNA and methylation: a multifaceted liaison. Chembiochem. 2015;16:195–203.
40. Wang Y, Li Y, Toth JI, Petroski MD, Zhang Z, Zhao JC. N6-methyl adenosine modification destabilizes developmental regulators in embryonic stem cells. Nat Cell Biol. 2014;16:191–8.
41. Wang Y, Zhao JC. Update: mechanisms underlying N6-Methyladenosine modification of eukaryotic mRNA. Trends Genet. 2016;32:763–73.
42. Boissel S, Reish O, Proulx K, Kawagoe-Takaki H, Sedgwick B, Yeo GS, Meyre D, Golzio C, Molinari F, Kadhom N, et al. Loss-of-function mutation in the dioxygenase-encoding FTO gene causes severe growth retardation and multiple malformations. Am J Hum Genet. 2009;85:106–11.
43. Fischer J, Koch L, Emmerling C, Vierkotten J, Peters T, Brüning JC, Rüther U. Inactivation of the Fto gene protects from obesity. Nature. 2009;458:894–8.
44. Church C, Moir L, McMurray F, Girard C, Banks GT, Teboul L, Wells S, Brüning JC, Nolan PM, Ashcroft FM, et al. Overexpression of Fto leads to increased food intake and results in obesity. Nat Genet. 2010;42:1086–92.
45. Gao X, Shin YH, Li M, Wang F, Tong Q, Zhang P. The fat mass and obesity associated gene FTO functions in the brain to regulate postnatal growth in mice. PLoS One. 2010;5:e14005.
46. Speakman JR. The 'Fat Mass and Obesity related' (FTO) gene: mechanisms of impact on obesity and energy balance. Curr Obes Rep. 2015;4:73–91.
47. Berulava T, Horsthemke B. The obesity-associated SNPs in intron 1 of the FTO gene affect primary transcript levels. Eur J Hum Genet. 2010;18:1054–6.
48. Zhao X, Yang Y, Sun BF, Shi Y, Yang X, Xiao W, Hao YJ, Ping XL, Chen YS, Wang WJ, et al. FTO-dependent demethylation of N6-methyladenosine regulates mRNA splicing and is required for adipogenesis. Cell Res. 2014;24:1403–19.
49. Kim YJ, Lee HS, Kim YK, Park S, Kim JM, Yun JH, Yu HY, Kim BJ. Association of metabolites with obesity and type 2 diabetes based on FTO genotype. PLoS One. 2016;11:e0156612.
50. Liu ZW, Zhang JT, Cai QY, Zhang HX, Wang YH, Yan HT, Wu HM, Yang XJ. Birth weight is associated with placental fat mass- and obesity-associated gene expression and promoter methylation in a Chinese population. J Matern Fetal Neonatal Med. 2016;29:106–11.
51. Dayeh T, Volkov P, Salö S, Hall E, Nilsson E, Olsson AH, Kirkpatrick CL, Wollheim CB, Eliasson L, Rönn T, et al. Genome-wide DNA methylation analysis of human pancreatic

islets from type 2 diabetic and non-diabetic donors identifies candidate genes that influence insulin secretion. PLoS Genet. 2014;10:e1004160.

52. Toperoff G, Kark JD, Aran D, Nassar H, Ahmad WA, Sinnreich R, Azaiza D, Glaser B, Hellman A. Premature aging of leukocyte DNA methylation is associated with type 2 diabetes prevalence. Clin Epigenetics. 2015;7:35.

53. Rönn T, Ling C. DNA methylation as a diagnostic and therapeutic target in the battle against type2 diabetes. Epigenomics. 2015;7:451–60.

54. Howell JJ, Ricoult SJ, Ben-Sahra I, Manning BD. A growing role for mTOR in promoting anabolic metabolism. Biochem Soc Trans. 2013;41:906–12.

55. Gulati P, Cheung MK, Antrobus R, Church CD, Harding HP, Tung YC, Rimmington D, Ma M, Ron D, Lehner PJ, et al. Role for the obesity-related FTO gene in the cellular sensing of amino acids. Proc Natl Acad Sci U S A. 2013;110:2557–62.

56. Gulati P, Yeo GS. The biology of FTO: from nucleic acid demethylase to amino acid sensor. Diabetologia. 2013;56:2113–21.

57. Manifava M, Smith M, Rotondo S, Walker S, Niewczas I, Zoncu R, Clark J, Ktistakis NT. Dynamics of mTORC1 activation in response to amino acids. elife. 2016;5:e19960.

58. Cao H, Wang L, Chen B, Zheng P, He Y, Ding Y, Deng Y, Lu X, Guo X, Zhang Y, et al. DNA demethylation upregulated Nrf2 expression in Alzheimer's disease cellular model. Front Aging Neurosci. 2016;7:244.

59. Bendavit G, Aboulkassim T, Hilmi K, Shah S, Batist G. Nrf2transcriptionfactorcandirectly regulate mTOR: linking cytoprotective gene expression to a major metabolic regulator that generates redoox activity. J Biol Chem. 2016;291:25,476–88.

60. Zheng L, Zhang W, Zhou Y, Li F, Wie H, Peng J. Recent advances in understanding amino acid sensing mechanisms that regulate mTORC1. Int J Mol Sci. 2016;17:E1636.

61. Shibata T, Saito S, Kokubu A, Suzuki T, Yamamoto M, Hirohashi S. Global downstream pathway analysis reveals a dependence of oncogenic NF-E2-related factor 2 mutation on the mTOR growth signaling pathway. Cancer Res. 2010;70:9095–105.

62. Kurinna S, Schäfer M, Ostano P, Karouzakis E, Chiorino G, Bloch W, Bachmann A, Gay S, Garrod D, Lefort K, et al. A novel Nrf2-miR-29-desmocollin-2 axis regulates desmosome function in keratinocytes. Nat Commun. 2014;5:5099.

63. Kurinna S, Werner S. NRF2 and microRNAs: new but awaited relations. Biochem Soc Trans. 2015;43:595–601.

64. Dibble CC, Cantley LC. Regulation of mTORC1 by PI3K signaling. Trends Cell Biol. 2015;25:545–55.

65. Kuroda A, Rauch TA, Todorov I, Ku HT, Al-Abdullah IH, Kandeel F, Mullen Y, Pfeifer GP, Ferreri K. Insulin gene expression is regulated by DNA methylation. PLoS One. 2009;4:e6953.

66. Dooley J, Garcia-Perez JE, Sreenivasan J, Schlenner SM, Vangoitsenhoven R, Papadopoulou AS, Tian L, Schonefeldt S, Serneels L, Deroose C, et al. The microRNA-29 family dictates the balance between homeostatic and pathological glucose handling in diabetes and obesity. Diabetes. 2016;65:53–61.

67. Qin LQ, He K, Xu JY. Milkconsumptionandcirculatinginsulin-likegrowthfactor-Ilevel:Asystematic literature review. Int J Food Sci Nutr. 2009;60(Suppl. 7):330–40.

68. Hoppe C, Mølgaard C, Michaelsen KF. Cow's milk and linear growth in industrialized and developing countries. Annu Rev Nutr. 2006;26:131–73.

69. Ouni M, Gunes Y, Belot MP, Castell AL, Fradin D, Bougnères P. The IGF1 P2 promoter is an epigenetic QTL for circulating IGF1 and human growth. Clin Epigenetics. 2015;7:22.

70. Ouni M, Belot MP, Castell AL, Fradin D, Bougnères P. The P2 promoter of the IGF1 gene is a major epigenetic locus for GH responsiveness. Pharmacogen J. 2016;16:102–6.

71. Tahir SA, Yang G, Goltsov A, Song KD, Ren C, Wang J, Chang W, Thompson TC. Caveolin-1-LRP6 signaling module stimulates aerobic glycolysis in prostate cancer. Cancer Res. 2013;73:1900–11.

72. Tang W, Feng X, Zhang S, Ren Z, Liu Y, Yang B, Iv B, Cai Y, Xia J, Ge N. Caveolin-1 confers resistance of hepatoma cells to anoikis by activating IGF-1 pathway. Cell Physiol Biochem. 2015;36:1223–36.

73. Palacios-Ortega S, Varela-Guruceaga M, Martínez JA, deMiguel C, Milagro FI. Effects of high glucose on caveolin-1 and insulin signaling in 3T3-L1 adipocytes. Adipocytes. 2015;5:65–80.

74. Palacios-Ortega S, Varela-Guruceaga M, Milagro FI, Martínez JA, deMiguel C. Expression of caveolin1 is enhanced by DNA demethylation during adipocyte differentiation. Status of insulin signaling. PLoS One. 2014;9:e95100.

75. Palomares O, Yaman G, Azkur AK, Akkoc T, Akdis M, Akdis CA. Role of Treg in immune regulation of allergic diseases. Eur J Immunol. 2010;40:1232–40.

76. Pellerin L, Jenks JA, Bégin P, Bacchetta R, Nadeau KC. Regulatory T cells and their roles in immune dysregulation and allergy. Immunol Res. 2014;58:358–68.

77. Alroqi FJ, Chatila TA. T regulatory cell biology in health and disease. Curr Allergy Asthma Rep. 2016;16:27.

78. Huehn J, Beyer M. Epigenetic and transcriptional control of Foxp3+ regulatory T cells. Semin Immunol. 2015;27:10–8.

79. Polansky JK, Kretschmer K, Freyer J, Floess S, Garbe A, Baron U, Olek S, Hamann A, von Boehmer H, Huehn J. DNA methylation controls Foxp3 gene expression. Eur J Immunol. 2008;38:1654–63.

80. Polansky JK, Schreiber L, Thelemann C, Ludwig L, Krüger M, Baumgrass R, Cording S, Floess S, Hamann A, Huehn J. Methylation matters: binding of Ets-1 to the demethylated Foxp3 gene contributes to the stabilization of Foxp3 expression in regulatory T cells. J Mol Med. 2010;88:1029–40.

81. Paparo L, Nocerino R, Cosenza L, Aitoro R, D'Argenio V, DelMonaco V, DiScala C, Amoroso A, Di Costanzo M, Salvatore F, et al. Epigenetic features of FoxP3 in children with cow's milk allergy. Clin Epigenetics. 2016;8:86.

82. Janson PC, Winerdal ME, Marits P, Thörn M, Ohlsson R, Winqvist O. FOXP3 promoter demethylation reveals the committed Treg population in humans. PLoS One. 2008;3:e1612.

83. Bacchetta R, Gambineri E, Roncarolo MG. Role of regulatory T cells and FOXP3 in human diseases. J Allergy Clin Immunol. 2007;120:227–35.

84. Nadeau K, McDonald Hyman C, Noth EM, Pratt B, Hammond SK, Balmes J, Tager I. Ambient air pollution impairs regulatory T-cell function in asthma. J Allergy Clin Immunol. 2010;126:845–52.

85. Hinz D, Bauer M, Röder S, Olek S, Huehn J, Sack U, Borte M, Simon JC, Lehmann I, Herberth G, LINA Study Group. Cord blood Tregs with stable FOXP3 expression are influenced by prenatal environment and associated with atopic dermatitis at the age of one year. Allergy. 2012;67:380–9.

86. Lal G, Bromberg JS. Epigenetic mechanisms of regulation of Foxp3 expression. Blood. 2009;114:3727–35.

87. Lal G, Zhang N, vander Touw W, Ding Y, Ju W, Bottinger EP, Reid SP, Levy DE, Bromberg JS. Epigenetic regulation of Foxp3 expression in regulatory T cells by DNA methylation. J Immunol. 2009;182:259–73.

88. Melnik BC, John SM, Schmitz G. Milk: an exosomal microRNA transmitter promoting thymic regulatory T cell maturation preventing the development of atopy? J Transl Med. 2014;12:43.

89. Melnik BC, John SM, Schmitz G. Milk: an epigenetic inducer of FoxP3 expression. J Allergy Clin Immunol. 2016;138:937–8.

90. Parigi SM, Eldh M, Larssen P, Gabrielsson S, Villablanca EJ. Breast milk and solid food shaping intestinal immunity. Front Immunol. 2015;6:415.

91. Petrus NC, Henneman P, Venema A, Mul A, vanSinderen F, Haagmans M, Mook O, Hennekam RC, Sprikkelman AB, Mannens M. Cow's milk allergy in Dutch children: an epigenetic pilot survey. Clin Transl Allergy. 2016;6:16.

92. Tooley KL, El-Merhibi A, Cummins AG, Grose RH, Lymn KA, DeNichilo M, Penttila IA. Maternal milk, but not formula, regulates the immune response to beta-lactoglobulin in allergy-prone rat pups. J Nutr. 2009;139:2145–51.

93. Lopez-Pastrana J, Shao Y, Chernaya V, Wang H, Yang XF. Epigenetic enzymes are the therapeutic targets for CD4(+)CD25(+/high)Foxp3(+) regulatory T cells. Transl Res. 2015;165:221–40.

94. Bluestone JA. FOXP3, the transcription factor at the heart of the rebirth of immune tolerance. J Immunol. 2017;198:979–80.

95. Ranhotra HS. The NR4A orphan nuclear receptors: mediators in metabolism and diseases. J Recept Signal Transduct Res. 2015;35:184–8.

96. Sekiya T, Kashiwagi I, Yoshida R, Fukaya T, Morita R, Kimura A, Ichinose H, Metzger D, Chambon P, Yoshimura A. Nr4a receptors are essential for thymic regulatory T cell development and immune homeostasis. Nat Immunol. 2013;14:230–7.

97. Won HY, Hwang ES. Transcriptional modulation of regulatory T cell development by novel regulators NR4As. Arch Pharm Res. 2016;39:1530–6.

98. Sekiya T, Kondo T, Shichita T, Morita R, Ichinose H, Yoshimura A. Suppression of Th2 and Tfh immune reactions by Nr4a receptors in mature T reg cells. J Exp Med. 2015;212:1623–40.

99. Sekiya T, Nakatsukasa H, Lu Q, Yoshimura A. Roles of transcription factors and epigenetic modifications in differentiation and maintenance of regulatory T cells. Microbes Infect. 2016;18:378–86.

100. Bandukwala HS, Rao A. 'Nurr'ishing Treg cells: Nr4a transcription factors control Foxp3 expression. Nat Immunol. 2013;14:201–3.

101. Zhang Y, Fatima N, Dufau ML. Coordinated changes in DNA methylation and histone modifications regulate silencing/derepression of luteinizing hormone receptor gene transcription. Mol Cell Biol. 2005;25:7929–39.

102. Yeh CM, Chang LY, Lin SH, Chou JL, Hsieh HY, Zeng LH, Chuang SY, Wang HW, Dittner C, Lin CY, et al. Epigenetic silencing of the NR4A3 tumor suppressor, by aberrant JAK/STAT signaling, predicts prognosis in gastric cancer. Sci Rep. 2016;6:31690.

103. Zhao Y, Nomiyama T, Findeisen HM, Qing H, Aono J, Jones KL, Heywood EB, Bruemmer D. Epigenetic regulation of the NR4A orphan nuclear receptor NOR1 by histone acetylation. FEBS Lett. 2014;588:4825–30.

104. ElOsta A, Wolffe AP. DNA methylation and histone de acetylation in the control of gene expression: basic biochemistry to human development and disease. Gene Expr. 2000;9:63–75.

105. Dobosy JR, Selker EU. Emerging connections between DNA methylation and histone acetylation. Cell Mol Life Sci. 2001;58:721–7.

106. Fuks F, Hurd PJ, Wolf D, Nan X, Bird AP, Kouzarides T. The methyl-CpG-binding protein MeCP2 links DNA methylation to histone methylation. J Biol Chem. 2003;278:4035–40.

107. Drewell RA, Goddard CJ, Thomas JO, Surani MA. Methylation-dependent silencing at the H19 imprinting control region by MeCP2. Nucleic Acids Res. 2002;30:1139–44.

108. Sisk PM, Lovelady CA, Dillard RG, Gruber KJ, O'Shea TM. Early human milk feeding is associated with a lower risk of necrotizing enterocolitis in very low birth weight infants. J Perinatol. 2007;27:428–33.

109. Wang W, Xue L, Ma T, Li Y, Li Z. Non-intervention observation: dynamic evolution laws of inflammatory response in necrotizing enterocolitis. Exp Ther Med. 2016;12:1770–4.

110. Labrie V, Buske OJ, Oh E, Jeremian R, Ptak C, Gasiunas G, Maleckas A, Petereit R, Žvirbliene A, Adamonis K, et al. Lactase nonpersistence is directed by DNA-variation-dependent epigenetic aging. Nat Struct Mol Biol. 2016;23:566–73.

111. Swallow DM, Troelsen JT. Escape from epigenetic silencing of lactase expression is triggered by a single-nucleotide change. Nat Struct Mol Biol. 2016;23:505–7.

112. Olds LC, Sibley E. Lactase persistence DNA variant enhances lactase promoter activity in vitro: functional role as a cis regulatory element. Hum Mol Genet. 2003;12:2333–40.

113. Troelsen JT, Olsen J, Møller J, Sjöström H. An upstream polymorphism associated with lactase persistence has increased enhancer activity. Gastroenterology. 2003;125:1686–94.

114. Lewinsky RH, Jensen TG, Møller J, Stensballe A, Olsen J, Troelsen JT. T-13910 DNA variant associated with lactase persistence interacts with Oct-1 and stimulates lactase promoter activity in vitro. Hum Mol Genet. 2005;14:3945–53.
115. Wang Z, Maravelias C, Sibley E. Lactase gene promoter fragments mediate differential spatial and temporal expression patterns in transgenic mice. DNA Cell Biol. 2006;25:215–22.
116. Roszkowska R, Taranta-Janusz K, Wasilewska A. Rola wczesnego programowania metabolicznego w patogenezie chorób cywilizacyjnych [The role of early-life metabolic programming in the pathogenesis of lifestyle diseases]. Dev Period Med. 2014;18(4):477–82. Polish.
117. Melnik BC, Schmitz G. MicroRNAs: milk's epigenetic regulators. Best Pract Res Clin Endocrinol Metab. 2017;31(4):427–42. https://doi.org/10.1016/j.beem.2017.10.003. Epub 2017 Oct 20.

The Metabolome of Breast Milk and Its Potential Long-Term Effects on the Child

Özlem Naciye Şahin, Despina D. Briana, and Gian Carlo Di Renzo

1 Introduction

Current recommendations suggest that the optimal way to feed a neonate is by breastfeeding alone. Human breast milk supplies the complete nutritional requirements of the rapidly growing and developing infant up to the age of 6 months [1]. In accordance with this view, the recommendations from both the World Health Organisation (WHO) and the United Nations Children's Fund (UNICEF) are for infants up to the age of 6 months to receive exclusively breast milk, with other foods being gradually introduced alongside continuing breast milk until the child's second birthday. The time from initial conception up to the second birthday, often referred to as the first 1000 days, is a vital period influencing the metabolic programming of the child thereafter. During the period for which the mother is lactating, the composition of breast milk alters significantly, which may reflect the changing nutritional needs of the child [2].

Breast milk has been the subject of intensive research for several decades now. It is known to contain both the macro- and micronutrients necessary for infant growth as well as other molecules which are biologically active. The constituents of breast

Ö. N. Şahin (✉)
Department of Child Health and Diseases, Arel University, Medical Faculty, Istanbul, Türkiye

D. D. Briana
NICU, Third Department of Pediatrics, National and Kapodistrian University of Athens, University General Hospital "ATTIKON", Athens, Greece

G. C. Di Renzo
Centre of Perinatal Medicine of the University of Perugia, Perugia, Italy

Sechenov University, Moscow, Russia
e-mail: giancarlo.direnzo@unipg.it

Ö. N. Şahin et al. (eds.), *Breastfeeding and Metabolic Programming*, https://doi.org/10.1007/978-3-031-33278-4_13

milk supply the basic molecular building blocks for the child's development [3] and provide a suitable environment in the maturing gut for an optimal microbiome to establish [3–6].

2 The Breast Milk Metabolome

Metabolomic studies focus on the entirety of metabolites in a particular fluid. Human milk is one such fluid. The metabolites are typically of relatively low molecular mass. There have been studies of the composition of the metabolome, the intermolecular interactions and its relation to other factors, in particular gestational age, the stage of lactation and the health of the mother, including her nutritional intake, use of medication or illicit drugs. There has also been research focusing on metabolism in the infant, including metabolomic studies of the infant urine and faeces. The former is helpful in understanding the metabolic fate of milk constituents, whilst the latter provides information about microbial involvement in the overall handling of nutrients within the body [7–11].

Marincola et al. [12] were amongst the first to conduct metabolomic research into breast milk. This study relied on nuclear magnetic resonance (NMR) spectroscopy and gas chromatography-mass spectrometry techniques and was published in 2012. A more complete analysis was subsequently performed and the results published by Smilowitz et al. and Praticò et al., in 2013 and 2014, respectively [13, 14]. These last two studies both used NMR analysis and examined milk from mothers whose offspring were born at full-term. Smilowitz and colleagues analysed milk from mothers 90 days after lactation commenced and identified 65 different constituents. Praticò and colleagues used samples from mothers who had been breast-feeding for a month and identified 43 separate constituents. The constituents included a number of different amino acids, and metabolites thereof, substrates for energy generation, products of the citric acid cycle, short chain aliphatic acids, lactose and oligosaccharides. The component present in the largest quantity was lactose. Next in abundance were the human milk oligosaccharides, citric acid, urea and glutamate. It is generally agreed that the two key determinants responsible for the varied composition between breast milk from different mothers are the mother's Lewis gene type and secretor status. These differences are expressed by the number and structural type of fucosylated HMOs present in the sample [14–16].

There have also been metabolomic investigations comparing the metabolomes of breast milk and baby formula. Qian et al. [16] provide a detailed review of this research. By comparing milk in this way, it has been possible to discover how breast milk is unique. In particular, breast milk contains HMOs, decanoates, octanoates and aliphatic acids lacking esterification. Baby formula, in contrast, contains abundant sugars (fructose and glucose), benzamidoacetic acid, ethanoate, 2-oxopropanoate, phenylalanine and intermediate products of the citric acid cycle [16, 17].

Thus, in metabolomic terms, baby formula and breast milk are markedly different. The metabolomic studies comparing the consequences of breastfeeding versus use of baby formula have been reviewed twice [18, 19].

2.1 Breast Milk and Its Metabolome

In the initial months after birth, breast milk can supply the nutritional requirements of the child, whilst also nourishing a healthy gastrointestinal microbiome. Not only does milk supply the building blocks for the growing and developing infant, namely both the macro- and micronutrients, but it also delivers a range of cytokines and other immunologically active signals to the baby. These constituents are reviewed by Bardanzellu et al. [20] and Slupsky [21].

There is considerable variation in the composition of breast milk over the period of breastfeeding. Colostrum, for example, contains the highest levels of immunologically active molecules and oligosaccharides. Concentrations of these molecules reduce over time. There are also other compositional changes over the course of lactation, affecting amino acids, sugars, aliphatic acids and certain other molecules [21–25] (see Table 1).

Oligosaccharide levels follow a general trend of reduction over time, whereas lactose, a number of amino acids and free aliphatic acids of various lengths all tend to increase. Thus, milk does not consist of a fixed ratio of components. The regulation of which molecules are present and at what level lies with the breast tissue and depends on maternal genetic factors. The alterations in composition are continuous in response to the infant's changing need for particular metabolites and is instrumental in preparing the growth of a healthy microbiome, potentially throughout life. There is a much greater degree of similarity in the microbial flora and faecal metabolites of different infants fed artificial milk than between infants breastfed by different mothers. This dissimilarity stems from the differences in the contents of breast milk over the course of breastfeeding. The composition of artificial milk is fixed, however. The choice of breastfeeding or artificial milk seems to play a vital role in determining the eventual composition of the gut microbiome [20, 25].

Table 1 How the composition of milk varies at different stages of lactation in mothers with a secretor phenotype (adapted from reference [21])

	Molecules, the concentration of which rises during the period of breastfeeding	Molecules, the concentration of which falls during the period of breastfeeding	Molecules, the concentration of which exhibits no significant alteration during the period of breastfeeding
Sugars	Lactose 3-Fucosyllactose Glucose	2′-Fucosyllactose 3′-Galactosyllactose 3′-Sialyllactose 6′-Sialyllactose Fucose Lacto-N-tetraose Lacto-N-neotetraose Lacto-N-fucopentaose I Lacto-N-fucopentaose III Sialic acid Myoinositol	Galactose Lactodifucotetraose Lacto-N-fucopentaose II
Amino acids	Alanine Glutamate Glutamine Phenylalanine Threonine Valine	Leucine Lysine Proline	Asparagine Aspartate Histidine I Soleucine Methionine Tyrosine
Free aliphatic acids and derivatives thereof	Ethanone Azelaic acid Butyrate Carnitine Decanoate Octanoate	Ethanoate	
Glycolysis		Lactate pyruvate	
Intermediate products of citric acid cycle	*Cis*-Aconitate	Citric acid Fumarate Succinate	2-Oxoglutarate
Others	2-Aminobutyrate Choline Glycerophosphocholine Urea	Ascorbate Betaine Creatine Methanoic acid Benzamidoacetic acid Hypoxanthine phosphocholine Taurine	Pantothenate Methanol Creatine phosphate creatinine Ethanolamine Uridine

3 Human Milk Responds to the Needs of the Neonate

Breast milk has a unique composition exactly tailored to the requirements for growth in the neonate. When breast milk is substituted with milk from other species, this deeply affects the metabolism of the neonate. For instance, baby formula-fed infants have raised circulating levels of amino acids and this high level potentially interferes with normal signalling by insulin [26]. The persistently high levels of plasma amino acids may prevent the mitochondria in the liver from functioning properly. This then potentially causes obesity, insulin insensitivity and dyslipidaemias [27].

The molecules within breast milk may also produce direct interactions with particular metabolic processes. An example is modulation of the action of the mechanistic target of rapamycin (mTOR) molecule, which guides optimal development [28]. mTOR forms a complex (mTORC1) which performs a kinase function depending on nutrient levels and regulates various processes affecting cellular growth, protein manufacture and lipid assembly, alongside deposition of fat within adipose tissues. MTORC1 is especially significant in regulating growth and metabolism of osseous tissues, voluntary muscle, the brain and spinal cord, gut, blood cellular components and certain other systems [29]. The amino acid level also controls the activity of mTORC1. The level of leucine in the whey portion of breast milk correlates with the circulating level of leucine in breastfed children [30]. In fruit flies (Drosophila spp.), the way nutrient levels can be detected by the TOR system is also affected by the presence of *Lactobacillus plantarum*, amongst other bacteria. A recent study found that *L. plantarum* may actually be passed from the mother to the infant during feeding [31, 32]. It seems likely, therefore, that the microbiome in the infant has an effect on the way the mTOR network functions, although this has not yet been decisively proven.

4 Metabolites Originating from the Microbiota at Different Times

The effect of breast feeding or bottle feeding at different points on how the gut flora metabolises amino acids with aromatic residues is another topic to be considered.

5 Being Bottle-Fed Results in More Secondary Metabolites of Bile Salts Produced by Microbial Action

There is a significant effect of being bottle-fed versus breastfed on the bile salts identifiable in faeces. Approximately 20 metabolites of bile salts have been detected, as well as cyprinol sulphate, the metabolic precursor. Bile acids exhibiting primary and secondary conjugation, as well as bound to glycine, taurine and sulphate moieties have been noted. The bile compound most strongly associated with breastfeeding is cyprinol sulphate, the faecal level of which rises up to the age of 7 months in exclusively breastfed infants. The molecule glycochenodeoxycholate is present in characteristic amounts depending on the type of feeding, as some bile acids are conjugated to a sulphate group, such as sulphated chenodeoxycholate. Surprisingly, however, the metabolite lithocholate was barely detectable in faeces from infants below the age of 1 year. In any case, secondary bile metabolites are present in lower levels in children's faeces than in those of adults [33].

Infants who are breastfed have higher levels of 4-hydroxyphenyllactate and indolelactate in their faeces up to the age of 1 year. There is no difference in the levels of these compounds between infants who are exclusively breastfed and those who receive supplemental formula milk; however, children who are given additional supplementation with bifidobacteria have been shown to have higher levels. It has been noted in the literature already that the amino acids possessing an aromatic residue (phenylalanine, tyrosine and tryptophan) are metabolised by bifidobacteria to phenyllactate, 4-hydroxyphenyllactate and indolelactate, respectively [34–36]. Bifidobacteria represent the most important bacterial flora in children receiving breast milk. It is not clear what happens to the aromatic amino acids in the gut by assessing their concentrations in faeces, and this likely results from their having multiple metabolic fates. Phenyllactate stands out in this respect. The infant diet does not appear to affect its level, which always appears to increase as the infant gets older. One explanation for this is colonisation of the gastrointestinal tract by other bacterial genera that are also capable of converting phenylalanine to phenyllactate. In contrast, once weaning had begun at the second birthday, the levels of 4-hydroxyphenyllactate and indolelactate became virtually undetectable. Brink et al. have noted that tryptophan can be metabolised into kyneurate, indole-3-lactate and indole-3-ethanoate. These products were detected at higher levels in faecal samples from children receiving breast milk compared to those consuming dairy or soy milk formula [37].

Children aged between 1 and $1\frac{1}{2}$ years are already colonised by bacterial species capable of synthesising lithocholate by 7α-dehydroxylation of bile acids [38]. Indeed, according to Hammons et al., lithocholate can even be detected in faeces from 3 months old children, albeit the levels vary considerably [39]. It was more common in faecal samples from these very young children to identify other secondary metabolites of bile salts, such as 7-keto lithocholate, 3-dehydrochenodeoxycholate, Ursodeoxycholate, 7,12-dioxolithocholate, 7-ketodeoxycholate, 3-dehydrocholate and 7-epicholate. The existence of unexpected metabolites in faeces has already been noted by Lester et al., in reference to ursodeoxycholate [40]. Infants who received formula alone or with breast milk had higher faecal levels of 7-keto lithocholate, 3-dehydrochenodeoxy-cholate, Ursodeoxycholate and 7-epicholate. These metabolites may be indicative of a more varied gut microflora in children fed formula than in those exclusively fed breast milk [41]. Hammons *et al.* have also noted that secondary metabolites of bile salts were more abundant in infants receiving baby formula [39]. In research using young pigs, the faeces also contained raised amounts of the secondary metabolite, deoxycholate.

6 Conclusion

The microbial flora of the gastrointestinal tract, metabolism and the immune system all undergo important alterations in response to a person's diet. The fact that breast milk affects all these processes suggests that it is a highly evolved and sophisticated nutritional and communication system that exists to offer the neonate the greatest chance to be healthy. The alterations in the constituents of breast milk over the course of lactation are probably reflective of the infant's developing requirements and the evolutionary advantage of a particular type of gut flora. Metabolomics is an important type of phenotypical investigation and is vital in any research examining the metabolic consequences of changes in diet. Metabolomic studies on faeces help to establish the roles played by microbial gut flora. If values are established in healthy individuals, metabolomic analysis of peripheral blood, urine and faeces can be used to assess short- and long-term consequences of dietary interventions.

There is a need for further research on various aspects of breast milk on the child's growth and development. This research should also encompass metabolic programming and immunological effects. The health status of the mother and the effects of the environment also need to be factored in. In order to fully comprehend how a dietary change affects specific individuals and their microbiome, there is a need to also consider genetic and epigenetic aspects. The application of nutrigenomics and microbiomics together will elucidate how milk and the various compounds it contains modulate genetic expression in the infant, either directly or via microbial activity. This is an ambitious aim, and will take many more years, but ultimately such research can only lead to a much more effective use of dietary manipulations to promote health.

References

1. Poulsen KO, Sundekilde UK. The metabolomic analysis of human milk offers unique insights into potential child health benefits. Curr Nutr Rep. 2021;10(1):12–29. https://doi.org/10.1007/s13668-020-00345-x. Epub 2021 Feb 8.
2. Ballard O, Morrow AL. Human milk composition. Nutrients and bioactive factors. Pediatr Clin N Am. 2013;60:49–74.
3. Pacheco AR, Barile D, Underwood MA, Mills DA. The impact of the milk glycobiome on the neonate gut microbiota. Annu Rev Anim Biosci. 2015;3:419–45.
4. Kunz C, Rudloff S, Baier W. Oligosaccharides in human milk: structural, functional, and metabolic aspects. Annu Rev Nutr. 2000;20:699–722.
5. Ten-Doménech I, Ramos-Garcia V, Piñeiro-Ramos JD, Gormaz M, Parra-Llorca A, Vento M, et al. Current practice in untargeted human milk metabolomics. Meta. 2020;10:43.
6. Sundekilde UK, Downey E, O'Mahony J, O'Shea C-A, Ryan C, Kelly A, et al. The effect of gestational and lactational age on the human milk metabolome. Nutrients. 2016;8:304.
7. Spevacek AR, Smilowitz JT, Chin EL, Underwood MA, German JB, Slupsky CM. Infant maturity at birth reveals minor differences in the maternal milk metabolome in the first month of lactation. J Nutr. 2015;145:1698–708.

8. Shoji H, Shimizu T. Effect of human breast milk on biological metabolism in infants. Pediatr Int. 2019;61:6–15.

9. Martin FP, Sprenger N, Montoliu I, Rezzi S, Kochhar S, Nicholson JK. Dietary modulation of gut functional ecology studied by fecal metabonomics. J Proteome Res. 2010;9:5284–95.

10. Nicholson JK, Holmes E, Kinross J, Burcelin R, Gibson G, Jia W, et al. Host-gut microbiota metabolic interactions. Science (80-). 2012;336:1262–7.

11. Urbaniak C, McMillan A, Angelini M, Gloor GB, Sumarah M, Burton JP, et al. Effect of chemotherapy on the microbiota and metabolome of human milk, a case report. Microbiome. 2014;2:2.

12. Marincola FC, Noto A, Caboni P, Reali A, Barberini L, Lussu M, et al. A metabolomic study of preterm human and formula milk by high resolution NMR and GC/MS analysis: preliminary results. J Matern Fetal Neonatal Med. 2012;25:62–7.

13. Smilowitz JT, O'Sullivan A, Barile D, German JB, Lönnerdal B, Slupsky CM. The human milk metabolome reveals diverse oligo- saccharide profiles. J Nutr. 2013;143:1709–18.

14. Praticò G, Capuani G, Tomassini A, Baldassarre ME, Delfini M, Miccheli A. Exploring human breast milk composition by NMR-based metabolomics. Nat Prod Res. 2014;28:95–101.

15. Dessì A, Briana D, Corbu S, Gavrili S, Marincola FC, Georgantzi S, et al. Metabolomics of breast milk: the importance of phenotypes. Meta. 2018;8:8. https://doi.org/10.3390/metabo8040079.

16. Qian L, Zhao A, Zhang Y, Chen T, Zeisel SH, Jia W, et al. Metabolomic approaches to explore chemical diversity of human breast-milk, formula milk and bovine milk. Int J Mol Sci. 2016;17:17. https://doi.org/10.3390/ijms17122128.

17. Scano P, Murgia A, Demuru M, Consonni R, Caboni P. Metabolite profiles of formula milk compared to breast milk. Food Res Int. 2016;87:76–82.

18. Phan M, Momin SR, Senn MK, Wood AC. Metabolomic insights into the effects of breast milk versus formula milk feeding in in- fants. Curr Nutr Rep. 2019;8:295–306. https://doi.org/10.1007/s13668-019-00284-2.

19. Li K, Jiang J, Xiao H, Wu K, Qi C, Sun J, et al. Changes in the metabolite profile of breast milk over lactation stages and their relationship with dietary intake in Chinese women: HPLC-QTOFMS based metabolomic analysis. Food Funct. 2018;9:5189–97.

20. Bardanzellu F, Fanos V, Reali A. "Omics" in human colostrum and mature milk: looking to old data with new eyes. Nutrients. 2017;9:843.

21. Slupsky CM. Metabolomics in human milk research. Nestle Nutr Inst Workshop Ser. 2019;90:179–90. https://doi.org/10.1159/000490305. Epub 2019 Mar 13.

22. Munblit D, Peroni DG, Boix-Amorós A, et al. Human milk and allergic diseases: an un- solved puzzle. Nutrients. 2017;9:894.

23. Smilowitz JT, O'Sullivan A, Barile D, et al. The human milk metabolome reveals diverse oligosaccharide profiles. J Nutr. 2013;143:1709–18.

24. Spevacek AR, Smilowitz JT, Chin EL, et al. Infant maturity at birth reveals minor differ- ences in the maternal milk metabolome in the first month of lactation. J Nutr. 2015;145:1698–708.

25. Sundekilde UK, Downey E, O'Mahony JA, et al. The effect of gestational and lactational age on the human milk metabolome. Nutrients. 2016;8:E304.

26. Hyde R, Taylor PM, Hundal HS. Amino acid transporters: roles in amino acid sensing and signalling in animal cells. Biochem J. 2003;373:1–18.

27. Morán-Ramos S, Ocampo-Medina E, Gutierrez-Aguilar R, et al. An amino acid signature associated with obesity predicts 2-year risk of hypertriglyceridemia in school-age children. Sci Rep. 2017;7:5607.

28. Melnik BC. Milk—a nutrient system of mammalian evolution promoting mTORC1-dependent translation. Int J Mol Sci. 2015;16:17048–87.

29. Semba RD, Trehan I, Gonzalez-Freire M, et al. Perspective: the potential role of essential amino acids and the mechanistic target of rapamycin complex 1 (mTORC1) pathway in the pathogenesis of child stunting. Adv Nutr. 2016;7:853–65.

30. Melnik BC. Excessive leucine-mTORC1-signalling of cow milk-based infant formula: the missing link to understand early childhood obesity. J Obes. 2012;2012:197653.
31. Storelli G, Defaye A, Erkosar B, et al. Lacto-bacillus plantarum promotes drosophila systemic growth by modulating hormonal signals through TOR-dependent nutrient sensing. Cell Metab. 2011;14:403–14.
32. Sillner N, Walker A, Lucio M, Maier TV, Bazanella M, Rychlik M, Haller D, Schmitt-Kopplin P. Longitudinal profiles of dietary and microbial metabolites in formula- and breastfed infants. Front Mol Biosci. 2021;8:660456. https://doi.org/10.3389/fmolb.2021.660456.
33. Huang CTL, Rodriguez JT, Woodward WE, Nichols BL. Comparison of patterns of fecal bile acid and neutral sterol between children and adults. Am J Clin Nutr. 1976;29:1196–203. https://doi.org/10.1093/ajcn/29.11.1196.
34. Beloborodov NV, Khodakova AS, Bairamov IT, Olenin AY. Microbial origin of Phenylcarboxylic acids in the human body. Biochem Mosc. 2009;74:1350–5. https://doi.org/10.1134/s0006297909120086.
35. Beloborodova N, Bairamov I, Olenin A, Shubina V, Teplova V, Fedotcheva N. Effect of phenolic acids of microbial origin on production of reactive oxygen species in mitochondria and neutrophils. J Biomed Sci. 2012;19:89. https://doi.org/10.1186/1423-0127-19-89.
36. Aragozzini F, Ferrari A, Pacini N, Gualandris R. Indole-3-lactic acid as a tryptophan metabolite produced by Bifidobacterium Spp. Appl Environ Microbiol. 1979;38:544–6. https://doi.org/10.1128/aem.38.3.544-546.1979.
37. Brink LR, Mercer KE, Piccolo BD, Chintapalli SV, Elolimy A, Bowlin AK, et al. Neonatal diet alters fecal microbiota and metabolome profiles at different ages in infants fed breast Milk or formula. Am J Clin Nutr. 2020;111:1190–202.
38. Eyssen H. Role of the gut microflora in metabolism of lipids and sterols. Proc Nutr Soc. 1973;32:59–63. https://doi.org/10.1079/pns19730016.
39. Hammons JL, Jordan WE, Stewart RL, Taulbee JD, Berg RW. Age and diet effects on fecal bile acids in infants. J Pediatr Gastroenterol Nutr. 1988;7:30–8. https://doi.org/10.1097/00005176-198801000-00008.
40. Lester R, Pyrek JS, Little JM, Adcock EW. Diversity of bile acids in the fetus and newborn infant. J Pediatr Gastroenterol Nutr. 1983;2:355–64. https://doi.org/10.1097/00005176-198302020-00026.
41. Bazanella M, Maier TV, Clavel T, Lagkouvardos I, Lucio M, Maldonado-Gòmez MX, et al. Randomized controlled trial on the impact of early-life intervention with bifidobacteria on the healthy infant fecal microbiota and metabolome. Am J Clin Nutr. 2017;106:1274–86.

The Infant–Mother Molecular Conversation Involving Breast Milk mRNA

Özlem Naciye Şahin and Despina D. Briana

1 Introduction

In mammalian species, there is an ongoing biological dialogue between the mother and offspring from the moment the blastocyst first implants up to the end of breast-feeding. In utero, signals pass via the placenta, whilst postpartum signalling occurs via milk to the gut. MicroRNAs (miRNAs) are brief unpaired sequences of RNA, around 22 nucleotides in total, which feature in many aspects of normal physiology and development. This chapter looks at the part played by miRNAs in the complex molecular dialogue shaping the development of the child, from the moment of implantation up to birth and beyond. The fact that miRNAs can be identified in so many body fluids, including amniotic fluid, the blood of the cord and in human milk means that a new way to understand normal and abnormal physiological processes in development has appeared, and raises the hope that one day new, non-invasive biomarkers will be found [1].

In mammalian species, both in utero and postpartum the offspring are at risk of overwhelming infection due to their undeveloped immune systems. The mother supplies protective factors which enter the foetus through the placenta or amniotic fluid prior to birth, and afterwards via lactation [2, 3].

This biological dialogue commences from implantation, via the placenta/tropho-blast [3]. The blastocyst communicates with the reproductive system of the mother [4]. In utero, the placental role in developmental control is vital, and involves the transfer of endocrine signals, growth factors and cytokines [4], in addition to several other molecules capable of eliciting a response, such as miRNA [5, 6]. The

Ö. N. Şahin (✉)
Department of Child Health and Diseases, Arel University, Medical Faculty, Istanbul, Türkiye

D. D. Briana
NICU, Third Department of Pediatrics, National and Kapodistrian University of Athens, University General Hospital "ATTIKON", Athens, Greece

Ö. N. Şahin et al. (eds.), *Breastfeeding and Metabolic Programming*, https://doi.org/10.1007/978-3-031-33278-4_14

bioactivity occurs on both a local and systemic level, enabling co-ordination of the physiological and metabolic parameters to enable the foetus to develop properly within the womb [3–5]. Not only do the conditions prevailing in the uterus affect how the foetus grows and develops, they also influence how healthy the mother and offspring remain for a prolonged period after delivery [6–9].

The gut is unusually permeable whilst the foetus is in utero, and this may permit amniotic fluid to be absorbed into the foetal circulation. Amniotic fluid shares some similarities with breast milk in terms of containing nutrients, protective and regulatory factors [10]. It is noteworthy that premature piglets who were given amniotic fluid postpartum exhibited a similar response to those fed colostrum. In both cases, the effect was to regulate gut inflammatory processes, raise body mass, change the microbiome of the intestine and alter RNA transcription of regions encoding molecules responsible for inflammation [11].

Postpartum, breast milk assumes the role of molecular communicator with the offspring that was previously played by amniotic fluid [1, 2]. Breast milk supplies complete nutrition to the neonate, enabling him or her to develop and grow healthily. However, it also goes beyond providing the raw materials needed for healthy metabolism to occur. It also fulfils protective and molecular programming roles with long-term consequences [11]. It has been suggested that a suitable term to refer to the multiple signals emanating from the breast and transferred to the infant in milk is 'lactocrine' signalling [12].

The existence of a complex molecular dialogue between the mother and offspring both in utero and postpartum is believed to date back to the beginning of lactation in mammalian species, with further development related to the evolving placental organ [13, 14]. Compared to other primates, human beings are born in a less mature state and call for more maternal care. Indeed, proteomic comparison of breast milk with the milk of rhesus macaques demonstrated that breast milk had a greater abundance of proteins destined to aid in maturation of the gut, immune defences and central nervous system [15]. Evolutionary forces have shaped the form lactation takes as well as the constituents found in milk, explaining both the variety between species and that seen between animals of the same species [16, 17]. This chapter first addresses the evidence base for the existence and physiological role of specific miRNAs in milk, then reviews the latest evidence pointing towards involvement of miRNAs in an ongoing biological dialogue between mother and offspring, both in utero and whilst being breastfed.

2   A Short Introduction to the Short Sequences Known as miRNAs

A typical miRNA is approximately 22 nucleotides long, does not code for any gene and consists of an unpaired strand. Transcription of nuclear miRNA genes results in formation of primary miRNAs, which contain a hairpin twist and are subsequently truncated by Drosha, an endoribonuclease enzyme, resulting in formation of precursor miRNA. The exportin-5 molecule transports the precursor miRNAs into the cytoplasm for further modification. Dicer, another endoribonuclease, modifies the precursor molecule to produce miRNA as a duplexed strand [18, 19]. In this form the miRNA is made up of a guide and messenger strand. The messenger strand undergoes degradation, at which point the miRNA is finally in its mature form. MiRNAs bind to argonaute proteins, which form part of the RNA-induced silencing complex (RISC). The miRNAs partially match the 3′ untranslated segment of specific mRNAs and this allows RISC to process the mRNA [18], either preventing them being translated into protein or causing the mRNA to be degraded. This effectively knocks down gene expression selectively [19]. It is possible for a particular miRNA to detect several different mRNAs, or for several miRNAs to all detect the same mRNA [20, 21]. The expression of genetic expression by miRNAs may be termed 'meta-regulation', since it acts to limit transcription and translation events and assists in degradation of synthesised protein products of genes [22]. Of special significance is the ability of miRNAs to perform epigenetic modifications, with important consequences for the metabolic programming of the foetus [23, 24]. These alterations to target tissues persist within the developing human for lengthy periods [24, 25]. Epigenetic factors and miRNAs have reciprocal roles in regulating each other [24, 25]. It has been proven that miRNAs affect the physiology and development of eukaryotic organisms in many different aspects, including cellular division and differentiation, tissue-specificity, programmed cell death, immune maturation and immune reactions. They have also been demonstrated to be of significance in the pathophysiology of neoplasia [26], circulatory disorders [27, 28] and diabetes mellitus [24, 29].

There is an online database, miRBase, currently located at http://www.mirbase. org/, which contains useful information about primary miRNA sequences, the nomenclature to use, and mature miRNA sequences that have been confirmed to exist through experiments. As of October 2016, this database listed 28,645 hairpin precursor sequences for miRNAs, identified across multiple species of animals and plants. There were 1881 hairpin sequences and 2588 mature miRNAs listed as known to occur in humans. This site also links to TarBase, a repository for confirmed targets of miRNA, as well as to sites reporting in silico predictions of which mRNAs are the probable targets (DIANA-microT, tools4mirs.org, miRDB, RNA22, TargetMiner, PicTar-vertebrates). There are a number of applications now suitable for analysing the probable function of miRNAs, such as MAGIA (miRNA And Genes Integrated Analysis), which can be downloaded from http://gencomp.bio. unipd.it/magia/start/. This software compares the way miRNA and mRNA levels of expression are correlated and thus provides key insights to enable the complex underlying regulatory mechanisms to be unravelled. It is also possible to learn how miRNAs are typically expressed in specific diseases using the miR2 disease database, located at http://www.mir2disease.org/. Ingenuity Pathway Analysis (QIAGEN) is an application routinely employed to predict in silico which mRNA specific miRNA sequences may target.

MiRNAs are ubiquitous, not just intracellular or within the tissues, but in every body, fluid examined so far, namely breast milk, blood, urine, saliva, sweat, semen and amniotic fluid [4]. They have also been identified in the blood of the umbilical cord [30]. It was previously thought that RNA was inherently short-lived, since there are ribonucleases (RNases) ever-present as a defence against nucleic acids belonging to bacteria or viruses. More recently it has become clear that RNA is in fact preserved well in body fluids [4]. The role of the RNases has been elucidated in ensuring immunity (both innate and acquired), in triggering the immune system to attack and in preserving the barrier function of mucosae [31]. The idea that RNA may play a role as a messenger outside the cell was first voiced by Benner in 1988. In proposing that intercellular communication might occur via RNA, he put forward the theory that RNA regulates the balance between RNA degradation and RNA preservation. The suggestion was also that RNA played a pathophysiological role, especially in malignancy and formation of new blood vessels [32]. In the two decades following the announcement of Benner's theory, there was an ongoing research effort to understand how RNA influences the expression of particular genes [33] and where it may perform an intercellular communicative function [34]. Currently it is clear that there are forms of RNA that do not code for genes but have other key functions. Examples include miRNA and long non-coding RNA (lncRNA). These non-coding sequences act as signals between cells and orchestrate development of the child. They are prevented from being degraded by being bound by RNA-binding proteins or by being packaged into vesicles that are then released by the cell into the extracellular environment [35–37].

Over the last 10 years, there has been intensive research into the biosynthesis, functional role and contents of extracellular vesicles (EV). EVs are used to package proteins, lipids and nucleic acids, not least miRNA and lncRNAs [35]. They are now known to be key players in cell-to-cell signalling, whether in eukaryotic or bacterial species [38]. Their functional role encompasses the development of mature sperm capable of motion, growth of follicles, meiosis of the oocyte, the synthesis of steroid hormones and inhibition of polyspermy after the zygote has formed. Within the uterine cavity, communication between the developing embryo and the endometrial lining at the time of implantation occurs via EVs [39], and this communicative role persists for the entire pregnancy [40, 41].

3 Recent Appreciation of how Important miRNAs Really Are

A significant role in the physiological regulation of pregnancy seems to be played by miRNAs acting as signals between mother and foetus [5]. In eutherian mammals, miRNAs regulate how ready the endometrium becomes for implantation, implantation itself, the way the placenta works and labour [42, 43]. Following formation of the zygote, miRNAs within the seminal fluid or spermatocyte may regulate genetic expression, which influences the success rate for implantation of the zygote. Exactly what levels and kind of miRNAs are found in single sperm cells are still not known

[2]. miRNAs help to ensure the conceptus is not targeted by the maternal immune system [44]. A survey of 48 patients showed that the outcomes of the later stages of pregnancy appear linked to particular miRNAs with ability to modulate immune function present before conception occurs and in the first trimester [44]. As the placenta grows, miRNAs may attach to genetic regions coding for genes involved in invasion, cellular division, programmed cell death and new vessel formation [43]. There are also characteristic miRNAs present in the placental tissues and mother's systemic circulation [45]. It is common for the miRNAs to be grouped on the basis of synergy, and their expression may depend on common promoters, which are principally active during pregnancy [46]. The fact that these clusters of miRNAs largely cease being expressed following delivery is suggestive of their being synthesised by the foetus or placenta and thus specific to the pregnant state [47]. It is not yet established why certain miRNAs are continuously synthesised whereas other miRNAs are only produced in particular tissues when specific environmental conditions pertain. It is noteworthy that both normal delivery at full term and premature delivery have been linked to miRNAs. A study involving 17 women, 8 of whom had a pregnancy at full term and 9 of whom were undergoing spontaneous delivery at term, found that microRNA223 and microRNA34 were expressed by cervical tissues during birth [47]. In mice, the microRNA200 family of transcripts act on the progesterone receptor and ZEB1 and 2 (transcription factors) to make the uterus remain relaxed or begin to contract. This finding was confirmed in human beings by examining myometrial tissue obtained whilst a Caesarean section was being undertaken, in women who were active in labour and in those where active labour had not yet commenced [48]. Furthermore, the foetus may be the source of miRNAs which pass via the placenta or amniotic fluid into the mother's bloodstream [49]. Alongside these sources of miRNA within the mother and foetus, there are also non-coding RNAs in the mother's diet and these may enter the foetal circulation via the placenta [50]. miRNA identified in amniotic fluid plays roles as diverse as guiding the path axons take, intercellular adhesion and the signals regulated by the mitogen-activated protein kinase. Thus, they regulate how the nervous system and other foetal organs develop [51]. There has been research examining miRNA expression in blood taken from women who delivered vaginally versus those undergoing Caesarean section, but this comparison has not been repeated for breast milk or amniotic fluid levels. It would be illuminating to see whether the levels in breast milk vary according to how delivery occurred, so hopefully such research will be undertaken soon [52].

Enteral feeding from an early age may cause epigenetic modification of the genome, with consequences for the health of the child later in life. In a murine model, it was found that providing mice with a protein-depleted diet following weaning resulted in changes to the levels of several miRNAs, the majority playing a role in the division of cells. The miRNAs involved were miR-98, miR-199, miR-21, lethal-7 and miR-210 [53]. It has recently been discovered that miRNA plays a role in the remodelling of chromatin. Genetic expression is potentially controlled by the complex interactions between miRNAs, (de)methylation of particular regions and alterations to the histone proteins [53]. Formerly, many of the studies concerning the methylation of particular genes took diet as the key variable. More recent studies have examined how dietary changes alter the expression of particular miRNAs [54]. An ovine model examined the effect of maternal undernourishment at the time of conception. The foetuses expressed a different miRNA profile in voluntary muscle from usual, which also appeared to be found in sheep developing insulin insensitivity [55]. Moreover, in an ovine model of obese mothers, the foetus expressed miRNA in muscle in a pattern which appeared to predispose them to laying down fat within the muscles [56]. The altered pattern of miRNA expression may result from maternal signalling to the foetus via the amniotic fluid. Nonetheless, this research is still at a relatively early stage and further research will be needed to clarify how the mother's state of health influences miRNA expression in the foetus and newborn animal.

4 Potentially Significant miRNA Biomarkers in Human Milk

The neonatal period and infancy are when very significant growth and development occurs in mammals, particularly in humans. Breast milk has been definitively shown to provide immune benefits as well as other advantages, both immediate and in the future. Breastfed infants have lower rates of illness and death and their cognitive development is more advanced [57–59]. At least 12 different body fluids have been evaluated for their RNA content, but the highest level is found in breast milk. Indeed, breast milk RNA concentration exceeds that of amniotic fluid 80-fold [4]. Human milk contains over 1400 fully matured miRNAs [60]. The origin of this RBA is believed to be the lactocytes [61]. When skimmed preparations are examined, it is seen that miRNAs are bound to specific proteins (Ago2, plus other specialised proteins), which protect them [61, 62]. They may also be in lactocytes within the milk [63] or packaged into the many different types of vesicles found in milk, such as fat globules or exosomes [64–66]. It is believed that the exosomes bearing miRNA resist gastric acid degradation and are absorbed, such that they can enter the plasma and then be taken up by particular tissues in the infant [67]. An experimental model has been employed to demonstrate that exosomes in cow milk are not degraded by the severe conditions of the gastrointestinal tract [68]. Several miRNAs which only occur in human lactocytes or in fat globules during lactation have either been characterised or are known to exist [69]. miRNAs originating in the diet have apparent stability within the mouth and the gut and are absorbed into the adult circulation, where they seem to have epigenetic effects [70–72]. It has recently been shown that exosomes derived from cows' milk are endocytosed by the lining cells of the gut and blood vessels. Although this occurs in adults, it has not yet been conclusively demonstrated that miRNAs can be absorbed intact from the infant gut [73, 74]. Recently it has been shown in an in vitro study that temperature plays a role in endocytosis of cows' milk exosomes by the gut and that this also affects how much degradation actually occurs. An even newer study has demonstrated the ability of miRNAs from sows' milk to influence genetic expression and to encourage gut cells to divide, both in the animal itself and in the laboratory. miRNAs may either provide a nutritional benefit or perform a regulatory function. Theories stipulating a functional role for miRNAs suggest that the miRNAs act to better regulate particular aspects of infant physiology, such as through modulating T lymphocytic behaviour, controlling the maturation of B lymphocytes and obstructing the development of allergic hypersensitivity. Theories of miRNA as a nutritional resource, by contrast, imply that miRNA cannot be absorbed into the infant circulation intact and merely provide the building blocks the infant requires [73, 74].

What physiological function is performed by miRNAs and other types of RNA not destined for translation, as well as their fate, has not yet been fully elucidated. Human milk has an abundance of miRNAs known to be involved in immune regulations. Other miRNAs with varied physiological roles, such as cellular phenotypical maturation and development, tissue specificity, metabolism and developmental guidance have also been identified [69]. Certain miRNAs contained in breast milk have a role in neural development and potentially modulate the way the brain develops. An example of this is miR-118.2, which regulates expression of the Teneurin Transmembrane Protein 2. This protein is widely expressed within the brain and spinal cord and has a significant role in how neurones work. There are also miRNAs in breast milk which target particular tissues, e.g. miR-142-5p [70]. miR-142-5p is involved in the generation of new blood cells. It appears probable, therefore, that miRNA in breast milk does in fact play a regulatory role on particular physiological systems in the infant as they develop. Moreover, miRNAs also influence the way metabolism develops. Postnatally, the mTORC1 signalling pathways are regulated to a significant extent by miR-21 [70, 72, 74], whereas members of the let-7 RNA family play a role in how the infant handles glucose, including the setting of glycaemic levels and the degree to which the body responds to insulin [70, 72, 75]. A group of miRNAs which exist in large amounts in the lipid portion and exosomes of breast milk, namely miR-33, miR-122, miR-370, miR-378-3p, and miR-125a-5p, play possible major roles in how the infant handles lipids, as well as potentially regulating the way the lactating breast functions [72–75].

miRNAs which are involved in epigenetic modification of gene expression produce effects that are chronic and endure. One miRNA in particular, miR-148-3p, which exists at an especially high level in breast milk [72], takes DNA methyltransferase 3b as its target. This enzyme plays an essential role in the developing infant [75] and is a vital agent for DNA methylation in the gut lining [76]. Breastfed infants may obtain benefit from regulation of maturation of specific physiological systems, such as the gut, thanks to the miRNAs contained in breast milk. There is a never-ending regeneration of the crypt-villus axis in the intestine, a process modulated through epigenetic alterations to DNA and transcription factors [77]. The addition of methyl or acetyl moieties to the histone proteins are key events in shaping the way the crypt cells multiply and mature [77]. In the stem cells of the gut the DNA has specific regions where methylation acts as an epigenetic regulatory mechanism.

It seems that miRNAs within breast milk may take as their target molecules which methylate DNA or modify histones, and this would then explain how milk helps the gastrointestinal tract to mature [78–80].

The levels of mRNA and miRNA is breast milk vary at different times of day, which may be indicative of a further physiological role. This circadian fluctuation in miRNA levels has a potential role in setting up or governing circadian rhythmicity in the infant, especially within the gut. This type of control is currently referred to as lactocrine circadian signalling [78–81].

For the period of lactation, the amounts of specific miRNAs synthesised, especially miR-25, miR-155, miR-182, miR-191, miR-221 and miR-223, vary in bovine, porcine, rodent and human mammary glands [79–81]. The lactocytes in cows respond to the presence of lactogenic endocrine signals, such as the prolactin level, by altering the level of miRNA found both inside and outside the cell [82]. This variation supports the notion that miRNA is a normal component of physiological lactation in healthy animals. It is significant that abnormal levels of miRNAs correlate with breast pathology, which may mean they can be used in the future as biomarkers indicating how well the breast is functioning in breastfeeding and whether disease is present [78, 79]. The plasma level of miRNA has been employed in calculating the risk of malignancy in the breast, as well as other pathological conditions, such as mastitis [83–85]. In an analogous way, miRNA evaluation in milk may be a useful proxy for the presence of pathological conditions in neonates and infants. In any case, the unique molecular communicative mechanism between breastfeeding mother and child is worthy of deeper investigation.

5 Conclusion

In mammalian species, there is an ongoing biological dialogue between the mother and offspring from the moment the blastocyst first implants up to the end of breastfeeding. In utero, signals pass via the placenta. At present, there is a deepening appreciation of the way miRNA functions to modulate and govern both physiological and pathophysiological mechanisms in the mother and child, through the molecular communicative medium of the placenta and breast milk. miRNAs are found very widely expressed in both the intracellular and extracellular spaces of both the mother and her offspring. This chapter has examined how miRNAs may direct development of the foetus and infant. More specifically, we have looked at the evidence indicating that miRNAs in breast milk have a role beyond merely providing nutrition for the growing human, through their being absorbed and acting as regulators of specific gene expression.

References

1. Floris I, Kraft JD, Altosaar I. Roles of MicroRNA across prenatal and postnatal periods. Int J Mol Sci. 2016;17(12):1994. https://doi.org/10.3390/ijms17121994.
2. Power ML, Schulkin J. Maternal regulation of offspring development in mammals is an ancient adaptation tied to lactation. Appl Transl Genom. 2013;2:55–63.
3. Fazeli A, Holt WV. Cross talk during the periconception period. Theriogenology. 2016;86:438–42.
4. Petraglia F, Pasquale F, Wylie WV. Placental expression of neurohormones and other neuro-active molecules in human pregnancy. In: Power ML, Schulkin J, editors. Birth, distress and disease. Cambridge: Cambridge University Press; 2005. p. 16–73.
5. Weber JA, Baxter DH, Zhang S, Huang DY, Huang KH, Lee MJ, Galas DJ, Wang K. The microRNA spectrum in 12 body fluids. Clin Chem. 2010;56:1733–41.
6. Forbes K. IFPA Gabor than award lecture: molecular control of placental growth: the emerging role of microRNAs. Placenta. 2013;34:S27–33.
7. Thornburg KL, Marshall N. The placenta is the center of the chronic disease universe. Am J Obstet Gynecol. 2015;213:S14–20.
8. Janssen AB, Kertes DA, McNamara GI, Braithwaite EC, Creeth HDJ, Glover VI, John RM. A role for the placenta in programming maternal mood and childhood behavioural disorders. J Neuroendocrinol. 2016;28:1–6.
9. Tung J, Archie EA, Altmann J, Alberts SC. Cumulative early life adversity predicts longevity in wild baboons. Nat Commun. 2016;7:11,181.
10. Underwood MA, Gilbert WM, Sherman MP. Amniotic fluid: not just fetal urine anymore. J Perinatol. 2005;25:341–8.
11. Siggers J, Ostergaard MV, Siggers RH, Skovgaard K, Mølbak L, Thymann T, Schmidt M, Møller HK, Purup S, Fink LN, et al. Postnatal amniotic fluid intake reduces gut inflammatory responses and necrotizing enterocolitis in preterm neonates. Am J Physiol Gastrointest Liver Physiol. 2013;304:G864–75.
12. Altosaar I, Siggers J. Micromolecules to nanoparticles-human milk: more than nutrition. In: German B, Rhine W, editors. Proceedings of the 3rd annual international conference on human milk science and innovation. Prolacta Bioscience, City of Industry, CA: Pasadena, CA; 2015, pp. 6–8.
13. Bartol FF, Wiley AA, Bagnell CA. Epigenetic programming of porcine endometrial function and the lactocrine hypothesis. Reprod Domest Anim. 2008;43:273–9.
14. Vorbach C, Capecchi MR, Penninger JM. Evolution of the mammary gland from the innate immune system? BioEssays News Rev Mol Cell Dev Biol. 2006;28:606–16.
15. Sale S, Pavelic K. Mammary lineage tracing: the coming of age. Cell Mol Life Sci. 2015;72:1577–83.
16. Beck KL, Weber D, Phinney BS, Smilowitz JT, Hinde K, Lönnerdal B, Korf I, Lemay DG. Comparative proteomics of human and macaque milk reveals species-specific nutrition during postnatal development. J Proteome Res. 2015;14:2143–57.
17. Hinde K, Milligan LA. Primate milk: proximate mechanisms and ultimate perspectives. Evol Anthropol. 2011;20:9–23.
18. Hinde K, German JB. Food in an evolutionary context: insights from mother's milk. J Sci Food Agric. 2012;92:2219–23.
19. Finnegan EF, Pasquinelli AE. MicroRNA biogenesis: regulating the regulators. Crit Rev Biochem Mol Biol. 2013;48:51–68.
20. Guo H, Ingolia NT, Weissman JS, Bartel DP. Mammalian microRNAs predominantly act to decrease target mRNA levels. Nature. 2010;466:835–40.
21. Krol J, Loedige I, Filipowicz W. The widespread regulation of microRNA biogenesis, function and decay. Nat Rev Genet. 2010;11:597–610.
22. Lewis BP, Burge CB, Bartel DP. Conserved seed pairing, often flanked by adenosines, indicates that thousands of human genes are microRNA targets. Cell. 2005;120:15–20.

23. Enright AJ, John B, Gaul U, Tuschl T, Sander C, Marks DS. MicroRNA targets in drosophila. Genome Biol. 2003;5:R1.
24. Sookoian S, Gianotti TF, Burgueño AL, Pirola CJ. Fetal metabolic programming and epigenetic modifications: a systems biology approach. Pediatr Res. 2013;73:531–42.
25. Floris I, Descamps B, Vardeu A, Mitic T, Posadino AM, Shantikumar S, Sala-Newby G, Capobianco G, Mangialardi G, Howard L, et al. Gestational diabetes mellitus impairs fetal endothelial cell functions through a mechanism involving microRNA-101 and histone methyltransferase enhancer of zester homolog-2. Arterioscler Thromb Vasc Biol. 2015;35:664–74.
26. Pasquinelli AE. MicroRNAs and their targets: recognition, regulation and an emerging reciprocal relationship. Nat Rev Genet. 2012;13:271–82.
27. Xue Z, Yilan D, Ping J, Fei M. Bioinformatic analysis of cancer-related microRNAs and their target genes. Yi Chuan. 2015;37:855–64.
28. Spinetti G, Fortunato O, Caporali A, Shantikumar S, Marchetti M, Meloni M, Descamps B, Floris I, Sangalli E, Vono R, et al. MicroRNA-15a and microRNA-16 impair human circulating proangiogenic cell functions and are increased in the proangiogenic cells and serum of patients with critical limb ischemia. Circ Res. 2013;112:335–46.
29. Ovchinnikova ES, Schmitter D, Vegter EL, Ter Maaten JM, Valente MAE, Liu LCY, van der Harst P, Pinto YM, de Boer RA, Meyer S, et al. Signature of circulating microRNAs in patients with acute heart failure. Eur J Heart Fail. 2016;18:414–23.
30. Shantikumar S, Caporali A, Emanueli C. Role of microRNAs in diabetes and its cardiovascular complications. Cardiovasc Res. 2012;93:583–93.
31. Merkerova M, Vasikova A, Belickova M, Bruchova H. MicroRNA expression profiles in umbilical cord blood cell lineages. Stem Cells Dev. 2010;19:17–26.
32. Rosenberg, H.F. Vertebrate secretory (RNAse A) ribonucleases and host defense. In *Ribonucleases*; Nicholson, A.W., Ed.; Springer: Berlin/Heidelberg, Germany, 2011; Volume 26, pp. 35–53.
33. Benner SA. Extracellular "communicator RNA". FEBS Lett. 1988;233:225–8.
34. Diederichs S, Bartsch L, Berkmann JC, Fröse K, Heitmann J, Hoppe C, Iggena D, Jazmati D, Karschnia P, Linsenmeier M, et al. The dark matter of the cancer genome: aberrations in regulatory elements, untranslated regions, splice sites, non-coding RNA and synonymous mutations. EMBO Mol Med. 2016;8:442–57.
35. Karlsson O, Baccarelli AA. Environmental health and long non-coding RNAs. Curr Environ Health Rep. 2016;3:178–87.
36. Karlsson O, Rodosthenous RS, Jara C, Brennan KJ, Wright RO, Baccarelli AA, Wright RJ. Detection of long non-coding RNAs in human breastmilk extracellular vesicles: implications for early child development. Epigenetics. 2016;11:721–9.
37. Mitchell PS, Parkin RK, Kroh EM, Fritz BR, Wyman SK, Pogosova-Agadjanyan EL, Peterson A, Noteboom J, O'Briant KC, Allen A, et al. Circulating microRNAs as stable blood-based markers for cancer detection. Proc Natl Acad Sci U S A. 2008;105:10,513–8.
38. Valadi H, Ekström K, Bossios A, Sjöstrand M, Lee JJ, Lötvall JO. Exosome-mediated transfer of mRNAs and microRNAs is a novel mechanism of genetic exchange between cells. Nat Cell Biol. 2007;9:654–9.
39. Yáñez-Mó M, Siljander PR-M, Andreu Z, Zavec AB, Borràs FE, Buzas EI, Buzas K, Casal E, Cappello F, Carvalho J, et al. Biological properties of extracellular vesicles and their physiological functions. J Extracell Vesicles. 2015;4:27,066.
40. Machtinger R, Laurent LC, Baccarelli AA. Extracellular vesicles: roles in gamete maturation, fertilization and embryo implantation. Hum Reprod Update. 2016;22:182–93.
41. Nardi Fda S, Michelon TF, Neumann J, Manvailer LFS, Wagner B, Horn PA, Bicalho Mda G, Rebmann V. High levels of circulating extracellular vesicles with altered expression and function during pregnancy. Immunobiology. 2016;221:753–60.
42. Burnett LA, Nowak RA. Exosomes mediate embryo and maternal interactions at implantation and during pregnancy. Front Biosci. 2016;8:79–96.

43. Mouillet J-F, Chu T, Sadovsky Y. Expression patterns of placental microRNAs. Birth Defects Res A Clin Mol Teratol. 2011;91:737–43.
44. Bidarimath M, Khalaj K, Wessels JM, Tayade C. MicroRNAs, immune cells and pregnancy. Cell Mol Immunol. 2014;11:538–47.
45. Winger EE, Reed JL, Ji X. First-trimester maternal cell microRNA is a superior pregnancy marker to immunological testing for predicting adverse pregnancy outcome. J Reprod Immunol. 2015;110:22–35.
46. Chim SSC, Shing TKF, Hung ECW, Leung T-Y, Lau T-K, Chiu RWK, Lo YMD. Detection and characterization of placental microRNAs in maternal plasma. Clin Chem. 2008;54:482–90.
47. Morales-Prieto DM, Ospina-Prieto S, Chaiwangyen W, Schoenleben M, Markert UR. Pregnancy- associated miRNA-clusters. J Reprod Immunol. 2013;97:51–61.
48. Hassan SS, Romero R, Pineles B, Tarca AL, Montenegro D, Erez O, Mittal P, Kusanovic JP, Mazaki-Tovi S, Espinoza J, et al. MicroRNA expression profiling of the human uterine cervix after term labor and delivery. Am J Obstet Gynecol. 2010;202(80):e1–80.e8.
49. Williams KC, Renthal NE, Condon JC, Gerard RD, Mendelson CR. MicroRNA-200a serves a key role in the decline of progesterone receptor function leading to term and preterm labor. Proc Natl Acad Sci U S A. 2012;109:7529–34.
50. Wong FCK, Lo YMD. Prenatal diagnosis innovation: genome sequencing of maternal plasma. Annu Rev Med. 2016;67:419–32.
51. Li J, Zhang Y, Li D, Liu Y, Chu D, Jiang X, Hou D, Zen K, Zhang C-Y. Small non-coding RNAs transfer through mammalian placenta and directly regulate fetal gene expression. Protein Cell. 2015;6:391–6.
52. Morisaki S, Miura K, Higashijima A, Abe S, Miura S, Hasegawa Y, Yoshida A, Kaneuchi M, Yoshiura K, Masuzaki H. Effect of labor on plasma concentrations and postpartum clearance of cell-free, pregnancy-associated, placenta-specific microRNAs. Prenat Diagn. 2015;35:44–50.
53. Cabrera-Rubio R, Collado MC, Laitinen K, Salminen S, Isolauri E, Mira A. The human milk microbiome changes over lactation and is shaped by maternal weight and mode of delivery. Am J Clin Nutr. 2012;96:544–51.
54. Cretoiu D, Xu J, Xiao J, Suciu N, Cretoiu SM. Circulating microRNAs as potential molecular biomarkers in pathophysiological evolution of pregnancy. Dis Markers. 2016;2016:1–7.
55. Lillycrop KA, Burdge GC. Epigenetic mechanisms linking early nutrition to long term health. Best Pract Res Clin Endocrinol Metab. 2012;26:667–76.
56. Vickers MH. Early life nutrition, epigenetics and programming of later life disease. Nutrients. 2014;6:2165–78.
57. Isaacs EB, Fischl BR, Quinn BT, Chong WK, Gadian DG, Lucas A. Impact of breast milk on intelligence quotient, brain size, and white matter development. Pediatr Res. 2010;67:357–62. https://doi.org/10.1203/PDR.0b013e3181d026da.
58. Luby JL, Belden AC, Whalen D, Harms MP, Barch DM. Breastfeeding and childhood IQ: the mediating role of gray matter volume. J Am Acad Child Adolesc Psychiatry. 2016;55:367–75. https://doi.org/10.1016/j.jaac.2016.02.009.
59. Parylak SL, Deng W, Gage FH. Mother's milk programs offspring's cognition. Nat Neurosci. 2014;17:8–9. https://doi.org/10.1038/nn.3611.
60. Alsaweed M, Hartmann PE, Geddes DT, Kakulas F. MicroRNAs in breastmilk and the lactating breast: potential immunoprotectors and developmental regulators for the infant and the mother. Int J Environ Res Public Health. 2015;12:13,981–4,020. https://doi.org/10.3390/ijerph121113981.
61. Alsaweed M, Lai CT, Hartmann PE, Geddes DT, Kakulas F. Human milk miRNAs primarily originate from the mammary gland resulting in unique miRNA profiles of fractionated milk. Sci Rep. 2016;6:20680. https://doi.org/10.1038/srep20680.
62. Floris I, Billard H, Boquien CY, Joram-Gauvard E, Simon L, Legrand A, Boscher C, Roze JC, Bolanos-Jimenez F, Kaeffer B. miRNA analysis by quantitative PCR in preterm human breast milk reveals daily fluctuations of hsa-miR-16–5p. PLoS One. 2015;10:e0140488. https://doi.org/10.1371/journal.pone.0140488.

63. Alsaweed M, Lai CT, Hartmann PE, Geddes DT, Kakulas F. Human milk cells contain numerous miRNAs that may change with milk removal and regulate multiple physiological processes. Int J Mol Sci. 2016;17:956. https://doi.org/10.3390/ijms17060956.

64. Munch EM, Harris RA, Mohammad M, Benham AL, Pejerrey SM, Showalter L, Hu M, Shope CD, Maningat PD, Gunaratne PH, et al. Transcriptome profiling of microRNA by next-gen deep sequencing reveals known and novel miRNA species in the lipid fraction of human breast milk. PLoS One. 2013;8:e50564. https://doi.org/10.1371/journal.pone.0050564.

65. Kosaka N, Iguchi H, Ochiya T. Circulating microRNA in body fluid: a new potential biomarker for cancer diagnosis and prognosis. Cancer Sci. 2010;101:2087–92. https://doi.org/10.1111/j.1349-7006.2010.01650.x.

66. Zhou Q, Li M, Wang X, Li Q, Wang T, Zhu Q, Zhou X, Wang X, Gao X, Li X. Immune-related microRNAs are abundant in breast milk exosomes. Int J Biol Sci. 2012;8:118–23. https://doi.org/10.7150/ijbs.8.118.

67. Hassiotou F, Beltran A, Chetwynd E, Stuebe AM, Twigger A-J, Metzger P, Trengove N, Lai CT, Filgueira L, Blancafort P, et al. Breastmilk is a novel source of stem cells with multilineage differentiation potential. Stem Cells. 2012;30:2164–74. https://doi.org/10.1002/stem.1188.

68. Benmoussa A, Lee CHC, Laffont B, Savard P, Laugier J, Boilard E, Gilbert C, Fliss I, Provost P. Commercial dairy cow milk microRNAs resist digestion under simulated gastrointestinal tract conditions. J Nutr. 2016;146:2206–15. https://doi.org/10.3945/jn.116.237651.

69. Alsaweed M, Lai CT, Hartmann PE, Geddes DT, Kakulas F. Human milk cells and lipids conserve numerous known and novel miRNAs, some of which are differentially expressed during lactation. PLoS One. 2016;11:e0152610. https://doi.org/10.1371/journal.pone.0152610.

70. Zhang L, Hou D, Chen X, Li D, Zhu L, Zhang Y, Li J, Bian Z, Liang X, Cai X, et al. Exogenous plant MIR168a specifically targets mammalian LDLRAP1: evidence of cross-kingdom regulation by microRNA. Cell Res. 2012;22:107–26. https://doi.org/10.1038/cr.2011.158.

71. Baier SR, Nguyen C, Xie F, Wood JR, Zempleni J. MicroRNAs are absorbed in biologically meaningful amounts from nutritionally relevant doses of cow milk and affect gene expression in peripheral blood mononuclear cells, HEK-293 kidney cell cultures, and mouse livers. J Nutr. 2014;144:1495–500. https://doi.org/10.3945/jn.114.196436.

72. Zempleni J, Baier SR, Howard KM, Cui J. Gene regulation by dietary microRNAs. Can J Physiol Pharmacol. 2015;93:1097–102. https://doi.org/10.1139/cjpp-2014-0392.

73. Kusuma RJ, Manca S, Friemel T, Sukreet S, Nguyen C, Zempleni J. Human vascular endothelial cells transport foreign exosomes from cow's milk by endocytosis. Am J Physiol Cell Physiol. 2016;310:C800–7. https://doi.org/10.1152/ajpcell.00169.2015.

74. Melnik BC, Kakulas F, Geddes DT, Hartmann PE, John SM, Carrera-Bastos P, Cordain L, Schmitz G. Milk miRNAs: simple nutrients or systemic functional regulators? Nutr Metab. 2016;13:1–5. https://doi.org/10.1186/s12986-016-0101-2.

75. Duursma AM, Kedde M, Schrier M, le Sage C, Agami R. miR-148 targets human DNMT3b protein coding region. RNA. 2008;14:872–7. https://doi.org/10.1261/rna.972008.

76. Elliott EN, Sheaffer KL, Kaestner KH. The 'de novo' DNA methyltransferase Dnmt3b compensates the Dnmt1-deficient intestinal epithelium. elife. 2016;5:e12975. https://doi.org/10.7554/eLife.12975.

77. Roostaee A, Benoit YD, Boudjadi S, Beaulieu J-F. Epigenetics in intestinal epithelial cell renewal. J Cell Physiol. 2016;231:2361–7. https://doi.org/10.1002/jcp.25401.

78. Maningat PD, Sen P, Rijnkels M, Sunehag AL, Hadsell DL, Bray M, Haymond MW. Gene expression in the human mammary epithelium during lactation: the milk fat globule transcriptome. Physiol Genomics. 2009;37:12–22. https://doi.org/10.1152/physiolgenomics.90341.2008.

79. Li Z, Liu H, Jin X, Lo L, Liu J. Expression profiles of microRNAs from lactating and non-lactating bovine mammary glands and identification of miRNA related to lactation. BMC Genomics. 2012;13:731. https://doi.org/10.1186/1471-2164-13-731.

80. Gu Y, Li M, Wang T, Liang Y, Zhong Z, Wang X, Zhou Q, Chen L, Lang Q, He Z, et al. Lactation-related microRNA expression profiles of porcine breast milk exosomes. PLoS One. 2012;7:e43691. https://doi.org/10.1371/journal.pone.0043691.
81. Izumi H, Kosaka N, Shimizu T, Sekine K, Ochiya T, Takase M. Time-dependent expression profiles of microRNAs and mRNAs in rat milk whey. PLoS One. 2014;9:e88843. https://doi.org/10.1371/journal.pone.0088843.
82. Muroya S, Hagi T, Kimura A, Aso H, Matsuzaki M, Nomura M. Lactogenic hormones alter cellular and extracellular microRNA expression in bovine mammary epithelial cell culture. J Anim Sci Biotechnol. 2016;7:8. https://doi.org/10.1186/s40104-016-0068-x.
83. Singh R, Mo Y-Y. Role of microRNAs in breast cancer. Cancer Biol Ther. 2013;14:201–12. https://doi.org/10.4161/cbt.23296.
84. Chen X, Ba Y, Ma L, Cai X, Yin Y, Wang K, Guo J, Zhang Y, Chen J, Guo X, et al. Characterization of microRNAs in serum: a novel class of biomarkers for diagnosis of cancer and other diseases. Cell Res. 2008;18:997–1006. https://doi.org/10.1038/cr.2008.282.
85. Taga I, Lan CQ, Altosaar I. Plant essential oils and mastitis disease: their potential inhibitory effects on pro-inflammatory cytokine production in response to bacteria related inflammation. Nat Prod Commun. 2012;7:675–82.

Genetic Causes of Obesity and Bioactive Substances

Özlem Naciye Şahin, Samim Ozen, and Despina D. Briana

1 Introduction

Obesity has many different causes. Although rates of obesity are higher in developed countries, its incidence has recently undergone a sharp rise in developing countries [1, 2]. Unless the current trend alters, it appears that, by the year 2030, there will be 1.12bn obese people globally, representing one in five of the world's population, whilst 2.16bn people will be overweight, a further 38% of all humans on Earth [2, 3]. There are genetic factors that have favoured this positive energy imbalance during the last few decades [4]. Genetic mutations in a number of different genes cause increased appetite and altered metabolism. There have been a number of techniques in use within the last 20 years in an attempt to identify genetic factors implicated in obesity, with an emphasis on severely affected individuals, including both genome-wide linkage studies (GWLS) and genome-wide association studies (GWAS), in addition to a detailed investigation of specific genes. The current state of knowledge from GWAS reveals around 127 locations on the human genome that have a connection with obesity. This approach has been active since 2005 and has revealed key information about the role of genetic factors in common obesity. Evidence from animal studies as well as single nucleotide polymorphism (SNP) screens point to the need to examine the entire genome in order to understand how obesity occurs. SNP screens look for non-synonymous SNPs (nsSNPs) which

Ö. N. Şahin (✉)
Department of Child Health and Diseases, Arel University, Medical Faculty, Istanbul, Türkiye

S. Ozen
Department of Pediatrics, Pediatric Endocrinology Division, Medical Faculty, Ege University, Izmir, Türkiye

D. D. Briana
NICU, Third Department of Pediatrics, National and Kapodistrian University of Athens, University General Hospital "ATTIKON", Athens, Greece

© The Author(s), under exclusive license to Springer Nature Switzerland AG 2023
Ö. N. Şahin et al. (eds.), *Breastfeeding and Metabolic Programming*, https://doi.org/10.1007/978-3-031-33278-4_15

may help identify mutations, which lead to functionally altered protein products. It is anticipated that contemporary genetic investigations and deeper research will enable further elucidation of the genetic factors controlling obesity, paving the way for new and successful treatment approaches [4–6].

Up to now, the gene found to be associated with the highest risk of obesity is FTO (fat mass and obesity-associated protein). Possession of any of the risk-associated allelic variants of FTO correlated with a rise in body mass of between 1 and 1.5 kg and an elevation of between 20% and 30% in the risk of becoming obese [7, 8]. Interactions between an individual's genes and the environment (known as GEIs) result in obesity and the development of a number of metabolic disorders [8, 9]. Epigenetic changes are heritable alterations to the way a gene functions that do not involve mutation of the DNA sequence [9]. The mechanisms by which epigenetic modifications occur include DNA methylation, remodelled chromatin, altered DNA packing around the nucleosomes and alteration of histone proteins. Each of these epigenetic modifications, in concert with a GEI, may lead to obesity and metabolic problems [10–13].

The hypothalamus is known to play a significant role in regulating the use of energy in the body. In the 1950s, the scientific consensus was that storage of fat was intimately connected to the level of energy intake. However, the role of specific molecules in regulating the feeling of satiety, especially glucagon (from the pancreas), bombesin and cholecystokinin, began to be appreciated from the latter half of the 1970s and into the 1990s [14, 15].

A series of molecules that fulfil a signalling function and influence the hypothalamic control of feeding will be discussed.

2 Leptin

The name 'leptin' derives from the Greek adjective λεπτός (leptos), signifying 'thin'. Discovery was due to Zhang et al., who noted in 1994 [16, 17] that it was the protein product of the ob (LEP) gene. Leptin is a protein composed of 167 amino acid residues and principally expressed by fat tissues, at a level corresponding to the body's adipose volume [18]. Leptin also occurs in breast milk and has a regulatory function in energy metabolism [19–21]. The circulating level of leptin corresponds to the body mass and it is capable of traversing the blood-brain barrier to inform the CNS about the energy reserves held by the body [22, 23].

Leptin has its own dedicated receptor, expressed in the arcuate nucleus. It modulates the expression of orexin by neurons which have their cell bodies within the lateral hippocampus [22, 24, 25]. Miralles demonstrated in 2006 that leptin had a significant effect on how the hypothalamus developed after birth, a finding highlighting the need to control feeding in the infant. Infants who feed excessively lay down additional fat and have a raised body mass index. Their circulating leptin level is raised and they begin to be insensitive to the presence of this molecular signal [22].

Stimulation of leptin receptors on the hypothalamic arcuate nucleus results in decreased appetite. Leptin also inhibits the activity of orexigenic neurons. The overall result is that feeding reduces and energy expenditure goes up [21]. Adipose tissue also expresses the leptin receptor. Stimulation of these receptors results in breakdown of lipids and decreased lipid formation [26]. Moreover, in addition to its role in energy balance, leptin acts on the reproductive and immune systems and affects bone metabolism [27–29]. It has been postulated by some experts that leptin in breast milk is involved in programming the metabolism into childhood and even adulthood, by virtue of its leading the infant to feel quickly satiated [22, 27]. According to Schuster, leptin is present at a raised level in human milk for the first month post-partum. If maternal BMI is within the average range, there is a correlation between breast milk leptin, circulating leptin levels, the degree of fat laid down and BMI. The circulating leptin titre is higher in breastfeeding mothers than in those whose infants were bottle-fed (1.16 ± 0.99 vs 0.68 ± 1.11 ng/mL, respectively), although why this should be so is unknown. It is theorised that leptin in breast milk enters the bloodstream of the infant [27]. In any case, data clearly demonstrate that leptin in breast milk plays a key role in the infant feeling satiated. The role of leptin in this respect is of special concern in developed countries, where obesity has already reached epidemic proportions [30, 31].

Leptin is expressed by a variety of organs, namely adipose tissue, stomach, placenta and breast [31, 32]. The discovery of this hormone fills in many gaps in the current understanding of how appetite is regulated in the longer term. It is notable, however, that in the majority of patients suffering from obesity, there is still a high level of leptin, and administration of extraneous leptin does not affect appetite [33, 34]. This is also the case when lean individuals are treated in this way [35, 36]. There are, however, some reports suggesting that extraneous leptin is of value in treating obesity [37, 38]. Bado et al. found that leptin was expressed in murine gastric mucosae and was readily absorbed into circulation when cholecystokinin was present, making the animals stop eating [39]. Another study revealed that leptin could produce both endocrine and exocrine effects when the contents of the stomach were mixed into the circulation [32, 40]. Nonetheless, it has subsequently been demonstrated that leptin entering the bloodstream via the gastric wall is less effective than endogenous leptin expressed by adipose tissue [41]. Leptin is principally released by the stomach in response to the presence of a food bolus [42]. Two different studies, both dating from 1997, have demonstrated that human milk contains leptin. Not only was leptin synthesised in the mammary gland itself, but it also passed from maternal bloodstream into breast milk. At present, it is still unknown which of these two sources of the hormone is the major one [43]. The perinatal period, including the weeks leading up to delivery, plays a key role in how metabolism is programmed in later life. Malnutrition at this stage predisposes to activation of certain metabolic switches. Likewise, if the mother is overweight or obese, this also alters the metabolic programming, predisposing the infant to obesity and its metabolic complications as he or she grows into adulthood [44, 45]. It has been shown that breastfeeding encourages much more favourable metabolic programming as compared to bottle-feeding.

3   Adiponectin

The expression of adiponectin is regulated at the gene expression level by factors including IGF-1. It has a regulatory function in metabolism [46, 47]. This molecule both stimulates beta oxidation of lipids by skeletal muscle and inhibits the release of glucose by the liver. Adiponectin regulates plasma levels of various metabolic substrates, in particular the aliphatic acids. It has also been shown to influence appetite-related behaviour [47, 48]. One study found that premature infants expressed lower levels of the hormone than those born at full term [49]. It is also present in breast milk and can traverse the intestinal wall to enter the bloodstream, where it has a direct effect on infantile metabolism [50–52]. The level of adiponectin is inversely correlated to specific anthropometric measurements of the neonate and young infant [48, 53–56]. Nonetheless, breast milk contains falling levels of adiponectin over the course of lactation. It has been hypothesised that breastfed individuals are less prone to obesity in adult life due to the presence of adiponectin in breast milk. During the early stages of weaning, adiponectin has an important role in ensuring catabolism occurs [57, 58].

4   Insulin

Insulin is a hormone playing a vital role in the handling of carbohydrates by the body. Its main effects are anabolic. The release of insulin is rapidly stimulated by food intake. The level of insulin released corresponds to the fat mass of the individual. Insulin, therefore, plays a central role in how glucose is metabolised by promoting cellular uptake of glucose and stimulating glycogenesis [59, 60].

Insulin acts on the hypothalamus to reduce appetite (i.e. it is anorexigenic), and it also participates in processes related to satiety. When insulin is bound by its receptor, a cascade of pathways is activated and the FOXP-1 protein (Forkhead box protein 1), a transcription factor, enters its phosphorylated form. Insulin also influences neurotransmitter release. POMC expression is increased, whereas agouti-related peptide levels fall. This hormone also has major effects during pregnancy. Pregnant mothers may exhibit raised plasma glucose, elevated insulin levels and insulin resistance, but these metabolic abnormalities usually revert to normal 5 days after delivery if the mother is otherwise healthy [60, 61]. In the presence of maternal diabetes mellitus or obesity, the hyperglycaemia does not spontaneously remit and the level of insulin also remains outside the normal range. These endocrine alterations can also affect the foetus adversely, resulting in low birthweight, and the mother may express less milk post-partum [62]. Jovanovic-Peterson was the first to identify insulin within breast milk, approximately 20 years ago, but how the presence of this hormone in human milk affects the neonate is still not fully understood [62]. Nonetheless, there is evidence from a number of studies that insulin in human milk affects the health and functional development of the infant [60, 61]. A study using a rodent model discovered a potential role for insulin in milk in guiding the development of the intestinal epithelium and regulating amylase synthesis by the pancreas at the stage when the rat was weaned [63]. The concentration of insulin in breast milk is correlated to the maternal circulating level of this hormone [63]. Mothers with obesity were noted to have a plasma insulin concentration sevenfold that of their healthy peers at 6 months after delivery [64]. It has been noted by some researchers that breast milk insulin levels do not correlate with maternal body mass index. High breast milk insulin levels may be harmful to the breastfed infant. Indeed, Whitmore's 2012 study found that a raised insulin level had potentially adverse effects on infantile body composition during the first months of life [60].

5   Ghrelin

Greenberg was the first to demonstrate that ghrelin is secreted by the breast [65, 66]. This hormone enters the central nervous system from the circulation by traversing the blood-brain barrier. It then acts on the arcuate nucleus, where it stimulates NPY and AgRP secretion, which activates a rise in the levels of orexin A and B. Ghrelin release is stimulated by feeding and has a wide range of actions, including how glucose is handled by the body, energy balance, the motility of the gut, release of stomach acid, circulatory functioning and immune activity [56]. Ghrelin is a competitive antagonist to leptin at receptors on the tenth cranial nerve. It stimulates the neurons of the tractus solitarius and increases dorsomotor activity, thereby stimulating increased stomach acid release [21]. Circulating ghrelin levels correlate to maternal age, height and weight, as well as infantile length and weight. Research has shown that ghrelin levels rise over the course of lactation, being highest in mature milk [55]. Bottle-fed infants have a more elevated circulating level of ghrelin and weigh more than infants who are breastfed [56]; however, the precise mechanisms of action are still not known and need to be investigated.

6   Obestatin

Obestatin produces the opposite action to ghrelin. This hormone facilitates cellular uptake of glucose, regardless of whether insulin is present or not. This is believed to occur by the hormone prompting translocation of the GLUT4 transporter protein. This probably occurs through a signalling process, since inhibition of the signals prevents glucose from being taken up into the cell in the presence of obestatin [67, 68]. This molecule is also present in breast milk, although, according to Aydın et al. (2008), the level is higher in colostrum than in mature milk [69].

7   Resistin

Amongst several other actions, resistin also increases appetite, particularly if body mass is low or metabolism is perturbed in some way. The mechanism appears closely linked to the expressed levels of a number of neuropeptides, in particular NPY and AMPK [17]. There is a strong association of resistin with being obese, insensitive to insulin and acquiring diabetes mellitus [70]. The peak circulating level of resistin in the infant occurs in the initial three post-partum days, declining thereafter [71]. It has been observed that breast milk contains resistin, but the level gradually declines over the course of breastfeeding. In any case, there is only a very weak correlation between circulating resistin levels in the infant and breast milk concentrations [72].

8   PPARγ

PPARγ (peroxisome proliferator-activated receptor-gamma), together with the associated co-activator, form a myokine, the release of which is under the control of PGC-1α. This complex regulates oxygen intake, mitochondrial synthetic activity and expression of UCP1 (uncoupling protein 1), the net effect of which is to regulate heat production and energy use by the mitochondria. Exactly what role PPARγ plays in foetal growth and development is not fully understood, but one major role is to stimulate adipose tissue deposition in utero [73]. The peak level of PPARγ occurs within the initial month post-partum [74, 75].

9   Copeptin

Copeptin appears to have numerous roles, involving both acid-base balance and acting as a growth factor [76, 77]. Dobsa and Cullen [78] report that copeptin has an indirect effect on the excretion of water and thus the circulatory system, as well as muscular contraction occurring during labour and breastfeeding [78]. There is an association of circulating copeptin level with obesity, and thus this molecule may also exert indirect effects on feeding behaviour [77]. The connection is likely to occur through the association of raised arginine vasopressin with higher levels of cortisol. This then leads to increased adipose deposition, especially in the area of the trunk, provoked by the orexigenic effects of cortisol [79]. Circulating copeptin concentration is independent of both glucose and insulin levels in patients with type 2 diabetes mellitus [43, 80]. Aydın et al. discovered in 2013 [74] that the concentration of copeptin in breast milk rose alongside the plasma level and showed an increasing trend over the course of breastfeeding [74].

10 Apelin

High levels of both insulin and apelin have been reported in obese patients. Apelin levels are dysregulated in obese individuals and it has been proposed that if insulin rises, so must apelin [81]. Research has revealed that there is a correlation between obesity and apelin, but no research so far has addressed how apelin levels relate to food intake [82]. Given this association of apelin with obesity, it seems reasonable to hypothesise that this hormone has effects on both metabolism and the circulatory system. Further research is called for, however, before the relationship can be fully understood [83]. Habata was the first to discover apelin in mammalian colostrum (in mice) in 1990, and it was identified in breast milk in 2010 [84]. The level of apelin in milk increases over the course of breastfeeding, being highest in mature milk. The fact that the hormone is present in breast milk and that it has an altered level in cases of obesity probably confirms its role in promoting neonatal gain weight.

11 Nesfatin

Dong (2014) demonstrated an association of raised hypothalamic levels of nesfatin-1 with lower food intake because of earlier satiety. Weight loss was also observed as adipose mass had also decreased. Aydın et al. were the first to examine nesfatin levels in breast milk [85], concluding that mature milk has a higher concentration of this hormone than colostrum. Mothers suffering from gestational diabetes but otherwise healthy expressed a lower level of nesfatin than healthy controls. This decreased level meant the mothers with gestational diabetes had a larger appetite than usual and anorexigenic mechanisms were impaired. There may be similar effects on the foetus or infant, too [85].

12 Glucagon-like Peptide (GLP-1)

GLP-1 is transcribed from the pro-glucagon gene. Its effect is anorexigenic [86]. GLP-1 has a brief half-life (around 2 min) since it is degraded by dipeptidases. The levels of carbohydrates, lipids and protein influence the secretion of GLP-1 [87]. The principal role of this hormone is glucose homeostasis, in addition to stimulating the release of insulin (i.e. insulinotropic). Where GLP-1 is present, the pancreatic alpha and beta cells become more sensitive to glucose levels. The insulinotropic effect occurs only when there is hyperglycaemia [88]. Glucagon mainly serves to signal satiety.

13 Insulin-like Growth Factor-1 (IGF-1)

The way serum IGF-1 level and body composition are interrelated may differ between adults and children. Whilst some research has been able to demonstrate that IGF-1 levels are inversely related to the degree of body fat, when children were examined, IGF-1 levels and BMI were directly linked [39, 89]. There is a slow rise in IGF-1 concentration in breast milk over the course of lactation. Since neonates have deficient levels of growth factors, it has been suggested that growth factors might be absorbed from breast milk to remedy this deficit [53]. Indeed, IGF-1 does appear to undergo active uptake from breast milk and can enter circulation. Accordingly, breastfed infants have higher circulating levels of IGF-1 than bottle-fed infants. A putative action of IGF-1 is weight gain. According to Ohkawa et al., obesity in adults may be caused by elevated IGF-1 levels [78]. There have been calls for more studies addressing the relationship between the level of IGF-1 in breast milk and how the infant develops [50, 90].

14 Cortisol

Breast milk performs an essential physiological role by carrying bioactive molecules of maternal origin to the developing infant. Cortisol is one such bioactive molecule. This transfer allows the regulation of infant growth and the expression of particular phenotypes [91]. Cortisol carries out multiple physiological functions related to metabolism, immunity and the development of the nervous system. It plays an important role in regulating levels of glucose and lipids in the circulation to match energy requirements [92]. Cortisol also activates the conversion of the inactive hormone, cortisone, to bioactive cortisol through the action of 11-beta hydroxysteroid dehydrogenase [93]. Cortisol also appears in breast milk when the mother is well-nourished. Cortisol in breast milk correlates with having a normal birthweight and gaining weight in the neonate [94]. According to a study by Van der Voon (2016), the level of glucocorticoids expressed in breast milk was higher if the child had been born at term than if born prematurely [95].

15 IL-6

IL-6 is a cytokine that has a pleiotropic effect. It acts on inflammatory processes, immune response and haemopoiesis. Adipose tissue accounts for 15–35% of the expression of this cytokine [96]. In humans, this molecule is a protein formed of 212 amino acid residues with a signalling peptide composed of 28 residues. The IL-6 gene is located on Chromosome 7. IL-6 is generated at the site of inflammation and transported via the bloodstream to the liver, where it triggers the expression of C-reactive protein, serum amyloid A (SAA), haptoglobin, alpha-1-antichymotrypsin and fibrinogen [97]. IL-6 simultaneously raises the levels of cytokines but inhibits the synthesis of transferrin, albumin and fibronectin. A-type amyloidosis occurs due to the accumulation of SAA in particular tissues [98]. Although the pro-inflammatory role is what IL-6 is best known for, paradoxically it also participates in the suppression of inflammation and in regeneration [99]. Notably, IL-6 expression is higher in cases of obesity than in healthy controls [100]. Whilst it is not yet proven whether an elevated level of IL-6 expression exerts a damaging or a protective effect in obesity, it has been established that insulin insensitivity and inflammation do increase through the upgraded expression of SOCS3 (suppressor of cytokine signalling 3) [101]. IL-6 stimulates a pro-inflammatory response by binding to soluble IL-6Rα in the circulation, which then interacts with glycoprotein-130 on the cell's outer membrane, so-called 'trans-signalling'. It performs its anti-inflammatory role through the classic signalling mechanism activated when IL-6 interacts with membrane-bound IL-6Rα and glycoprotein-130 [102]. Inflammation, as indicated by infiltration of macrophages into white adipose tissue, was less active in a murine model involving feeding the animals high fat whilst selectively blocking the actions of IL-6 on fat tissue [103]. Il-6 stimulates osteoclasts, cells implicated in osteoporosis and in physiological osseous resorption. Furthermore, it acts on RANKL (receptor activator of nuclear factor kappa-B ligand) [104]. By stimulating a higher level of VEGF (vascular endothelial growth factor) secretion, IL-6 causes the formation of new blood vessels and increases endothelium permeability. This effect is seen in the synovium in cases of rheumatoid arthritis and is part of the pathophysiological mechanisms of the disease [105].

IL-6 has a molecular mass of 28 kDa and is a glycoprotein. It contains four helical structures. The molecular region interacting with the receptor is denoted as Zone 1. Three binding sites have been identified on the molecule. The human herpesvirus 6 (HHV-6) also synthesises an IL-6, which has an identical sequence to the human type in regions 2 and 3. The IL-6R molecule is soluble in circulating blood and can perform a regulatory role in inflammation, in common with other soluble receptors, which may act agonistically or antagonistically in cytokine signalling events. The antagonistic function depends on the inhibition of IL-1α and TNF-α. The soluble IL-6 receptor amplifies the signal produced by IL-6. There are, in fact, only certain cell populations that express a membrane-bound IL-6 receptor, specifically macrophages, neutrophils, some types of T-lymphocytes and hepatocytes.

A number of researchers have reported that IL-6 has metabolic effects. For example, there is a significant release of IL-6 from muscles during exercise [106, 107]. In a different study, there was a connection between body fat mass of obese individuals and IL-6 levels released by adipose tissue [108]. Obesity is thus classified as a condition involving a persistent low level of inflammation. One study reported that homozygous IL-6 knockout mice were obese at an advanced age, but this finding has not been replicated elsewhere [109]. Another study noted that homozygous IL-6 knockout mice demonstrated both insulin resistance and glucose intolerance [110].It is noteworthy that the mice involved had a form of hepatitis that was dampened by inhibiting TNF-α, a finding which suggests a direct connection between the activity of IL-6 and TNF-α. In patients receiving tocilizumab, which neutralises the IL-6 receptor, there was around a 4 kg increase in body mass (i.e. 7% change) and severe hypertriglyceridaemia, accompanied by hypercholesterolaemia. These findings led to the hypothesis that IL-6 was somehow implicated in metabolic disorders in humans. In studies involving transgenic mice which overexpress IL-6 and IL-6R, the transgenic animals were smaller than the non-transgenic mice and their adipose tissue mass was lower, an effect mediated through the signalling pathway. In mice that lack IL-6, the IL6 receptor is still expressed by hepatocytes. IL-6 is believed to moderate the sensitivity of the liver to insulin and control glucose tolerance, both effects being mediated via the classical IL-6 signalling pathway. When IL-6 is present at a high concentration, lipolysis occurs and fatty acids are oxidised. IL-6Rα mediates lipolysis by releasing fatty acids stored around the viscera. Nonetheless, this mobilisation of fatty acids may cause the liver and heart to accumulate adipose tissue and may result in insulin insensitivity.

16   Other Cytokines

There has been research examining the level of cytokines present in breast milk. Measurements were undertaken in breast milk samples from 15 mothers at 1, 4, 8 and 12 weeks post-partum. The cytokines measured were monocyte chemoattractant protein, epithelial neutrophil-activating factor-78, hepatocyte growth factor and insulin-like growth factor binding protein-1. There has also been the study of interleukins 6 and 8, colony stimulating factor-1, osteoclastogenesis inhibitory factor and metalloproteinase tissue inhibiting factor-2 amongst others. It was noted that these cytokines demonstrated a time-related decline in expression. Cytokines are responsible for producing inflammatory and neoplastic alterations within the breast and thus they have been proposed as potential biomarkers for disease [80]. However, research indicates that cytokine levels in breast milk do not increase with time, and there appears to be no correlation between parity and the levels of cytokines. The short-term expression of particular cytokines during breastfeeding may influence changes in the breast. Whilst animal models have been extensively and successfully employed to inform knowledge about cytokine levels in the mammary gland during the process after delivery, as well as during neoplastic changes, there is a lack of agreement on how to interpret breast milk cytokine levels due to considerable heterogeneity in study methods employed. These reports mainly study the potential effects of cytokines on an infant's health, as well as the functions of cytokines implicated in mastitis.

Autocrine rather than endocrine signalling appears to be the dominant mode at an early stage of lactation. In this initial phase, milk production is governed by how much milk is already being discharged and how frequently the infant tugs on the breast. Given their established role in secretion and signalling, cytokine levels have been suspected to be linked to how quickly milk is produced.

However, whilst there are several studies that have found an association between IL-6 and IL-8 expression and neoplasia of the mammary gland, involution or inflammation, only one study so far has addressed the relationship between pregnancy and the levels of cytokines in breast milk.

17 Tumour Necrosis Factor-Alpha (TNF-α)

TNF-α was named after its ability to cause necrosis in tumours. However, it is widely expressed, for example, by macrophages and adipose tissue. This molecule reduces the uptake of glucose in response to insulin and inhibits the actions of lipoprotein lipase. It contributes to normal development and functioning of the immune system in infants. TNF-α is secreted into breast milk by macrophages and the epithelium of the breast. The contribution of TNF-α to maturation of infant immunity is essential. The immunoprotectivity of breast milk stems from its containing few inflammatory mediators and producing a general effect of suppressing inflammation [109]. Rudloff was the first to report on the level of TNF-α in breast milk one and 2 days after delivery [89]. In the initial 2 days of breastfeeding, infants are exposed to 60 ng of TNF-α. The levels of this factor have been compared in colostrum and mature milk by Meki [110]. Colostrum was found to contain 402.8 ± 29.7 pg/mL, whereas mature milk contained 178.3 ± 14.4 pg/mL. However, studies of how TNF-α levels correlate to the health of the infant have been very infrequent. One finding of significance, however, is that TNF-α levels and lean mass are negatively correlated at 1 month of age [19].

References

1. Singh RK, Kumar P, Mahalingam K. Molecular genetics of human obesity: a comprehensive review. C R Biol. 2017;340(2):87–108. https://doi.org/10.1016/j.crvi.2016.11.007. Epub 2017 Jan 13.
2. Ng M, Fleming T, Robinson M, Thomson B, Graetz N, Margono C, et al. Global, regional, and national prevalence of overweight and obesity in children and adults during 1980–2013: a systematic analysis for the Global Burden of Disease Study 2013. Lancet. 2014;384(9945):766–81. https://doi.org/10.1016/S0140-6736(14)60460-8. Epub 2014 May 29. Erratum in: Lancet. 2014 Aug 30;384(9945):746.

3. Kelly T, Yang W, Chen C-S, Reynolds K, He J. Global burden of obesity in 2005 and projections to 2030. Int J Obes. 2008;32:1431–7. https://doi.org/10.1038/ijo.2008.102.

4. Erlichman J, Kerbey AL, James WPT. Physical activity and its impact on health outcomes, paper 2: prevention of unhealthy weight gain and obesity by physical activity: an analysis of the evidence. Obes Rev. 2002;3:273–87.

5. Alonso R, Faras M, Alvarez V, Cuevas A. The genetics of obesity. In: Rodriguez-Oquendo A, editor. Translational cardiometabolic genomic medicine. Elsevier; 2016. p. 161–77. http://linkinghub.elsevier.com/retrieve/pii/B978012799961600007X.

6. Lyon HN, Hirschhorn JN. Genetics of common forms of obesity: a brief overview. Am J Clin Nutr. 2005;82:215S–7S.

7. Scuteri A, Sanna S, Chen W-M, Uda M, Albai G, Strait J, et al. Genome-wide association scan shows genetic variants in the FTO gene are associated with obesity-related traits. PLoS Genet. 2007;3:e115. https://doi.org/10.1371/journal.pgen.0030115.

8. Frayling TM, Timpson NJ, Weedon MN, Zeggini E, Freathy RM, Lindgren CM, et al. A common variant in the FTO gene is associated with body mass index and predisposes to childhood and adult obesity. Science. 2007;316:889–94.

9. Ordovas JM, Shen J. Gene-environment interactions and susceptibility to metabolic syndrome and other chronic diseases. J Periodontol. 2008;79:1508–13. https://doi.org/10.1902/jop.2008.080232.

10. Bird A. Perceptions of epigenetics. Nature. 2007;447:396–8. https://doi.org/10.1038/nature05913.

11. Barres R, Zierath JR. DNA methylation in metabolic disorders. Am J Clin Nutr. 2011;93:897S–900S. https://doi.org/10.3945/ajcn.110.001933.

12. Campion J, Milagro FI, Martınez JA. Individuality and epigenetics in obesity. Obes Rev. 2009;10:383–92. https://doi.org/10.1111/j.1467-789X.2009.00595.x.

13. Dolinoy DC, Jirtle RL. Environmental epigenomics in human health and disease. Environ Mol Mutagen. 2008;49:4–8.

14. Hetherington AW, Ranson SW. Hypothalamic lesions and adiposity in the rat. Anat Rec. 1940;78:149–72. https://doi.org/10.1002/ar.1090780203.

15. Minokoshi Y, Kim Y-B, Peroni OD, Fryer LGD, Müller C, Carling D, Kahn BB. Leptin stimulates fatty-acid oxidation by activating AMP activated protein kinase. Nature. 2002;415:339–43. https://doi.org/10.1038/415339a.

16. Zhang Y, Chua S Jr. Leptin function and regulation. Compr Physiol. 2017;8(1):351–69. https://doi.org/10.1002/cphy.c160041.

17. Zhang Y, Proenca R, Maffei M. Positional cloning of the mouse obese gene and its human homologue. Nature. 1994;372(2):425–32.

18. Friedman JM, Halaas JL. Leptin and the regulation of body weight in mammals. Nature. 1998;3(95):763–70.

19. Schuster S, Hechler C, Gebauer C, Kiess W, Kratzsch J. Leptin in maternal serum and breastmilk: association with infants' body weight gain in a longitudinal study over 6 months of lactation. Pediatr Res. 2011;70(6):633–7.

20. Smith-Kirwin S, O'Connor D, Johnston J, de Lancy E, Hassink S, Funanage V. Leptin expression in human mammary epithelial cells and breastmilk. J Clin Endocrinol Metab. 1998;83(5):1810.

21. Bonnet M, Gourdou I, Leroux C, Chilliard Y, Djiane J. Leptin expression in the ovine mammary gland: putative sequential involvement of adipose, epithelial and myoepithelial cells during pregnancy and lactation. J Amin Sci. 2002;80(3):723–8.

22. Miralles O, Sanchez J, Paolou A. A physiological role of breast milk leptin in body weight control in developing infants. Obesity (Silver Spring). 2006;14:1371–7.

23. Casabiell X, Pineiro V, Tomeo M, Peino R, Dieguez C, Casanueva F. Presence of leptin in colostrum and/or breast milk from lactating mothers: a potential role in the regulation of neonatal food intake. J Clin Endocrinol Metab. 1997;82(12):1470–3.

24. Schwartz MW. Central nervous system regulation of food intake. Obesity. 2006;14(2):1–8.

25. Savino F, Fissore M, Grassino E, Nanni G, Oggero R, Silvestro L. Ghrelin, leptin and IGF-1 levels in breast-fed and formula-fed infants in the first years of life. Acta Paediatr. 2005;9 4(5):531–7.

26. Minokoshi Y, Kim YB, Peroni OD, et al. Leptin stimulates fatty–acid oxidation by activating amp-activated protein kinase. Nature. 2002;415:339–43.

27. Quiros-Gonzalez I, Yadav VK. Central genes, pathways and modules that regulate bone mass. Arch Biochem Biophysic. 2014;561:130–6.

28. Garcia-Galiano D, Allen SJ, Elias CF. Role of adipocyte-derived hormone leptin in reproductive control. Horm Mol Biol Clin Investig. 2014;19:141–9.

29. Abella V, Scotece M, Conde J. Leptin in the interplay of inflammation, metabolism and immune system disorders. Nat Rev Rheumatol. 2017;13:100–9.

30. Pico C, Oliver P, Sanchez J. The intake of physiological doses of leptin during lactation in rats improves insulin sensitivity and affects food preferences later in life. Endorionology. 2008;149:733–40.

31. Bado A, Levasseur S, Attoub S. The stomach is a source of leptin. Nature. 1998;394:790–3.

32. Cinti S, Matteis rd, Pico C. Secretory granules of endocrine and chief cells of human stomach mucosa contain leptin. Int J Obes. 2000;24:789–93.

33. Maffei M, Halaas J, Ravussin E. Leptin levels in human and rodent: measurement of plasma leptina and ob RNA obese and weight-reduced subjects. Nat Med. 1995;1:1155–61.

34. Lonnqvist F, Arner P, Nordfors L, Schalling M. Overexpression of the obese (ob) gene in adipose tissue of human obese subjects. Nat Med. 1995;1:950–3.

35. Heymsfield SB, Greenberg AS, Fujikooka K, et al. Recombinant leptin for weight loss in obese and lean adults: a randomized, controlled, dose-escalation trial. JAMA. 1999;282:1568–75.

36. Hukshorn CJ, van Dielen FM, Buurman WA. The effect of pegylated recombinant human leptin (PEG-OB) on weight loss and inflammatory status in obese subjects. Int J Obes. 2002;26:504.

37. Farooqi IS, Jebb SA, Langmack G, et al. Effects of recombinant leptin therapy in a child with congenital leptin deficiency. N Engl J Med. 1999;341:879–84.

38. Farooqi IS, Matarese G, Lord GM. Beneficial effects of leptin on obesity, T cell hyporesponsiveness, and neuroendocrine/metabolic dysfunction of human congenital leptin deficiency. J Clin Invest. 2002;110:1093–103.

39. Stanley T, Feldpausch M, Murphy C, Grinspoon S, Makimura H. Discordance of IGF-1 and GH stimulation testing for altered GH secretion in obesity. Growth Hormon IGF Res. 2014;24(1):10–5.

40. Cinti S, de Matteis R, Ceresi E, et al. Leptin in human stomach. Gut. 2001;49:155.

41. Pico C, Oliver P, Sanchez T. Gastric leptin a putative role in the short term regulation of food intake. Br J Nutr. 2003;90:735–41.

42. Pico C, Sanchez J, Oliver P. Leptin production by the stomach is upregulated in obese (*fa/fa*) Zucker rats. Obes Res. 2002;10:932–8.

43. Morgenthaler N. Assay for the measurement of copeptin a stable peptide from the precursor of vasopressin. Clin Chem. 2006;52(1):112–9.

44. Barker DJI, Erikson JG, Forsen T. Fetal origins of hyperphagia, obesity, and hypertension and postnatal amplification by hypercaloric nutrition. Am J Physiol Endocrinol Metab. 2000;279:83–7.

45. Martorell R, Stein AD, Schroeder DG. Early nutrition and later adiposity. J Nutr. 2001;131:8745–800.

46. Perry B, Wang Y. Appetite regulation and weight control: the role of gut hormone. Nutr Diabetes. 2012;2(1):e26.
47. Lopez M, Tovar S, Vazquez M, Williams L, Dieguez C. Peripheral tissue-brain interactions in the regulation of food intake. Proc Nutr Soc. 2007;66(1):131–55.
48. Newburg D, Woo J, Morrow A. Characteristics and potential functions of human milk adiponectin. J Pediatr. 2010;156(2):41–6.
49. Andreas N, Hyde M, Gale C, Parkinson J, Jeffries S, Holmes E. Effect of maternal body mass index on hormones in breast milk: a systematic review. PLoS One. 2014;9(12):1–25.
50. Savino F, Lupica M, Benetti S, Petrucci E, Liguor S, Cordero Di Montezemolo L. Adiponectin in breast milk: relation to serum adiponectin concentration in lactating mothers and their infants. Acta Paediatr. 2012;101(10):1058–62.
51. Woo J, Guerrero M, Guo F, Martin L, Davidson BS, Ortega H. Human milk adiponectin affects infant weight trajectory during the second year of life. J Pediatr Gastroenterol Nutr. 2012;54(4):532–9.
52. Ozarda Y, Gunes Y, Tuncer G. The concentration of adiponectin in breast milk is related to maternal hormonal and inflammatory status during 6 months of lactation. Clin Chem Lab Med. 2012;50:911.
53. Kon I, Shilina N, Gmoshinskaya M, Ivanushkina T. The study of breastmilk IGF-1, leptin, ghrelin and adiponectin levels as possible reasons of high weight gain in breast-fed infants. Ann Nutr Metab. 2014;65(4):317–23.
54. Dundar N, Dundar B, Cesur G, Yilmaz N, Sutcu R, Ozguner F. Ghrelin and adiponectin levels in colostrum, cord blood and maternal serum. Pediatr Int. 2010;52(4):622–5.
55. Steculorum S, Collden G, Coupe B, Croizier S, Lockie S, Andrews Z. Neonatal ghrelin programs development of hypothalamic feeding circuits. J Clin Investig. 2015;125(2):846–58.
56. Whatmore AJ, Hall CM, Jones J, Westwood M, Clayton PE. Ghrelin concentrations in healthy children and adolescents. Clin Endocrinol. 2003;59(5):649–54.
57. Haschke F, Ziegler Grathwohl D. Fast growth of infants of overweight mothers :can it be slowed down? Ann Nutr Metab. 2014;64(1):19–24.
58. Catli G, Olgac N, Dündar B. Adipokines in breastmilk: an update. J Clin Res Pediatr Endocrinol. 2014;65(1):19–24.
59. Kronborg H, Vaeth M, Rasmussen K. Obesity and early cessation of breastfeeding in Denmark. Eur J Pub Health. 2012;3(2):316–22.
60. Whitmore T, Trengove N, Graham D, Hartman P. Analysis of insulin in human breast milk in mothers with type 1 and type 2 diabetes mellitus. Int J Endocrinol. 2012;1:1–9.
61. Ahuja S, Boylan M, Hart S, Shriver R, Spallholz J, Pence B. Glucose and insulin levels are increased in obese and overweight mothers' breast-milk. Food Nutr Sci. 2011;2(3):201–6.
62. Jovanovic-Peterson L, Fuhrmann K, Hedden K, Walker L, Peterson C. Maternal milk and plasma glucose and insulin levels: studies in normal and diabetic subjects. J Am Coll Nutr. 1989;8(2):125–31.
63. Kirk S, Samuelsson A, Argenton M. Maternal obesity induced by diet in rats permanently influences central processes regulating food intake in offspring. PLoS One. 2009;4(6):e5870.
64. Friedman JM, Halaas JL. Leptin and the regulation of body weight in mammals. Nature (Lond). 1998;395:763–70.
65. Grönberg M, Tsolakis A, Magnusson L, Janson E, Saras J. Distribution of obestatin and ghrelin in human tissues immunoreactive cells in the gastrointestinal tract, pancreas and mammary glands. J Histochem Cytochem. 2008;56(9):793–801.
66. Dundar N, Dundar B, Cesur G, Yilmaz N, Sutcu R, Ozguner F. Ghrelin and adiponectin levels in colostrum, cord blood and maternal serum. Paediatr Int. 2010;52:622–5.
67. Granata R, Gallo D, Luque RM, Baragli A, Scarlatti F, Grande C. Obestatin regulates adipocyte function and protects against diet induced insulin resistance and inflammation. Fed Am Soc Exp Biol J. 2012;26(8):3393–411.

68. Savino F, Benetti S, Lupica MM, Petrucci E, Palumeri E, Cordero Di Montezemolo L. Ghrelin and obestatin in infants, lactating mothers and breastmilk. Horm Res Paediatr. 2012;78(56):297–303.

69. Aydin S, Ozkan Y, Erman F, Gurates B, Kilic N, Colak R. Presence of obestatin in breastmilk: relationship among obestatin, ghrelin and leptin in lactating women. Nutrition. 2008;24(78):689–93.

70. Jamaluddin M, Weakley S, Yao Q, Chen C. Resistin: functional roles and therapeutic considerations for cardiovascular disease. Br J Pharmacol. 2012;165(3):622–32.

71. Ilcol Y, Hizli Z, Eroz E. Resistin is present in human breast milk and it correlates with maternal hormonal status ND serum level of c-reactive protein. Clin Chem Lab Med. 2008;46(1):118–24.

72. Savino F, Sorrenti M, Benetti S, Lupica M, Liguori S, Oggero R. Resistin and leptin in breast milk in infants in early life. Early Hum Dev. 2012;88:779–882.

73. Kelly DP. Medicine. Irisin light may fire. Science. 2012;336(6077):42–3.

74. Aydin S, Kuloglu T, Aydin S. Copeptin adropin and irisin concentrations in breastmilk and plasma of healthy women and those with gestational diabetes mellitus. Peptides. 2013;47:66–70.

75. Mora I, Espinoza A, Lopez N, Acevo P, Romero FM, Montero P. Indicadores de riesgo cardiovascular, patrones de lactancia y estilo de vida de la madre durante el proceso de crecimiento y desarrollo fetal e infantile. Nutr Clin Diet Hosp. 2015;35(2):91–100.

76. Repaske D, Medlei R, Gultekin E, Krishnamani M, Halaby G, Findling j. Heterogeneity in clinical manifestation of autosomal dominant of neurohypophyseal diabetes insipidus caused by a mutation encoding Ala-1->Val in the signa peptide of arginine vasopressin/neurophysin II/copeptin precursor. J Clin Endocrinol Metab. 1997;82(1):51–6.

77. Khan S, Dhillon O, O'Brien R, Struck J, Quinn P, Morgenthaler N. C-terminal provasopressin (copeptin) as a novel and prognostic marker in acute myocardial infarction: Leicester acute myocardial infarction peptide (LAMP) study. Circulation. 2007;115(16):2013–5.

78. Ohkawa N, Shoji H, Kitamura T, Suganuma H, Yoshikawa N, Suzuki M. IGF-leptin and active ghrelin levels in very low birth weight infants during the first 8 weeks of life. Acta Paediatr. 2009;99:37–41.

79. Dobsa L, Cullen K. Copeptin and its potential role in diagnosis and prognosis of various diseases. Biochem Med. 2013;23(2):172–90.

80. Enhorning S, Struck J, Wirfalt E, Hedblad B, Morgenthaler N, Melander O. Plasma copeptin unifying factor behind the metabolic syndrome. J Clin Endocrinol Metab. 2011;967(7):1065–72.

81. Boucher J, Masri B, Daviaud D, Gesta S, Guigne C, Mazzucotelli A, Apelin A. Newly identified adipokine upregulated by insulin and obesity. Endocrinology. 2006;146(4):1764–71.

82. Saleem U, Khaleghi M, Morgenthaler N, Bergmann A, Struck J, Mosley T. Plasma carboxyterminal provasopressin (copeptin): a novel marker of insulin resistance and metabolic syndrome. J Clin Endocrinol Metab. 2009;94(7):2558–64.

83. Castan-Laurell I, Daviaud VM, Dray C, Kovacikova M, Kovacikova Z, Hejnova J, Stich V, Valet P. Effect of hypocaloric diet-induced weight loss in obese women on plasma apelin and adipose tissue expression of apelin and APJ. Eur J Endocrinol. 2008;158(6):905–10.

84. Habata Y, Fuji R, Hosova M, Fukusumi S, Kwamata Y, Hinuma S. Apelin, the natural ligand of the orphan receptor APJ, is abundantly secreted in the colostrum BBA. Biochim Biophys Acta, Mol Cell Res. 1999;1452(1):25–35.

85. Aydin S. The presence of the peptides apelin, ghrelin and nesfatin 1 in the human breastmilk and the lowering of their levels in patients with gestational diabetes mellitus. Peptides. 2010;31(12):2236–40.

86. Schueler J, Alexander B, Hart A, Austin K, Larson E. Presence and dynamics of leptin. GLP-1, and PYY in human breast milk at early post-partum. Obesity. 2013;21(7):1451–8.

87. Schira J, Burkhard G. The physiological role of GLP-1 in human incretin, ileal break or more? Regul Pept. 2005;128(2):109–15.
88. Schuelere J, Alexander B, Hart A, Austin K, Larson E. Presence and dynamics of leptin, GLP-1 and PYY in human breastmilk at early post-partum. Obesity. 2013;21(7):1451–8.
89. Elmlinger M, Hochhaus F, Loui A, Frommer K, Obladen M, Ranke K. Insulin-like growth factors and binding proteins in early milk from mothers of preterm and term infants. Horm Res Paediatr. 2007;68(3):124–31.
90. Stanley T, Feldpausch M, Murphy C, Grinspoon S, Makimura H. Discordance of IGF-I and GH stimulation testing for altered GH secretion in obesity. Growth Hormon IGF Res. 2014;24(1):10–5.
91. Hinde K, Skibiel A, Foster A, Del Rosso L, Mendoza S, Capitanio J. Cortisol in mothers's milk across lactation reflects maternal life history and predicts infant temperament. Behav Ecol. 2014;26:269–81.
92. Jwa S, Fujiwara T, Kondo N. Latent protective effects of breastfeeding on late childhood overweight and obesity: a nationwide prospective study. Obesity. 2014;22:1527–37.
93. Carter M, Dudley D, Nathanielsz P. Fetal cortisol is evaluated in maternal obesity. Reprod Sci. 2011;18:139 A.
94. Entringer S. Impact of stress and stress physiology during pregnancy on child metabolic function and obesity risk. Curr Opin Clin Nutrit Metab Care. 2013;16:1320–7.
95. Van der Voorn B, de Waard M, van Goudoever JB, Rotteveel J, Heijboer AC, Finken MJ. Breastmilk cortisol and cortisone concentrations follow the diurnal rhythm of maternal hypothalamus-pituitary-adrenal axis activity. J Nutr. 2016;146(11):2174–9.
96. Fruhbeck G, Gomez-Ambrosi J, Muruzabal FJ, Burrel MA. The adipocyte: a model for integration of endocrine and metabolic signaling in energy metabolism regulation. Am J Physiol Endocrinol Metab. 2001;280(6):E827–47.
97. Heinrich PC, Castell JV, Andus T. Interleukin-6 and the acute phase response. Biochem J. 1990;1990(265):621–36.
98. Gillmore JD, Lovat LB, Persey MR, Pepys MB, Hawkins PN. Amyloid load and clinical outcome in AA amyloidosis in relation to circulating concentration of serum amyloid A protein. Lancet. 2001;358(24):299.
99. Scheller J, Chalaris A, Schmidt-Arras D, Rose-John S. The pro- and anti-inflammatory properties of the cytokine interleukin-6. Biochim Biophys Acta. 2011;1813:878–88.
100. MohamedAli VS, Goodrick A, Katz RDR, Miles JM, Yudkin JS, Klein S, Koppack SW. Subcutaneous adipose tissue releases interleukin-6 but not tumor necrosis factor alpha in vivo. J Clin Endocrinol Metab. 1997;82(12):4196.
101. Lazar MA. How obesity causes diabetes: not a tall tale. Science. 2005;307(5708):373–5.
102. Scheller J, Chalaris A, Schmidt-Arras D, Rose-John S. The pro- and anti-inflammatory properties of the the cytokine interleukin-6. Biochem Biophys Acta. 2011;1813(5):878–88.
103. Kraakman MJ, Kammoun HI, Allen TI, Desvaerte V, Henstrige DC, Estevez E, et al. Blocking IL-6 trans-signaling prevents high-fat diet induced adipose tissue macrophage recruitment but does not improve insulin resistance. Cell Metab. 2015;21(3):403–16.
104. Hashizume M, Hayakawa N, Mihara M. IL-6 transsignalling directly induces RANKL on fibroblast-like synovial cells and is involved in RANKL induction by TNF-α and IL-17. Rheumatology (Oxford). 2008;47:1635–40.
105. Hashizume M, Hayakawa N, Suzuki M, Mihara M. IL-6/sIL-6R trans signaling, but not TNF-α induced angiogenesis in huvec and synovial cell co-culture system. Rheumatol Int. 2009;29:1449–54.
106. Pedersen BK, Febbrario MA. Muscle as an endocrine organ: focus on muscle derived interleukin-6. Physiol Rev. 2008;88:1379–406.
107. Pedersen BK, Steensberg A, Fischer C, Keller C, Keller P, Plomgaard P, Febbraio M, Saltin B. Searching for the exercise factor: is IL-6 a candidate? J Muscle Res Cell Motil. 2003;24:113–9.

108. Skurk T, Alberti-Huber C, Herder C, Hauner H. Relationship between adipocyte size and adipokine expression and secretion. J Clin Endocrinol Metab. 2007;92(3):1023–33.
109. Wallenius V, Wallenius K, Ahren B, Rudling M, Carlsten H, Dickson SL, Ohlsson C, Jansson JO. Interleukin-6-defficient mice develop mature-onset obesity. Nat Med. 2002;8(8):75–9.
110. Wunderlich FT, Ströhle P, Könner AC, Gruber S, Tovar S, Brönneke HS, Juntti-Berggren L, Li LS, van Rooijen N, Libert C, Berggren PO, Brüning JC. Interleukin-6 signaling in liver-parenchymal cells suppresses hepatic inflammation and improves systemic insulin action. Cell Metab. 2010;12:237–49.

Epigenetic Causes of Obesity

Özlem Naciye Şahin, Samim Ozen, and Despina D. Briana

1   Introduction

Obesity is a multifactorial disorder in which genetics, epigenetics and the environment all act and interact with each other. Through a number of investigative techniques, including linkage analysis, genome-wide association studies and large-scale sequencing of either the entire genome or the exon-containing component, a large number of genes have been implicated in the processes predisposing to severe obesity [1, 2]. At present, the number of locations on the genome with established associations with obesity exceeds 200 [3, 4]. Nonetheless, genetic variability is insufficient to account for the patterns of inheritance observed in obese individuals, and clustering in families also indicates epigenetic factors. Epigenetic modifications are also caused by changes in the environment, such as overfeeding [5, 6], and a proportion of epigenetic alterations appear irreversible.

Epigenetic modifications are mechanisms for altering the expression of particular genes that do not result in alteration of the sequence of bases in DNA, but do persist through both mitotic and meiotic cell divisions [6]. Epigenetic alterations may be accomplished by methylation of DNA sequences, by the action of miRNA transcripts not destined for translation and through changes to histones. They are crucial in understanding differences between individuals and are potential candidates for explaining various complex phenotypes, including obesity. In

Ö. N. Şahin (✉)
Department of Child Health and Diseases, Arel University, Medical Faculty, Istanbul, Türkiye

S. Ozen
Department of Pediatrics, Pediatric Endocrinology Division, Medical Faculty, Ege University, Izmir, Türkiye

D. D. Briana
NICU, Third Department of Pediatrics, National and Kapodistrian University of Athens, University General Hospital "ATTIKON", Athens, Greece

Ö. N. Şahin et al. (eds.), *Breastfeeding and Metabolic Programming*, https://doi.org/10.1007/978-3-031-33278-4_16

population studies, DNA methylation is the most commonly used investigative technique, mainly because the modifications are somewhat stable and can be readily assessed by high-throughput assays. The usual way methylation occurs is by the addition of a methyl residue at the 5′ position on a cytosine bound via a phosphate group to a guanine, i.e. on a CpG dinucleotide [6]. CpG methylations have been confirmed to influence cell differentiation and fate in mammalian species. DNA methyltransferase enzymes (DNMTs) largely preserve the methylation of specific DNA regions that originally occurred at specific stages of development [6]. A molecular cellular mechanism should mediate the ability of phenotypes to be shaped by changes in the environment. The epigenome is thus capable of being modified in utero, during the neonatal period, at puberty and as the individual grows older. If epigenetic modifications in particular DNA regions already exist prior to gastrulation, specific cell lineages exhibit differences between otherwise genetically identical individuals. These changes are designated metastable epialleles. Such epialleles are believed to be especially sensitive to environmental changes[7, 8]. There may be also epigenetic modifications at other points in the genome, resulting from interaction with the environment. This type of epigenetic changes, however, are specific to a particular tissue and only happen in adulthood [9, 10].

MicroRNAs (miRNAs) are short sequences of RNA that do not code for a product. They are between 21 and 25 nucleotides in length. miRNAs play a vital role as modulators of genetic expression at the post-transcriptional level. Through attachment to cis-elements in the 3′ untranslated region of messenger RNAs, miRNAs render the mRNAs less stable and they are unable to be translated into protein [11, 12]. The majority of miRNAs have the capability of targeting multiple mRNAs. In addition, a single mRNA may become the target of several different miRNAs [13].

This chapter discusses the principal epigenetic modifications of the genome achieved through DNA methylation and the miRNA expression profiles observed in obese individuals. Generally, the results of human studies will be compared alongside experiments in animal models.

2 How DNA Methylation Occurring In Utero and in the Neonatal Period Affects Obesity

There is a range of epidemiological evidence supporting the notion that in utero events contribute to the development of diseases in adulthood. The risk of becoming obese and developing metabolic problems is increased where a foetus has been both under- and over-nourished as a result of maternal diet during pregnancy [14, 15]. There are two especially well-documented examples of this phenomenon, viz the Hunger Winter of 1944–1945 in the Netherlands [16] and the 1959–1961 famine in China [17], both of which showed that foetal exposure to under-nutrition increased the likelihood of types 2 diabetes and cardiovascular disease in later life. The fact that this effect occurs through epigenetic modifications in early life is suggested by various findings. The IGF2 gene was less subject to DNA methylation in cells derived from peripheral blood taken from individuals born during the Hunger Winter when compared with their siblings of the same sex born earlier. This association was especially strong for the time around which conception must have occurred; thus, epigenetic modifications may occur even at the very earliest stages of development [15].

Although genetic factors significantly affect the risk of a person becoming obese, there is still a major part of the risk that is attributable to the environment and to how genes interact with it. Epigenetics help to explain why the number of obese individuals has expanded so rapidly despite the relative stability of the human genome. Organisms other than unicellular ones carry the same genome throughout their different tissues, yet the genes expressed vary between cell populations. Epigenetics induce alterations in the phenotype which may be inherited yet do not involve any alteration in the DNA bases [18]. Epigenetic changes may be conceptualised as involving different ways to pack the cellular DNA, meaning that some genes are accessible for expression, whereas others remain quiescent. The environment, including nutrition and the microbiome, may induce epigenetic alterations in the germ cells of the parents, the foetal cells or those of an infant, resulting in a different epigenetic programme being followed. Some changes can also occur later in life [19].

3   Mechanisms for Epigenetic Alterations

The following processes are now known to operate to produce epigenetic changes: methylation of DNA, alteration of histones and miRNA-mediated post-transcriptional modifications. These epigenetic changes can be inherited in somatic cells by mitotic division or passed down through meiotic divisions.

4   Methylation of DNA

The enzymes that catalyse the transfer of a methyl group to a CpG site (see earlier for definition) are the DNA methyltransferases. CpG sites commonly occur in regions of the gene acting as promoters. When a methyl group is attached, transcription factors cannot easily attach to the target sequence due to conformational change in the DNA helix. Thus, the gene's expression is hindered. Accordingly, a significant degree of methylation effectively prevents the expression of the gene, whereas in the absence of methylation, transcription will usually occur [18]. A number of processes appear to be under epigenetic control via methylation, in particular excess weight gain, orexigenesis, energy balance, insulin signalling, immune function, inflammatory responses, growth and timing of physiological events by circadian rhythm [19]. One study used genome-wide analysis to evaluate the methylation status in CpG sites in 479 adult volunteers, all of European origin. It was found that the HIF3A gene (hypoxia-inducible factor 3α) was hypermethylated in blood and fat cells [20]. Since hypoxic responses are implicated in obese patients, there are grounds to hypothesise that alterations in HIF function occur in obesity and its complications, including metabolic complications [21]. Leptin (LEP) and POMC genes also contain abundant CpG sequences, which make them liable to epigenetic modifications via methylation. Both genes are highly significant in regulating body mass. Lesseur et al. evaluated the level of methylation of the leptin gene in blood cells taken from mothers, the placenta and the umbilical cord. In cases mothers had been obese prior to conception, their blood cells were hypermethylated. Maternal tobacco use prior to conception and low birth weight were associated with hypermethylated cord blood cells. Furthermore, hypermethylation of the maternal LEP gene strongly correlated with hypermethylation of this gene in neonatal blood [22]. Likewise, the leptin gene was highly methylated in males born to mothers who went through the Netherlands Hunger Winter, when compared with brothers who were not exposed to this situation [23]. Researchers investigating obesity and metabolic disorders have also examined a number of other genes, notably ADIPOQ (adiponectin), PGC1α (peroxisome proliferator-activated receptor coactivator 1α), IGF-2 (insulin-like growth factor 2), IRS-1 (insulin receptor substrate 1) and LY86 (lymphocyte antigen 86) [18, 19]. The presence of epigenetic modifications as a biomarker for a chronic reduction in body mass (or its reversal) has also been investigated. Crujeiras et al. evaluated 18 adult males who lost at least 5% of their body mass following a special diet lasting 8 weeks. Men who were able to keep the weight off were those who had a more highly methylated POMC and a less methylated NPY gene region prior to the intervention [24]. There is currently research underway looking at whether the methylation status of the POMC region can identify those at risk of metabolic syndrome at an early stage [25]. The investigation of DNA methylation is still ongoing in humans and animal models and is beginning to elucidate the interactions between genes and the environment.

5 Modification of Histones

5.1 *miRNA*

DNA within the cell is wrapped around specific proteins, known as histones. These proteins contain a globular and tail domain, the latter found at the N-terminal end. The tail region of histones has a high pH and sticks out from the nucleosome. Thus, it is accessible to modification by the addition of a methyl, acetyl, ubiquitin or phosphoryl moiety. If these modifications occur, the DNA becomes exposed, meaning its genes can be expressed, repaired, copied or used in recombination [26]. The epigenetic regulation of adipose tissue formation and thus obesity occurs through modification of the scaffolding histones. There are five genes, in particular, where histone-level modifications play a key role in regulating their behaviour during adipogenesis, namely pre-adipocyte factor-1 (Pref-1), CCAAT-enhancer-binding protein β (C/EBP β), C/EBPα, PPARγ and adipocyte protein 2 (aP2) [27]. A group of enzymes termed HDACs (histone deacetylases) play a crucial role in regulating gene expression in stressful situations. One study used an animal model and examined chromatin structure in two situations: a high fat or a normal diet. The hepatocytes of those animals with a high fat intake had chromatin that had been reshaped through the activity of HDAC, the changes then producing differential expression of the liver transcription factors HNFα, CCAAT/enhancer binding protein α (CEBP/α) and FOXA1 [28]. This study also noted that the histone modification remained even after the high fat diet was stopped, at least in one species under study. A different species, however, underwent histone remodelling that reverted later. These alterations in the reversibility of histone modification were attributed to genetic differences between species [29]. The levels of HDAC in the hypothalamus have also been noted to vary between fasting and fed states and in cases a fat-rich diet led to obesity [30].

MicroRNAs, as described earlier, are RNA sequences of no longer than 25 nucleotides in length which do not encode a gene product. Instead, they perform an epigenetic role by preventing genes from being expressed or by changing synthetic events after mRNA has been transcribed [31]. It has been proven that miRNAs feature in numerous physiological and pathophysiological mechanisms, one of which is the division and maturation of adipocytes. They are also implicated in insulin insensitivity and the chronic mild inflammatory response that accompanies obesity [32]. A study noted that paediatric patients who were obese had a significant association between their body mass and the levels of specific miRNAs, in particular miR-486-5p, miR-486-3p, miR-142-3p, miR-130 b and miR-423-5p. When weight was gained or lost, 10 miRNAs altered in level [18]. Zhao et al. were able to associate miRNA expression with an increase in body mass and noted that eight specific miRNAs, if raised, led to a three times increase in the likelihood of obesity [19]. The expression of miRNAs in exosomes produced by fat cells has also been noted to change when loss of body mass and raised sensitivity to insulin were achieved following gastric bypass surgery [20]. Thus, evidence accumulating from a wide variety of different investigations points to the fact that miRNAs are significant factors in obesity and obesity-associated metabolic alterations. There is potential for miRNAs to be employed as useful biomarkers or even as drug targets in the future.

6 Epigenetic Modifications Triggered In Utero and in Early Development

The conditions pertaining to in utero are vitally important in foetal development. The intrauterine environment may induce epigenetic changes with long-term consequences for the child's metabolism. There is valuable evidence for this phenomenon from epidemiological data gathered on two populations, both subjected to severe under-nutrition at the same period in history (the 1940s), but whose later nourishment differed considerably. The two populations in question are those children born following the Hunger Winter in the Netherlands, whose nutrition reverted to a satisfactory level afterwards [21], and the children born during the siege of Leningrad [22, 23]. In the latter case, under-nutrition persisted for a long time after the siege. The children in the Dutch cohort had a lower degree of DNA methylation in the region of the IGF2 gene than their siblings of the same gender who were not undernourished in utero. Furthermore, these individuals also suffered from greater susceptibility to metabolic disorders than the survivors of the Leningrad siege. The findings support the notion that intrauterine events programme the metabolism through epigenetic modifications. Further support for this hypothesis comes from animal models of metabolism. In a murine model, the offspring of nutrition-depleted mothers, which were then fed a fat-rich diet, developed circulatory and metabolic disorders [24]. However, it is not just foetal under-nutrition that increases the risk of future obesity. This also applies to situations where the mother suffers from obesity and related metabolic disorders. Furthermore, it appears that transgenerational transmission of obesogenic programming is possible, which raises the disturbing possibility that the cycle of obesity and metabolic disorders may remain unbroken between generations [25].

7 Obesogens—Endocrine Disrupting Chemicals (EDCs)

Whilst considering epigenetic modifications, the part played by the so-called 'obesogens', i.e. chemicals capable of interfering with endocrine signalling, should be considered. These EDCs play a putative role in the cellular biology of adipocytes, endocrine signalling and the homeostatic regulation of body mass. There is evidence from epidemiological research to suggest that maternal exposure to EDCs is linked to a predisposition to become obese and develop metabolic disorders in later life. This effect is potentially due to epigenetic modifications. In animal studies, maternal exposure to polycyclic aromatic hydrocarbons whilst pregnant leads to increased body and adipose tissue mass in the offspring, in addition to raised levels of PPARγ, C/EBPα, Cox2, FAS and adiponectin. The PPARγ region was also relatively demethylated. These epigenetic modifications were also observed in the second generation [26, 27]. A study that examined the whole genome for epigenetic modifications found that female adult mice which were exposed at the time of birth to bisphenol A (at a dose that causes physiological effects in humans) had a different pattern from unexposed mice in terms of methylation in genes responsible for metabolism. A specific metabolic phenotype has been linked to the degree of methylation of DNA for the following genes: Janus kinase-2 (Jak-2), retinoid X receptor (Rxr), regulatory factor x-associated protein (Rfxap), and transmembrane protein

238 (Tmem 238). Whilst a detailed overview of how EDCs are implicated in obesity and the evidence from human and animal studies is beyond the aims of this chapter, there do appear to be compelling reasons for linking EDC exposure to obesity in childhood and the development of metabolic complications [29, 33].

8   Conclusion

Obesity is a disorder that is both highly complex and can present differently in different patients. This heterogeneity is partly caused by epigenetic factors. Obesity can develop in childhood, adolescence or young adulthood due to interactions between genes and the environment. When caring for obese patients, it is necessary to take into consideration the genetic and epigenetic factors that underlie the disorder, as this helps illuminate possible options for treatment.

Knowledge about methylation in the genome and patterns of miRNA expression is in its infancy, and there is still an incomplete understanding of what the growing experimental data are telling us. At present, and especially in research using human subjects, the data regarding methylation or miRNA expression cannot pinpoint how exactly these changes influence gene expression. Thus, the exact ways genes are promoted in particular organs, the modifications to metabolic pathways and the influence on body mass remain a matter of conjecture. Deeper research using animals or biopsy samples from humans will be required.

It is already clear, however, that epigenetic modifications mostly originate in early development. To what extent epigenetic modification is susceptible to alteration is not known. Research using a longitudinal design will be needed to clarify how far and how epigenetic changes may be undone. Future epigenetic studies may help to quantify risk for particular individuals and may allow more precise targeting of specific interventions. It is possible that such epigenetic studies may allow clusters of miRNA or methylation patterns to be grouped into phenotypes of clinical significance. The effects of exercise on such phenotypical expression have already been noted in the literature. There may be benefits for individuals with particular phenotypes from particular diets, intermittent fasting or other treatments. However, before such benefits can be investigated, there is a need for the following to occur:

- Studies enrolling high numbers with extensive clinical details
- New methods that can pick up the entirety of epigenetic alterations
- Animal data to confirm the likely disease mechanisms in humans
- Assessment of the reversibility of specific epigenetic modifications
- Studies with long-term follow-up treatments
- Bioinformatics applications capable of summarising and analysing the wealth of data generated

References

1. Apalasamy YD, Mohamed Z. Obesity and genomics: role of technology in unraveling the complex genetic architecture of obesity. Hum Genet. 2015;134:361–74. https://doi.org/10.1007/s00439-015-1533-x.
2. Tam V, Turcotte M, Meyre D. Established and emerging strategies to crack the genetic code of obesity. Obes Rev. 2019;20:212–40. https://doi.org/10.1111/obr.12770.
3. Fall T, Mendelson M, Speliotes EK. Recent advances in human genetics and epigenetics of adiposity: pathway to precision medicine? Gastroenterology. 2017;152:1695–706. https://doi.org/10.1053/j.gastro.2017.01.054.
4. Yengo L, et al. Meta-analysis of genome-wide association studies for height and body mass index in approximately 700000 individuals of European ancestry. Hum Mol Genet. 2018;27:3641–9. https://doi.org/10.1093/hmg/ddy271.
5. van Dijk SJ, Molloy PL, Varinli H, Morrison JL, Muhlhausler BS. Members of EPIS epigenetics and human obesity. Int J Obes. 2015;39:85–97. https://doi.org/10.1038/ijo.2014.34.
6. Weber M, Schubeler D. Genomic patterns of DNA methylation: targets and function of an epigenetic mark. Curr Opin Cell Biol. 2007;19:273–80. https://doi.org/10.1016/j.ceb.2007.04.011.
7. Dolinoy DC, Das R, Weidman JR, Jirtle RL. Metastable epialleles, imprinting, and the fetal origins of adult diseases. Pediatr Res. 2007;61:30R–7R. https://doi.org/10.1203/pdr.0b013e31804575f7.
8. Finer S, Holland ML, Nanty L, Rakyan VK. The hunt for the epiallele. Environ Mol Mutagen. 2011;52:1–11. https://doi.org/10.1002/em.20590.
9. Jirtle RL, Skinner MK. Environmental epigenomics and disease susceptibility. Nat Rev Genet. 2007;8:253–62. https://doi.org/10.1038/nrg2045.
10. Saussenthaler S, et al. Epigenetic regulation of hepatic Dpp4 expression in response to dietary protein. J Nutr Biochem. 2019;63:109–16. https://doi.org/10.1016/j.jnutbio.2018.09.025.
11. Bartel DP. MicroRNAs: genomics, biogenesis, mechanism, and function. Cell. 2004;116:281–97. https://doi.org/10.1016/s0092-8674(04)00045-5.
12. Guo H, Ingolia NT, Weissman JS, Bartel DP. Mammalian microRNAs predominantly act to decrease target mRNA levels. Nature. 2010;466:835–40. https://doi.org/10.1038/nature09267.
13. Doench JG, Sharp PA. Specificity of microRNA target selection in translational repression. Genes Dev. 2004;18:504–11. https://doi.org/10.1101/gad.1184404.
14. Fernandez-Twinn DS, Hjort L, Novakovic B, Ozanne SE, Saffery R. Intrauterine programming of obesity and type 2 diabetes. Diabetologia. 2019;62:1789–801. https://doi.org/10.1007/s00125-019-4951-9.
15. Heijmans BT, et al. Persistent epigenetic differences associated with prenatal exposure to famine in humans. Proc Natl Acad Sci U S A. 2008;105:17,046–9. https://doi.org/10.1073/pnas.0806560105.
16. Kyle UG, Pichard C. The Dutch famine of 1944–1945: a pathophysiological model of long-term consequences of wasting disease. Curr Opin Clin Nutr Metab Care. 2006;9:388–94. https://doi.org/10.1097/01.mco.0000232898.74415.42.
17. Li C, Lumey LH. Exposure to the Chinese famine of 1959–61 in early life and long-term health conditions: a systematic review and meta-analysis. Int J Epidemiol. 2017;46:1157–70. https://doi.org/10.1093/ije/dyx013.
18. Jaenisch R, Bird A. Epigenetic regulation of gene expression: how the genome integrates intrinsic and environmental signals. Nat Genet. 2003;33:245–54.
19. Lopomo A, Burgio E, Migliore L. Epigenetics of obesity. Prog Mol Biol Transl Sci. 2016;140:151–84.
20. Dick KJ, Nelson CP, Tsaprouni L, et al. DNA methylation and body-mass index: a genome-wide analysis. Lancet. 2014;383(9933):1990–8.
21. Pan H, Lin X, Wu Y, et al. HIF3A association with adiposity: the story begins before birth. Epigenomics. 2015;7(6):937–50.

22. Lesseur C, Armstrong DA, Paquette AG, Koestler DC, Padbury JF, Marsit CJ. Tissue-specific leptin promoter DNA methylation is associated with maternal and infant perinatal factors. Mol Cell Endocrinol. 2013;381(1–2):160–7.
23. Tobi EW, Lumey LH, Talens RP, et al. DNA methylation differences after exposure to prenatal famine are common and timing- and sex-specific. Hum Mol Genet. 2009;18(21):4046–53.
24. Crujeiras AB, Campion J, Díaz-Lagares A, et al. Association of weight regain with specific methylation levels in the NPY and POMC promoters in leukocytes of obese men: a translational study. Regul Pept. 2013;186:1–6.
25. Yoo JY, Lee S, Lee HA, et al. Can proopiomelanocortin methylation be used as an early predictor of metabolic syndrome? Diabetes Care. 2014;37(3):734–9.
26. Bannister AJ, Kouzarides T. Regulation of chromatin by histone modifications. Cell Res. 2011;21(3):381–95.
27. Zhang Q, Ramlee MK, Brunmeir R, Villanueva CJ, Halperin D, Xu F. Dynamic and distinct histone modifications modulate the expression of key adipogenesis regulatory genes. Cell Cycle. 2012;11(23):4310–22.
28. Leung A, Parks BW, Du J, et al. Open chromatin profiling in mice livers reveals unique chromatin variations induced by high fat diet. J Biol Chem. 2014;289(34):23,557–67.
29. Leung A, Trac C, Du J, Natarajan R, Schones DE. Persistent chromatin modifications induced by high fat diet. J Biol Chem. 2016;291(20):10,446–55.
30. Funato H, Tsai AL, Willie JT, et al. Enhanced orexin receptor-2 signaling prevents diet-induced obesity and improves leptin sensitivity. Cell Metab. 2009;9(1):64–76.
31. Pasquinelli AE. MicroRNAs and their targets: recognition, regulation and an emerging reciprocal relationship. Nat Rev Genet. 2012;13(4):271–82.
32. Cruz KJC, Oliveira ARS, de Morais JBS, Severo JS, Marreiro D, do N. The role of microRNAs on adipogenesis, chronic low grade inflammation and insulin resistance in obesity. Nutrition. 2017;35:28–35.
33. Leung A, Parks BW, Du J, et al. Open chromatin profiling in mice livers reveals unique chromatin variations induced by high fat diet. J Biol Chem. 2014;289(34):23557–67.

Gestational Diabetes and Variety in the Composition of Breast Milk

Özlem Naciye Şahin and Gian Carlo Di Renzo

1 Introduction

Diabetes commonly occurs in pregnant women and may cause a number of complications both for the mother and the child, including in the neonatal period. The effects that abnormal maternal metabolism may have on the newborn and infant in terms of nutrition supplied and effects on metabolic programming are important subjects for research since it is already known that individuals born to women with either gestational or pre-existing diabetes mellitus (DM) are at raised risk of developing type 2 diabetes eventually, albeit epidemiological data also demonstrate that being breastfed in infancy protects in the longer term against both becoming obese and suffering from type 2 DM. Since maternal and neonatal metabolic abnormalities are so strongly associated, an understanding of how DM affects the composition of breast milk is especially valuable, particularly given the fact that breast milk is the medium through which protective benefit is conferred on neonates [1–3].

Milk is a biological fluid of dynamic composition, with features that make it unique to each species and to the mother from whom it comes. In humans, breast milk composition is under continuous change during lactation, stimulated by the requirements of the growing infant. This change is also the result of the way the breast matures in pregnancy, under control by the placenta. The American Academy of Pediatrics (AAP) states very clearly its view that 'Breastfeeding and human milk

Ö. N. Şahin (✉)
Department of Child Health and Diseases, Arel University, Medical Faculty, Istanbul, Türkiye

G. C. Di Renzo
Centre of Perinatal Medicine of the University of Perugia, Perugia, Italy

Sechenov University, Moscow, Russia
e-mail: giancarlo.direnzo@unipg.it

Ö. N. Şahin et al. (eds.), *Breastfeeding and Metabolic Programming*, https://doi.org/10.1007/978-3-031-33278-4_17

are the normative standards for infant feeding and nutrition'. Furthermore, according to the AAP, even premature infants should receive mainly breast milk, albeit supplemented as required. The rationale behind recommending breast milk as the primary diet also involves recognition of the way breastfeeding offers both immediate and longer term benefits to mother and child [1–3].

One theory advocates the idea that nutritional signals received by the infant in the postpartum period alter the development of metabolism, causing irreversible changes in metabolic programming, which then raise or lower the risk of metabolic abnormalities. Evidence for this theory includes the observation that being breastfed can protect against both becoming obese and developing type 2 DM later in life. This protective effect occurs due to breast milk containing certain bioactive molecules capable of modulating how the neonatal organ systems develop and grow [4–8].

These bioactive molecules in breast milk include hormones, antibodies, lysozyme, lactoferrin, sugars, nucleotide growth factors and antioxidant enzymes. They play significant roles in immunity and control of metabolism and are believed to regulate how the infant grows and develops. Breast milk has a dynamic composition, with the precise constituents and their levels affected by various factors, including the gestational age at which delivery occurred, the mother's diet and the extent to which the maternal metabolism is healthy or unhealthy [9–11].

Maternal DM may either pre-date the pregnancy (in the form of type 1, i.e. insulin dependent, or type 2 DM) or may only develop once the woman is pregnant, in which case the term 'gestational diabetes mellitus' (GDM) is appropriate. The latter is a frequently occurring complication in pregnant women. In cases of GDM, the mother displays carbohydrate intolerance, which ranges in the degree of severity. The definition precludes pre-existing DM of either type. Being diabetic exposes the mother and child to various risks in both the short and the long term. The second phase of lactogenesis occurs late in diabetic mothers and breast milk composition is altered. There have been a number of studies investigating the composition of breast milk in an attempt to unravel the mechanisms by which breast milk protects the neonate and also exposes the child to the risk of future metabolic complications [12].

2 Gestational Diabetes

2.1 *Energetic Value*

There have been two studies that specifically noted the calorific value of breast milk in mothers with GDM. However, they obtained conflicting results. In one of the studies, the calorific value exceeded that of milk from healthy mothers throughout the course of lactation. However, the other study noted that mature milk samples from mothers with GDM had a lower than usual calorific value. In both investigations, the same analyser was employed (manufactured by Miris). The way the breast milk was gathered and stored did, however, differ between studies [13, 14].

2.2 Protein Content

There have been three investigations into the amount of protein contained in the breast milk of diabetic versus healthy mothers. These studies all concluded that the protein level in colostrum did not differ depending on the presence of diabetes. However, there was some disagreement about the findings in transitional and mature milk samples. Whilst the study undertaken by Saphira et al. noted the levels did not differ significantly, Dritsaku et al. found the protein level was reduced in breast milk from mothers with diabetes [13–15].

2.3 Endocrinological Differences

The insulin content of both colostrum and mature breast milk has been investigated several times. According to Ley et al., whose method utilised an immunoassay with electrogenerated chemiluminescence, insulin is present at a higher concentration in early than mature breast milk. There was an association between certain maternal factors and a raised insulin level in mature milk. These factors included a raised BMI prior to conception, hyperglycaemia whilst pregnant, reduced sensitivity to insulin and a raised level of circulating adiponectin. There were no associations between these factors and insulin concentration in early milk. Two different investigations utilised ELISA to calculate insulin levels in breast milk. Both studies compared milk from women with gestational DM with milk from healthy mothers. Whilst Nunes et al. concluded that insulin levels were the same, whether in colostrum or in mature milk, Yu et al. noted that insulin was raised in both types in the samples from diabetic mothers, an effect that was particularly pronounced if the mother was being administered injectable insulin [16–18].

There is also disagreement on how GDM affects adiponectin levels in breast milk. Although two studies concluded that GDM made no difference to the adiponectin concentration in breast milk, Yu et al. noted that adiponectin levels were decreased in milk from mothers with GDM on days 3 (i.e. colostrum) and 90 (i.e. mature milk), but were normal on day 42 [16–18].

The data for ghrelin levels, however, are in agreement with each other. In milk from mothers with GDM, the ghrelin level is decreased in colostrum and mature milk, albeit it is present at a normal level in transitional milk [17, 19, 20].

When milk (colostrum and transitional) from mothers with GDM was investigated in two different studies, the level of irisin was determined as decreased below normal. However, in mature breast milk, one study found a reduced level (Fatima et al.), whilst the other did not (Aydın et al.). Furthermore, in the latter study, a trend of increasing irisin was ascertained as milk matured from colostrum to mature via transitional, regardless of whether the mother's glucose tolerance was normal or not [21, 22].

Aydın et al. also evaluated a number of other bioactive molecules in milk that can fulfil an endocrine function. The subjects in this research were not receiving extraneous insulin, had an uncomplicated pregnancy and had delivered at full-term. In samples from mothers with GDM, the levels of apelin and nesfatin-1 were decreased compared to those from glucose normotolerant controls. Moreover, mature milk contained more of these compounds than colostrum [19]. Three molecules with endocrine activity involved in energy balance and diabetes are copeptin, adropin and irisin. The study revealed that colostrum contains a significantly greater level of copeptin than transitional milk, with mature milk having the greatest amount, regardless of the mother's glucose tolerance status. By contrast, mature milk contained the lowest levels of adropin, regardless of the mother's glucose tolerance status, whilst transitional milk and colostrum both contain a higher level, but the transitional milk level is above that found in colostrum. The study also assessed the levels of several other bioactive compounds over the course of lactation, specifically preptin, salusin-α, salusin-β, pro-hepcidin and hepcidin-25. It was discovered that there were elevated levels of certain of these molecules in the samples from mothers with GDM: in colostrum, preptin, pro-hepcidin and hepcidin-25 were raised, the latter two molecules also being present at an increased concentration in transitional milk. However, colostrum from the mothers with GDM contained reduced levels of salusin-α and salusin-β. The analysis of SREBP1-c indicated that its concentration was very low in colostrum and unable to be detected in mature milk [19–23].

2.4 Proteins Involved in Immunity

The concentration of IgA in breast milk from subjects who were healthy or with GDM has been investigated in two different studies, one focusing on colostrum and the other on transitional milk [15, 24]. The colostrum did not differ in terms of IgA, but in transitional milk the total protein and the level of glycosylated protein were both discovered to be lower. Only the study undertaken by Smilowitz et al. evaluated lactoferrin levels. It was noted that transitional milk contains an unusually high level of glycosylation in the samples from GDM mothers. These findings support the notion that maternal hyperglycaemia may have enduring consequences on the development of immune function in infants [24].

An analysis undertaken by Ustebay et al. focused on the levels of chemerin and dermcidin throughout the stages of lactation, noting that these were raised in the milk of mothers with GDM. The levels peaked in colostrum, whilst the lowest levels were in samples of mature milk [25].

One study assessed the concentrations of neutrophil gelatinase-associated lipocalin (NGAL), together with the complexed form containing matrix metalloproteinase-9 (MMP-9) in colostrum. In samples taken from mothers with diabetes, the complexed form was present in greater amounts than in breast milk from normal subjects [26].

2.5 Proteomic Profile

Two studies generated a proteomic profile for breast milk from mothers with GDM. One study utilised high-performance liquid chromatography, whilst the other employed high-sensitivity, label-free, semi-quantitative mass spectrometry [27, 28]. Klein and colleagues examined the levels of 11 different free amino acids in breast milk samples (colostrum and mature milk) from both healthy and diabetic mothers. A trend of increasing levels of free amino acids was observed in both groups, whilst there was no significant difference between the groups in terms of any of the amino acids tested [27].

The study undertaken by Grapov et al. concentrated on colostrum alone. Some 601 proteins were found to be present. For 260 of these proteins, quantification was carried out. By means of an orthogonal partial least-squares discriminant analysis, a group of 27 proteins was determined to have the highest predictive power for the presence of GDM. It was also ascertained that there was a statistically significant difference between the levels of 10 of these proteins in milk from healthy versus diabetic mothers. This analysis depended on use of the power law global error model, with correction for multiple testing. These findings reveal that maternal glucose intolerance affects the levels of proteins found in colostrum, with knock-on effects on immune function and nutrition [28].

2.6 Sugars

Two studies have evaluated the total level of sugars in breast milk, comparing milk from healthy and diabetic mothers. These studies noted that the sugar content in colostrum and transitional milk did not differ significantly, although this was not the case in the mature milk samples. Whilst Saphira et al. found the saccharide content lower in the GDM samples, Dritsaku et al. identified no systematic difference [13, 14].

A single study has examined lactose and glucose levels in breast milk in GDM. The samples involved were all of the colostrum. Whilst GDM was associated with decreased levels of lactose, the glucose level did not differ significantly between milk from healthy and diabetic mothers [15].

Only one study has evaluated the levels of oligosaccharides in transitional milk in women with GDM and the authors concluded that GDM does not significantly affect these levels [24].

2.7 Lipids

Three studies have measured the lipid levels in breast milk in cases of GDM, with results that somewhat contradicted each other. According to Kaushik et al. [15], in cases of maternal GDM, the lipid content in colostrum is reduced. However, both

Dritsaku's and Saphira's studies indicated no significant difference in lipids in colostrum. There is also some disagreement about lipids in mature milk, with Saphira et al. reporting lowered levels, but Dritsaku et al. failing to find any systematic difference. However, all three studies were in agreement that there is no difference between groups in the lipid content of mature milk [13, 14].

The study conducted by Kaushik et al. also measured the level of triacylglycerides and cholesterol in colostrum, noting that the groups did not differ significantly [15].

The research undertaken by Azular Certok et al. evaluated how maternal diabetes affected the fatty acid content of colostrum. The main difference was that four aliphatic acids, in particular, were present at raised levels in the colostrum of diabetic mothers, i.e. γ-linolenic, eicosatrienoic, arachidonic and docosatetraenoic acid. These acids are all of the omega-6 unsaturated type [29].

2.8 Electrolyte Content

In colostrum from diabetic mothers, the sodium level was raised, according to two studies [15, 30]. Galipau, furthermore, noted that insulin administration also caused sodium to rise. Kaushik et al. [15] note that the levels of potassium, phosphate and calcium do not differ significantly between samples of colostrum gathered from diabetic or healthy mothers.

2.9 MicroRNA

There has recently been research into the levels of particular microRNAs (miRNAs) in breast milk with an established role in the development of adipose tissue. The miRNAs involved were let-7a, miRNA-30B and miRNA-378. Levels of the first and last of these differed significantly between samples from diabetic and healthy mothers. Nonetheless, if the mother's body mass index was factored in, this result became statistically insignificant, since body mass index alone predicts the risk of metabolic problems in pregnant women [31].

2.10 Metabolome

The metabolomic profile of breast milk has been investigated by Wen et al. They noted the presence of 187 metabolic compounds in human milk, amongst which there were 4 alkanes, 17 molecules derived from amino acid precursors, 21 amino acids, 22 aliphatic acids of saturated type, 29 aliphatic acids with double bonds, 8 metabolites found in the citric acid cycle, 3 co-factors or vitamins, 3 oxoacids and metabolites thereof, 1 compound in the glycolytic pathway, 43 organic acids and 36 carbon-containing other compounds. There were many features of the metabolomic profile of breast milk that were common to samples from both healthy and diabetic mothers. Nonetheless, when colostrum, transitional milk and mature milk were all examined, 28 metabolites were present at concentrations that differed at the level of statistical significance [32].

3 Type 1 Diabetes Mellitus

There are eight studies in the literature that examine breast milk in mothers with type 1 DM, the disease having had its onset prior to the pregnancy. All of these studies are more than 20 years old. The studies investigate the effects of length of diagnosis and the effects of different interventions. Four of the studies have the same design.

3.1 *Proteins*

According to three published studies, the overall protein level does not differ significantly between milk from diabetic and non-diabetic mothers [33–35]. A single study [33] assessed the levels of lactoferrin and secreted IgA in breast milk. Being diabetic did not result in a statistically significant difference in milk protein levels.

One study measured the level of prolactin in breast milk in healthy or type 1 diabetic mothers and ascertained that, 1 week after delivery, the prolactin level was decreased in the milk from diabetic mothers, as determined by immunoassay [36]. This decrease in prolactin level may be attributable to hyperglycaemia in the diabetic mothers since elevated capillary glucose measurements correlated well with the prolactin level in breast milk from the diabetic mothers. Those mothers whose blood glucose level had been well controlled during the pregnancy and shortly after birth tended to have a greater prolactin concentration in breast milk. The level of prolactin is inversely related to the milk lactose level, which was demonstrable in milk samples from healthy controls on the second day after birth. This inverse relationship did not appear until 2 weeks after birth in the diabetic group. Thus, the data confirm that lactogenesis is retarded and lactation delayed in cases of maternal type 1 diabetes [36].

3.2 *Lipids*

The macronutrient constituent of breast milk from diabetic mothers that has attracted the most research interest is lipid. There are four published studies addressing this topic. However, the studies do not agree with their conclusions. Whilst three studies concluded that diabetes had no significant effect on the overall lipid content, the study by Bitman et al. found that breast milk from diabetic mothers contained only two thirds the level seen in milk from controls.

The topic of breast milk aliphatic acids in type 1 diabetes has been addressed by three studies. According to van Beusekom, the aliphatic acid content overall was normal in milk from diabetic mothers. Bitman et al. noted that medium length aliphatic acid synthesis was lower in diabetic samples, pointing to reduced manufacture of these acids by the breast, whilst oleic acid and polyunsaturated aliphatic acids were raised, which implied metabolism favoured lengthening of the hydrocarbon tail in diabetes. Ferris et al., by contrast, noted that the milk from diabetic mothers actually contained a level of medium length aliphatic acids that was always above that found in the control group, but still within the normal reference range. This study also found that the lengthier aliphatic acids were, in fact, present at decreased concentrations in the diabetic group, when assessed at 2 weeks and 12 weeks after delivery [34–37].

3.3   Carbohydrates

There have been three published investigations into carbohydrate levels in the breast milk of diabetic mothers. These studies all conclude that lactose levels do not significantly differ from normal samples. However, whilst Butte et al. noted the level of glucose 2.3-fold higher than normal in the diabetic samples, van Beusekom did not detect such a difference. A single study assessed the inositol concentration in breast milk and found it normal in diabetic mothers' milk [35].

3.4   Electrolytes

Two separate investigations into electrolyte levels in breast milk from diabetic mothers found that potassium, calcium and magnesium levels were all normal in the diabetic samples. However, there is no consensus regarding sodium levels, since Butte et al. noted a 1.2-fold elevation in level, whilst Bitman et al. reported the level as normal.

One investigation noted that phosphate, zinc, copper and iron levels in breast milk remained normal regardless of diabetic status, whilst another found the chlorite and citrate levels also normal in both groups [33, 34].

3.5   Vitamins

The sole vitamin investigated so far in the breast milk of diabetic mothers is vitamin E. The concentration of this vitamin fell by half at 7–14 days after delivery, irrespective of diabetic status [38].

4 Conclusion

There has been relatively little detailed research into breast milk from diabetic mothers and those studies published so far have only addressed a limited number of breast milk constituents, involving variables of various types. Thus, given the evidence base that exists currently, it is challenging to draw conclusions on how diabetes affects the composition of breast milk or what benefits breastfeeding still offers in such cases. More research is called for to flesh out the picture. In particular, studies should follow a case-control design methodology and should address the effects of premature birth and gestational age. Studies of the impact on breast milk produced by the various treatments available in diabetes are required. Moreover, since cases of type 2 DM are steadily increasing, research into breast milk from mothers with this condition is also a necessity. The results of all these studies should lead to the situation in which nutritional support for the mother and premature infants can be more precisely and effectively targeted.

References

1. Peila C, Gazzolo D, Bertino E, Cresi F, Coscia A. Influence of diabetes during pregnancy on human milk composition. Nutrients. 2020;12(1):185. Published 2020 Jan 9. https://doi.org/10.3390/nu12010185.
2. World Health Organization global strategies for infant and young child feeding. http://www.who.int/child_adolescent_health/documents/9789241595193/en/index.html. Accessed 10 Feb 2022.
3. Horta B.L., Victora C.G., World Health Organization long-term effects of breastfeeding: a systematic review. https://apps.who.int/iris/bitstream/handle/10665/79198/9789241505307_eng.pdf?sequence=1. Accessed 10 Feb 2022.
4. Lucas A, Fewtrell MS, Cole TJ. Fetal origins of adult disease—the hypothesis revisited. Br Med J. 1999;319:245–9. https://doi.org/10.1136/bmj.319.7204.245.
5. Plagemann A. A matter of insulin: developmental programming of body weight regulation. J Matern Fetal Neonatal Med. 2008;21:143–8. https://doi.org/10.1080/14767050801929869.
6. Owen CG, Martin RM, Whincup PH, Smith GD, Cook DG. Does breastfeeding influence risk of type 2 diabetes in later life? A quantitative analysis of published evidence. Am J Clin Nutr. 2006;84:1043–54. https://doi.org/10.1093/ajcn/84.5.1043.
7. Hamosh M. Bioactive factors in human milk. Pediatr Clin N Am. 2001;48:69–86. https://doi.org/10.1016/S0031-3955(05)70286-8.
8. Adair LS. Methods appropriate for studying the relationship of breastfeeding to obesity. J Nutr. 2009;139:S408–11. https://doi.org/10.3945/jn.108.097808.
9. Hawkes J, Bryan DL, Gibson R. Cells from mature human milk are capable of cytokine production following in vitro stimulation. Adv Exp Med Biol. 2004;554:467–70.
10. McGill HC Jr, Mott GE, Lewis DS, McMahan CA, Jackson EM. Early determinants of adult metabolic regulation: effects of infant nutrition on adult lipid and lipoprotein metabolism. Nutr Rev. 1996;54:S31–40. https://doi.org/10.1111/j.1753-4887.1996.tb03868.x.
11. Ballard O, Morrow AL. Human milk composition: nutrients and bioactive factors. Pediatr Clin N Am. 2013;60:49–74. https://doi.org/10.1016/j.pcl.2012.10.002.
12. Hartmann P, Cregan M. Lactogenesis and the effects of insulin-dependent diabetes mellitus and prematurity. J Nutr. 2001;131:3016S–20S. https://doi.org/10.1093/jn/131.11.3016S.

13. Dritsakou K, Liosis G, Valsami G. The impact of maternal- and neonatal-associated factors on human milk's macronutrients and energy. J Matern Fetal Neonatal Med. 2017;30:1302–8. https://doi.org/10.1080/14767058.2016.1212329.

14. Shapira D, Mandel D, Mimouni FB, Moran-Lev H, Morom R, Mangel L, Lubetzky R. The effect of gestational diabetes mellitus on human milk macronutrients content. J Perinatol. 2019;39:820–3. https://doi.org/10.1038/s41372-019-0362-5.

15. Kaushik S, Trivedi SS, Jain A, Bhattacharjee J. Unusual changes in colostrum composition in lactating indian women having medical complications during pregnancy—a pilot study. Indian J Clin Biochem. 2002;17:68–73. https://doi.org/10.1007/BF02867974.

16. Ley SH, Hanley AJ, Sermer M, Zinman B, O'Connor DL. Associations of prenatal metabolic abnormalities with insulin and adiponectin concentrations in human milk. Am J Clin Nutr. 2012;95:867–74. https://doi.org/10.3945/ajcn.111.028431.

17. Yu X, Rong SS, Sun X, Ding G, Wan W, Zou L, Wu S, Li M, Wang D. Associations of breast milk adiponectin, leptin, insulin and ghrelin with maternal characteristics and early infant growth: a longitudinal study. Br J Nutr. 2018;120:1380–7. https://doi.org/10.1017/S0007114518002933.

18. Nunes M, da Silva CH, Bosa VL, Bernardi JR, Werlang ICR, Goldani MZ. NESCA group could a remarkable decrease in leptin and insulin levels from colostrum to mature milk contribute to early growth catch-up of SGA infants? BMC Pregnancy Childbirth. 2017;17:410. https://doi.org/10.1186/s12884-017-1593-0.

19. Aydin S. The presence of the peptides apelin, ghrelin and nesfatin-1 in the human breast milk, and the lowering of their levels in patients with gestational diabetes mellitus. Peptides. 2010;31:2236–40. https://doi.org/10.1016/j.peptides.2010.08.021.

20. Aydin S, Geckil H, Karatas F, Donder E, Kumru S, Kavak EC, Colak R, Ozkan Y, Sahin I. Milk and blood ghrelin level in diabetics. Nutrition. 2007;23:807–11. https://doi.org/10.1016/j.nut.2007.08.015.

21. Fatimaa SS, Khalidb E, Ladakc AA, Ali SA. Colostrum and mature breast milk analysis of serum irisin and sterol regulatory element-binding proteins-1c in gestational diabetes mellitus. J Matern Fetal Neonatal Med. 2019;32:2993–9. https://doi.org/10.1080/14767058.2018.1454422.

22. Aydin S, Kuloglu T, Aydin S. Copeptin, adropin and irisin concentrations in breast milk and plasma of healthy women and those with gestational diabetes mellitus. Peptides. 2013;47:66–70. https://doi.org/10.1016/j.peptides.2013.07.001.

23. Aydin S, Celik O, Gurates B, Sahin I, Ulas M, Yilmaz M, Kalayci M, Kuloglu T, Catak Z, Aksoy A, et al. Concentrations of preptin, salusins and hepcidins in plasma and milk of lactating women with or without gestational diabetes mellitus. Peptides. 2019;49:123–30. https://doi.org/10.1016/j.peptides.2013.09.006.

24. Smilowitz JT, Totten SM, Huang J, Grapov D, Durham HA, Lammi-Keefe CJ, Lebrilla C, German JB. Human milk secretory immunoglobulin A and lactoferrin N-Glycans are altered in women with gestational diabetes mellitus. J Nutr. 2013;143:1906–12. https://doi.org/10.3945/jn.113.180695.

25. Ustebay S, Baykus Y, Deniz R, Ugur K, Yavuzkir S, Yardim M, Kalayci M, Çaglar M, Aydin S. Chemerin and dermcidin in human milk and their alteration in gestational diabetes. J Hum Lact. 2019;35:550–8. https://doi.org/10.1177/0890334419837523.

26. Metallinou D, Lykeridou K, Karampas G, Liosis GT, Skevaki C, Rizou M, Papassotiriou I, Rizos D. Postpartum human breast milk levels of neutrophil gelatinase-associated lipocalin (NGAL) and matrix metalloproteinase-9 (MMP-9)/NGAL complex in normal and pregnancies complicated with insulin-dependent gestational diabetes mellitus. A prospective pilot case-control study. J Obstet Gynaecol. 2019;29:1–7.

27. Klein K, Bancher-Todesca D, Graf T, Garo F, Roth E, Kautzky-Willer A, Worda C. Concentration of free amino acids in human milk of women with gestational diabetes mellitus and healthy women. Breastfeed Med. 2013;8:111–5. https://doi.org/10.1089/bfm.2011.0155.

28. Grapov D, Lemay DG, Weber D, Phinney BS, Azulay Chertok IR, Gho DS, German JB, Smilowitz JT. The human colostrum whey proteome is altered in gestational diabetes mellitus. J Proteome Res. 2015;14:512–20. https://doi.org/10.1021/pr500818d.
29. Azulay Chertok IR, Haile ZT, Eventov-Friedman S, Silanikove N, Argov-Argaman N. Influence of gestational diabetes mellitus on fatty acid concentrations in human colostrum. Nutrition. 2017;36:17–21. https://doi.org/10.1016/j.nut.2016.12.001.
30. Galipeau R, Goulet C, Chagnon M. Infant and maternal factors influencing breastmilk sodium among primiparous mothers. Breastfeed Med. 2012;7:290–4. https://doi.org/10.1089/bfm.2011.0022.
31. Xi Y, Jiang X, Li R, Chen M, Song W, Li X. The levels of human milk microRNAs and their association with maternal weight characteristics. Eur J Clin Nutr. 2016;70:445–9. https://doi.org/10.1038/ejcn.2015.168.
32. Wen L, Wu Y, Yang Y, Han TL, Wang W, Fu H, Zheng Y, Shan T, Chen J, Xu P, et al. Gestational diabetes mellitus changes the metabolomes of human colostrum, transition milk and mature milk. Med Sci Monit. 2019;25:6128–52. https://doi.org/10.12659/MSM.915827.
33. Butte NF, Garza C, Burr R, Goldman AS, Kennedy K, Kitzmiller JL. Milk composition of insulin-dependent diabetic women. J Pediatr Gastroenterol Nutr. 1987;6:936–41. https://doi.org/10.1097/00005176-198711000-00020.
34. Bitman J, Hamosh M, Hamosh P. Milk composition and volume during the onset of lactation in a diabetic mother. Am J Clin Nutr. 1989;50:1364–9. https://doi.org/10.1093/ajcn/50.6.1364.
35. Van Beusekom CM, Zeegers TA, Martini IA, Velvis HJ, Visser GH, van Doormaal JJ, Muskiet FA. Milk of patients with tightly controlled insulin-dependent diabetes mellitus has normal macronutrient and fatty acid composition. Am J Clin Nutr. 1993;57:938–43. https://doi.org/10.1093/ajcn/57.6.938.
36. Ostrom KM, Ferris AM. Prolactin concentrations in serum and milk of mothers with and without insulin-dependent diabetes. Am J Clin Nutr. 1993;58:49–53. https://doi.org/10.1093/ajcn/58.1.49.
37. Jackson MB, Lammi-Keefe CJ, Jensen RG. Total lipid and fatty acid composition of milk from women with and without insulin-dependent diabetes mellitus. Am J Clin Nutr. 1994;60:353–61. https://doi.org/10.1093/ajcn/60.3.353.
38. Lammi-Keefe CJ, Jonas CR, Ferris AM, Capacchione CM. Vitamin E in plasma and milk of lactating women with insulin-dependent diabetes mellitus. J Pediatr Gastroenterol Nutr. 1995;20:305–9. https://doi.org/10.1097/00005176-199504000-00007.

Maternal PUFA Supplementation and Epigenetic Influences on Fat Tissue

Özlem Naciye Şahin and Aysel Özpınar

1 Introduction

Brown adipose tissue (BAT) has the unique ability amongst fat cells of generating heat without causing muscular movement (i.e. shivering). It achieves this by converting surplus chemical energy into heat via UCP1 (uncoupling protein 1), located within mitochondria. At present, research is focusing on BAT due to its essential role in regulating energy balance through the consumption of calories to generate body heat. Although the majority of children, adolescents and healthy adults have extensive deposits of BAT [1–4], adults suffering from obesity do not possess this tissue, which implies a role in how individuals become obese. Children who are obese and are susceptible to metabolic disorders are at risk of continuing to be obese in adulthood and of developing type 2 diabetes mellitus. Accordingly, ways to prevent children becoming obese and a knowledge of the factors governing the development of an excessive body mass index are vital for interventions to halt the vast numbers of adults who are now obese. How BAT grows in utero and shortly after birth is crucial to the longer term persistence of BAT in children and adults [5, 6]. Up to now, however, researchers have not addressed in detail how the mother's diet may affect the maturation of foetal BAT. Although it is clear that the presence or absence of BAT has a major impact on the development of obesity, the relationship between the quantity of BAT present neonatally, the speed with which BAT is lost and the risk of becoming obese at a later stage has not yet been elucidated. It is known, however, that BAT is lost either through degeneration or a switch in

Ö. N. Şahin (✉)
Department of Child Health and Diseases, Arel University, Medical Faculty, Istanbul, Türkiye

A. Özpınar
Department of Basic Sciences, Medical Biochemistry, Medical Faculty, Acibadem Mehmet Ali Aydinlar University, Istanbul, Türkiye
e-mail: aysel.ozpinar@acibadem.edu.tr

Ö. N. Şahin et al. (eds.), *Breastfeeding and Metabolic Programming*,
https://doi.org/10.1007/978-3-031-33278-4_18

phenotype to white adipose. Specifically, the potential for reducing obesity in her children by manipulating the mother's diet in pregnancy remains unknown [6–9].

There are areas of BAT at a deep level in the neck, above the clavicles, lying alongside the vertebrae, around the kidneys and in the axilla. BAT is 50-fold more metabolically active than white adipose tissue. BAT makes up 1.5% of the entire body mass, but 5% of the mass consisting of adipocytes. Approaching 90% of BATs are in a state of activation. A study using imaging to identify anatomical regions where rodents have BAT demonstrated that the deposition of BAT in humans and rodents is in the same anatomical locations; hence, rodent BAT is considered analogous to human BAT in experimental studies. In terms of thermogenesis and activity by the mitochondria, BAT located above the clavicle in humans was similar to interscapular BAT in rodents. The crucial period for BAT to be laid down is in the third trimester, i.e. during the last stage of pregnancy. In humans, interscapular BAT quickly disappears postnatally. BAT degenerates and its place is taken by white fat cells, or the brown fat alters its phenotype to become white fat. The BATs found at a deep level in the cervical region and above the clavicle do not degenerate in this way and are still functioning in adolescents and adults. BAT thermogenesis does, however, cease to be functional eventually as the individual ages, or if obesity and type 2 diabetes occur. Since rodents and humans demonstrate similar features in terms of BAT function and development, interscapular BAT in rodents is a reasonable model for cervical and supraclavicular BAT in humans [10–18].

There is epigenetic control over the development of BAT. Epigenetic refers to mechanisms that can reversibly alter genetic expression in a heritable manner without fundamentally altering the sequence of bases in DNA. Thus, epigenetic mechanisms include the addition of methyl groups to particular regions, modification of histones (i.e. chromatic restructuring) and expression of microRNAs, which do not encode a gene product but modify expression of mRNA [19]. There are around ten miRNAs which are known to affect the expression of genes involved in BAT development [20]. Modification of histones involves addition of methyl or acetyl moieties to the lysine residues on the tail portion of the histone, specifically at position H3K9 or H3K27. These modifications affect which genetic sequences are expressed or silenced [21, 22]. The mother's diet plays a major role in influencing epigenetic modifications and thus foetal growth. At present, it has not been established whether the epigenetic mechanisms controlling the development of BAT can be modified by dietary interventions.

There is a growing volume of data to indicate that n-3 PUFA encourages the development of BAT and thermogenic function [23–27]. It has been shown in mice that the stimulation of BAT development by eicosapentaenoic acid occurs via an epigenetic mechanism, namely miRNA function [28]. Thus, it is reasonable to enquire whether supplying the pregnant mother with n-3 PUFA may lead the foetus to increase its deposition of BAT. A study has examined whether administration of n-3 PUFA to the mother in early pregnancy affects the way the foetus develops BAT. It noted that n-3 PUFAs could stimulate the transcription of genes related to

BAT formation by means of chromatic remodelling and miRNA expression, i.e. an epigenetic mechanism. Taking these findings into consideration, there does appear to be benefit in a strategy for combatting childhood obesity through stimulation of BAT development. BAT thermogenesis can rapidly consume calories and prevent storage of excess energy as white adipose.

2 How Being Exposed to n-3 PUFAs in the Mother's Diet Causes Epigenetic Changes Modulating the Development of BAT in the Foetus

MicroRNAs are brief sequences of RNA which do not encode a gene product, but serve to regulate genetic transcription events. They are of major importance in the development of BAT [1, 28, 29]. If the dicer endoribonuclease prevents miRNA being expressed, adipocyte precursors are prevented from differentiating into brown adipocytes [30]. One particular miRNA, miR-193b/365, acts on Myf5+ cells to prevent their differentiation into muscle, and instead causes them to express a brown adipocytic phenotype [31]. Another miRNA, miR-30b also stimulates the expression of genes giving a brown adipocytic phenotype, in this case leading to greater mitochondrial respiratory metabolism by means of encouraging the transcriptional co-repressor receptor-interacting protein 140 (Rip140) to be degraded. n-3 PUFAs also act on the undifferentiated precursors of brown adipocytes to raise the levels of other miRNAs particular to the BAT type, namely miR-30b and miR-193b/365 [28]. It has been shown experimentally (both in vitro and in vivo) that animals whose mothers were administered n-3 PUFAs whilst pregnant expressed miRNA in a pattern favouring BTA formation, such as expression of miR-30b and miR-193/365.

Increased heat generation by BAT is associated with raised expression of the Drosha gene and its protein product. Drosha is a ribonuclease enzyme which plays an essential part in cleaving primary transcript RNA into stem loop precursor miRNA. This operation is carried out by the so-called 'microprocessor'. Potentially the level of n-3 PUFAs modulates how the microprocessor functions, thereby increasing precursor miRNAs within interscapular brown fat and altering the miRNA expression profile. Some evidence confirming this hypothesis is that knockout mice lacking adipose-specific Dgcr8 do not lay down functional levels of BAT and are unable to tolerate any type of cold. Dgcr8 forms a subunit within the microprocessor capable of recognition of primary transcript miRNA and processing it to the precursor form. There is research ongoing into the effect of increased dietary intake in the mother on foetal miRNA processing, especially the conversion of primary miRNA to precursor miRNA [30–32].

A further key way in which genetic transcription may be modified epigenetically is through the modification of the histones in chromatin. This influences cellular differentiation and the genes expressed by particular tissues. There is growing evidence to link the growth of BAT to epigenetic modifications produced by addition of acetyl or methyl groups to the N-terminal tail of histones [22]. Overall, chromatin adopts a looser conformation and is less positively charged when acetyl groups are added to lysine residues on histones, which enables a higher level of transcription. The numbers of acetyl groups added depend on how active two groups of enzymes with opposing actions are i.e. histone acetyltransferases (HAT) and histone deacetylases (HDACs). It has been demonstrated that one HAT in particular, Gen5/PCAF, enhances the development of BAT [33]. When the activity of HDAC1 or 9 is inhibited, transcription-level events activating BAT can be observed [30, 34, 35]. Thermogenesis by BAT depends on HDAC3 being active. The addition of a methyl functional group to histones can occur on lysine or arginine residues in the polypeptide chain. The conformational change this induces renders DNA more or less easy for various transcription factors or epigenetically controlled molecules to access. The addition of a methyl group at the H3K9 position by the G9a methyltransferase prevents cells differentiating into BAT [36], whereas methylation by EHMT1 activates thermogenic activity in BAT [34]. Loss of the JMJD1a histone demethylase, which acts at the H3K9 site, has been alleged to cause obesity. A further key location on histones where methylases act is H3K27. The removal of the three methyl groups at position H3K27 by the enzymes UTX or JMJD3 is necessary for BAT to develop. Recent evidence has shown that there are alternating additions of acetyl and methyl groups at position H3K27 as BAT is growing. When the beta3-adrenoceptor was stimulated, HDAC1 detached from its position and the H3K27 site was acetylated and then three methyl groups were removed. These events permitted transcription events associated with the development of BAT to occur.

3   Conclusion

The majority of the evidence for how BAT develops has come from animal models or cell cultures where specific genes for epigenetic writers or erasers had been knocked out. Epigenetic writers add epigenetic markers to DNA or chromatin, whereas epigenetic erasers delete such markers. These are surprisingly few data in existence showing the effect of dietary alterations on epigenetic events linked to the development of BAT. It is known, however, that transcription is altered in a specific way by n3-PUFAs. The epigenetic markers are increased acetylation at H3K27 and reduced trimethylation at the same point. This occurs via the action of the enzymes HDAC1 and JMJD3. Furthermore, n-3 PUFAs result in increased dimethylation at H3K9, which activates the epigenetic writer enzyme EHMT1, but does not affect the activity of the demethylator enzyme JMJD1. In conclusion, then, foetal exposure to n3-PUFAs modifies epigenetic marking, which increases the development of BAT capable of thermogenesis [33–37].

References

1. Fan R, Toney AM, Jang Y, Ro SH, Chung S. Maternal n-3 PUFA supplementation promotes fetal brown adipose tissue development through epigenetic modifications in C57BL/6 mice. Biochim Biophys Acta Mol Cell Biol Lipids. 2018;1863(12):1488–97. https://doi.org/10.1016/j.bbalip.2018.09.008. Epub 2018 Sep 25.
2. Zhong Y, Catheline D, Houeijeh A, Sharma D, Du L, Besengez C, Deruelle P, Legrand P, Storme L. Maternal omega-3 PUFA supplementation prevents hyperoxia-induced pulmonary hypertension in the offspring. Am J Physiol Lung Cell Mol Physiol. 2018;315(1):L116–32. https://doi.org/10.1152/ajplung.00527.2017. Epub 2018 Mar 29.
3. De Giuseppe R, Roggi C, Cena H. N-3 LC-PUFA supplementation: effects on infant and maternal outcomes. Eur J Nutr. 2014;53(5):1147–54. https://doi.org/10.1007/s00394-014-0660-9. Epub 2014 Jan 22.
4. Harms M, Seale P. Brown and beige fat: development, function and therapeutic potential. Nat Med. 2013;19:1252–63.
5. Gilsanz V, Hu HH, Kajimura S. Relevance of brown adipose tissue in infancy and adolescence. Pediatr Res. 2013;73:3–9.
6. Cypess AM, Kahn CR. The role and importance of brown adipose tissue in energy homeostasis. Curr Opin Pediatr. 2010;22:478–84.
7. Cypess AM, Lehman S, Williams G, Tal I, Rodman D, Goldfine AB, Kuo FC, Palmer EL, Tseng YH, Doria A, Kolodny GM, Kahn CR. Identification and importance of brown adipose tissue in adult humans. N Engl J Med. 2009;360:1509–17.
8. Chechi K, Nedergaard J, Richard D. Brown adipose tissue as an anti-obesity tissue in humans. Obesity Rev. 2014;15:92–106.
9. Symonds ME, Pope M, Budge H. Adipose tissue development during early life: novel insights into energy balance from small and large mammals. Proc Nutr Soc. 2012;71:363–70.
10. Symonds ME, Pope M, Sharkey D, Budge H. Adipose tissue and fetal programming. Diabetologia. 2012;55:1597–606.
11. Zingaretti MC, Crosta F, Vitali A, Guerrieri M, Frontini A, Cannon B, Nedergaard J, Cinti S. The presence of UCP1 demonstrates that metabolically active adipose tissue in the neck of adult humans truly represents brown adipose tissue. FASEB J. 2009;23:3113–20.
12. Porter C, Herndon DN, Chondronikola M, Chao T, Annamalai P, Bhattarai N, Saraf MK, Capek KD, Reidy PT, Daquinag AC, Kolonin MG, Rasmussen BB, Borsheim E, Toliver- Kinsky T, Sidossis LS. Human and mouse Brown adipose tissue mitochondria have comparable UCP1 function. Cell Metab. 2016;24:246–55.
13. Leitner BP, Huang S, Brychta RJ, Duckworth CJ, Baskin AS, McGehee S, Tal I, Dieckmann W, Gupta G, Kolodny GM, Pacak K, Herscovitch P, Cypess AM, Chen KY. Mapping of human brown adipose tissue in lean and obese young men. Proc Natl Acad Sci U S A. 2017;114:8649–54.
14. Zhang F, Hao G, Shao M, Nham K, An Y, Wang Q, Zhu Y, Kusminski CM, Hassan G, Gupta RK, Zhai Q, Sun X, Scherer PE, Oz OK. An adipose tissue atlas: an image-guided identification of human-like BAT and beige depots in rodents. Cell Metab. 2018;27:252–262.e253.
15. Symonds ME, Pope M, Budge H. The ontogeny of brown adipose tissue. Annu Rev Nutr. 2015;35:295–320.
16. Campos EI, Reinberg D. Histones: annotating chromatin. Annu Rev Genet. 2009;43:559–99.
17. Fedorova E, Zink D. Nuclear architecture and gene regulation. Biochim Biophys Acta. 2008;1783:2174–84.
18. Handy DE, Castro R, Loscalzo J. Epigenetic modifications: basic mechanisms and role in cardiovascular disease. Circulation. 2011;123:2145–56.
19. Chen Y, Pan R, Pfeifer A. Regulation of brown and beige fat by microRNAs. Pharmacol Ther. 2017;170:1–7.

20. Lecoutre S, Petrus P, Rydén M, Breton C. Transgenerational epigenetic mechanisms in adipose tissue development, trends in endocrinology & metabolism, (2018). Emerging evidence and mechanisms. Biochim Biophys Acta. 2018;29:675.
21. Kim J, Okla M, Erickson A, Carr T, Natarajan SK, Chung S. Eicosapentaenoic acid potentiates brown thermogenesis through FFAR4-dependent up-regulation of miR-30b and miR-378. J Biol Chem. 2016;291:20551–62.
22. Sambeat A, Gulyaeva O, Dempersmier J, Sul HS. Epigenetic regulation of the thermogenic adipose program. Trends Endocrinol Metab. 2017;28:19–31.
23. Okla M, Kim J, Koehler K, Chung S. Dietary factors promoting Brown and Beige fat development and thermogenesis, vol. 8. Adv Nutr (Bethesda, MD); 2017. p. 473–83.
24. Bargut TC, Silva-e-Silva AC, Souza-Mello V, Mandarim-de-Lacerda CA, Aguila MB. Mice fed fish oil diet and upregulation of brown adipose tissue thermogenic markers. Eur J Nutr. 2016;55:159–69.
25. Pahlavani M, Razafimanjato F, Ramalingam L, Kalupahana NS, Moussa H, Scoggin S, Moustaid-Moussa N. Eicosapentaenoic acid regulates brown adipose tissue metabolism in high-fat-fed mice and in clonal brown adipocytes. J Nutr Biochem. 2017;39:101–9.
26. Zhao M, Chen X. Eicosapentaenoic acid promotes thermogenic and fatty acid storage capacity in mouse subcutaneous adipocytes. Biochem Biophys Res Commun. 2014;450:1446–51.
27. Fan R, Koehler K, Chung S. Adaptive thermogenesis by dietary n-3 polyunsaturated fatty acids: emerging evidence and mechanisms. Biochim Biophys Acta. 2018;
28. Trajkovski M, Lodish H. MicroRNA networks regulate development of brown adipocytes. Trends Endocrinol Metab. 2013;24:442–50.
29. Arner P, Kulyte A. MicroRNA regulatory networks in human adipose tissue and obesity, nature reviews. Endocrinology. 2015;11:276–88.
30. Karbiener M, Scheideler M. MicroRNA functions in Brite/Brown fat—novel perspectives towards anti-obesity strategies. Comput Struct Biotechnol J. 2014;11:101–5.
31. Mori MA, Thomou T, Boucher J, Lee KY, Lallukka S, Kim JK, Torriani M, Yki-Järvinen H, Grinspoon SK, Cypess AM. Altered miRNA processing disrupts brown/white adipocyte determination and associates with lipodystrophy. J Clin Invest. 2014;124:3339–51.
32. Sun L, Xie H, Mori MA, Alexander R, Yuan B, Hattangadi SM, Liu Q, Kahn CR, Lodish HF. Mir193b–365 is essential for brown fat differentiation. Nat Cell Biol. 2011;13:958.
33. Jin Q, Wang C, Kuang X, Feng X, Sartorelli V, Ying H, Ge K, Dent SY. Gcn5 and PCAF regulate PPARγ and Prdm16 expression to facilitate brown adipogenesis. Mol Cell Biol. 2014; MCB. 00622–00614.
34. Emmett MJ, Lim H-W, Jager J, Richter HJ, Adlanmerini M, Peed LC, Briggs ER, Steger DJ, Ma T, Sims CA. Histone deacetylase 3 prepares brown adipose tissue for acute thermogenic challenge. Nature. 2017;546:544.
35. Tateishi K, Okada Y, Kallin EM, Zhang Y. Role of Jhdm2a in regulating metabolic gene expression and obesity resistance. Nature. 2009;458:757.
36. Swanson D, Block R, Mousa SA. Omega-3 fatty acids EPA and DHA: health benefits throughout life. Adv Nutr. 2012;3:1–7.
37. Inagaki T, Tachibana M, Magoori K, Kudo H, Tanaka T, Okamura M, Naito M, Kodama T, Shinkai Y, Sakai J. Obesity and metabolic syndrome in histone demethylase JHDM2a-deficient mice. Genes Cells. 2009;14:991–1001.

Breast Milk Proteases

Özlem Naciye Şahin and Despina D. Briana

1 Introduction

The proteins contained in milk carry out a broad array of complicated biological functions. Some proteins in milk have one function in their intact form, whilst also containing a sequence of latent function that becomes active following splitting of the main peptide chain. This bioactivity may involve attacking harmful microbes in the gut as well as regulating the infant's immune response. Thus, they may confer an evolutionary advantage. Current evidence suggests that this unmasking of latent bioactivity actually begins even, whilst milk is still within the breast. A range of proteolytic enzymes (proteases) in milk act on proteins in the milk to produce these bioactive peptide sequences. Furthermore, these same enzymes retain their functionality in the infant's intestine, potentially performing a more important catalytic function than even the proteases secreted by the infant's developing gut. This may reflect the fact that newborn infants are somewhat inefficient in digesting milk unless assisted by the proteases present in milk. The bioactive sequences latent in certain milk protein precursors are released through a series of steps involving both milk-derived proteases and proteases secreted by the infant gut. One of the aims of research is to understand how this release of latent bioactivity orchestrated through protease activity contributes to an evolutionary advantage for the mother and child [1, 2].

Ö. N. Şahin (✉)
Department of Child Health and Diseases, Arel University, Medical Faculty, Istanbul, Türkiye

D. D. Briana
NICU, Third Department of Pediatrics, National and Kapodistrian University of Athens, University General Hospital "ATTIKON", Athens, Greece

Ö. N. Şahin et al. (eds.), *Breastfeeding and Metabolic Programming*, https://doi.org/10.1007/978-3-031-33278-4_19

2 Milk as a Complex Biofluid

There has been a growing awareness amongst researchers investigating lactation in mammals and the unique nature of milk as a complete nutritional system for mammalian offspring that the use of the single term 'milk' for this entire dynamic system understates its true complexity. Referring to milk might suggest that there is a simple archetype for this biofluid and that it can be readily defined in terms of typical constituents. This simple picture is now known to be erroneous. The composition of milk varies continuously over the course of breastfeeding. Thus, researchers need to develop paradigms that reflect this dynamic change in milk. Not only is there a need to catalogue how composition alters, but also what effects this alteration results in. The goal is to comprehend both the nutritional benefits of varying composition and how milk exerts a protective role in the offspring. Milk is a complex fluid and the constituents are also complex. Alongside enzymes there are immunoglobulins, entire cells and several microbes. This wider appreciation of milk's constituents has often been overlooked, resulting in methods for storing breast milk and processing it, which lead to a loss of bioactivity by both molecules and microbes. Thus, its benefits may be lost if consumed following storage rather than directly. None of the artificial baby milks now on the market offer the range of bioactivity possessed by fresh, natural breast milk.

The full development of lactation in mammals has been shaped by the constant influence of selective evolutionary pressure, ensuring maximum success for the mother and offspring. Milk can be seen as the outcome of a more than 200-million-year old process of evolutionary pressures [3]. Any addition to milk comes at maternal biological cost, potentially reducing her own survival. Thus, unless the additional constituent confers some selective advantage for the infant, it is unlikely to be preserved by evolution. It is obvious that those constituents that offer complete nourishment to the infant have been selected by evolution, but the constituents which offer a protective rather than nutritional role have also been subject to the same evolutionary pressure. Only now is the rich protein chemistry of milk beginning to be appreciated, as providing both nutrition and protection to the developing baby and varying to match the developmental stage reached by the infant. This system has a previously unsuspected complexity. Proteins, specifically, perform a wider set of roles than initially believed.

3 Functions of Proteins in Intact and Truncated Form

Proteins are biological polymers which possess specific characteristics. This applies to both their intact and truncated (partially proteolyzed) forms. The truncated sequence may be more active than, or carry out a separate role from, its intact precursor. Truncation occurs through proteolytic degradation by proteases originating in milk or secreted by the infant gut. Research is currently focusing on why evolution has favoured this way of activating peptide sequences. The bioactive role of the latent sequences is already known to include attacking harmful microbes, regulating immunity and carrying out other roles that prevent infection, regulate growth and provide the breastfed infant with a greater chance of survival to reproductive age [1–3].

4   A New Way to Understand Protein Nutrition

The currently accepted model for how proteins are digested in human beings envisages several stages in the process. First, gastric acid causes denaturation of ingested proteins, which are then subject to initial proteolysis within the gastric cavity. As the chyme continues into the small intestine, hydrolytic degradation at a more neutral pH is the next step. The proteins are thus broken up into separate amino acids, capable of absorption via the gut epithelium.

5   Protein Digestion by Infants

This model requires adaptation when considering neonates. At this stage the gut is still undergoing development and there is a less acidic environment within the stomach as well as decreased proteolysis. Despite this situation, infants can still absorb proteins within milk in an efficient manner. Thus, the standard model requires the addition of a range of maternally-derived proteases present in milk, which are capable of performing proteolysis in the infant gut in a specific manner. These proteases then supplement the infant's endogenous digestive capabilities. It appears from current evidence that this process is so well orchestrated that these proteases can not only reduce proteins into absorbable fragments (i.e. individual amino acids) but can ensure that truncated proteins are released with an active, specific, biological function that helps ensure immunity, healthy metabolism or normal development.

The investigation of protein digestion within the gut took many years but ultimately yielded a detailed understanding of how this process occurs. There are also studies which have looked at how these gut enzymes affect the proteins in milk. The peptides formed by hydrolysis have also been examined [3, 4]. Several studies running alongside each other have assessed how peptides derived from milk can exert an antimicrobial action, control inflammation, promote mucosal repair, decrease hypertension, inhibit thrombus and transport calcium [5]. There is now an increasing array of techniques emerging from chemical, genomic, computational biological and clinical investigations suitable for investigating infant digestion in vivo. These techniques may be used for the identification of individual peptides in the gut of breastfed children as well as to confirm which enzymes actually truncate the protein to expose the bioactive peptide. The bioactivity of the released peptides is also under investigation. The multidisciplinary approach has been used in studies conducted in infants fed via an indwelling gastric tube, whether born at full term or prematurely. These studies used highly advanced analytical techniques such as mass spectrometry combined with similarity searching in silico [6–8].

Several hundred previously unknown peptides have now been characterised thanks to advances in the field of peptide analytical chemistry [9]. There now remains the significant task of matching individual peptides to specific roles, such as control of microbial flora or regulation of the immune system [9]. The roles that have been assigned to some of these peptides include protection, nutrition and developmental regulation of the child, as well as preventing pathogenic infection of the mother's breast.

Developments in the field of milk protein chemistry continue to elucidate peptide structures and their roles and this will hopefully translate into advances in infant nutrition. Advancing scientific understanding of the molecular and physiological mechanisms involved has the potential to improve the clinical and nutritional management of premature neonates, elderly patients or those whose intestinal function is impaired by drug actions. In neonates, the mature expression of digestive enzymes has not yet developed, whereas in elderly patients the ability to digest is impaired. There is considerable hope amongst researchers that the lessons learned will be applicable to health interventions across the entire age range.

6 Which Proteases Are Present in Milk?

A study by Demers-Mathieu et al. detected several functional proteases in breast milk from mothers whose infants were born before full term. These proteases included kallikrein, carboxypeptidase, plasmin, thrombin, elastase and cytosol aminopeptidase. In addition, cathepsin D was found in an inactive form. There was minimal effect of gestational age or time elapsed since delivery on how active the proteases were, their level or that of protease inhibitors. It appears that most studies of breast milk have only used antibody methods to detect a limited number of peptides (procathepsin D and elastase), but studies on cows' milk have extensively employed immunodetection to identify these two peptides plus plasmin and several other peptides of interest. Although several studies have been able to measure the concentration of plasmin in breast milk, the detection of elastase has so far only been qualitative [10–14].

Studies investigating how active plasmin and elastase are in cows' milk have also been published [15, 16]. Other studies have examined plasmin activity in breast milk in cases where delivery occurred at term and prematurely. Due to differences in the units employed while reporting on these studies, comparisons are complicated or impossible. It has also been established that the pro-enzyme, plasminogen, plasmin itself and both activator enzymes (namely urokinase and tissue-type plasminogen activators) and inhibitors are present in breast milk. Further research is needed to confirm exactly how these various molecules interact in milk [15–17].

Although plasmin is the most extensively studied of the proteases present in milk, it is, in fact, kallikrein which is present at the highest concentration and has the highest activity. One reason for the research focus on plasmin is that this protease is of particular interest to the dairy industry. Plasmin in bovine milk is active in cheese ripening, helping to generate its specific textures and taste. Thus, the quality of the resulting product depends on plasmin activity. Furthermore, in cases of mastitis, plasmin demonstrates enhanced activity, which speeds up the breakdown of milk proteins and spoils the milk [18, 19].

Kallikrein is a protease present at high concentration in blood, but which has also been identified in proteomic studies as a constituent of breast milk [9]. Its exact function in milk is currently unknown, although it is evidently involved in coagulation, degradation of fibrin and production of kinin. An investigation of the transcriptome of epithelial cells in cow udders indicates these cells release kallikrein into milk. There are therefore two potential origins for kallikrein in breast milk—either production from the epithelial cells of the breast or absorption from the circulation into milk [20, 21].

The level of kallikrein and its activity both differ significantly in milk produced following premature birth, but is steady after term, regardless of how much time has elapsed since birth. The varying levels may result from alterations in the synthesis of kallikrein and its precursor, how permeable the glandular epithelium of the breast is or variation in the expression levels of protease inhibitors. The experimental data do not indicate that the levels of protease inhibitors differ according to gestational age at delivery or time elapsed since birth, but there remains a lack of evidence pertaining to the level of α_2-Macroglobulin, a known inhibitor of kallikrein present in milk. Proteomic studies have shown that this molecule is present in breast milk, but its concentration is too low to be reliably quantified using ELISA [12]. In unpasteurised cows' milk the level of α_2-macroglobulin is relatively high at 126.8 mg L^{-1} [21–23].

7 Implications for the Health of the Breastfed Infant

One of the most well-established functions of milk is its ability to supply highly nutritious proteins to the neonate. Research carried out over the last one hundred years has identified many hundred different proteins, which collectively perform numerous physiological functions, including antimicrobial and immuno-regulatory roles. The proteins in milk originate from the epithelium of the breast, absorption from the circulation (either by passive diffusion or by assisted transfer) or are released by maternal immunocytes. To the present knowledge of milk protein chemistry must also be added the role of proteases in releasing encrypted peptide sequences. In this way, a complete picture can be constructed of how milk assists in healthy infant development.

There is a large number of different factors contributing to the control of enzymatic activity in milk, including that of the proteases. The components involved include inhibitory molecules, activating molecules, pre-enzymes, proteases, acidity, precise location in the gut and the conformation of the protein substrate. The proteases present in milk act specifically on particular proteins, such as the caseins, but do not hydrolyse lactoferrin, antibodies or certain other types of protein. Thus, within the infant gut, certain proteins are unaffected and retain bioactivity, including the release of specific peptide sequences at the required microlocation.

Further studies are needed to elucidate protease activity within the infant gut. It is already apparent that proteases in milk play a very significant role in digestion, and it has been calculated that most breakdown of protein in the infant's gastric cavity occurs in this way [5, 6]. The evidence so far supports the notion that proteases in milk have arisen due to selective evolutionary pressure, since that confer a health advantage to the infant through more efficient intestinal digestion and release of peptides with specific functions. It used to be thought that the fact that proteolysis in the infant stomach develops slowly was a weakness, but this may be an incorrect conclusion. Infants certainly digest less efficiently than adults, but this inefficiency is partly balanced by proteases in milk, which help to meet physiological needs. Evolution may have favoured a solution to infant digestion where the mother continues to control nutrition during the first stages of life of her offspring.

8 Conclusion

Recent technological advancements mean that some of the more surprising functions of milk as a complex and bioactive fluid are becoming known. From now on, researchers need to view infant nutrition as part of a system where the mother and child interact through milk. The dynamic features of milk, its varied composition and bioactivity all require further elucidation.

Proteases in milk carry out several functions, amongst which is the release of specific peptide sequences at particular points, both in the breast and when milk enters the infant gut. This function involves the specific proteases in milk and the fact that particular locations in the infant gut trigger particular forms of hydrolysis. Not only is an understanding of this system of value in managing infants, but it has also potential implications for patients of all ages and in all types of illness.

References

1. Dallas DC, German JB. Enzymes in human milk. Nestle Nutr Inst Workshop Ser. 2017;88:129–36. https://doi.org/10.1159/000455250. Epub 2017 Mar 27.
2. Gopalakrishna KP, Hand TW. Influence of maternal milk on the neonatal intestinal microbiome. Nutrients. 2020;12(3):823. https://doi.org/10.3390/nu12030823.
3. Oftedal OT. The mammary gland and its origin during synapsid evolution. J Mammary Gland Biol Neoplasia. 2002;7(3):225–52.

4. Lonnerdal B. Human milk: bioactive proteins/peptides and functional properties. Nestle Nutr Inst Workshop Ser. 2016;86:97–107.
5. Dallas D, et al. Extensive in vivo human milk peptidomics reveals specific proteolysis yielding protective antimicrobial peptides. J Proteome Res. 2013;12(5):2295–304.
6. Clare DA, Swaisgood HE. Bioactive milk peptides: a prospectus. J Dairy Sci. 2000;83(6):1187–95.
7. Dallas DC, et al. A peptidomic analysis of human milk digestion in the infant stomach reveals protein-specific degradation patterns. J Nutr. 2014;144(6):815–20.
8. Holton TA, et al. Following the digestion of milk proteins from mother to baby. J Proteome Res. 2014;13(12):5777–83.
9. Guerrero A, et al. Mechanistic peptidomics: factors that dictate specificity in the formation of endogenous peptides in human milk. Mol Cell Proteomics. 2014;13(12):3343–51.
10. Korycha-Dahl M, Dumas BR, Chene N, Martal J. Plasmin activity in milk. J Dairy Sci. 1983;66:704–11.
11. Armaforte E, Curran E, Huppertz T, Ryan CA, Caboni MF, O'Connor PM, Ross RP, Hirtz C, Sommerer N, Chevalier F. Proteins and proteolysis in pre-term and term human milk and possible implications for infant formulae. Int Dairy J. 2010;20:715–23.
12. Lindberg T, Ohlsson K, Westrom B. Protease inhibitors and their relation to protease activity in human milk. Pediatr Res. 1982;16:479–83.
13. Větvicka V, Vagner J, Baudys M, Tang J, Foundling S, Fusek M. Human breast milk contains procathepsin—detection by specific antibodies. Biochem Mol Biol Int. 1993;30:921–8.
14. Borulf S, Lindberg T, Mansson M. Immunoreactive anionic trypsin and anionic elastase in human milk. Acta Paediatr Scand. 1987;76:11–5.
15. Politis I, Lachance E, Block E, Turner J. Plasmin and plasminogen in bovine milk: a relationship with involution? J Dairy Sci. 1989;72:900–6.
16. Considine T, Healy A, Kelly A, McSweeney P. Proteolytic specificity of elastase on bovine α s1-casein. Food Chem. 2000;69:19–26.
17. Larsen LB, Benfeldt C, Rasmussen LK, Petersen TE. Bovine milk procathepsin D and cathepsin D: coagulation and milk protein degradation. J Dairy Res. 1996;63:119–30.
18. Heegaard CW, Larsen LB, Rasmussen LK, Højberg K-E, Petersen TE, Andreasen PA. Plasminogen activation system in human milk. J Pediatr Gastroenterol Nutr. 1997;25:159–66.
19. Lu DD, Suzanne NS. Isolation and characterization of native bovine milk plasminogen activators. J Dairy Sci. 1993;76:3369–83.
20. Barbano D, Rasmussen R, Lynch J. Influence of milk somatic cell count and milk age on cheese yield. J Dairy Sci. 1991;74(2):369–88.
21. Dallas DC, et al. Current peptidomics: applications, purification, identification, quantification and functional analysis. Proteomics. 2015;15:1026–38.
22. Khaldi N, et al. Predicting the important enzymes in human breast milk digestion. J Agric Food Chem. 2014;62(29):7225–32.
23. Wickramasinghe S, et al. Transcriptional profiling of bovine milk using RNA sequencing. BMC Genomics. 2012;13(1):45–58.

Breast Milk and Leptin Resistance

Özlem Naciye Şahin and Muhittin Abdülkadir Serdar

1 Introduction

Leptin, an endocrine signalling molecule released by fat tissue in proportion to the body fat mass, was discovered in 1994. It is a protein with a molecular mass of 160 kDa. The investigative focus following discovery was principally on the effects of the hormone on energy balance through its actions on the brain. The fact that leptin plays a key part in controlling energy balance came from observing patients lacking leptin. These individuals eat excessively and become obese as children. However, if leptin is replaced by artificial means, their appetite diminishes and they expend larger amounts of energy. This discovery led to the decision to try treating obese adults in general by leptin replacement or supplementation. This strategy is flawed, however, since the majority of obese individuals do not have any abnormality in the leptin alleles. Surprisingly, obese individuals actually have higher plasma concentrations of leptin than non-obese controls, yet they become obese. Thus, it appears they develop an insensitivity to leptin, meaning they are predisposed to weight gain and are unable to lose this extra weight. How leptin insensitivity occurs has not yet been fully elucidated, although several theories have been put forward, in particular the involvement of increased C-reactive protein, reduced transduction of signals triggered by leptin or lowered levels of activity by histone deacetylases [1–5]. At present the picture is incomplete, but it appears that the transportation of leptin across the blood-brain barrier is compromised in some way, and this is a key factor in pathogenesis [6–8].

Ö. N. Şahin (✉)
Department of Child Health and Diseases, Arel University, Medical Faculty, Istanbul, Türkiye

M. A. Serdar
Department of Basic Sciences, Medical Biochemistry, Medical Faculty, Acibadem Mehmet Ali Aydinlar University, Istanbul, Türkiye
e-mail: maserdar@acibadem.com.tr

Ö. N. Şahin et al. (eds.), *Breastfeeding and Metabolic Programming*,
https://doi.org/10.1007/978-3-031-33278-4_20

Evidence is accumulating, both from epidemiological and experimental research, to show that the environment has a critical effect on the likelihood of individuals becoming obese or developing metabolic abnormalities as adults. These environmental effects occur at specific stages in development, especially in utero and during breastfeeding. These alterations in an individual's metabolic tendencies are termed 'metabolic programming'. The programming consists of epigenetic alterations to the genome through such mechanisms as methylation of particular DNA sequences or chromatin remodelling through acetylation of histones. A recently published study in rats demonstrated that feeding a lipid-enhanced diet to rats in pregnancy and during lactation meant the offspring had a raised body mass, became obese and had hypothalamic insensitivity to leptin [9–11].

It has been shown in a number of studies that rats born in small litters, which therefore have access to more milk, are prone to becoming obese and over-eating. They are also relatively insensitive to leptin's effects on the hypothalamus as well as insulin's effects on the liver. The liver, furthermore, exhibits signs of oxidative stress [9, 12, 13]. However, whilst over-suckling may cause such problems, other studies demonstrate that breastfeeding confers a lower risk of becoming obese and/or diabetic at a later stage. It has recently been demonstrated that animals transferred to different mothers from those in which obesity had been induced using monosodium l-glutamate went back to a normal body mass, were not hyperphagic and resumed normal leptin responses. However, the details of how this occurs and the relevance to human physiology are not yet fully clear. Furthermore, there needs to be research into what happens if the dams are given other kinds of diet resulting in obesity and only during lactation. In particular, the effects of such an intervention on the mother's fat mass, metabolic programme and type of breast milk need to be noted, alongside how these changes impact energy usage in the young and the sensitivity to insulin and leptin as adults [14–18].

In rats, differentiated structures within the central nervous system which regulate or exigenesis and energy balance, notably the arcuate nucleus of the hypothalamus, begin to form at the end of the in utero period (the final 7 days) and keep progressing whilst lactation continues [19, 20]. There are several factors influencing how these structures mature and develop, one of which is the composition of milk. The existence of a pathway under control by leptin is demonstrable around 6–14 days postpartum. At that time, the blood level of leptin is raised to the point where it is referred to as the 'postnatal leptin surge'. It appears, therefore, that the concentration of leptin whilst the animal is still suckling affects the way the central nervous system develops [21, 22].

It was noted by Harder et al. that an excessive level of insulin around the time of birth results in an abnormal neuroanatomy and physiology of the hypothalamus. Other studies note how hyper-insulinaemia during breastfeeding cause the offspring to become overweight, intolerant to glucose and hypertensive [23]. When rats born to obese mothers were administered a lipid-enhanced diet or overfed shortly after birth, they later became prone to overeating, obesity, excessive circulating lipid levels and their glucose tolerance was impaired. These features are potentially due to insensitivity of the hypothalamus to leptin and insulin [9, 24, 25].

There is therefore considerable research interest in exactly how maternal obesity relates to later obesity in offspring, abnormal metabolism of glucose and reduced hypothalamic responsiveness to leptin and insulin.

2   How Does Metabolic Programming Happen?

Rats born to mothers with experimentally-induced obesity have been used to assess the potential for metabolic programming to occur. These animals develop a raised body mass in conjunction with being intolerant of glucose and insensitive to insulin. There is abnormality of action of the hypothalamus in response to leptin or insulin, and overfeeding is always present at all ages. It has thus been shown in an animal model that an abnormal maternal diet induces maladaptive metabolic programming in offspring at the stage of suckling.

When female rodents were administered a lipid-enhanced died during pregnancy or lactation, they became obese and the metabolism of both lipids and carbohydrates developed abnormalities [3, 26, 27]. Breast milk ensures that infants develop normally and may provide immunity against a number of pathogens [19, 28]. If the child is weaned prematurely, this may trigger pathological development [29]. Accordingly, there are tight limits to the composition of breast milk if these functions are to be fulfilled. If any of the macronutrients (carbohydrates, lipids or proteins) is out of balance or the levels of endocrine signalling molecules, such as insulin or leptin, are abnormal, there may be enduring changes to the physiology and metabolism of the offspring [7, 13]. It has been noted recently that if insulin levels in the offspring are lowered during feeding, the incidence of metabolic disorders linked to overfeeding is reduced [26]. Animals with experimentally-induced obesity produce mature milk which has elevated concentrations of glucose, proteins, cholesterol and triacylglycerides. The same changes in milk were also noted by Franco et al., who employed rats fed a lipid-enriched diet from a period 2 months before mating until the end of lactation. The offspring of these rat dams had abnormally high circulating levels when weaned, alongside a raised body fat mass and body mass overall [16]. In contrast, Guarda et al. demonstrated, in 2014, how administering linseed oil to rats with suckling offspring changed the composition of milk and resulted in a healthier amount of adipose tissue in offspring of either sex. It seems, therefore, that the composition of breast milk does play a key role at this early stage [13].

After feeding, there is a rise in the circulating glucose level, resulting in a corresponding rise in insulin. The surplus energy is stored in the form of triacylglycerides in fat tissues, and this process raises the circulating leptin level. Both insulin and leptin act on the arcuate nucleus of the hypothalamus, resulting in a fall in secretion of NPY (neuropeptide Y) and a rise in secreted POMC (proopiomelanocortin). This combination of signals induces satiety and encourages the use of energy [27–30]. The offspring of animals where obesity had been experimentally induced fed continuously, which is expected if NPY levels are high and POMC levels low.

A number of molecules have been investigated in experiments aiming to understand how insulin and leptin interact in their effects on the hypothalamus. These molecules include the IRβ and ObRb receptors, as well as IRS-2, PI3K, Akt, JAK-2 and STAT-3. They were also quantified in adult animals. Where the dam had been rendered obese through administration of a diet with excess sugar, the levels of all of these molecules were below normal, implying the hypothalamus is relatively insensitive to leptin and insulin, a condition leading to obesity in adulthood.

In a study by Rodrigues et al. [31], rats born to dams fed an excessive diet during the period of lactation demonstrated abnormal action of leptin on the hypothalamus and an ongoing tendency to overfeed. Additionally, it has been found that milk from dams with small litters has a raised level of triacylglycerides. It was also noted in earlier studies that the action of leptin on the hypothalamus is abnormal in rats born to mothers fed a lipid-enhanced diet during pregnancy [27–31].

There is a relative paucity of experimental evidence regarding the effects of unusual diet solely during lactation. It appears from the evidence gathered so far that a maternal diet containing an excess level of sugar not only produces obesity but also sets up abnormal metabolic programming.

The offspring of these mothers had an increased fat mass and the fat cells were hypertrophic. The circulating leptin concentration was also raised. It has already been established that the synthesis of leptin increases as fat mass rises [16]. A recent study also showed that undernourished dams produced offspring which were obese and demonstrated hyperleptinaemia as adults [30]. According to a study undertaken by Franco et al. in 2012, these abnormalities were also detectable at the stage of weaning (i.e. at day 21) in offspring where the maternal diet had been lipid-enriched. The body adipose was greater in extent than normal. Alongside a raised fat mass, the inguinal fat cells also expressed an increased level of mRNA coding for leptin and the circulating level was also above normal [16, 24]. A further study [32] using a rat animal model also linked obesity and abnormally raised leptin levels in adulthood to a metabolic programme induced by feeding the mother rats a lipid-enriched diet whilst pregnant and lactating [32].

The offspring of mothers with experimentally-induced obesity also exhibited insulin insensitivity in peripheral tissues, which was apparent from an abnormally raised circulating insulin level and increased HOMA (homeostatic model assessment) index. Furthermore, the rate at which glucose levels fell in an insulin tolerance test was retarded, which confirms that insensitivity to insulin was present. If there was maternal obesity in animals, the offspring put on excess weight, laid down more fat tissue and exhibited hyperphagia. The effects of insulin, both centrally and peripherally, were impaired and there was evidence that inflammation had been initiated [33, 34]. The existence of hyperinsulinaemia in conjunction with obesity and insulin insensitivity was also demonstrated by Ashino et al. in their 2012 study of rats born to dams oversupplied with lipids in pregnancy and lactation [27].

3   Conclusion

Thus, experimental data indicate that various kinds of physiological stress on lactating mothers set up abnormal metabolic programming in their offspring. Furthermore, the period of breastfeeding is highly significant in terms of whether the offspring eventually develops obesity during adulthood [33–34]. The findings so far highlight lactation as a key moment in the development of an abnormal metabolic programme, with dietary abnormalities at this point reflected in epigenetic alterations in the offspring, especially during the leptin surge that follows birth. This process occurs because the central nervous system is especially sensitive to environmental insults at a very young age, such as when breastfeeding takes place. The offspring of mothers whose obesity was due to excess sugar intake are especially at risk of metabolic abnormalities initiated during lactation. A maternal diet very rich in sugar is especially risky for making offspring eat excessively and become obese. The mechanism for this pathology involves the hypothalamus losing its normal responses to leptin and insulin and the peripheral tissues becoming insensitive to insulin.

References

1. Izquierdo AG, Crujeiras AB, Casanueva FF, Carreira MC. Leptin, obesity, and leptin resistance: where are we 25 years later? Nutrients. 2019;11(11):2704. https://doi.org/10.3390/nu11112704.
2. Zhang Y, Proenca R, Maffei M, Barone M, Leopold L, Friedman JM. Positional cloning of the mouse obese gene and its human homologue. Nature. 1994;372:425–32. https://doi.org/10.1038/372425a0.
3. Farooqi IS, Jebb SA, Langmack G, Lawrence E, Cheetham CH, Prentice AM, Hughes IA, McCamish MA, O'Rahilly S. Effects of recombinant leptin therapy in a child with congenital leptin deficiency. N Engl J Med. 1999;341:879–84. https://doi.org/10.1056/NEJM199909163411204.
4. Woods SC, Schwartz MW, Baskin DG, Seeley RJ. Food intake and the regulation of body weight. Annu Rev Psychol. 2000;51:255–77. https://doi.org/10.1146/annurev.psych.51.1.255.
5. Considine RV, Sinha MK, Heiman ML, Kriauciunas A, Stephens TW, Nyce MR, Ohannesian JP, Marco CC, McKee LJ, Bauer TL, et al. Serum immunoreactive-leptin concentrations in normal-weight and obese humans. N Engl J Med. 1996;334:292–5. https://doi.org/10.1056/NEJM199602013340503.
6. Bjorbaek C, Elmquist JK, Frantz JD, Shoelson SE, Flier JS. Identification of SOCS-3 as a potential mediator of central leptin resistance. Mol Cell. 1998;1:619–25. https://doi.org/10.1016/S1097-2765(00)80062-3.
7. Chen K, Li F, Li J, Cai H, Strom S, Bisello A, Kelley DE, Friedman-Einat M, Skibinski GA, McCrory MA, et al. Induction of leptin resistance through direct interaction of C-reactive protein with leptin. Nat Med. 2006;12:425–32. https://doi.org/10.1038/nm1372.
8. Kabra DG, Pfuhlmann K, Garcia-Caceres C, Schriever SC, Casquero GV, Kebede AF, Fuente-Martin E, Trivedi C, Heppner K, Uhlenhaut NH, et al. Hypothalamic leptin action is mediated by histone deacetylase 5. Nat Commun. 2016;7:10782. https://doi.org/10.1038/ncomms10782.
9. Gomes RM, Bueno FG, Schamber CR, de Mello JCP, de Oliveira JC, Francisco FA, Moreira VM, Junior MDF, Pedrino GR, de Freitas Mathias PC, Miranda RA, de Moraes SMF, Natali MRM. Maternal diet-induced obesity during suckling period programs offspring obese pheno-

type and hypothalamic leptin/insulin resistance. J Nutr Biochem. 2018;61:24–32. https://doi.org/10.1016/j.jnutbio.2018.07.006. Epub 2018 Jul 25.

10. Barker DJ. The developmental origins of adult disease. J Am Coll Nutr. 2004;23:588S–95S.

11. Larsson MW, Lind MV, Larnkjær A, et al. Excessive weight gain followed by catch-down in exclusively breastfed infants: an exploratory study. Nutrients. 2018;10(9):1290. Published 2018 Sep 12. https://doi.org/10.3390/nu10091290.

12. Howie GJ, Sloboda DM, Kamal T, Vickers MH. Maternal nutritional history predicts obesity in adult offspring independent of postnatal diet. J Physiol. 2009;587:905–15.

13. Guarda DS, Lisboa PC, de Oliveira E, Nogueira-Neto JF, de Moura EG, Figueiredo MS. Flaxseed oil during lactation changes milk and body composition in male and female suckling pups rats. Food Chem Toxicol. 2014;69C:69–75.

14. Breton C. The hypothalamus-adipose axis is a key target of developmental programming by maternal nutritional manipulation. J Endocrinol. 2013;216:R19–31.

15. Burdge GC, Hanson MA, Slater-Jefferies JL, Lillycrop KA. Epigenetic regulation of transcription: a mechanism for inducing variations in phenotype (fetal programming) by differences in nutrition during early life? Br J Nutr. 2007;97:1036–46.

16. Franco JG, Fernandes TP, Rocha CP, Calvino C, Pazos-Moura CC, Lisboa PC, et al. Maternal high-fat diet induces obesity and adrenal and thyroid dysfunction in male rat offspring at weaning. J Physiol. 2012;590:5503–18.

17. Rodrigues AL, de Moura EG, Passos MC, Dutra SC, Lisboa PC. Postnatal early overnutrition changes the leptin signalling pathway in the hypothalamic-pituitary-thyroid axis of young and adult rats. J Physiol. 2009;587:2647–61.

18. Conceição EP, Franco JG, Oliveira E, Resende AC, Amaral TA, Peixoto-Silva N, et al. Oxidative stress programming in a rat model of postnatal early overnutrition—role of insulin resistance. J Nutr Biochem. 2013;24:81–7.

19. von Kries R, Koletzko B, Sauerwald T, von Mutius E, Barnert D, Grunert V, et al. Breast feeding and obesity: cross sectional study. BMJ. 1999;319:147–50.

20. Grunewald M, Hellmuth C, Demmelmair H, Koletzko B. Excessive weight gain during full breast-feeding. Ann Nutr Metab. 2014;64:271–5.

21. Rodekamp E, Harder T, Kohlhoff R, Franke K, Dudenhausen JW, Plagemann A. Long-term impact of breast-feeding on body weight and glucose tolerance in children of diabetic mothers: role of the late neonatal period and early infancy. Diabetes Care. 2005;28:1457–62.

22. Stocker CJ, Cawthorne MA. The influence of leptin on early life programming of obesity. Trends Biotechnol. 2008;26:545–51.

23. Harder T, Plagemann A, Rohde W, Dorner G. Syndrome X-like alterations in adult female rats due to neonatal insulin treatment. Metabolism. 1998;47:855–62.

24. Chen H, Simar D, Morris MJ. Hypothalamic neuroendocrine circuitry is programmed by maternal obesity: interaction with postnatal nutritional environment. PLoS One. 2009;4:e6259.

25. Conceicao EP, Carvalho JC, Manhaes AC, Guarda DS, Figueiredo MS, Quitete FT, et al. Effect of early overfeeding on palatable food preference and brain Dopam inergic reward system at adulthood: role of calcium supplementation. J Neuroendocrinol. 2016;28

26. Samuelsson AM, Matthews PA, Argenton M, Christie MR, McConnell JM, Jansen EH, et al. Diet-induced obesity in female mice leads to offspring hyperphagia, adiposity, hypertension, and insulin resistance: a novel murine model of developmental programming. Hypertension. 2008;51:383–92.

27. Ashino NG, Saito KN, Souza FD, Nakutz FS, Roman EA, Velloso LA, et al. Maternal high-fat feeding through pregnancy and lactation predisposes mouse offspring to molecular insulin resistance and fatty liver. J Nutr Biochem. 2012;23:341–8.

28. Troina AA, Figueiredo MS, Moura EG, Boaventura GT, Soares LL, Cardozo LFMF, et al. Maternal flaxseed diet during lactation alters milk composition and programs the offspring body composition, lipid profile and sexual function. Food Chem Toxicol. 2010;48:697–703.

29. Younes-Rapozo V, de Moura EG, Lima ND, Barradas PC, Manhaes AC, de Oliveira E, et al. Early weaning is associated with higher neuropeptide Y (NPY) and lower cocaine—and

amphetamine-regulated transcript (CART) expressions in the paraventricular nucleus (PVN) in adulthood. Brit J Nutr. 2012;108:2286–95.

30. Malta A, Souza AA, Ribeiro TA, Francisco FA, Pavanello A, Prates KV, et al. Neonatal treatment with scopolamine butylbromide prevents metabolic dysfunction in male rats. Sci Rep. 2016;6:30,745.

31. Morton GJ, Cummings DE, Baskin DG, Barsh GS, Schwartz MW. Central nervous system control of food intake and body weight. Nature. 2006;443:289–95.

32. Morrison CD, Huypens P, Stewart LK, Gettys TW. Implications of crosstalk between leptin and insulin signaling during the development of diet-induced obesity. BBA-Mol Basis Dis. 2009;1792:409–16.

33. Cunha AC, Pereira RO, Pereira MJ, Soares Vde M, Martins MR, Teixeira MT, et al. Long-term effects of overfeeding during lactation on insulin secretion—the role of GLUT-2. J Nutr Biochem. 2009;20:435–42.

34. Rodriguez EM, Blazquez JL, Guerra M. The design of barriers in the hypothalamus allows the median eminence and the arcuate nucleus to enjoy private milieus: the former opens to the portal blood and the latter to the cerebrospinal fluid. Peptides. 2010;31:757–76.

The Effects of Metabolic Alteration on Embryonic Stem Cells

Özlem Naciye Şahin and Muhittin Abdülkadir Serdar

Stem cells exist in multicellular organisms as a reservoir of precursor cells which are pluripotent and can renew themselves multiple times. More differentiated cell types develop from these stem cells. In the majority of somatic cells, the lifespan is relatively fixed and if they are severely damaged, they can only be replaced from less differentiated cell types. Thus, for tissue integrity, a pool of stem cells is generally essential. Since stem cells possess these valuable capabilities of regeneration and differentiation, they have become the subject of considerable research interest. Areas where stem cells have been studied include in regenerative medicine and as a way to understand how humans develop and age [1, 2].

The way stem cells regenerate themselves and differentiate into specific cell types has been investigated using metabolomic and transcriptomic approaches. The eventual path a stem cell takes towards differentiation is governed by a number of morphogens, growth factors and pathways linked to metabolism. The eventual fate of stem cells is determined by the degree of glycolysis and oxidative phosphorylation as well as by epigenetic modifications within the cells, such as the addition of methyl or acetyl groups to the histones around which DNA is packaged. It is becoming increasingly evident that the metabolic conditions in the surrounding environment also play a role in the fate of stem cells. The metabolic settings of stem cells reflect both the individual cell's metabolic requirements and the limits imposed by the metabolic environment in which it finds itself [1, 3].

Ö. N. Şahin (✉)
Department of Child Health and Diseases, Arel University, Medical Faculty, Istanbul, Türkiye

M. A. Serdar
Medical Faculty, Department of Basic Sciences, Medical Biochemistry, Acibadem Mehmet Ali Aydinlar University, Istanbul, Türkiye
e-mail: maserdar@acibadem.com.tr

Ö. N. Şahin et al. (eds.), *Breastfeeding and Metabolic Programming*, https://doi.org/10.1007/978-3-031-33278-4_21

235

1 Metabolic Conditions Supporting Pluripotent Stem Cells

Oxidative phosphorylation is the term used to describe the metabolic process occurring in mitochondria whereby energy substrates are oxidised in the tricarboxylic acid cycle and other reactions, generating electrons via the oxidation and reduction of NADH which are fed in to the electron transport chain and ultimately used to generated ATP via ATP synthases. In the majority of cells in mammals, this is the preferred method of generating energy, although a few cell populations do utilise a mechanism whereby ATP is generated at substrate level, despite its relative inefficiency.

The capacity to give rise to different cell lineages (pluripotency) appears within the embryonic epiblast prior to implantation. Pluripotent stem cells (PSCs) are found in the epiblast prior to implantation and are designated naive. After implantation occurs, the PSCs become committed to producing particular lineages [4]. Epiblasts obtained before implantation from rats may be cultured in vitro, where they are referred to as embryonic stem cells (ESCs). They may be halted in the PSC stage for as long as required by use of a cell culture medium providing LIF, GSK3β and MEK inhibitors. This experimental setup is frequently termed '2iL conditions' [5]. There are several key ways in which PSCs in their naive or primed states differ from each other, in particular: their ability to produce PSCs destined for the germline; the epigenomic composition; whether they express genes associated with pluripotent naivety or particular lineages; the signals they need to receive to keep regenerating themselves; and how they metabolise energetic substrates [6]. PSCs in their naive state typically prefer oxidative phosphorylation to generate energy, whereas PSCs which have undergone priming are virtually dependent on glycolysis alone [7–9]. It is not yet established whether these metabolic preferences expressed in vitro represent the situation in vivo, i.e. whether oxidative phosphorylation occurs before implantation but anaerobic glycolysis is the preferred modality once the embryo implants itself in the uterus [10, 11]. One recently published study came to the conclusion that the switch between anaerobic and aerobic metabolism mainly depended on culture conditions, rather than representing an intrinsic difference in the cells themselves [7]. There is, nonetheless, also evidence to show that the choice of method used to generate ATP depends on intrinsic factors within the stem cells, whether primed or naive. This intrinsic preference may be expressed through epigenetic alterations [8]. Candidate transcription factors involved in switching from one form of energy generation to another are LIF-induced Stat3, which increases the level of mitochondrial genetic expression [7], and Esrrb, which increases expression of genes involved in aerobic metabolism [7, 12, 13]. During aerobic metabolism, NAD+ is constantly regenerated, as it is needed in the tricarboxylic acid cycle. This form of metabolism also ensures a steady supply of α-ketoglutarate (αKG), a co-factor involved in epigenetic alterations, such as the Jumonji domain- containing (JmjC) histone demethylases and ten-eleven translocation (TET) methyl cytosine dioxygenases. TETs also require ferrous ions to perform their role of demethylating histones and DNA, which are both mechanisms used in epigenetic regulation.

Changing the cell culture conditions can alter how stem cells handle glucose and glutamine. The 2i conditions, which involve addition of inhibitors for both GSK3β and MEK, result in an alteration in the level of alpha-ketoglutarate [13], an intermediate product in the tricarboxylic acid cycle. This results in increased levels of succinate. Alpha-ketoglutarate acts as co-factor for the dioxygenases responsible for epigenetic modifications, whereas succinate competes to inhibit the same enzymes. If the level of alpha-ketoglutarate rises relative to succinate, the dioxygenase enzymes act to reverse the epigenetic silencing achieved by trimethylation of the histones at positions H3K9, H3K27 and H4K20, as well as methylation of DNA sequences themselves. This then means the stem cells retain their naive pluripotency [13]. Indeed, supplementing the alpha-ketoglutarate level caused the cells to express a naive pluripotent phenotype, whereas they began to differentiate when the succinate level was supplemented. Alpha-ketoglutarate alone does not guarantee retention of pluripotent naivety, however, as it may also affect demethylation of histones and thus lead to a more differentiated phenotype [14].

The evidence, therefore, favours assigning a key role to alpha-ketoglutarate and the dioxygenases which depend on its co-presence with ferrous ions for their action in setting the epigenetic switches resulting in a naive pluripotent or more differentiated phenotype. This role may explain the fact that aerobic metabolism involving the mitochondria is seen in PSCs of naive type and those in the process of differentiation, but not in primed PSCs, where anaerobic metabolism is normal. The picture, nonetheless, is still incomplete and further research is needed to assign definite connections between different pluripotent states and preferred modality of metabolism. As long as there is a lack of consensus about the ideal cell culture conditions for studying PSCs, conclusions about metabolism are likely to remain tentative.

There is one more co-factor required for the action of the dioxygenases alongside alpha-ketoglutarate and ferrous ions, i.e. ascorbic acid (vitamin C). This co-factor's presence can change the phenotype of somatic cells into that of an induced PSC, through removal of the methyl group on 5-methylcytosine in DNA or removing the three methyl groups found at position K9 on the H3 histone [15, 16]. However, whereas alpha-ketoglutarate is found in all mammalian cells, ascorbic acid is not synthesised intrinsically by humans and must come from the diet. The fact that the dioxygenases depend for their epigenetic function on both endogenous metabolic by-products and molecules of exogenous origin means they combine inputs from both the embryo itself and the environment in determining how stem cells will differentiate [17, 18].

Glycolysis occurs via a sequence of cytosolic reactions of redox type and results in the six-membered glucose ring being split to form two pyruvic acid molecules, each containing three carbon atoms. This generates two extra ATP molecules. The generation of ATP in this way is known as substrate level phosphorylation. In the majority of cells, pyruvic acid can be subsequently converted into lactic acid through the action of lactic acid dehydrogenase or into acetyl-CoA through the action of pyruvic acid dehydrogenase.

Glycolytic intermediate products may also be utilised in synthesis of macromolecules at times of rapid cell division. The advantages of anaerobic metabolism/

glycolysis are that it can synthesise ATP swiftly and produce smaller molecules needed to assemble macromolecules for growth. However, it has the disadvantage that it fails to generate as much ATP from each glucose molecule as is possible through oxidative phosphorylation [1].

In the murine model, stem cells which are differentiating into a primed pluripotent phenotype from the naive type automatically decrease reliance on oxidative phosphorylation and rely instead on substrate level phosphorylation to generate ATP. Accordingly, they express large numbers of glucose transporters, resulting in increased volumes of glucose uptake and greater glycolytic activity [7, 19]. Furthermore, the increased glucose utilisation also fuels the pentose phosphate pathway by which nucleotides can be manufactured in the cell [20, 21]. These changes can be understood as intended to facilitate rapid cell division of the pluripotent stem cells. Similar metabolic alterations are seen in the so-called 'Warburg effect', which occurs in neoplasia [22]. This effect occurs in cells that undergo rapid proliferation, especially in malignancy. It involves the stockpiling of intermediate molecules in the glycolytic pathway, which are then utilised in cellular division, at the same time as injury resulting from the production of reactive oxygen species is minimised. The accumulated intermediates may be utilised in various synthetic pathways: to generate amino acids via 3-phosphoglycerate; to generate lipids via dihydoxyacetone phosphate and acetyl CoA; and to form nucleotides and NADPH through glucose-6-phosphate and the pentose phosphate pathway. Thus, the metabolic needs of rapidly dividing cells, whether in neoplasia or in the normal physiological differentiation of pluripotent stem cells, can be supplied.

2 Conclusion

There is increasing evidence to implicate numerous metabolic pathways in regulating the type of differentiation undergone by many stem cells. Although a significant number of metabolic adaptations in stem cells reflect the local environment around the cell, this does not mean that such metabolic adaptations have no long-term programming effects on cells. In the same way that cells may be reprogrammed through signalling by growth factors; so, too, different metabolic preferences may induce epigenetic alterations, changes in the rate of division and expression of different phenotypes. Furthermore, the evidence also shows that there are intrinsic preferences for specific metabolic settings in specific states of differentiation. The metabolic state of specific cells reflects the outcome of different factors operating simultaneously, i.e. intrinsic preferences attached to a phenotype and the surrounding microenvironmental conditions. When this interplay of different factors is better understood, it will be possible to change the conditions in a targeted way to achieve particular aims both for tissue engineering in the laboratory and for regenerative procedures in human patients [1].

References

1. Shyh-Chang N, Ng HH. The metabolic programming of stem cells. Genes Dev. 2017 Feb 15;31(4):336-346.
2. Lamberto F, Peral-Sanchez I, Muenthaisong S, Zana M, Willaime-Morawek S, Dinnyés A. Environmental Alterations during Embryonic Development: Studying the Impact of Stressors on Pluripotent Stem Cell-Derived Cardiomyocytes. Genes (Basel). 2021;12(10):1564.
3. Diamante L, Martello G. Metabolic regulation in pluripotent stem cells. Curr Opin Genet Dev. 2022;75:101923.
4. Boroviak T, Loos R, Lombard P, Okahara J, Behr R, Sasaki E, Nichols J, Smith A, Bertone P. Lineage-specific profiling delineates the emergence and progression of naïve pluripotency in mammalian embryogenesis. Dev Cell. 2015;35:366–82.
5. Ying QL, Wray J, Nichols J, Batlle-Morera L, Doble B, Woodgett J, Cohen P, Smith A. The ground state of embryonic stem cell self-renewal. Nature. 2008;453:519–23.
6. Zhang WC, Shyh-Chang N, Yang H, Rai A, Umashankar S, Ma S, Soh BS, Sun LL, Tai BC, Nga ME, et al. Glycine decarboxylase activity drives non-small cell lung cancer tumor-initiating cells and tumorigenesis. Cell. 2012;148:259–72.
7. Zhou W, Choi M, Margineantu D, Margaretha L, Hesson J, Cavanaugh C, Blau CA, Horwitz MS, Hockenbery D, Ware C, et al. HIF1α induced switch from bivalent to exclusively glycolytic metabolism during ESC-to-EpiSC/hESC transition. EMBO J. 2012;31:2103–16.
8. Takashima Y, Guo G, Loos R, Nichols J, Ficz G, Krueger F, Oxley D, Santos F, Clarke J, Mansfield W, et al. Resetting transcription factor control circuitry toward ground-state pluripotency in human. Cell. 2014;158:1254–69.
9. Sperber H, Mathieu J, Wang Y, Ferreccio A, Hesson J, Xu Z, Ficher KA, Devi A, Detraux D, Gu H, et al. The metabolome regulates the epigenetic landscape during naive-to-primed human embryonic stem cell transition. Nat Cell Biol. 2015;17:1523–35.
10. Barbehenn EK, Wales RG, Lowry OH. Measurement of metabolites in single preimplantation embryos; a new means to study metabolic control in early embryos. J Embryol Exp Morphol. 1978;43:29–46.
11. Brinster RL, Troike DE. Requirements for blastocyst development in vitro. J Anim Sci. 1979;49(Suppl. 2):26–34.
12. Carbognin E, Betto RM, Soriano ME, Smith AG, Martello G. Stat3 promotes mitochondrial transcription and oxidative respiration during maintenance and induction of naïve pluripotency. EMBO J. 2016;35:618–34.
13. Carey BW, Finley LWS, Cross JR, Allis CD, Thompson CB. Intracellular α-ketoglutarate maintains the pluripotency of embryonic stem cells. Nature. 2015;518:413–6.
14. TeSlaa T, Chaikovsky AC, Lipchina I, Escobar SL, Hochedlinger K, Huang J, Graeber TG, Braas D, Teitell MA. α-Ketoglutarate accelerates the initial differentiation of primed human pluripotent stem cells. Cell Metab. 2016;24:485–93.
15. Chen C-T, Shih Y-RV, Kuo TK, Lee OK, Wei Y-H. Coordinated changes of mitochondrial biogenesis and antioxidantenzymes during osteogenic differentiation of human mesenchymal stem cells. Stem Cells. 2008a;26:960–8.
16. Chen C, Liu Y, Liu R, Ikenoue T, Guan KL, Liu Y, Zheng P. TSC-mTOR maintains quiescence and function of hematopoietic stem cells by repressing mitochondrial biogenesis and reactive oxygen species. J Exp Med. 2008b;205:2397–408.
17. Chen C, Liu Y, Liu Y, Zheng P. mTOR regulation and therapeutic rejuvenation of aging hematopoietic stem cells. Sci Signal. 2009;2:ra75.
18. Chen J, Guo L, Zhang L, Wu H, Yang J, Liu H, Wang X, Hu X, Gu T, Zhou Z, et al. Vitamin C modulates TET1 function during somatic cell reprogramming. Nat Genet. 2013;12:1504–9.
19. Leese HJ. Metabolic control during preimplantation mammalian development. Hum Reprod Update. 1995;1:63–72.

20. Varum S, Rodrigues AS, Moura MB, Momcilovic O, Easley CA IV, Ramalho-Santos J, Van Houten B, Schatten G. Energy metabolism in human pluripotent stem cells and their differentiated counterparts. PLoS One. 2011;6:e20914.
21. Manganelli G, Fico A, Masullo U, Pizzolongo F, Cimmino A, Filosa S. Modulation of the pentose phosphate pathway induces endodermal differentiation in embryonic stem cells. PLoS One. 2012;7:e29321.
22. Vander Heiden MG, Cantley LC, Thompson CB. Understanding the Warburg effect: the metabolic requirements of cell proliferation. Science. 2009;324:1029–33.

Part III
Breastfeeding and Neuro-developmental Programming

Neural Maturation of Breastfed Infants

Özge Serçe Pehlevan, Bülent Kara, and Despina D. Briana

1   Introduction

Brain development starts from fetal life, and proceeds well into adolescence [1]. Brain structures and functioning develop sequentially [2]. Caudal to rostral progression occurs in brain development [2]. This progression starts from the rhombencephalon followed by the diencephalon and telencephalon. Cortical growth goes behind primary cortical structure formation [2, 3]. Neuronal maturation also occurs in a hierarchical progression. It starts from the "primitive" brainstem, and progresses to form "advanced" cortical and cognitive functions. This process proceeds beyond the first weeks of postnatal life [2–4]. The "triune brain" evolutionary hypothesis supports this hierarchical fashion of neuronal development. In this hypothesis, the early primitive brain, the intermediate brain, and the most advanced brain structure develop consecutively. The role of the early primitive brain is an arrangement of movement, vital functions, and self-preservation. The intermediate brain is associated with hunger, instincts, emotions, fight or flight, and memory and sensory input, and the last developed brain structures play roles in reasoning, motor functions, and perception [2, 5]. Neural structures grow rapidly and peak

Ö. S. Pehlevan (✉)
Faculty of Medicine, Department of Pediatrics, Division of Neonatology, Kocaeli University, Kocaeli, Türkiye
e-mail: ozge.serce@kocaeli.edu.tr

B. Kara
Faculty of Medicine, Department of Pediatrics, Division of Pediatric Neurology, Kocaeli University, Kocaeli, Türkiye
e-mail: bulent.kara@kocaeli.edu.tr

D. D. Briana
NICU, Third Department of Pediatrics, National and Kapodistrian University of Athens, University General Hospital "ATTIKON", Athens, Greece

Ö. N. Şahin et al. (eds.), *Breastfeeding and Metabolic Programming*, https://doi.org/10.1007/978-3-031-33278-4_22

synaptogenesis of the medulla presents during the last weeks of gestation [2, 4, 6]. The one-third of brain growth takes place during the last 2 months of gestation [2, 7]. Therefore, preterm neonates have nearly 60% of the brain volume of a full-term neonate at birth. This smaller brain will continue to grow after birth [2, 7, 8]. Preterm infants also have decreased corpus callosum, white matter, and cortical gray matter volume in the adolescent period [9–13].

The average newborn brain weight is 350 g. It will have rapidly tripled its birth weight size by age 1 and quadrupled its birth weight size by age 3 [14, 15]. After this year, the brain grows slowly, and it approaches the quintuple mark by age 15 [14, 16]. The dentate gyrus of the hippocampus is responsible for memory. Neuron proliferation also takes place in this area. It is the most vulnerable process to environmental factors during the first several weeks of life [14, 17]. In this period, the proliferation of the other forms of neural tissue occurs concordantly in the brain [14]. The accelerated tempo of postnatal myelination and neuron migration to the various parts of the brain presents during the first 2 years of life [14, 18, 19]. Dramatic growth in synapse formation is the key element of these years [14, 17]. Pruning, an example of programmed cell death, leads to a decline in synaptic density. It is necessary for appropriate neurodevelopment [14, 17, 20–22]. Inadequate pruning is one of the proposed etiologic factors for autism spectrum disorders [14, 23]. The permeability and vulnerability to neurotoxins of the blood-brain barrier (BBB) are higher in the first years of life than later [14, 17]. Building brain architecture via cells and connections formation and creating a selectively permeable barrier within the brain and the environment are the summary of neurodevelopmental procedures during infancy. An infant's diet presents key elements required for optimum brain development during this process.

2 The Composition of Breast Milk

The content and interactions of the milk bioactive components are adapted to the growth velocity of infants, and dependent on specific target points of each species [24–26]. In humans, these target points are mainly the central nervous system (CNS), the immune system, and the achievement of affiliative behavior [26]. Human milk is an essential nutrition for the infant's development contributing to survival and life quality that can extend to adulthood [25, 27–32]. So, the main health policies recommend exclusive breastfeeding as the most appropriate type of feeding during the first 6 months of life, and continuation of breastfeeding along with complementary foods for at least 2 years [32–37].

Human milk contains a variety of nutrients that potentially have synergistic effects [14]. Breast milk composition does not have a uniform character as infant formula. It is a dynamic liquid that rapidly adapts to the nutritional requirements of infants [24, 25, 36]. Its composition changes within a day, during lactation, and according to infantile demand (Table 1) [24–28, 37]. For example, the protein content is higher in breast milk from mothers of preterm infants than in term infants

Table 1 Content of breast milk from mothers of preterm and term infants [27]

	1st week		2nd week		3rd–4th week		10th–12th week	
	Preterm	Term	Preterm	Term	Preterm	Term	Preterm	Term
Energy (Kcal/dL)	60(45–75)	60(44–77)	71(49–94)	67(47–86)	77(61–92)	66(48–85)	66(39–94)	68(50–86)
Protein (g/dL)	2.2(0.3–4.1)	1.8(0.4–3.2)	1.5(0.8–2.3)	1.3(0.8–1.8)	1.4(0.6–2.2)	1.2(0.8–1.6)	1.0(0.6–1.4)	0.9(0.6–1.2)
Lipid (g/dL)	2.6(0.5–4.7)	2.2(0.7–3.7)	3.5(1.6–5.5)	3.0(1.2(4.8)	3.5(1.6–5.5)	3.3(1.6–5.1)	3.7(0.8–6.5)	3.7(0.8–6.5)
Lactose (Kcal/dL)	5.7(3.9–7.5)	5.8(4.2–7.4)	5.7(4.1–7.3)	6.2(5–7.3)	6.0(5–7)	6.7(5.3–8.1)	6.8(6.2–7.2)	6.7(5.3–8.1)
Oligosaccharides (g/dL)	2.1(1.3–2.9)	1.9(1.1–2.7)	2.1(1.1–3.1)	1.9(1.1–2.7)	1.7(1.1–2.3)	1.6(1–2.2)	No data	No data

(Table 1) [24, 26, 38]. Another example is lactoferrin which decreases during the first several days of lactation [26]. Colostrum, the milk of the first 5 days of postnatal life, evolves through transitional milk between 6 and 13 days. Then, mature milk presents for 14 days and beyond [25, 26].

2.1 Breast Milk Proteins

Proteins in human milk exert various physiological activities that include the promotion of the immune and gastrointestinal systems [26]. Casein supplies amino acids and supports calcium and phosphorus absorption [26]. The whey-to-casein percentage in breast milk changes during lactation [26, 39]. Lactoferrin and alpha-lactalbumin are the main contents of whey proteins. Alpha-lactalbumin is a valuable nutritional element and has antitumor activity [26, 40–42]. Lactoferrin, an iron-binding protein, supports the growth of gut epithelium and has bacteriocidal properties. Brain-derived neurotrophic factor (BDNF) is another protein in human milk. Its serum level is associated with neuronal development in infants [32, 43]. However, the persistence of BDNF levels do not extend to prepubertal age [32]. The main expression of this protein is in the hippocampus [32, 44]. It supports synaptic connections, it is associated with the development and growth of the brain, and is responsible for dendrite formation and differentiation, as well as plasticity [32, 45–47].

2.2 The Non-protein Nitrogen Content of Breast Milk

The nonprotein nitrogen fraction of breast milk contains peptide hormones, polyamines, urea, uric acid, carnitine, ammonia, free amino acids, creatine, creatinine, choline, amino alcohols of phospholipids, amino sugars, growth factors such as nerve growth factor, nucleotides, and nucleic acids [14, 25, 26]. Nucleotides play roles in the immune system and gut environment regulation, as well as in the absorption and digestion of foods [26]. Carnitine is involved in long-chain polyunsaturated fatty acids (LC-PUFA) metabolism that is important for favoring neurodevelopment [14, 20]. Breast milk provides nearly 9% of the creatine intake [25, 46]. The brain is significantly vulnerable to creatine deficiency which leads to worse neurodevelopmental outcomes like mental retardation and autism [25].

2.3 Carbohydrates in Breast Milk

The principal carbohydrate in human milk is lactose [26]. Lactose inhibits enteropathogen binding to host cell receptors and enhances calcium absorption [26]. Besides these benefits, it has a significant role in rapid brain development in early life [26]. Galactolipids are the key elements of myelination [26]. The infant's liver is unable to synthesize all of the galactolipid requirements [26]. Fortunately, milk galactose is an excellent source of galactolipids [26]. Human milk has higher lactose levels than other species' milk [26]. A correlation between the volume of the brain and the lactose content in the milk is considered [26].

The integral part of the plasma membranes of nerves contains sialic acid. It locates mainly in the nerve endings and dendrites [14, 26, 48]. Sialic acid is present in gangliosides, glycoproteins, and oligosaccharides [49]. Oligosaccharides are biologically active carbohydrates, and one of the main largest solid elements of breast milk [24, 26, 50]. They favor the colonization of the infant's intestinal microbiota [24]. Gangliosides are glycosphingolipids that take part in neuronal migration and maturation, myelin, and synapse formation [49–52]. Sialic acid fortification supports learning performance in animals by increasing its amount in the frontal cortex [26, 49, 53]. The human brain has the highest sialic acid quantity in the world. In humans, breastfeeding leads to higher amounts of sialic acid than formula feeding [26, 49, 54].

2.4 Lipids in Breast Milk

Lipids supply 50% of the calories in milk. The fat content of human milk changes dynamically to various factors (Table 1) [24, 26, 55, 56]. Specifically, human breast milk provides an abundance of lipid components, especially cholesterol and essential fatty acids that are vital for brain and retina development [15, 28, 57–60].

2.4.1 The Sterols in Breast Milk

The sterol content of breast milk rises over the lactation period. Serum cholesterol levels are higher in breastfed infants than in formula-fed ones [14, 26]. Cholesterol, the major component of sterol content, is an essential part of all membranes. Nerve conduction in the brain requires the laying down of the myelin sheaths, and this process needs cholesterol [14, 25, 26]. It is also important for glial cells [14]. Cholesterol has been implicated in adult cognitive performance [15, 60].

2.4.2 The Fatty Acids in Breast Milk

Docosahexaenoic acid (DHA; polyunsaturated omega-3 fatty acid) and arachidonic acid (AA; polyunsaturated omega-6 fatty acid) forms nearly 20% of the fatty acid ingredient of the brain. They are mainly located in phospholipids of neural membranes, particularly in the cerebral cortex and other gray matter regions [2, 15, 28, 57, 61–66]. They play an important role in the early neurodevelopmental process including cortical maturation, neuronal growth, repair, and myelination [9, 15, 66–70]. An infant's immature liver synthesize capacity cannot meet the LC-PUFAs needs of the developing brain without a dietary source [15, 26, 58, 71, 72]. These lipid-rich components of human milk may contribute to advanced cognitive and psychomotor development in breastfed children compared with formula-fed children [9, 26, 71]. The main fatty acid content of the brain is DHA, but DHA content in milk or brain tissue is significantly correlated with the mother's diet and their biosynthesis from precursors [14, 27, 73]. Therefore, their concentrations in breast milk are highly variable. The amount of fatty acid in the diet is important due to its impact on the neural tissue, both gray and white matter structure [14]. These fatty acids also modulate the inflammatory response and energetic metabolism in adipose tissue, and muscle [57, 74, 75]. The last trimester of pregnancy and the first 2 years of life are characterized by accelerated brain growth. The brain has the most abundant accretion of main fatty acids in these periods [2, 15, 61, 76–78]. Preterm infants are devoid of this significant transplacental transfer of fatty acids during the last trimester of pregnancy. Therefore, they are prone to fatty acid deficiency. The impact of DHA levels in the brain on the clinical outcomes of preterm infants is unknown [2, 77]. Several studies reported positive correlations between PUFA levels in red blood cells and maturation of white matter, cerebral cortex volume, thalamus, and basal ganglia in late preterm infants [62, 76, 79]. Despite opposing views of some authors, there have been reports stating encouraging outcomes on the visual and cognitive function of supplementation with PUFAs [15, 35, 61, 71, 80–89]. Therefore, PUFA fortification of the preterm infant may be a neurorestorative intervention [61]. Fortunately, breast milk is an excellent source of fatty acids, and preterm mothers' milk contains higher DHA values compared with term human milk [26, 61].

Various amounts of LC-PUFAs are added to formulas [26]. Although infant formulas try to mimic human milk, infant formulas have quite different fatty acid profiles and shapes which are not used by the brain in the same way [26, 36, 90, 91]. These differences lead to a discrepancy in the fatty acid composition of cell membranes and alter gene expression within those cells, leading to subsequent changes in brain structure and function. LC-PUFA dietary intake promotes the development of dendritic spines and the formation of synaptic membranes, thus bringing out neurotransmission and cell-to-cell signaling [14, 15, 92]. Rat pups fed a diet not containing n-3 fatty acids that have much less DHA, and more n-6 fatty acids in their brain [93]. This diet leads to learning and memory disorders in adult rats, and more depression scores [14, 94, 95]. Mothers with higher dietary intake of n-6 and a lower dietary intake of n-3 PUFAs during the last month of pregnancy and lactation transfer less DHA to their offspring [96]. The neuronal plasma membrane manages signal transduction of neuronal growth and migration, synapse formation, and plasticity. This decreased transfer of DHA can influence the fluidity of this membrane [57, 89]. Therefore, the amount of PUFAs and the proportion between n-6 and n-3 PUFAs in diet may influence infants' speech-language skills [14].

2.4.3   The Milk Fat Globule Membrane (MFGM)

The milk fat globule membrane in human milk has various bioactive elements [25, 35, 49, 90]. The ratio of lipid and protein weight of the MFGM is 1:1 [49, 97, 98]. The lipid component of the MFGM is composed mainly of cholesterol and phospholipids [35, 36, 49]. Thirty percent of the total phospholipid composition in MFGM consists of sphingomyelin, phosphatidylcholine, and phosphatidylethanolamine [25, 49, 97]. Several trials report the promising impact of MFGM supplements on children's microbiota, defense against infections, and neurodevelopment [25, 35, 49, 99–107]. Feeding by infant formula supplemented with bovine MFGM supplementation leads to similar cognitive outcomes with breastfed infants, and higher cognitive outcomes than standard formula-fed infants [25, 107].

2.5   The Vitamins in Breast Milk

The water-soluble vitamins in breast milk are ascorbic acid, pyridoxine, thiamin, folate, riboflavin, biotin, niacin, choline, pantothenate, and vitamin B12. Breast milk contains fat-soluble vitamins such as A, D, E, and K [14, 24, 26, 108, 109]. The number of water-soluble vitamins in human milk changes by various factors like the dietary intake of mothers, the stage of lactation, and preterm birth [24, 26].

2.5.1   Choline

Choline (vitamin B4), is abundant in human milk. The biosynthesis of the membrane constituents, phosphatidylcholine, sphingomyelin, choline plasmalogens, and the neurotransmitter acetylcholine requires choline as a precursor [48]. Choline plays a significant role in neurodevelopment, and neural tube closure like folate [14, 49, 110–112]. Choline supplementation influences memory and learning in animal studies [14, 49, 113]. Neurogenesis and synaptogenesis are the two sensitive periods to choline supplementation in rats that result in positive outcomes in brain function. This period in rats reflects the time period from in utero to 4 years of age in humans [49, 114]. The infants of mothers who have diminished choline levels during the first months of pregnancy have poor cognitive functions at 18 months [49, 115]. Sphingomyelin and its metabolites have roles in cell signaling and proliferation, apoptosis as well as inflammation [48, 116–118]. Oral sphingomyelin increases myelination in rats [49, 117]. It promotes the maturation of the intestine and inhibits intestinal absorption of cholesterol [49, 118, 119]. Very low birth weight infants who take the sphingomyelin fortification had better neurodevelopmental outcomes between 6 and 18 months of age [120].

2.5.2 Folate

Folate is an essential cofactor in various biological pathways, including nucleotide synthesis [111, 121]. Folate deficiency leads to sensory axonal neuropathy, cognitive impairment, depression, and schizophrenia [111, 122–126]. Folate and vitamin B12 deficiencies additively disrupt memory function in rats who have Alzheimer's disease by blunting hippocampal insulin signaling and altering the intestinal microbial environment [127].

2.5.3 Vitamin D

Active vitamin D has antioxidant properties. It influences brain development. Furthermore, it plays a significant role in neuron development and neuroprotection [111, 128, 129]. Vitamin D regulates immunity against certain bacteria, and the intestinal microbiota [111]. Vitamin D deficiency leads to aging and behavioral, social, motor, and sensory impairments [111, 130–133].

2.5.4 Vitamin A

Vitamin A deficiency influences gut microbiota by increasing the population of *Bacteroides vulgatus* [111, 134]. In recent years, the impact of carotenoids, especially lutein in the development and functions of the brain, has been investigated [15, 135]. The main accumulation of lutein is in the brain. Carotenoid-supplemented formulas increase brain carotenoids particularly in the hippocampus, occipital cortex, and striatum [15, 135]. Lutein promotes cell communication and neuroprotection through antioxidant mechanisms [15, 135]. The formula-fed preterm decedents have lower brain lutein quantity than breastfed ones. On the other hand, formula-fed term decedents do not show this difference [15, 136]. Lutein absorption is also higher in human milk than in infant formula [15, 137, 138]. Further studies investigating the impact of carotenoids on psychomotor outcomes are required.

2.6 Micronutrients and Trace Elements in Breast Milk

Breast milk consists of micronutrients and trace elements that have active roles in CNS development and functioning [24, 26]. Magnesium (Mg) regulates neuronal transmission and neuromuscular coordination. It is a cofactor for various enzymes. Moreover, Mg is responsible for RNA, DNA, and protein stability [110, 139, 140]. Mg inhibits the calcium channel in the N-methyl-D-aspartate (NMDA) receptor. Therefore, it preserves excitotoxicity, and neuronal apoptosis [111, 139, 141–143]. Brain Mg levels promote synaptic plasticity, and therefore affect learning and memory skills [111, 144, 145]. Mg deficiency is associated with inflammation and oxidative response [111].

Zinc is located in structures of various proteins. It is a cofactor of a variety of enzymes that regulate many cellular functions and signaling pathways [111, 146]. Zinc is one of the trace elements that have neuroprotective functions [111, 147–150]. Zinc is also located in synaptic vesicles, particularly in glutamatergic terminals [111, 151–153]. Furthermore, Zinc is responsible for neuronal activity, and influences the activity of N-methyl-D-aspartate (NMDA), amino-3-hydroxyl-5-methyl-4-isoxazole-propionate (AMPA), GABA-A, glycine inotropic, and GPR39 receptors [111, 153–155].

2.7 The Role of Breast Milk in the Regulation of Immune Functions

Persistent inflammation is a well-known factor that causes neurodevelopmental disorders. Diet in the early period of life influences the regulation of inflammation in a long-term manner [14, 156]. Shorter breastfeeding duration dysregulates immune functions and may lead to neuroinflammation as the predisposing etiology of autism spectrum disorders [14, 157].

2.8 Effects of Breastfeeding on Mother-Child Interactions

Maternal care is important in the early neurodevelopment and epigenetic programming of their offspring's CNS [158–161]. Breastfeeding affects both mothers and their infants by altering the maternal hormones [14]. Human milk consists of oxytocin, which is a neuropeptide in the brain. Oxytocin is released in response to sucking and stimulates the let-down of milk [158, 162, 163]. It is associated with affiliation and bonding [158, 164, 165]. Therefore, it may influence mother–infant relations [14, 158, 166, 167]. Genetic variations in the oxytocin pathway lead to alterations in limbic regions [167, 168]. Negative central constituent in the event-related brain potential occurs from frontal cortical regions, especially the anterior cingulate cortex [157, 169]. Therefore, chronic modulation of the oxytocin pathway can alter the brain structures which are responsible for mediating attention and emotions [158]. Lactation can improve maternal stress levels [14, 169]. Lactating mothers had greater brain activation than formula-feeding ones during the first postpartum month. This difference was correlated with improved maternal sensitivity when their offsprings were 3–4 months old [169, 170]. Maternal sensitivity during infancy is associated with language development [171]. In the study of Hardin et al., infants of depressed and breastfeeding mother had no dysregulation of the behavior or brain development in contrast to the depressed group who did not breastfeed [172]. Only infants of depressed and bottle-feeding mother had right frontal EEG asymmetry and more right along with less left hemisphere activity [173]. These findings demonstrate that breastfeeding may influence mother–child interactions in a long-term manner. Supporting this hypothesis, formula-fed infants have poorer speech processing [24, 26, 174].

2.9 Effects of Breastfeeding on Modulation of Gut-Brain Axis

Altering gut microbiota with breast milk may also promote brain and myelin development, resulting in improved brain function [67]. The gut-brain axis which represents the interactions between CNS and the intestinal microbiota is established in utero and grows through childhood [174, 175]. Bidirectional signals between the gastrointestinal tract and brain influence the sensory, motor, and secretory process of the gut, and also brain functions [111, 174]. This communication occurs continuously through hormonal, immune, neuronal, and other pathways that are generally determined by the microbiota, and the transition of bacterial products through the gut wall [174, 176, 177]. Lipopolysaccharides, present in the cell wall of Gram-negative bacteria, translocate from the gut mucosa to the systemic circulation and produce pro-inflammatory cytokines that are critically affecting the CNS [174, 178, 179]. On the other hand, probiotic microorganisms, for example, *Lactobacillus*, decrease the colonization of inflammatory microorganisms [174, 180]. Microbial gut-derived tryptophan metabolites modulate immunity by regulation of T cells [174, 181–183]. Furthermore, tryptophan metabolites increase kynurenine concentration. Engagement with kynurenine and aryl hydrocarbon receptors stimulates the differentiation of regulatory T cells. It rises the levels of indoleamine 2,3-dioxygenase up. Indoleamine 2,3-dioxygenase stimulates the catabolism of tryptophan [174, 183]. In mice, tryptophan metabolites that can transfer via the placenta impact CNS development in utero independently of the microbiota [174, 184]. Finally, tryptophan metabolites in systemic circulation influence the levels of serotonin and gamma-aminobutyric acid in the CNS and the production of neurotoxins in microglia and astrocytes [174, 185, 186]. Bacterial fermentation of complex polysaccharides in the colon is the source of short-chain fatty acids. These fatty acids alter mitochondrial function via the citric acid cycle and carnitine metabolism or have epigenetic effects [25, 174, 187]. The results of these factors are reversible behavioral, inflammatory, metabolic, electrographic, and epigenetic changes in brain function [174]. Some microbial products increase hydroxytryptamine (5-HT) in the colon and blood. Consequently, they promote neuronal cell division and differentiation in utero [188]. A decrease in 5-HT during the developmental process influences the maturation of cortical neurons, and barrel cortex development [189]. The blood-brain barrier (BBB) is a control region of the molecular transfer between the circulatory system and the brain parenchyma. GF mice have increased BBB permeability compared with non-GF ones with normal gut microbiota [190]. The interactions between the gut microbiota and the intestinal cells promote the production of peptides that activate afferent endings of the vagus nerve [13]. The transmission of signals to the CNS affects behavior and efferent neural activity as a pro-inflammatory response [174]. The brain receives information related to systemic inflammation, contributing to initiating behavioral responses [191]. Therefore, the gut microbiota is fundamental in the brain structure and modulation of function [174]. Therefore, dysbiosis may influence CNS development and functions during the most vulnerable brain development period, the first years of life [175].

Maternal transfer of commensal bacteria to the fetus takes place before birth via the placenta and the amniotic fluid. Colonization after birth is a complex and dynamic process and is dependent on the duration of gestation, mode of delivery, use of antibiotics, and type of feeding [24, 35, 174].

The gut microbiota is dominant of *Proteobacteria* and *Actinobacteria* in term infants born to healthy mothers with vaginal delivery, breastfeeding, and with no exposure to antibiotics [174]. With time, breast milk that contains high *Streptococci* and *Staphylococci* and complex oligosaccharides that stimulate the growth of *Staphylococci* and *Bifidobacteria,* also acquires *Firmicutes* and *Bacteroidetes* species [174]. By solid food intake, *Bacteroides* and *Clostridium* species enter the gut. The gut microbiota completes its final composition within 3 years [174]. A formula-fed infant has different gut microbiota with a wider microbiota composition than a breastfed infant [174]. *Clostridium* and *Streptococcus* species, *Bacillus subtilis, Lactobacillus acidophilus, Bacteroides vulgatus, Escherichia coli, Veillonella parvula,* and *Pseudomonas aeruginosa* are significantly higher in bottle-fed infants than in breastfed ones. On the contrary, *Lactobacillus rhamnosus* and *Staphylococci* are common in breastfed infants, whereas *Staphylococcus epidermidis* is almost absent in formula-fed infants [174]. Breast milk has also large amounts of oligosaccharides that act as prebiotics, promoting the beneficial probiotic microorganisms (Table 1) [192]. Dysbiosis alters synaptic maturation that influences motor control and anxiety-like behavior [193]. Healthy colonization of the gut microbiota supports myelin formation in animals. The absence of microbiota during early life promotes activity-related transcriptional pathways in the amygdala [194, 195]. Gut dysbiosis is related to significant neurological problems. Altered gut microbiota has a direct relationship with fine motor skills and childhood temperament at 18 months of age, cognition at 2 years of age, and communication, motor, personal, and social skills at 3 years of age [196–199]. All of these data confirm the significance of gut microbiota for appropriate CNS development and function. However, most of these data come from animal studies. Humans have greater expansion of the prefrontal cortex and the frontoinsular regions than animals. Because the human gut-brain axis has different characteristics from the axis of animals, these results cannot be generalized to humans [35].

2.10 The Impact of the Duration of Exclusive Breastfeeding on Neurodevelopment

Many neural outcomes, including white matter and total brain volume, and cortical thickness are associated with the duration of exclusive breastfeeding [9, 156]. There was a strict correlation between the extension of this duration and both increased parietal cortex thickness and higher cognitive scores in 571 adolescents [200]. Another study determined slower myelination in formula-fed children than in breastfed children [67]. Studies utilizing advanced magnetic resonance imaging (MRI) techniques reported that breastfed infants have better white matter maturation [34, 67, 201–203]. Deoni et al. compared white matter development by advanced MRI measures at age 10 months to 4 years between infants either exclusively breastfed for a mean of 413 days or exclusively formula-fed or fed a mixture of formula and breast milk [67]. Early exclusive breastfeeding leads to better development in relatively late-maturing white matter regions, including frontal and temporal white matter, corticospinal tracts, and superior longitudinal and occipitofrontal fasciculi. Breastfed infants have improved performance in some of these higher-order cognitive regions [61, 67, 204]. Better cognitive functions and the spatiotemporal formation of the myelin sheath require rapid and synchronized brain messaging that is facilitated by the white matter [205]. This process develops coordinated movement and improves social, emotional, and other behaviors [67, 206]. Breastfeeding duration has a positive correlation with the improved development and functioning of myelin water fraction in the internal capsule, superior orbital-frontal fasciculus, and left superior-parietal lobe of 1–4-year-old toddlers. These regions are responsible for executive and social-emotional behaviors, planning, and language skills in which breastfed infants were also advanced [67, 204]. A recent study has investigated nearly the same correlation between 4 and 8 years old children [9]. A remarkable association between the duration of breastfeeding and fractional anisotropy scores in left-lateralized white matter tracts, including the left superior longitudinal fasciculus and left angular bundle, which is indicative of greater intrahemispheric connectivity, and no correlation with corpus callosum size was reported [9]. The left angular bundle is associated with verbal episodic memory performance [207]. The largest white matter tract in the brain is the corpus callosum. It provides interhemispheric connectivity and is associated with developmental disorders [9, 208–210]. However, breast milk consumption is associated with the more global development of white matter volume or quality in other studies [9, 60, 67, 70]. The authors explained these by complex underlying mechanisms of significant association between breastfeeding duration and white matter connectivity [9]. Thus, breastfeeding could have neurorestorative potential through its impact on oligodendrocytes development and myelination [61]. Although not all findings are consistent, breastfeeding results in better intelligence quotient (IQ) scores, academic success, and neurocognitive, verbal, and language skills in later life [57, 60, 61, 200, 211–218]. Children with attention deficit and hyperactivity or autism spectrum disorder have shorter breastfeeding durations than their counterparts

[219–222]. The immature and small brain that has altered structural connectivity leads to preterm infants more vulnerable to adverse neurological outcomes than term infants [2, 6, 223, 224]. Both brain injury and immaturity result in neurocognitive, social, emotional, and behavioral deficits [225]. With the unique components not found in infant formula, human milk is essential in the development and protection of the preterm infant's brain [2, 202, 226–228]. Breastfed preterm infants have better IQ scores and cognitive functions than formula-fed ones [202]. Isaac et al. demonstrated a correlation between IQ, white matter volume, and breast milk intake in premature male infants, but not in females who were followed up during adolescence period [60]. Based on these data, the World Health Organization encourage feeding with breast milk for preterm infants as their term counterparts [229]. The underlying mechanisms of the various reported neurocognitive benefits of breastfeeding are largely unknown. Indeed, the impact of breastfeeding duration on child neurodevelopment is controversial [57, 212, 216, 230, 231]. Some studies stated that breastfeeding improves children's cognitive ability far into adult life [158, 212, 214, 232–239], while others reported no significant relationship between them [58, 231, 240–246].

3   Conclusion

Breast milk is an excellent nutritional source with its dynamic and rich content. It is a unique food that exactly fulfills the requirements of growing infants. It is qualified with complex content with various components that have different structures, amounts, and synergistic effects. Although the exact underlying mechanisms are largely unknown, the current data demonstrate that breastfeeding is a key element for optimal neurodevelopment. Lack of breast milk feeding has a lifelong impact on neurocognition and quality of life.

References

1. Barrera C, Mize KD, Jones N. Feeding patterns influence brain development in infancy. FAU Undergrad Res J. 2014;3:22–33.
2. Hallowell SG, Spatz DL. The relationship of brain development and breastfeeding in the late-preterm infant. J Pediatr Nurs. 2012;27:154–62.
3. Billiards SS, Pierson CR, Haynes RL, Folkerth RD, Kinney HC. Is the late preterm infant more vulnerable to gray matter injury than the term infant? Clin Perinatol. 2006;33:915–33.
4. Lan LM, Yamashita Y, Tang Y, et al. Normal fetal brain development: MR imaging with a half-fourier rapid acquisition with relaxation enhancement sequence. Radiology. 2000;215:205–10.
5. Darnall RA, Ariagno RL, Kinney HC. The late preterm infant and the control of breathing, sleep, and brainstem development: a review. Clin Perinatol. 2006;33:883–914.

6. Niu W, Xu X, Zhang H, et al. Breastfeeding improves dynamic reorganization of functional connectivity in preterm infants: a temporal brain network study. Med Biol Eng Comput. 2020;58:2805–19.

7. Kinney HC. The near-term (late preterm) human brain and risk forperiventricular leukomalacia: a review. Semin Perinatol. 2006;30:81–8.

8. Adams-Chapman I. Neurodevelopmental outcome of the late preterm infant. Clin Perinatol. 2006;33:947–64.

9. Bauer CE, Lewis JW, Brefczynski-Lewis J, et al. Breastfeeding duration is associated with regional, but not global, differences in white matter tracts. Brain Sci. 2019;10:19.

10. McNamara RK, Carlson SE. Role of omega-3 fatty acids in brain development and function: potential implications for the pathogenesis and prevention of psychopathology. Prostaglandins Leukot Essent Fatty Acids. 2006;75:329–49.

11. Stewart AL, Rifkin L, Amess PN, et al. Brain structure and neurocognitive and behavioral function in adolescents who were born very preterm. Lancet. 1999;353:1653–7.

12. Northam GB, Liégeois F, Chong WK, Wyatt JS, Baldeweg T. Total brain white matter is a major determinant of IQ in adolescents born preterm. Ann Neurol. 2011;69:702–11.

13. Peterson BS, Vohr B, Staib LH, et al. Regional brain volume abnormalities and long-term cognitive outcome in preterm infants. JAMA. 2000;284:1939–47.

14. Smith JM. Breastfeeding and language outcomes: a review of the literature. J Commun Disord. 2015;57:29–40.

15. Zielinska MA, Hamulka J, Grabowicz-Chądrzyńska I, Bryś J, Wesolowska A. Association between breastmilk LC PUFA, carotenoids and psychomotor development of exclusively breastfed infants. Int J Environ Res Public Health. 2019;16:1144.

16. Dekaban AS, Sadowsky D. Changes in brain weights during the span of human life: relation of brain weights to body heights and body weights. Ann Neurol. 1978;4:345–56.

17. Watson RE, DeSesso JM, Hurtt ME, Cappon GD. Postnatal growth and morphological development of the brain: a species comparison. Birth Defects Res B Dev Reprod Toxicol. 2006;77:471–84.

18. Matsuzawa J, Matsui M, Konishi T, et al. Age-related volumetric changes of brain gray and white matter in healthy infants and children. Cereb Cortex. 2001;11:335–42.

19. Sanai N, Nguyen T, Ihrie RA, et al. Corridors of migrating neurons in the human brain and their decline during infancy. Nature. 2011;478:382–6.

20. Zhang Z, Tran NT, Nguyen TS, et al. Impact of maternal nutritional supplementation in conjunction with a breastfeeding support program during the last trimester to 12 weeks postpartum on breastfeeding practices and child development at 30 months old. PLoS One. 2018;13:e0200519.

21. Prado EL, Dewey KG. Nutrition and brain development in early life. Nutr Rev. 2014;72:267–84.

22. Georgieff MK. Nutrition and the developing brain: nutrient priorities and measurement. Am J Clin Nutr. 2007;85:614–20.

23. Hill EL, Frith U. Understanding autism: insights from mind and brain. Philos Trans R Soc Lond Ser B Biol Sci. 2003;358:281–9.

24. Iglesia I, Moreno LA, Rodriguez-Martinez G. Feeding practices of infants. In: Vinciguerra M, Sanchez PC, editors. Moleculer nutrition: mother and infant. 1st ed. London: Elsevier; 2021. p. 57–86.

25. Garwolińska D, Namieśnik J, Kot-Wasik A, Hewelt-Belka W. Chemistry of human breast milk-A comprehensive review of the composition and role of milk metabolites in child development. J Agric Food Chem. 2018;66:11881–96.

26. Walker M. Breastfeeding management for the clinician: using the evidence. 5th ed. Burlington, Massachusetts: Jones and Bartlett Publishers; 2021.

27. Denne SC. Parenteral nutrition for the high-risk neonate. In: Gleason CA, Juul SE, editors. Avery's diseases of the newborn. 10th ed. Philadelphia, PA: Elsevier; 2018. p. 1023–31.

28. Movio C, de Oliveira SAN. Continued breastfeeding and the influence of fatty acids on infant neurological maturation: asystematic review. Health Sci. 2021;23:311–5.

29. Zhao X, Yang J. Longer breastfeeding duration, better child development? Evidence from a large-scale survey in China. Child Youth Serv Rev. 2022;133:1–18.

30. Khan JR, Hossain MB, Mistry SK. Breastfeeding is a protective factor for overweight/obesity among young children in Bangladesh: findings from a nationwide data. Child Youth Serv Rev. 2020;119:105525.

31. Lopez DA, Foxe JJ, Mao Y, Thompson WK, Martin HJ, Freedman EG. Breastfeeding duration is associated with domain-specific improvements in cognitive performance in 9-10-year-old children. Front Public Health. 2021;9:657422.

32. Berlanga-Macías C, Sánchez-López M, Solera-Martínez M, et al. Relationship between exclusive breastfeeding and brain-derived neurotrophic factor in children. PLoS One. 2021;16:e0248023.

33. World Health Organization. Infant and young child feeding. Geneva: World Health Organization; 2017.

34. Grace T, Oddy W, Bulsara M, Hands B. Breastfeeding and motor development: a longitudinal cohort study. Hum Mov Sci. 2017;51:9–16.

35. Cerdó T, Ruíz A, Acuña I, et al. A synbiotics, long chain polyunsaturated fatty acids, and milk fat globule membranes supplemented formula modulates microbiota maturation and neurodevelopment. Clin Nutr. 2022;41:1697–711.

36. Cilla A, Diego Quintaes K, Barberá R, Alegría A. Phospholipids in human milk and infant formulas: benefits and needs for correct infant nutrition. Crit Rev Food Sci Nutr. 2016;56:1880–92.

37. Agostoni C, Braegger C, Decsi T, et al. Breast-feeding: a commentary by the ESPGHAN committee on nutrition. J Pediatr Gastroenterol Nutr. 2009;49:112e25.

38. Lonnerdal B. Human milk proteins: key components for the biological activity of human milk. Adv Exp Med Biol. 2004;554:11e25.

39. Lonnerdal B. Nutritional and physiologic significance of human milk proteins. Am J Clin Nutr. 2003;77:1537–43.

40. Gustafsson L, Hallgren O, Mossberg AK, et al. HAMLET kills tumor cells by apoptosis: structure, cellular mechanisms, and therapy. J Nutr. 2005;135:1299–303.

41. Newburg DS. Innate immunity and human milk. J Nutr. 2005;135:1308–12.

42. Svensson M, Hakansson A, Mossberg AK, et al. Conversion of alpha-lactalbumin to a protein inducing apoptosis. Proc Natl Acad Sci U S A. 2000;97:4221–6.

43. Nassar MF, Younis NT, El-Arab SE, Fawzi FA. Neuro-developmental outcome and brain-derived neurotrophic factor level in relation to feeding practice in early infancy. Matern Child Nutr. 2011;7:188–97.

44. Binder DK, Scharfman HE. Brain-derived neurotrophic factor. Growth Factors. 2004;22:123–31.

45. Thoenen H. Neurotrophins and neuronal plasticity. Science. 1995;270:593–8.

46. Chapleau CA, Larimore JL, Theibert A, Pozzo-Miller L. Modulation of dendritic spine development and plasticity by BDNF and vesicular trafficking: fundamental roles in neurodevelopmental disorders associated with mental retardation and autism. J Neurodev Disord. 2009;1:185–96.

47. Edison EE, Brosnan ME, Aziz K, Brosnan JT. Br JNutr. 2013;110:1075–8.

48. Wang B. Sialic acid is an essential nutrient for brain development and cognition. Ann Rev Nutr. 2009;29:177–222.

49. Hernell O, Timby N, Domellöf M, Lönnerdal B. Clinical benefits of milk fat globule membranes for infants and children. J Pediatr. 2016;173(Suppl):S60–5.

50. Gabrielli O, Zampini L, Galeazzi T, et al. Preterm milk oligosaccharides during the first month of lactation. Pediatrics. 2011;128:e1520e31.

51. McJarrow P, Schnell N, Jumpsen J, Clandinin T. Influence of dietary gangliosides on neonatal brain development. Nutr Rev. 2009;67:451–63.

52. Palmano K, Rowan A, Guillermo R, Guan J, McJarrow P. The role of gangliosides in neuro-development. Nutrients. 2015;7:3891–913.
53. Wang B, Yu B, Karim M, et al. Dietary sialic acid supplementation improves learning and memory in piglets. Am J Clin Nutr. 2007;85:561–9.
54. Wang B, McVeagh P, Petocz P, Brand-Miller J. Brain ganglioside and glycoprotein sialic acid in breastfed compared with formula-fed infants. Am J Clin Nutr. 2003;78:1024–9.
55. Saarela T, Kokkonen J, Koivisto M. Macronutrient and energy contents of human milk fractions during the first six months of lactation. Acta Paediatr. 2005;94:1176e81.
56. Kent JC, Mitoulas LR, Cregan MD, et al. Volume and frequency of breastfeedings and fat content of breast milk throughout the day. Pediatrics. 2006;117:e387e95.
57. Amaro A, Baptista FI, Matafome P. Programming of future generations during breastfeeding: the intricate relation between metabolic and neurodevelopment disorders. Life Sci. 2022;298:120526.
58. Girard LC, Doyle O, Tremblay RE. Breastfeeding, cognitive and noncognitive development in early childhood: a population study. Pediatrics. 2017;139:e20161848.
59. Nyaradi A, Oddy WH, Hickling S, Li J, Foster JK. The relationship between nutrition in infancy and cognitive performance during adolescence. Front Nutr. 2015;2:2.
60. Isaacs EB, Fischl BR, Quinn BT, Chong WK, Gadian DG, Lucas A. Impact of breast milk on intelligence quotient, brain size, and white matter development. Pediatr Res. 2010;67:357–62.
61. Volpe JJ. Dysmaturation of premature brain: importance, cellular mechanisms, and potential interventions. Pediatr Neurol. 2019;95:42–66.
62. Innis SM. Perinatal biochemistry and physiology of long-chain polyunsaturated fatty acids. J Pediatr. 2003;143:S1eS58.
63. Xiao Y, Huang Y, Chen ZY. Distribution, depletion and recovery of docosahexaenoic acid are region-specific in the rat brain. Br J Nutr. 2005;94:544–50.
64. Innis SM. Fatty acids and early human development. Early Hum Dev. 2007;83:761–6.
65. Ribeiro ACAF, Batista TH, Veronesi VB, Giusti-Paiva A, Vilela FC. Cafeteria diet during the gestation period programs developmental and behavioral courses in the offspring. Int J Dev Neurosci. 2018;68:45–52.
66. Weiser MJ, Butt CM, Mohajeri MH. Docosahexaenoic acid and cognition throughout the lifespan. Nutrients. 2016;8:99.
67. Deoni SC, Dean DC 3rd, Piryatinsky I, et al. Breastfeeding and early white matter development: a cross-sectional study. NeuroImage. 2013;82:77–86.
68. Guesnet P, Alessandri JM. Docosahexaenoic acid (DHA) and the developing nervous system (CNS) - Implications for dietery recommendations. Biochimie. 2011;93:7–12.
69. Hadley KB, Ryan AS, Forsyth S, Gautier S, Salem N. The Essentiality of arachidonic acid in infant development. Nutrients. 2016;8:216.
70. Deoni S, Dean DI, Joelson S, O'Regan J, Schneider N. Early Nutrition influences developmental myelination and cognition in infants and young children. NeuroImage. 2018;178:649–59.
71. Bernard JY, Armand M, Peyre H, et al. Breastfeeding, polyunsaturated fatty acid levels in colostrum and child intelligence quotient at age 5-6 years. J Pediatr. 2017;183:43–50.
72. Andreas NJ, Kampmann B, Mehring L-DK. Human breast milk: a review on its composition and bioactivity. Early Hum Dev. 2015;91:629–35.
73. Innis SM. Dietary (n-3) fatty acids and brain development. J Nutr. 2007;137:855–9.
74. Sambra V, Echeverria F, Valenzuela A, Chouinard-Watkins R, Valenzuela R. Docosahexaenoic and arachidonic acids as neuroprotective nutrients throughout the life cycle. Nutrients. 2021;13:986.
75. Nakamura MT, Yudell BE, Loor JJ. Regulation of energy metabolism by long-chain fatty acids. Prog Lipid Res. 2014;53:124–44.
76. Kamino D, Studholme C, Liu M, et al. Postnatal polyunsaturated fatty acids associated with larger preterm brain tissue volumes and better outcomes. Pediatr Res. 2018;83:93–101.
77. Reynolds A. Breastfeeding and brain development. Pediatr Clin N Am. 2001;48:159–71.

78. Diau GY, Hsieh A, Sarkadi-Nagy E, Wijendran V, Nathanielsz P, Brenna JT. The influence of long chain polyunsaturate supplementation on docosahexaenoic acid and arachidonic acid in baboon neonate central nervous system. BMC Med. 2005;3:11.
79. Tam EW, Chau V, Barkovich AJ, et al. Early postnatal docosahexaenoic acid levels and improved preterm brain development. Pediatr Res. 2016;79:723–30.
80. Belfort MB, Ehrenkranz RA. Neurodevelopmental outcomes and nutritional strategies in very low birth weight infants. Semin Fetal Neonatal Med. 2017;22:42–8.
81. Makrides M, Gibson RA, McPhee AJ, et al. Neurodevelopmental outcomes of preterm infants fed high-dose docosahexaenoic acid: a randomized controlled trial. JAMA. 2009;301:175–82.
82. Jensen CL, Voigt RG, Llorente AM, et al. Effects of early maternal docosahexaenoic acid intake on neuropsychological status and visual acuity at five years of age of breast-fed term infants. J Pediatr. 2010;157:900–5.
83. Simmer K, Patole SK, Rao SC. Long-chain polyunsaturated fatty acid supplementation in infants born at term. Cochrane Database Syst Rev. 2011;4:CD000376.
84. Salas Lorenzo I, Chisaguano Tonato AM, de la Garza PA, et al. The effect of an infant formula supplemented with AA and DHA on fatty acid levels of infants with different FADS genotypes: the COGNIS study. Nutrients. 2019;11:602.
85. Koletzko B, Boey CCM, Campoy C, et al. E-mail current information and Asian perspectives on long-chain polyunsaturated fatty acids in pregnancy, lactation, and infancy: systematic review and practice recommendations from an early nutrition academy workshop. Ann Nutr Metab. 2014;65:49–80.
86. Wang Q, Cui Q, Yan C. The effect of supplementation of long-chain polyunsaturated fatty acids during lactation on neurodevelopmental outcomes of preterm infant from infancy to School age: a systematic review and metaanalysis. Pediatr Neurol. 2016;59:54–61.
87. Fu Y, Wang Y, Gao H, et al. Associations among dietary omega-3 polyunsaturated fatty acids, the gut microbiota, and intestinal immunity. Mediat Inflamm. 2021;2021:8879227.
88. Lien EL, Richard C, Hoffman DR. DHA and ARA addition to infant formula: current status and future research directions. Prostaglandins Leukot Essent Fatty Acids. 2018;128:26–40.
89. Carbone BE, Abouleish M, Watters KE, et al. Synaptic connectivity and cortical maturation are promoted by the ω-3 fatty acid docosahexaenoic acid. Cereb Cortex. 2020;30:226–40.
90. Sánchez-Hernández S, Esteban-Muñoz A, Giménez-Martínez R, Aguilar-Cordero MJ, Miralles-Buraglia B, Olalla-Herrera M. A comparison of changes in the fatty acid profile of human milk of Spanish lactating women during the first month of lactation using gas chromatography-mass spectrometry. A comparison with infant formulas. Nutrients. 2019;11:3055.
91. Nyaradi A, Li J, Hickling S, Foster J, Oddy WH. The role of nutrition in children's neuro-cognitive development, from pregnancy through childhood. Front Hum Neurosci. 2013;7:97.
92. Lauritzen L, Brambilla P, Mazzocchi A, Harsløf LB, Ciappolino V, Agostoni C. DHA effects in brain development and function. Nutrients. 2016;8:6.
93. Bourre J, Pascal G, Durand G, Masson M, Dumont O, Piciotti M. Alterations in the fatty acid composition of rat brain cells (neurons, astrocytes, and oligodendrocytes) and of sub-cellular fractions (myelin and synaptosomes) induced by a diet devoid of n-3 fatty acids. J Neurochem. 1984;43:342–8.
94. Greiner RS, Moriguchi T, Hutton A, Slotnick BM, Salem N. Rats with low levels of brain docosahexaenoic acid show impaired performance in olfactory-based and spatial learning tasks. Lipids. 1999;34:239–43.
95. DeMar JC, Ma K, Bell JM, Igarashi M, Greenstein D, Rapoport SI. One generation of n-3 polyunsaturated fatty acid deprivation increases depression and aggression test scores in rats. J Lipid Res. 2006;47:172–80.
96. Barrera C, Valenzuela R, Chamorro R, et al. The impact of maternal diet during pregnancy and lactation on the fatty acid composition of erythrocytes and breast milk of Chilean women. Nutrients. 2018;10:839.

97. Kanno C. Secretory membranes of the lactating mammary gland. Protoplasma. 1990;159:184–208.
98. Mather IH, Keenan TW. Origin and secretion of milk lipids. J Mammary Gland Biol Neoplasia. 1998;3:259–73.
99. Zavaleta N, Kvistgaard AS, Graverholt G, et al. Efficacy of an MFGM-enriched complementary food in diarrhea, anemia, and micronutrient status in infants. J Pediatr Gastroenterol Nutr. 2011;53:561–8.
100. Gurnida DA, Rowan AM, Idjradinata P, Muchtadi D, Sekarwana N. Association of complex lipids containing gangliosides with cognitive development of 6-month-old infants. Early Hum Dev. 2012;88:595–601.
101. Veereman-Wauters G, Staelens S, Rombaut R, et al. Milk fat globule membrane (INPULSE) enriched formula milk decreases febrile episodes and may improve behavioral regulation in young children. Nutrition. 2012;28:749–52.
102. Poppitt SD, McGregor RA, Wiessing KR, et al. Bovine complex milk lipid containing gangliosides for prevention of rotavirus infection and diarrhoea in northern Indian infants. J Pediatr Gastroenterol Nutr. 2014;59:167–71.
103. Timby N, Domellof E, Hernell O, L€onnerdal B, Domellof M. Neurodevelopment, nutrition, and growth until 12 months of age in infants fed a low-energy, low-protein formula supplemented with bovine milk fat globule membranes: a randomized controlled trial. Am J Clin Nutr. 2014;99:860–8.
104. Timby N, Hernell O, Vaarala O, Melin M, Leonnerdal B, Domellof M. Infections in infants fed formula supplemented with bovine milk fat M globule membranes. J Pediatr Gastroenterol Nutr. 2015;60:384–9.
105. Timby N, Lonnerdal B, Hernell O, Domellof M. Cardiovascular risk markers until 12 months of age in infants fed a formula supplemented with bovine milk fat globule membranes. Pediatr Res. 2014;6:394–400.
106. Billeaud C, Puccio G, Saliba E, et al. Safety and tolerance evaluation of milk fat globule membrane enriched infant formulas: a randomized controlled multicenter noninferiority trial in healthy term infants. Clin Med Insights Pediatr. 2014;8:51–60.
107. Timby N, Domellof E, Hernell O, Lonnerdal B, Domellof M. Neurodevelopment, nutrition, and growth until 12 mo of age in infants fed a low-energy, lowprotein formula supplemented with bovine milk fat globule membranes: a randomized controlled trial. Am J Clin Nutr. 2014;99:860–8.
108. Roschitz B, Plecko B, Huemer M, Biebl A, Foerster H, Sperl W. Nutritional infantile vitamin B12 deficiency: pathobiochemical considerations in seven patients. Arch Dis Child Fetal Neonatal Ed. 2005;90:F281–2.
109. Gartner LM, Morton J, Lawrence RA, et al. Breastfeeding and the use of human milk. Pediatrics. 2005;115:496–506.
110. Shaw GM, Carmichael SL, Yang W, Selvin S, Schaffer DM. Periconceptional dietary intake of choline and betaine and neural tube defects in offspring. Am J Epidemiol. 2004;160:102–9.
111. Daliry A. Pereira ENGDS. Role of maternal microbiota and nutrition in early-life neurodevelopmental disorders. Nutrients. 2021;13:3533.
112. Atta CA, Fiest KM, Frolkis AD, et al. Global birth prevalence of spina bifida by folic acid fortification status: a systematic review and meta-analysis. Am J Public Health. 2016;106:e24–34.
113. Zeisel SH. Choline: Critical role during fetal development and dietary requirements in adults. Ann Rev Nutr. 2006;26:229–50.
114. Zeisel SH. The fetal origins of memory: the role of dietary choline in optimal brain development. J Pediatr. 2006;149:131–6.
115. Wu BT, Dyer RA, King DJ, Richardson KJ, Innis SM. Early second trimester maternal plasma choline and betaine are related to measures of early cognitive development in term infants. PLoS One. 2012;7:e43448.
116. Wymann MP, Schneiter R. Lipid signalling in disease. Nat Rev Mol Cell Biol. 2008;9:162–76.

117. Oshida K, Shimizu T, Takase M, Tamura Y, Yamashiro Y. Effects of dietary sphingomyelin on central nervous system myelination in developing rats. Pediatr Res. 2003;53:589–93.
118. Nyberg L, Duan RD, Nilsson A. A mutual inhibitory effect on absorption of sphingomyelin and cholesterol. J Nutr Biochem. 2000;11:244–9.
119. Noh SK, Koo SI. Milk sphingomyelin is more effective than egg sphingomyelin in inhibiting intestinal absorption of cholesterol and fat in rats. J Nutr. 2004;134:2611–6.
120. Tanaka K, Hosozawa M, Kudo N, et al. The pilot study: sphingomyelin-fortified milk has a positive association with the neurobehavioural development of very low birth weight infants during infancy, randomized control trial. Brain and Development. 2013;35:45–52.
121. Depeint F, Bruce WR, Shangari N, Mehta R, O'Brien PJ. Mitochondrial function and toxicity: role of B vitamins on the one-carbon transfer pathways. Chem Biol Interact. 2006;163:113–32.
122. Reynolds EH. The neurology of folic acid deficiency. Handb Clin Neurol. 2014;120:927–43.
123. Koike H, Takahashi M, Ohyama K, et al. Clinicopathologic features of folate-deficiency neuropathy. Neurology. 2015;84:1026–33.
124. Hogervorst E, Kassam S, Kridawati A, et al. Nutrition research in cognitive impairment/dementia, with a focus on soya and folate. Proc Nutr Soc. 2017;76:437–42.
125. Bender A, Hagan KE, Kingston N. The association of folate and depression: a meta-analysis. J Psychiatr Res. 2017;95:9–18.
126. Cao B, Wang DF, Xu MY, et al. Lower folate levels in schizophrenia: a meta-analysis. Psychiatry Res. 2016;245:1–7.
127. Park S, Kang S, Sol KD. Folate and vitamin B-12 deficiencies additively impaired memory function and disturbed the gut microbiota in amyloid-beta infused rats. Int J Vitam Nutr Res. 2019;92:169–81.
128. Brown J, Bianco JI, McGrath JJ, Eyles DW. 1,25-dihydroxyvitamin D3 induces nerve growth factor, promotes neurite outgrowth and inhibits mitosis in embryonic rat hippocampal neurons. Neurosci Lett. 2003;343:139–43.
129. Garcion E, Wion-Barbot N, Montero-Menei CN, Berger F, Wion D. New clues about vitamin D functions in the nervous system. Trends Endocrinol Metab. 2002;13:100–5.
130. Burne TH, McGrath JJ, Eyles DW, Mackay-Sim A. Behavioural characterization of vitamin D receptor knockout mice. Behav Brain Res. 2005;157:299–308.
131. Kalueff AV, Lou YR, Laaksi I, Tuohimaa P. Impaired motor performance in mice lacking neurosteroid vitamin D receptors. Brain Res Bull. 2004;64:25–9.
132. Zou J, Minasyan A, Keisala T, et al. Progressive hearing loss in mice with a mutated vitamin D receptor gene. Audiol Neurootol. 2008;13:219–30.
133. Keisala T, Minasyan A, Lou YR, et al. Premature aging in vitamin D receptor mutant mice. J Steroid Biochem Mol Biol. 2009;115:91–7.
134. Hibberd MC, Wu M, Rodionov DA, et al. The effects of micronutrient deficiencies on bacterial species from the human gut microbiota. Sci Transl Med. 2017;9:eaal4069.
135. Johnson EJ. Role of lutein and zeaxanthin in visual and cognitive function throughout the lifespan. Nutr Rev. 2014;72:605–12.
136. Vishwanathan R, Kuchan MJ, Sen S, Johnson EJ. Lutein and preterm infants with decreased concentrations of brain carotenoids. J Pediatr Gastroenterol Nutr. 2014;59:659–65.
137. Lipkie TE, Banavara D, Shah B, et al. Caco-2 accumulation of lutein is greater from human milk than from infant formula despite similar bioaccessibility. Mol Nutr Food Res. 2014;58:2014–22.
138. Jeon S, Ranard KM, Neuringer M, et al. Lutein is differentially deposited across brain regions following formula or breast feeding of infant Rhesus Macaques. J Nutr. 2018;148:31–9.
139. Grober U, Schmidt J, Kisters K. Magnesium in prevention and therapy. Nutrients. 2015;7:8199–226.
140. Yamanaka R, Shindo Y, Oka K. Magnesium is a key player in neuronal maturation and neuropathology. Int J Mol Sci. 2019;20:3439.

141. Vink R, Nechifor M. Magnesium in the central nervous system. 1st ed. Adelaide: University of Adelaide Press; 2011. p. 342.
142. Castilho RF, Ward MW, Nicholls DG. Oxidative stress, mitochondrial function, and acute glutamate excitotoxicity in culture cerebellar granule cells. J Neurochem. 1999;72:1394–401.
143. Kirkland AE, Sarlo GL, Holton KF. The role of magnesium in neurological disorders. Nutrients. 2018;10:730.
144. Abumaria N, Yin B, Zhang L, et al. Effects of elevation of brain magnesium on fear conditioning, fear extinction, and synaptic plasticity in the infralimbic prefrontal cortex and lateral amygdala. J Neurosci. 2011;31:14871–81.
145. Slutsky I, Sadeghpour S, Li B, Liu G. Enhancement of synaptic plasticity through chronically reduced Ca2+ flux during uncorrelated activity. Neuron. 2004;44:835–49.
146. Takeda A. Movement of zinc and its functional significance in the brain. Brain Res Rev. 2000;34:137–48.
147. Choi DW, Yokoyama M, Koh J. Zinc neurotoxicity in cortical cell culture. Neuroscience. 1988;24:67–79.
148. Perry DK, Smyth MJ, Stennicke HR, et al. Zinc is a potent inhibitor of the apoptotic protease, caspase-3. A novel target for zinc in the inhibition of apoptosis. J Biol Chem. 1997;272:18530–3.
149. Cote A, Chiasson M, Peralta MR, Lafortune K, Pellegrini L, Toth K. Cell type-specific action of seizure-induced intracellular zinc accumulation in the rat hippocampus. J Physiol. 2005;566:821–37.
150. Plum LM, Rink L, Haase H. The essential toxin: impact of zinc on human health. Int J Environ Res Public Health. 2010;7:1342–65.
151. Frederickson CJ, Suh SW, Silva D, Thompson RB. Importance of zinc in the central nervous system: the zinc-containing neuron. J Nutr. 2000;130:1471–83.
152. Paoletti P, Vergnano AM, Barbour B, Casado M. Zinc at glutamatergic synapses. Neuroscience. 2009;158:126–36.
153. Sensi SL, Paoletti P, Koh JY, Aizenman E, Bush AI, Hershfinkel M. The neurophysiology and pathology of brain zinc. J Neurosci. 2011;31:16076–85.
154. Smart TG, Hosie AM, Miller PS. Zn2+ ions: modulators of excitatory and inhibitory synaptic activity. Neuroscientist. 2004;10:432–42.
155. Besser L, Chorin E, Sekler I, et al. Synaptically released zinc triggers metabotropic signaling via a zinc-sensing receptor in the hippocampus. J Neurosci. 2009;29:2890–901.
156. Wilson AC, Forsyth JS, Greene SA, Irvine L, Hau C, Howie PW. Relation of infant diet to childhood health: seven year follow up of cohort of children in Dundee infant feeding study. Br Med J. 1998;316:21–5.
157. Ashwood P, Wils S, van de Water J. The immune response in autism: a new frontier for autism research. J Leukoc Biol. 2006;80:1–15.
158. Krol KM, Rajhans P, Missana M, Grossmann T. Duration of exclusive breastfeeding is associated with differences in infants' brain responses to emotional body expressions. Front Behav Neurosci. 2015;8:459.
159. Cushing BS, Kramer KM. Mechanisms underlying epigenetic effects of early social experience: the role of neuropeptides and steroids. Neurosci Biobehav Rev. 2005;29:1089–105.
160. Masís-Calvo M, Sequeira-Cordero A, Mora-Gallegos A, Fornaguera-Trías J. Behavioral and neurochemical characterization of maternal care effects on juvenile Sprague-Dawleyrats. Physiol Behav. 2013;118:212–7.
161. Sarro EC, Wilson DA, Sullivan RM. Maternal regulation of infant brain state. Curr Biol. 2014;24:1664–9.
162. Lupoli B, Johansson B, Uvnäs-Moberg K, Svennersten-Sjaunja K. Effect of suckling on there lease of oxytocin, prolactin, cortisol, gastrin, cholecystokinin, somatostatin and insulin in dairy cows and their calves. J Dairy Res. 2001;68:175–87.

163. Dawood MY, Khan-Dawood FS, Wahi RS, Fuchs F. Oxytocin release and plasma anterior-pituitary and gonadal-hormones in women during lactation. J Clin Endocrinol Metab. 1981;52:678–83.

164. Young LJ, Wang Z. The neurobiology of pair bonding. Nat Neurosci. 2004;7:1048–54.

165. Feldman R. Oxytocin and social affiliation in humans. Horm Behav. 2012;61:380–91.

166. Feldman R, Weller A, Zagoory-Sharon O, Levine A. Evidence for a neuroendocrinological foundation of human affiliation: plasma oxytocin levels across pregnancy and the postpartum period predict mother-infant bonding. Psychol Sci. 2007;18:965–70.

167. Gordon I, Zagoory-Sharon O, Leckman JF, Feldman R. Oxytocin and the development of parenting in humans. Biol Psychiatry. 2010;68:377–82.

168. Tost H, Kolachana B, Hakimi S, et al. A common allele in the oxytocin receptor gene (OXTR) impacts prosocial temperament and human hypothalamic-limbic structure and function. Proc Natl Acad Sci. 2010;107:13936–41.

169. Kim P, Feldman R, Mayes LC, et al. Breastfeeding, brain activation to own infant cry, and maternal sensitivity. J Child Psychol Psychiatry. 2011;52:907–15.

170. Kim P, Leckman JF, Mayes LC, Feldman R, Wang X, Swain JE. The plasticity of human maternal brain: longitudinal changes in brain anatomy during the early postpartum period. Behav Neurosci. 2010;124:695–700.

171. Baumwell L, Tamis-LeMonda CS, Bornstein MH. Maternal verbal sensitivity and child language comprehension. Infant Behav Dev. 1997;20:247–58.

172. Hardin JS, Jones NA, Mize KD, Platt M. Affectionate touch in the context of breastfeeding and maternal depression influences infant neurodevelopmental and temperamental substrates. Neuropsychobiology. 2021;80:158–75.

173. Ferguson M, Molfese PJ. Breastfed infants process speech differently from bottle-fed infants: evidence from neuroelectrophysiology. Dev Neuropsychol. 2007;31:337–47.

174. Principi N, Esposito S. Gut microbiota and central nervous system development. J Infect. 2016;73:536–46.

175. Clarke G, O'Mahony SM, Dinan TG, Cryan JF. Priming for health: gut microbiota acquired in early life regulates physiology, brain and behaviour. Acta Paediatr. 2014;103:812–9.

176. Yang I, Corwin EJ, Brennan PA, Jordan S, Murphy JR, Dunlop A. The infant microbiome: implications for infant health and neurocognitive development. Nurs Res. 2016;65:76–88.

177. Latorre R, Sternini C, De Giorgio R, Greenwood-Van MB. Enteroendocrine cells: a review of their role in brain-gut communication. Neurogastroenterol Motil. 2016;28:620–30.

178. Theoharides TC, Asadi S, Patel A. Focal brain inflammation and autism. J Neuroinflammation. 2013;10:46.

179. Borre YE, O'Keeffe GW, Clarke G, et al. Microbiota and neurodevelopmental windows: implications for brain disorders. Trends Mol Med. 2014;20:509–18.

180. Bennett HA, Einarson A, Taddio A, Koren G, Einarson TR. Prevalence of depression during pregnancy: systematic review. Obstet Gynecol. 2004;103:698–709.

181. Qiu J, Heller JJ, Guo X, et al. The aryl hydrocarbon receptor regulates gut immunity through modulation of innate lymphoid cells. Immunity. 2012;36:92–104.

182. Veldhoen M, Hirota K, Westendorf AM, et al. The aryl hydrocarbon receptor links TH17-cell-mediated autoimmunity to environmental toxins. Nature. 2008;453:106–9.

183. Maes M, Rief W. Diagnostic classifications in depression and somatization should include biomarkers, such as disorders in the tryptophan catabolite (TRYCAT) pathway. Psychiatry Res. 2012;196:243–9.

184. de Aguero GM, Ganal-Vonarburg SC, Fuhrer T, et al. The maternal microbiota drives early postnatal innate immune development. Science. 2016;351:1296–302.

185. Nguyen N, Nakahama T, Le D, Van Son L, Chu H, Kishimoto T. Aryl hydrocarbon receptor and kynurenine: recent advances in autoimmune disease research. Front Immunol. 2014;5:551.

186. Barrett E, Ross R, O'Toole P, Fitzgerald G, Stanton C. g-Aminobutyric acid production by culturable bacteria from the human intestine. J Appl Microbiol. 2012;113:411–7.

187. Wong JM, de Souza R, Kendall CW, Emam A, Jenkins DJ. Colonic health: fermentation and short chain fatty acids. J Clin Gastroenterol. 2006;40:235–43.
188. Gaspar P, Cases O, Maroteaux L. The developmental role of serotonin: news from mouse molecular genetics. Nat Rev Neurosci. 2003;4:1002–12.
189. Vitalis T, Cases O, Passemard S, Callebert J, Parnavelas JG. Embryonic depletion of serotonin affects cortical development. Eur J Neurosci. 2007;26:331–44.
190. Braniste V, Al-Asmakh M, Kowal C, et al. The gut microbiota influences blood-brain barrier permeability in mice. Sci Transl Med. 2014;6:263ra158.
191. Miller AH, Maletic V, Raison CL. Inflammation and its discontents: the role of cytokines in the pathophysiology of majör depression. Biol Psychiatry. 2009;65:732–41.
192. Bezirtzoglou E, Tsiotsias A, Welling GW. Microbiota profile in feces of breast- and formula-fed newborns by using fluorescence in situ hybridization (FISH). Anaerobe. 2011;17:478–82.
193. Foster JA, Neufeld KAM. Gut-brain axis: how the microbiome influences anxiety and depression. Trends Neurosci. 2015;36:305–12.
194. Stilling RM, Ryan FJ, Hoban AE, et al. Microbes & neurodevelopment-Absence of microbiota during early life increases activity-related transcriptional pathways in the amygdala. Brain Behav Immun. 2015;50:209–20.
195. Erny D, de Angelis Hrabe AL, Jaitin D, et al. Host microbiota constantly control maturation and function of microglia in the CNS. Nat Neurosci. 2015;18:965–77.
196. Acuña I, Cerdó T, Ruiz A, et al. Infant gut microbiota associated with fine motor skills. Nutrients. 2021;13:1673.
197. Christian LM, Galley JD, Hade EM, Schoppe-Sullivan S, Kamp Dush C, Bailey MT. Gut microbiome composition is associated with temperament during early childhood. Brain Behav Immun. 2015;45:118–27.
198. Carlson AL, Xia K, Azcarate-Peril MA, et al. Infant gut microbiome associated with cognitive development. Biol Psychiatry. 2018;83:148–59.
199. Sordillo JE, Korrick S, Laranjo N, et al. Association of the infant gut microbiome with early childhood neurodevelopmental outcomes: an ancillary study to the VDAART randomized clinical trial. JAMA Netw Open. 2019;2:e190905.
200. Kafouri S, Kramer M, Leonard G, et al. Breastfeeding and brain structure in adolescence. Int J Epidemiol. 2013;42:150–9.
201. Elitt CM, Rosenberg PA. The challenge of understanding cerebral white matter injury in the premature infant. Neuroscience. 2014;276:216–38.
202. Belfort MB, Anderson PJ, Nowak VA, et al. Breast milk feeding, brain development, and neurocognitive outcomes: a 7-year longitudinal study in infantsborn at less than 30 weeks' gestation. J Pediatr. 2016;177:133–139.e1.
203. Ou X, Andres A, Cleves MA, et al. Sex-specific association between infant diet and white matter integrity in 8-y-old children. Pediatr Res. 2014;76:535–43.
204. Grossmann T, Johnson MH. The development of the social brain in human infancy. Eur J Neurosci. 2007;25:909–19.
205. Yakovlev PI, Lecours AR. The myelogenetic cycles of regional maturation of the brain. In: Minkowski A, editor. Regional development of the brain in early life. 1st ed. Oxford: Blackwell Scientific Publications; 1967. p. 3–65.
206. Wozniak JR, Lim KO. Advances in white matter imaging: a review of in vivo magnetic resonance methodologies and their applicability to the study of development and aging. Neurosci Biobehav Rev. 2006;30:762–74.
207. Ezzati A, Katz MJ, Lipton ML, Zimmerman ME, Lipton RB. Hippocampal volume and cingulum bundle fractional anisotropy are independently associated with verbal memory in older adults. Brain Imaging Behav. 2016;10:652–9.
208. Jarbo K, Verstynen T, Schneider W. In vivo quantification of global connectivity in the human corpus callosum. NeuroImage. 2012;59:1988–96.
209. Wol JJ, Gerig G, Lewis JD, et al. Altered corpus callosum morphology associated with autism over the first 2 years of life. Brain. 2015;138:2046–58.

210. Travers BG, Tromp DPM, Adluru N, et al. Atypical development of white matter microstructure of the corpus callosum in males with autism: a longitudinal investigation. Mol Autism. 2015;6:1–14.
211. Luby JL, Belden AC, Whalen D, Harms MP, Barch DM. Breastfeeding and Childhood IQ: the Mediating Role of Gray Matter Volume. J Am Acad Child Adolesc Psychiatry. 2016;55:367–75.
212. Mortensen EL, Michaelsen KF, Sanders SA, Reinisch JM. The association between duration of breastfeeding and adult intelligence. JAMA. 2002;287:2365–71.
213. Kim KM, Choi JW. Associations between breastfeeding and cognitive function in children from early childhood to school age: a prospective birth cohort study. Int Breastfeed J. 2020;15:83.
214. Quigley MA, Hockley C, Carson C, Kelly Y, Renfrew MJ, Sacker A. Breastfeeding is associated with improved child cognitive development: a population-based cohort study. J Pediatr. 2012;160:25–32.
215. Brion MJ, Lawlor DA, Matijasevich A, et al. What are the causal effects of breastfeeding on IQ, obesity and blood pressure evidence from comparing high-income with middle-income cohorts. Int J Epidemiol. 2011;40:670–80.
216. Kramer MS, Aboud F, Mironova E, et al. Breastfeeding and child cognitive development: new evidence from a large randomized trial. Arch Gen Psychiatry. 2008;65:578–84.
217. Gibbs BG, Forste R. Breastfeeding, parenting, and early cognitivedevelopment. J Pediatr. 2014;164:487–93.
218. Guzzardi MA, Granziera F, Sanguinetti E, Ditaranto F, Muratori F, Iozzo P. Exclusive breastfeeding predicts higher hearing-language development in girls of preschool age. Nutrients. 2020;12:2320.
219. Stadler DD, Musser ED, Holton KF, Shannon J, Nigg JT. Recalled initiation and duration of maternal breastfeeding among children with and without ADHD in a well characterized case-control sample. J Abnorm Child Psychol. 2016;44:347–55.
220. Huang S, Wang X, Sun T, et al. Association of breastfeeding for the first six months of life and autism spectrum disorders: a national multi-center study in China. Nutrients. 2021;14:45.
221. Ross MG, Desai M. Association of breastfeeding and child IQ score at age 5 years. Obstet Gynecol. 2021;138:135.
222. Tseng P-T, Yen C-F, Chen Y-W, et al. Maternal breastfeeding and attentiondeficit/hyperactivity disorder in children: a meta-analysis. Eur Child Adolesc Psychiatry. 2019;28:19–30.
223. Batalle D, Eixarch E, Figueras F, et al. Altered small-world topology of structural brain networks in infants with intrauterine growth restriction and its association with later neurodevelopmental outcome. NeuroImage. 2012;60:1352–66.
224. Van den Heuvel MP, Kersbergen KJ, de Reus MA, et al. Theneonatal connectome during preterm brain development. Cereb Cortex. 2014;25:3000–13.
225. Kerr-Wilson C, Mackay D, Smith G, Pell J. Meta-analysis of the association between preterm delivery and intelligence. J Publ Health. 2011;34:209–16.
226. Lucas A, Morley R, Cole TJ, Lister G, Leeson-Payne C. Breast milk and subsequent intelligence quotient in children born preterm. Lancet. 1992;339:261–4.
227. Bardanzellu F, Peroni DG, Fanos V. Human breast milk: bioactive components, from stem cells to health outcomes. Curr Nutr Rep. 2020;9:1–13.
228. Jimènez BC, Parada YA, Marin AV, de Pipaon Marcos MS. Short, medium and long term benefits of human milk intake in very low birth weightinfants. Nutr Hosp. 2017;34:1059–66.
229. Guideline: protecting, promoting and supporting breastfeeding in facilities providing maternity and newborn services. Geneva: World Health Organization; 2017.
230. Horwood LJ, Darlow BA, Mogridge N. Breast milk feeding and cognitive ability at 7-8 years. Arch Dis Child Fetal Neonatal Ed. 2001;84:F23–7.
231. Jiang M, Foster EM, Gibson-Davis CM. Breastfeeding and the child cognitive outcomes: a propensity score matching approach. Matern Child Health J. 2011;15:1296–307.

232. Oddy WH. Long-term health outcomes and mechanisms associated with breastfeeding. Expert Rev Pharmacoecon Outcomes Res. 2002;2:161–77.
233. Kramer MS, Guo T, Platt RW, et al. Infant growth and health outcomes associated with 3 compared with 6 mo of exclusive breastfeeding. Am J Clin Nutr. 2003;78:291–5.
234. Daniels MC, Adair LS. Breast-feeding influences cognitive development in Filipino children. J Nutr. 2005;135:2589–95.
235. Raju TN. Breastfeeding is a dynamic biological process--not simply a meal at the breast. Breastfeed Med. 2011;6:257–9.
236. Kim JI, Kim BN, Kim JW, et al. Breastfeeding is associated with enhanced learning abilities in school-aged children. Child Adolesc Psychiatry Ment Health. 2017;11:36.
237. Drane DL, Logemann JA. A critical evaluation of the evidence on the association between type of infant feeding and cognitive development. Paediatr Perinat Epidemiol. 2000;14:349–56.
238. Horwood LJ, Fergusson DM. Breastfeeding and later cognitive and academic outcomes. Pediatrics. 1998;101:E9.
239. Cai S, Pang WW, Low YL, GUSTO Study Group, et al. Infant feeding effects on early neuro-cognitive development in Asian children. Am J Clin Nutr. 2015;101:326–36.
240. Jain A, Concato J, Leventhal JM. How good is the evidence linking breastfeeding and intelligence? Pediatrics. 2002;109:1044–53.
241. Der G, Batty GD, Deary IJ. Effect of breast feeding on intelligence in children: prospective study, sibling pairs analysis, and meta-analysis. BMJ. 2006;333:945.
242. Holme A, MacArthur C, Lancashire R. The effects of breastfeeding on cognitive and neurological development of children at 9 years. Child Care Health Dev. 2010;36:583–90.
243. Borra C, Iacovou M, Sevilla A. The effect of breastfeeding on children's cognitive and non-cognitive development. Labour Econ. 2012;19:496–515.
244. Yang S, Martin RM, Oken E, et al. Breastfeeding during infancy and neurocognitive function in adolescence: 16-year follow-up of the PROBIT cluster-randomized trial. PLoS Med. 2018;15:e1002554.
245. Tumwine JK, Nankabirwa V, Diallo HA, et al. Exclusive breastfeeding promotion and neuro-psychological outcomes in 5-8 year old children from Uganda and Burkina Faso: results from the PROMISE EBF cluster randomized trial. PLoS One. 2018;13:e0191001.
246. Stelmach I, Kwarta P, Jerzyńska J, et al. Duration of breastfeeding and psychomotor development in 1-year-old children- Polish Mother and Child Cohort Study. Int J Occup Med Environ Health. 2019;32:175–84.

Breastfeeding and Motor Development in Preterm and Term Infants

Gülten Öztürk, Bülent Kara, and Gian Carlo Di Renzo

1 Introduction

Development is a term used for improvement in the functional capacity of body organs, and it is known that the development rate of a child is the fastest in the first 2 years of life [1]. Optimal neurodevelopment that includes cognitive and motor components are the keystone for healthy child growth and reflect central and peripheral nervous system maturation. Motor development is the progress in the coordination capacity of the musculoskeletal system and is a major indicator of postnatal healthy child growth [2–4].

Motor functions are subdivided into gross and fine motor skills. Gross motor functions like large body movements of the trunk and legs, allow achievement of walking, climbing, and running, whereas fine motor development reflects the improvement in the functional capacity of the shoulder, arm, and hand, which progresses to small hand and arm movements like pincer grasp and throwing [4].

G. Öztürk (✉)
Department of Pediatrics, Division of Pediatric Neurology, Marmara University Pendik Education and Research Hospital, İstanbul, Türkiye
e-mail: gulten@thomas.md

B. Kara
Faculty of Medicine, Department of Pediatrics, Division of Pediatric Neurology, Kocaeli University, Kocaeli, Türkiye
e-mail: bulent.kara@kocaeli.edu.tr

G. C. Di Renzo
Faculty of Medicine, Department of Pediatrics, Division of Pediatric Neurology, Kocaeli University, Kocaeli, Türkiye

Centre of Perinatal Medicine of the University of Perugia/Sechenov Universssity, Moscow, Russia
e-mail: giancarlo.direnzo@unipg.it

Ö. N. Şahin et al. (eds.), *Breastfeeding and Metabolic Programming*,
https://doi.org/10.1007/978-3-031-33278-4_23

"""

Gross motor improvement is followed by fine motor development, and this proceeds into the preschool years. It is known that healthy early motor development also reflects future cognitive development. Neurodevelopment is a dynamic process affected by multiple environmental and genetic factors some of which are still unclear [5].

Nutrition is the major known factor influencing infantile neurodevelopment. Nutrition is generally provided by maternal breast milk in the first months of life unless there is a contraindication and despite all the progress in the infant formula industry, World Health Organization (WHO) still recommends exclusive breastfeeding in the first 6 months of life [2, 6–8].

Typically, postnatal nutrition for babies is provided by maternal breast milk, infant formula, or a combination of them. It is known that maternal breast milk has a unique composition of nutrients, some of which have still not been copied by infant formulas.

The contribution of nutrition to neurodevelopment is now a proven fact, but there is still debate about the individual effects of nutritional content (human milk or formula) and type of feeding process (breastfeeding or bottle feeding) [9].

This chapter will focus on the effects of breastfeeding on the motor development of preterm and term infants. Human milk composition and the breastfeeding process will be discussed individually, regarding their contribution to the motor development of preterm and term infants.

2 Pathophysiology of Motor Development

Studies have shown that postnatal motor development is strongly related to myelination of the central nervous system's corticospinal, pyramidal, and corticobulbar tracts. Myelination is completed with a neuroanatomical arc followed by a well-described pattern from posterior to anterior and from center to outwards [10]. Myelination begins prenatally at 32 weeks of gestation and progresses rapidly in the first 2 years of life at a slower rate till puberty. As myelination is completed, the subcortical system, which is responsible for primitive reflexes, is gradually inhibited, and functional steps of motor development are achieved [11]. Regarding the complexity of its pathophysiology and the influence of psychosocial and socioeconomic factors, scientific information related to breastfeeding and neuromotor development is viewed with suspicion because of all the potential confounders [2].

The mother's nutritional status during pregnancy, the infant's birth weight, and the mother's education level are some known factors that contribute to neurodevelopment in addition to the nutrition type of the infant [12]. Some studies have focused on nutrition content, whereas others have studied the impact of the type of feeding process on neurodevelopment. The results of most studies about the effects of breastfeeding on motor development are controversial and difficult to compare because of the heterogeneity in study designs and the confounding factors. Most of the studies performed in the literature are based on recalls of the parents about the breastfeeding process. Although this raises suspicion about the reliability of the studies, it has been established that parental recall in the postnatal first 3 years of childhood about breastfeeding initiation and duration can be counted as reliable [13].

Prospective studies planned to evaluate the effects of human milk and the breastfeeding process on neuromotor development have mainly used Bayley Scales of Infant Development and Denver Developmental screening tests, which are universal but there are other adapted developmental tests used in the studies [14].

3 Composition of Human Milk

Human milk has a rough composition of 87% water, 1% protein, 4% lipid, and 7% carbohydrate. The constitutional distribution of human milk is affected by the physiological status of the mother. Gestational age and diet of the mother, the number of parities, and the stage of lactation are some known factors influencing the composition of human milk [7].

It is known that human milk has the lowest protein content among all mammalian milk, and this leads to a relatively lower growth rate in newborns. However, some specific components of human milk contribute directly to brain development and it is a challenge to imitate the optimal composition of these components in formulas as their ratio is affected by physiological changes in the body [7].

Hormones, antibodies, long-chain fatty acids, vitamins, minerals, growth factors, free amino acids, organic acids, oligosaccharides, and some other bioactive factors in human milk make it a unique and essential nutrient for newborn growth and development. Infant formulas contain similar nutritional content but still lack some physiological factors secreted by the human body, and studies have focused on the discovery of these unique factors and their effect on brain development.

4 Impact of Human Milk on Motor Development of Term Newborns

It is known that the constitution of human breast milk changes in different stages of lactation according to the needs of the neonate and is also affected by the mother's diet [15].

It has been shown that a large proportion of long-chain polyunsaturated fatty acids (LC-PUFA's) are derived from the essential fatty acid linoleic and alpha-linolenic acid. One of these fatty acids named 9,12-octadecadiynoic acid ($C18H28O2$) has been related to the development of adaptive behaviors in neonates [16].

Docosahexaenoic acid (DHA; 22:6n-3) and arachidonic acid (AA or ARA; 20:4n-6) are the long-chain polyunsaturated fatty acids (LC-PUFAs), which have been found rich in human milk but not in cow milk and most infant formulas;

accumulate in the human brain in the first months of life and have been found in greater amounts in breastfed infants' brain tissue. Animal studies have shown a positive impact of LC-PUFAs on cognitive development with higher IQ and resulting in better neuromotor performance scores. Rodent experiments have shown that LC-PUFA's have been found responsible for neurite growth and dendritic regeneration after cell injury and these findings also lead investigators for studies focused on genes involved in LC-PUFA metabolism to search the effects of breastfeeding in children's IQ [17]. A recent study has shown that n3 PUFA and n3-n6 PUFA concentration is higher in the mother's colostrum and infants fed with colostrum had higher scores on the Bayley's scales of infant development test at 14 months of evaluation [18].

A large number of oligosaccharides and the high cholesterol content of human milk specifically make a contribution to brain development. Sphingomyelin, iron, cholesterol, choline, and phospholipids of human milk are essential for myelin sheath formation in the brain [19]. Sialic acid in human milk is the building block of brain gangliosides [20]. Sialic acid is bound to oligosaccharides and after being absorbed from the newborn's gut, circulating sialylated oligosaccharides contribute to neonates' immune system and brain development [21].

Choline, myoinositol, and pantothenic acid, the major metabolites playing role in brain growth and cognitive functions have been found to have a time-dependent concentration in human milk, which makes it a challenge to provide infant formula with similar content [22].

Plasma concentrations of antioxidants found in human milk, which mainly are α- and β-carotenes, lutein, and α-tocopherol have been found higher in breastfed infants [15]. Lutein that is the main carotenoid of the human brain has been found to be related to gross motor skills [6, 23].

IgA and lactoferrin concentrations in human milk have been found inversely related to motor skills, whereas high lactalbumin concentration found in human milk had positive effects on motor functions [24].

Human breast milk contains 10–20% medium-chain fatty acids which can be converted directly to ketone bodies and 15–17% short-chain fatty acids which are the main energy supply of the brain in the form of ketone bodies [24]. Ketone bodies play an important role in a newborn's developing brain and studies have shown that the ketone transporter at blood-brain barriers is expressed at the highest level during breastfeeding and this level decreases with the cessation of breastfeeding [25]. Ketone body levels were found higher in term infants fed with human milk compared to formula-fed infants [26]. Some studies have shown a positive correlation between the docosahexaenoic acid (DHA) level in the mother's milk and better visual and neurological function in developing infants and it has been shown that DHA concentration in human milk is affected by the mother's diet. However, studies designed to evaluate the effects of DHA supplementation on the mother during lactation had controversial results regarding long-term neurodevelopmental outcomes [25].

Recently human milk has been found rich in miRNA which is non-coding RNA that takes part in the regulation of many developmental processes of the human body [27, 28]. A lipid bilayer enclosed extracellular vesicles and specifically, their milk exosome (MEX) subfraction which is released from mammary gland epithelial cells have been found to carry specific biomolecular information important for postnatal neurological programming. MEX and miRNAs are not found in infant formulas, and future studies are needed to clarify their unique functions [29]. It has been claimed that human milk miRNA that is synthesized endogenously by human lactating mammary epithelium takes important roles in the neonates' immune system and development after they enter the circulation [27]. miR-118.2 coded human milk miRNA has been shown to take a major role in neurodevelopment and connectivity of the central nervous system by targeting teneurin transmembrane protein 2 (TENM2), which is abundant in the central nervous system [30]. miRNA content in bovine milk and infant formula has been much less, compared to human milk and also difference has been detected in biological activity [21]. Donor milk has been shown to include more amount of miRNA content compared to infant formula or bovine milk and is preferred in cases of maternal human milk absence [30].

Alpha-tocopherol that is the biologically active form of vitamin E has been found essential for the development of Purkinje cells in the cerebellum and vitamin E deficiency has been related to the impairment of motor functions [6]. Human milk α-tocopherol level was correlated with the mother's total daily saturated fat intake and has been found to be sufficient for the infant's daily needs [31]. One study showed that total α-tocopherol that is naturally supplied by dietary intake of the mother from nuts, leafy green vegetables, almond oils, and sunflower seeds had a positive effect on motor skills [6]. However, a synthetic stereoisomer of RSR-α-tocopherol that is found in foods and supplements can accumulate in the liver and brain and negatively affect problem-solving. The alpha-tocopherol level has been found highest in colostrum and decreases in time during lactation. Infant formulas contain α-tocopherol levels similar to the 14th day of lactation, and as the concentration in breast milk changes at different stages of lactation, it stays stable in the formulas. One study found higher alpha-tocopherol concentration at 90 days of postnatal age in breastfed infants compared to formula-fed infants regardless of the gestational age [32]. Vitamin E supplementation has been suggested to formula-fed neonates who do not get colostrum in the first 2–3 days of life to prevent potential neurological effects of deficiency; however, these results have been controversial and need to be proven with larger studies [33]. The amount of γ-tocopherol isoform has increased in infant formulas in the last decades because of increased usage of soil oils, but the increased amount of this isomer is more related to proinflammatory properties and its high concentration might reverse the anti-inflammatory properties of alpha-tocopherol [34].

5 Impact of Human Milk on the Neurodevelopment of Preterm Newborns

Maternal milk is the best-recommended nutrient for preterm feeding [22]. There are differences in the composition of human milk between term and preterm newborns. It is known that the protein content of the mother's milk of preterms is higher by postnatal sixth weeks. The compositional difference also exists in free amino acids (valine, threonine, and arginine), lactoferrin, leptin, and albumin levels [15, 35]. Preterm milk has been found rich in IgA but deficient in leptin levels [15, 35]. Colostrum of the preterm has been found rich in myoinositol and is specifically recommended for better neurodevelopment [22].

Vitamin E deficiency has been detected specifically in preterm babies (<37 weeks of gestation), and the reason for this finding was explained as the reduction in the transfer of alfa tocopherol from the mother's blood through the placenta due to oxidative stress caused by preterm delivery. Low alpha-tocopherol levels have been associated with neurodevelopmental delay and spinocerebellar degeneration [32]. As colostrum contains the highest alpha-tocopherol, it is suggested that preterm newborns should be encouraged to be fed with their mother's milk or at least donor milk if their own mother's milk is not eligible [36].

One study demonstrated better cognitive functions in preterm infants fed with expressed breast milk compared to formula-fed infants [37]. The nutrition of preterm infants with expressed breast milk has been related to better scores in developmental tests [37]. However, there are also studies that showed better cognitive scores with human milk supplementation of preterms in the intensive care unit, but they reported no difference in motor function at 20 months of age evaluation [38].

A Cochrane review including nine studies comparing formula with donor breast milk reported no differences in neuromotor development at 18 months, but still the results were interpreted cautiously because of the need for replication of the studies in larger cohorts [39]. Some studies report similar growth and neurodevelopment rates with exclusive human milk compared to infant formula in extremely low-weight preterm infants [30, 40]. Supplementation of extremely low birth infants (ELBW) with α-tocopherol from 6 months to 24 months of age has been linked to better mental development at school ages [34].

One study compared brain volumes, and cognitive and motor function outcomes of extremely low or preterm infants (<30 GW or <1250 g) at term equivalents and at 7 years of age according to their postnatal nutrition types and reported that greater breast milk exposure was correlated with greater brain volume at term and better cognitive and motor functions at 7 years of age [41].

6 Effects of Breastfeeding on The Neurodevelopment of Term Newborns

Results of the studies focused on the relationship between breastfeeding and neuro-motor development are inconsistent, and most have an insufficient study design because of confounding factors. Some studies in the literature reported no clear association between breastfeeding and motor development [2, 6]. However, there are well-designed prospective studies that have shown the positive effect of breast-feeding on motor functions [11, 42].

One hypothesis about the role of breastfeeding on neuromotor development has claimed that the skin to skin contact during breastfeeding leads to increased mater-nal brain stimulation, which has positive benefits on neurodevelopment [37]. Breastfeeding is related to better problem-solving and gross motor functions at school ages. This was also associated with the higher education level of mothers who breastfed, as increased parental reading level contributed positively to the infant's cognitive development [11]. The higher parental reading level was consis-tent with better maternal awareness about the benefits of mother's milk to the new-born with greater motivation and effort for nursing with the breastfeeding process. It was also observed that parents with higher education levels provided a home environment with more stimulus for the child's neurodevelopment [6]. Skin-to-skin contact also causes emotional stimulation between the mother and the baby, which also contributes positively to the mental and motor development of the child [43–45].

Large epidemiological studies have shown better cognitive functions in exclu-sively breastfed infants compared to formula-fed infants, even when factors such as birth weight, gestational age, maternal education level, and socioeconomic status are taken into consideration [46]. White matter and cortex volumes have been found greater with better myelination in breastfed infants, which was correlated with bet-ter cognitive and verbal functions [6, 47].

Data about the duration of breastfeeding is inconsistent [48]. One study showed better cognitive and behavioral performance in longer-breastfed children [48]. Longer duration of breastfeeding has been linked to better performance in cognitive and behavioral domains, which suggests a positive effect of breastfeeding on frontal white matter areas. However, there are also studies in the literature that reject these findings [48]. One study that evaluated motor development at 4 months of age in term babies concluded that feeding differences do not impact motor achievements. Early solid food initiation, in addition to breastfeeding, might have an accelerating effect on motor functions in short term. However, there were still some confounding factors that might overshadow these results [40]. A counter-argument to refute these results could be the possibility that the reason for the early introduction of solid foods might be the readiness of the infants for this transition, which reflects their better neuromotor developmental status [49].

One study based on the child handbook records taken in infancy focused on the relationship between breastfeeding duration and brain regional volume during adolescence and showed a significant positive correlation between breastfeeding duration and gray matter volume in the dorsal and ventral striatum and the medial orbital gyrus. They also showed that the duration of breastfeeding had an impact on emotional behavior [50]. The optimal duration of exclusive breastfeeding or minimal total duration of breastfeeding was investigated through studies that measured neurobehavioral outcomes. A higher ratio of infants with optimal gross motor milestones was found among exclusively breastfed infants within 6 weeks postnatally [45, 48].

A Spanish study that was planned to evaluate the effects of breastfeeding in the first 4 months on mental and psychomotor development was conducted on 154 healthy infants who were followed from birth to 12 months of age and after excluding the confounding factors showed that infants who received breast milk for at least 4 months had higher results in psychomotor development index (PDI) at 6 and 12 months of age [51].

Another study showed that newborns who were ever breastfed showed better functions with 1.3 times better in gross and 1.6 times better in fine motor skills at 9 months of age compared to their age-matched controls who have never been breastfed. The confounding factors to be considered were the child's birth weight, maternal age, maternal education and smoking habits, ethnicity, household social class, and singleton status of the mother [52]. However, this study could not show any positive effect of the duration of exclusive breastfeeding on motor skills development, which conflicts with other studies supporting the positive impact of the duration of breastfeeding on motor development [46]. One debate about these conflicting results is that maternal IQ which has not been measured in the studies could be an important confounding factor claiming that intelligence is inheritable also mothers with higher IQ might be tending more to breastfeed and their kids with inherited higher IQ might have higher performance on motor function tests apart from breastfeeding process. The advantages of breastfeeding on cognition have been shown, but there are also some controversial debates claiming that breastfed children are born to parents with better educational status with higher motivation for the breastfeeding process and who also spend more effort to improve their kids' neuromotor development [52].

A Danish study performed on 1656 healthy infants focused on fine and general motor and language skills at 8 months of age and showed that an increase in the duration of breastfeeding is positively correlated with better scores in motor functions [53]. Another study performed by Angelson et al. showed that duration of breastfeeding has positive effects on cognitive scores in Bayley scales at 13 months of age and in Wechsler Preschool and Primary Scales of Intelligence-Revised (WPPSI-R) at 5 years of age, but they could not show any positive effects on motor scores of these scales after they adjusted the possible confounding factors like parental education and maternal age [54–56]. One more study performed in the US claimed that the duration of exclusive breastfeeding has protective effects against gross motor developmental delay with no overt effect on fine motor functions [14].

Methodological differences in the designs of these studies make it difficult to compare them. In a study, in addition to the positive contributions of the nutritional content of human milk to motor development and general cognitive abilities, which was evaluated at 2 years of age, the positive effect of intake of human milk by breastfeeding on memory was emphasized [37].

A cohort study with 14,000 newborns has shown 9% of gross motor delay and 6% of fine motor delay among babies who have never been breastfed and reported that they were 40–50% more prone to any kind of motor delay [9]. One study compared neurophysiological studies including flash visual evoked potential (VEP), brainstem auditory evoked potential (BAEP), and somatosensory evoked potential (SSEP) between breastfed and formula-fed infants and obtained better results in the breastfeeding group, which was interpreted as the positive impact of breastfeeding on brain myelination and maturation [9].

7 Effects of Breastfeeding on the Neurodevelopment of Preterm Newborns

Studies that focused on the effects of human milk on preterm infants have revealed that more exposure to breast milk resulted in larger brain volume and better maturity and less injury from prematurity in deep nuclear gray matter, amygdala, hippocampus, and cerebellum [57]. Human milk was found neuroprotective against the vulnerable brain regions of premature infants. Some studies have shown the beneficial effects of human milk on preterm infants against the disturbing environment of the neonatal intensive care unit (NICU) and led to better neurodevelopmental results at preschool ages [58]. Randomized studies have shown that early human milk intervention resulted in a shorter duration of NICU care and decreased risk for necrotizing enterocolitis and sepsis. Decreased neonatal morbidity results in long-term better neurodevelopmental outcomes [58].

Studies that focused on the effects of breastfeeding on preterm infants (<37 weeks of gestation) are limited with controversial results because of the low percentage of breastfeeding process due to immaturity and accompanying pathologies of newborns. Preterm infants are already born with a risk of neurodevelopmental delay due to the lack of positive influences of in utero environment on brain development and the negative effects of oxidative stress during premature delivery [40].

Feeding preterm neonates at the breast is usually a challenge for mothers, as neonates at intensive care units are first encouraged to be fed by expressed breast milk, donor milk or formulas are used when the mother's milk is not eligible. Transitioning from feeding with gavage or bottle to breastfeeding depends on the feeding capacity of the neonate and the motivation of the mother. Mothers of preterm neonates who breastfeed have been found to have more confidence and less risk of postpartum depression, which positively affects neurodevelopment [59, 60].

Most small for gestational age (SGA) newborns are fed with enriched formulas to enhance their growth and development. One multicenter randomized controlled study reported better linear growth with enriched formulas but reported no extra benefit in neurodevelopmental outcomes [40]. A study that performed 'Brazelton Neonatal Behavioral Assessment Scale' on SGA neonates on the ninth postnatal day showed fewer abnormal reflexes and depressive signs in breastfed infants, which was interpreted as the favorable effect of breastfeeding on neurobehavioral development [9, 61].

8   Conclusion

Motor functions are the cornerstone of a child's neuromotor development. Nutrition is the major known factor affecting the neuromotor development of a child. Despite all the rapid development in the infant formula industry, human milk is still the "gold standard" recommended unique nutrient for term and preterm neonates with major positive effects on motor development.

The breastfeeding process has a positive impact on the motor development of a child independently by allowing mother-child bonding and giving positive stimulation to the nursing mother. Despite the concerns about the need for fortification of preterm infants' nutrition, it has been shown that mother's milk is the most superiorly recommended nutrient with an acceptable positive impact on the neuromotor development of the infant. Concerning the positive impact of human milk on the motor development of the central nervous system, postnatal nursing strategies of term and preterm neonates should be focused on breastfeeding motivation unless there is a contraindication.

There are still many unknowns about the constitution of human milk and current studies are mainly focused on exploring these unique factors and their functions on development.

References

1. Aye T, Kuramoto-Ahuja T, Sato T, Sadakiyo K, Watanabe M, Maruyama H. Gross motor skill development of kindergarten children in Japan. J Phys Ther Sci. 2018;30:711–5.
2. Hernández Luengo M, Álvarez-Bueno C, Pozuelo-Carrascosa DP, Berlanga-Macías C, Martínez-Vizcaíno V, Notario-Pacheco B. Relationship between breast feeding and motor development in children: protocol for a systematic review and meta-analysis. BMJ Open. 2019;9:e029063.

3. de Onis M, Garza C, Victora CG, Onyango AW, Frongillo EA, Martines J. The WHO multicentre growth reference study: planning, study design, and methodology. Food Nutr Bull. 2004;25(Suppl 1):S15–26.
4. Lipkin PH. Motor development and dysfunction. In: Developmental -behavioral pediatrics: expert consult. 4th ed. Amsterdam: Elsevier; 2009. p. 643–52.
5. Ghassabian A, Sundaram R, Bell E, Bello SC, Kus C, Yeung E. Gross motor milestones and subsequent development. Pediatrics. 2016;138:1–8.
6. D'Souza EE, Vyas R, Sisitsky M, et al. Increased breastfeeding proportion is associated with improved gross motor skills at 3-5 years of age: a pilot study. Nutrients. 2022;14:2215.
7. Boquien CY. Human milk: An ideal food for nutrition of preterm newborn. Front Pediatr. 2018;16:295.
8. World Health Organization Breastfeeding; Available online: https://www.who.int/topics/breastfeeding/en/. Accessed 03 Oct 2022.
9. Gaber Rizk TM. Breast milk versus formula milk and neuropsychological development and sleep. J Pediatr Neonatal Care. 2014;1:00005.
10. Deoni S, Dean D 3rd, Joelson S, O'Regan J, Schneider N. Early nutrition influences developmental myelination and cognition in infants and young children. NeuroImage. 2018;178:649–59.
11. Allen MC, Capute AJ. Tone and reflex development before term. Pediatrics. 1990;85:393–9.
12. Rukanah R. Relationship of breastfeeding with gross and fine motor skills development in infant 6-12 months. J Vocation Nurs. 2021;2:25–31.
13. Li R, Scanlon KS, Serdula MK. The validity and reliability of maternal recall of breastfeeding practice. Nutr Rev. 2005;63:103–10.
14. Sacker A, Quigley MA, Kelly YJ. Breastfeeding and developmental delay: findings from the millennium cohort study. Pediatrics. 2006;118:e682–9.
15. Hanson C, Lyden E, Furtado J, Van Ormer M, Anderson-Berry A. A comparison of nutritional antioxidant content in breast milk, donor milk, and infant formulas. Nutrients. 2016;8:681.
16. Chen TC, Chao HR, Wu CY, et al. Effect of 9,12-octadecadiynoic acid on neurobehavioral development in *Caenorhabditis elegans*. Int J Mol Sci. 2021;22:8917.
17. Caspi A, Williams B, Kim-Cohen J. Moderation of breastfeeding effects on the IQ by genetic variation in fatty acid metabolism. Proc Natl Acad Sci U S A. 2007;104:18860–5.
18. Guxens M, Mendez MA, Molto´-Puigmartı´ C, et al. Breastfeeding, long chain polyunsaturated fatty acids in colostrum, and infant mental development. Pediatrics. 2011;128:e880–9.
19. Hadley KB, Ryan AS, Forsyth S, Gautier S, Salem N Jr. The essentiality of arachidonic acid in infant development. Nutrients. 2016;8:216.
20. Pang WW, Tan PT, Cai S, et al. Nutrients or nursing? Understanding how breast milk feeding affects child cognition. Eur J Nutr. 2020;59:609–19.
21. Lis-Kuberka J, Orczyk-Pawiłowicz M. Sialylated oligosaccharides and glycoconjugates of human milk. The impact on infant and newborn protection, development and well-being. Nutrients. 2019;11:306.
22. Peila C, Sottemano S, Cesare Marincola F, et al. Metabonomic profile of preterm human milk in the first month of lactation: from extreme to moderate prematurity. Foods. 2022;11:345.
23. Better J, Zimmer JP, Neuringer M, DeRusso PA. Serum lutein concentrations in healthy term infants fed human milk or infant formula with lutein. Eur J Nutr. 2010;49:45–51.
24. Jorgensen JM, Young R, Ashorn P, et al. Associations of human milk oligosaccharides and bioactive proteins with infant growth and development among Malawian mother-infant dyads. Am J Clin Nutr. 2020;113:209–20.
25. Innis SM. Impact of maternal diet on human milk composition and neurological development of infants. Am J Clin Nutr. 2014;99:734S–41S.
26. Cotter DG, d'Avignon DA, Wentz AE, Weber ML, Crawford PA. Obligate role for ketone body oxidation in neonatal metabolic homeostasis. J Biol Chem. 2011;286:6902–10.
27. Alsaweed M, Hartmann PE, Geddes DT, Kakulas F. MicroRNAs in breastmilk and the lactating breast: potential immunoprotectors and developmental regulators for the infant and the mother. Int J Environ Res Public Health. 2015;12:13981–4020.

28. Verduci E, Banderali G, Barberi S, et al. Epigenetic effects of human breast milk. Nutrients. 2014;6:1711–24.
29. Melnik BC, Stremmel W, Weiskirchen R, John SM, Schmitz G. Exosome-derived microRNAs of human milk and their effects on infant health and development. Biomol Ther. 2021;11:851.
30. Colacci M, Murthy K, DeRegnier RO, Khan JY, Robinson DT. Growth and development in extremely low birth weight infants after the introduction of exclusive human milk feedings. Am J Perinatol. 2017;34:130–7.
31. Antonakou A, Chiou A, Andrikopoulos NK, Bakoula C, Matalas AL. Breast milk tocopherol content during the first six months in exclusively breastfeeding Greek women. Eur J Nutr. 2011;50:195–202.
32. Assunção DGF, Silva LTPD, Camargo JDAS, Cobucci RN, Ribeiro KDDS. Vitamin E levels in preterm and full-term infants: a systematic review. Nutrients. 2022;14:2257.
33. Martysiak-Żurowska D, Szlagatys-Sidorkiewicz A, Zagierski M. Concentrations of alpha- and gamma-tocopherols in human breast milk during the first months of lactation and in infant formulas. Matern Child Nutr. 2013;9:473–82.
34. Kitajima H, Kanazawa T, Mori R, Hirano S, Ogihara T, Fujimura M. Long-term alpha-tocopherol supplements may improve mental development in extremely low birthweight infants. Acta Paediatr. 2015;104:e82–9.
35. Zhang Z, Adelman AS, Rai D, Boettcher J, Lönnerdal B. Amino acid profiles in term and preterm human milk through lactation: a systematic review. Nutrients. 2013;5:4800–21.
36. Chan GM, Chan MM, Gellermann W, et al. Resonance Raman spectroscopy and the preterm infant carotenoid status. J Pediatr Gastroenterol Nutr. 2013;56:556–9.
37. Bier JA, Oliver T, Ferguson AE, Vohr BR. Human milk improves cognitive and motor development of premature infants during infancy. J Hum Lact. 2002;18:361–7.
38. Patra K, Hamilton M, Johnson TJ, et al. NICU human milk dose and 20-month neurodevelopmental outcome in very low birth weight infants. Neonatology. 2017;112:330–6.
39. Michels KA, Ghassabian A, Mumford SL, et al. Breastfeeding and motor development in term and preterm infants in a longitudinal US cohort. Am J Clin Nutr. 2017;106:1456–62.
40. Hopperton KE, O'Connor DL, Bando N, et al. Nutrient enrichment of human milk with human and bovine milk-based fortifiers for infants born <1250 g: 18-month neurodevelopment follow-up of a randomized clinical trial. Curr Dev Nutr. 2019;3:nzz129.
41. Belfort MB, Anderson PJ, Nowak VA, et al. Breast milk feeding, brain development, and neurocognitive outcomes: a 7-year longitudinal study in infants born at less than 30 weeks' gestation. J Pediatr. 2016;177:133–139.e1.
42. Hermes L, Martins F, Righi NC. Seasonality and risk factors associated with motor development of full-term infants. Cad Bras Ter Ocup. 2021;29:1–17.
43. Baumgartel K, Jensen L, White SW, et al. The contributions of fetal growth restriction and gestational age to developmental outcomes at 12 months of age: a cohort study. Early Hum Dev. 2020;142:104951.
44. Dewey KG, Cohen RJ, Brown KH, Rivera LL. Effects of exclusive breastfeeding for four versus six months on maternal nutritional status and infant motor development: results of two randomized trials in Honduras. J Nutr. 2001;131:262–7.
45. Dee DL, Li R, Lee LC, Grummer-Strawn LM. Associations between breastfeeding practices and young children's language and motor skill development. Pediatrics. 2007;119(Suppl 1):S92–8.
46. Thorsdottir I, Gunnarsdottir I, Kvaran MA, Gretarsson SJ. Maternal body mass index, duration of exclusive breastfeeding and children's developmental status at the age of 6 years. Eur J Clin Nutr. 2005;59:426–31.
47. Deoni SC, Dean DC 3rd, Piryatinsky I, et al. Breastfeeding and early white matter development: a cross-sectional study. NeuroImage. 2013;82:77–86.
48. Bouwstra H, Boersma ER, Boehm G, Dijck-Brouwer DA, Muskiet FA, Hadders-Algra M. Exclusive breastfeeding of healthy term infants for at least 6 weeks improves neurological condition. J Nutr. 2003;133:4243–5.

49. Hernández-Luengo M, Álvarez-Bueno C, Martínez-Hortelano JA, Cavero-Redondo I, Martínez-Vizcaíno V, Notario-Pacheco B. The relationship between breastfeeding and motor development in children: a systematic review and meta-analysis. Nutr Rev. 2022;80:1827–35.
50. Koshiyama D, Okada N, Ando S, et al. Association between duration of breastfeeding based on maternal reports and dorsal and ventral striatum and medial orbital gyrus volumes in early adolescence. NeuroImage. 2020;220:117083.
51. Jardí C, Hernández-Martínez C, Canals J, et al. Influence of breastfeeding and iron status on mental and psychomotor development during the first year of life. Infant Behav Dev. 2018;50:300–10.
52. McCrory C, Murray A. The effect of breastfeeding on neuro-development in infancy. Matern Child Health J. 2013;17:1680–8.
53. Vestergaard M, Obel C, Henriksen TB, Sørensen HT, Skajaa E, Østergaard J. Duration of breastfeeding and developmental milestones during the latter half of infancy. Acta Paediatr. 1999;88:1327–32.
54. Angelsen NK, Vik T, Jacobsen G, Bakketeig LS. Breast feeding and cognitive development at age 1 and 5 years. Arch Dis Child. 2001;85:183–8.
55. Florey CDV, Leech AM, Blackhall A. Infant feeding and mental and motor development at 18 months of age in first born singletons. Int J Epidemiol. 1995;24(Suppl 1):S21–6.
56. Paine BJ, Makrides M, Gibson RA. Duration of breast-feeding and Bayley's mental developmental index at 1 year of age. J Paediatr Child Health. 1999;35:82–5.
57. Belfort MB, Inder TE. Human Milk and preterm infant brain development: a narrative review. Clin Ther. 2022;44:612–21.
58. Lechner BE, Vohr BR. Neurodevelopmental outcomes of preterm infants fed human milk: a systematic review. Clin Perinatol. 2017;44:69–83.
59. Buckley KM, Charles GE. Benefits and challenges of transitioning preterm infants to at-breast feedings. Int Breastfeed J. 2006;1:13.
60. Furman L, Minich N, Hack M. Correlates of lactation in mothers of very low birth weight infants. Pediatrics. 2002;109:e57.
61. Morley R, Fewtrell MS, Abbott RA, Stephenson T, MacFadyen U, Lucas A. Neurodevelopment in children born small for gestational age: a randomized trial of nutrient-enriched versus standard formula and comparison with a reference breastfed group. Pediatrics. 2004;113:515–21.

Breastfeeding, Intelligence, and Social-Language Development

İpek Dokurel Çetin and Bülent Kara

1 Introduction

Breastfeeding is a unique impulsive behavior of humanity that enhances the bond between mother and baby. Human milk is regarded as an optimal way of feeding infants because of its health benefits to infants and their mothers [1]. Promoting breastfeeding is the leading strategy to diminish the consequences of acquired infections, which results in infant mortality even in modern healthcare settings [2]. In the first several months after birth, breastfeeding is unquestionably the "gold standard" dietary source for humans [3]. Considering all of the evidence that indicates the favorable consequences of breastfeeding for the child and mother led the World Health Organization (WHO) and United Nations International Children's Emergency Fund (UNICEF) to encourage the global goal of exclusive breastfeeding for 4–6 months with the Innocenti Declaration [4]. The ideal strategy for breastfeeding is described as exclusive breastfeeding for 6 months and followed by continuing breastfeeding as long as the mother wishes while being introduced to complementary foods [5].

Mothers who are determined to breastfeed tend to have higher socioeconomic status and intelligence and to be older, more educated, and non-smokers [6]. Many mothers are willing to breastfeed in the first 6 months. However, just a minority of them can maintain breastfeeding for 2 years. Breastfeeding is a dynamic process

İ. D. Çetin (✉)
Faculty of Medicine, Division of Pediatric Neurology, Department of Pediatrics, Balikesir University, Balikesir, Türkiye
e-mail: ipek.cetin@balikesir.edu.tr

B. Kara
Faculty of Medicine, Division of Pediatric Neurology, Department of Pediatrics, Kocaeli University, Kocaeli, Türkiye
e-mail: bulent.kara@kocaeli.edu.tr

Ö. N. Şahin et al. (eds.), *Breastfeeding and Metabolic Programming*, https://doi.org/10.1007/978-3-031-33278-4_24

281

affected by socio-environmental factors and experiences. Common concerns for mothers dealing with daily life may affect a mother's decision to cease breastfeeding, like the perception of an infant's inadequate milk intake and insufficient workplace support [7]. Political and financial reinforcements are essential in promoting and supporting breastfeeding in favor of public health [8].

Existing researchers recognize the critical role of human milk, which provide nutrition, digestive enzymes, immunologic factors of many types, growth factors, hormones, and other bioactive factors that help to shape neurodevelopment and brain functions [9–11]. An immense number of studies are conducted to discover new components of human milk. Long-chain polyunsaturated fatty acids (LC-PUFAs), which are present in human milk but typically absent in formula, may be one of the nutrients related to these effects of breastfeeding on cognitive development. Docosahexaenoic acid (DHA) and arachidonic acid (ARA) are two important LCPUFAs that play a role in neurodevelopment by promoting healthy neuronal growth, repair, and myelination [12]. Infants produce a little amount of DHA during the first 2 weeks of life, but they are unable to produce enough of it on their own until they are about 6 months old. This raises the idea of a developmental window in which LC-PUFAs delivered during breastfeeding may be particularly sensitive to the development of the human brain. In accordance with Kafouri et al. [13], increasing the duration of exclusive breastfeeding—a result of more consumption of DHA—was significantly associated with improved cognitive abilities and a thicker parietal cortex. The *FADS* gene encodes an enzyme that directly impacts the metabolism of DHA and ARA. Two single nucleotide polymorphisms (SNPs) on the *FADS2* gene (rs174575 and rs1535) were investigated to evaluate the effect of individual differences in the metabolism and production of LC-PUFAs and breastfeeding on cognitive development [14]. As a result, all breastfed carriers having the *FADS2* genotype of the C allele on rs174575, which is linked to more effective fatty acid processing (i.e., LC-PUFAs), had resulted in the best IQ ratings. Zeisel et al. [15] stated that choline that is rich in human milk is an important determinant for neural tube closure in human fetuses and proposed that perinatal choline supplementation can have long-lasting effects on memory. Folate affects the embryogenesis of the brain and the supplementation of folate during the periconceptional period reduces the risk of serious defects in brain development [16]. Please refer to Table 1 for a brief explanation of the other nutrients, which affect early brain and neurocognitive development.

Epigenetics processes have been recognized as essential mediators in the origins of human health and disorders. Currently, the theoretical implications of the epigenetic process focus on DNA methylation [17]. There is some evidence to support these assumptions that breast milk influences DNA methylation. Moreover, breast milk contains long non-coding RNAs and small non-coding RNAs called microRNAs [18, 19]. These findings promote that the epigenetic effects of breast milk may not be restricted to DNA methylation. In breastfed individuals, higher gene expression levels of *LEP* gene (which encodes the anorexigenic hormone leptin), *POMC* gene (which encodes a precursor of many peptide hormones), and *SLC2A4* gene (which encodes the Glut-4 protein, an insulin-regulated glucose transporter) genes

Table 1 Micronutrients affect early brain and neurocognitive development

	Function	Results on metabolism/ disease	Supplementary
Iron [98]	Component of enzymes needed for neurotransmitters	Newborn iron deficiency	Lactoferrin binds free iron and possesses antimicrobial, anti-inflammatory, and immunomodulatory properties that serve to maintain homeostasis and control life-threatening diseases in the gut of newborns
Iodine [99]	Synthesis of thyroid hormone which is necessary for infant growth, mental development	Cretinism (prenatal deficiency) chronic iodine deficiency (postnatal deficiency)	Breast-milk iodine concentrations are related to current maternal iodine consumption rather than iodine status, depending on the geographic location.
Copper [100]	Due to its function as a cofactor for cuproenzymes and its involvement in signaling pathways, copper is an important nutrient	Copper-dependent anemia Childhood cirrhosis associated with copper Cirrhosis of Indian childhood	The processing of pro-neuropeptides, the metabolism of neurotransmitters, and the production of melanin are all carried out by copper-dependent enzymes found in the brain
Vitamin A [99]	Responsible for growth and development, normal vision and reproductive functions	Stunting, delayed puberty Xerophthalmia Anemia and weak resistance to infection, Upper respiratory or gastrointestinal diseases	Vitamin A levels are correlated with nocturnal growth hormone secretion
Thiamin [101] (Vitamin B1)	Coenzyme in the metabolism of carbohydrates and BCAAs Essential for synthesis of the primary neurotransmitter acetylcholine involved in nerve impulse transmission	Infantile beriberi Impairments in glucose tolerance in mother Increasing the risk of low birth-weight	Transketolase activity in erythrocytes, which represents the sufficiency of body reserves, is typically used to test thiamin nutritional status
Riboflavin [101] (Vitamin B2)	Involved in reactions of energy production and a free radical scavenge	Peripheral neuropathy, Poor growth, Impaired iron absorption	Riboflavin in stored milk is highly susceptible to photodegradation upon exposure to sunlight

(continued)

Table 1 (continued)

	Function	Results on metabolism/disease	Supplementary
Niacin [101]	Co-dehydrogenase in the oxidation of fuel molecules or as a hydrogen donor in reductive processes for the production of fatty acids Cofactor in oxidation-reduction reactions	Pellagra Insomnia Loss of appetite and exhaustion Painful tongue and mouth Indigestion	Niacin insufficiency is still a problem in countries with poor diets where corn and other grains are important food staples
Prydoxine [99] (Vitamin B6)	A cofactor for many enzymes of amino acid metabolism, glycolysis, and gluconeogenesis	Irritability Increased startle response Seizures	Plasma pyridoxal 5′-phosphate is the primary biomarker
Cobalamin [100] (Vitamin B12)	A cofactor in essential reactions of folate metabolism and DNA synthesis	Long-term cognitive and developmental retardation Apathy, muscle hypotonia, and anorexia Involuntary movements of the limbs/tongue	Vitamin B-12 is bound to apohaptocorrin, a cobalamin-binding protein in human milk
Vitamin D [98]	Essential in bone growth and immune system Induces the nerve growth factor, promotes neurite growth and inhibits neuronal apoptosis in the hippocampus	Rickets Poor development, delayed motor skills, and unusual excitability/irritability	For babies who are exclusively breastfed, vitamin D supplementation and sunshine exposure are advised to prevent vitamin D insufficiency. Maternal supplementation with 400–2000 IU per day can raise levels of vitamin D in breast milk.
Vitamin E [99] (Alpha-tocopherol)	Boost the development of the immune system Provide antioxidant defense against peroxidation		Preterm babies have lower levels of vitamin E (tocopherol), which makes them vulnerable to develop infections, thrombocytosis, hemolytic anemia, retrolental fibroplasia, intraventricular hemorrhage, bronchopulmonary dysplasia, spinocerebellar ataxia.

Table 1 (continued)

	Function	Results on metabolism/ disease	Supplementary
Folate [98, 102]	Necessary for protein, DNA, and RNA biosynthesis	neural tube defects (diminished periconceptual folate intake) risk factor for cardiovascular disease due to elevated plasma homocysteine cellular dysplasia, often the predecessor of cancerous lesions	The predominant form of folate in human milk is 5-methyltetrahydrofolate
Biotin [100]	Essential component of four carboxylase enzymes that are essential for gluconeogenesis, fatty acid biosynthesis, amino acid metabolism, and odd-chain fatty acid catabolism	Biotinidase deficiency Alopecia, dry scaly dermatitis, glossitis Pallor, mental depression Nausea, vomiting, and anorexia	Biotin regulates gene expression, cell growth, DNA damage repair, and the integrity of the chromatin structure through the biotinylation of histones
Choline [102]	A precursor of the neurotransmitter acetylcholine Involved in structural integrity of cell membranes Transmembrane signaling of lipid-cholesterol transport and metabolism Methyl group metabolism	Stunting Fatty liver Liver, muscle, and DNA damage	Choline is important in embryonic development, notably in the brain, where its availability appears to influence neural tube closure and cognition
LCPUFAs			
AA [103]	Regulate neuronal firing, long-term potentiation, and hippocampal plasticity		
DHA [103]	Helps neonates to achieve better developmental results, such as improved cognitive and visual acuity	Newborns fed with formula that devoid of DHA had a 15% lower concentration of DHA in their frontal cortex	DHA are structural components of cell membrane phospholipids (phosphatidylcholine, phosphatidylethanolamine, phosphatidylserine, and phosphatidylinositol) particularly in the central nervous system

BCAA branched chain amino acid, *LC-PUFAs* long-chain polyunsaturated fatty acids, *AA* arachidonic acid; *DHA* docosahexaenoic acid and lower expression levels of the NPY gene (which encodes the neuropeptide Y) were found to be in agreement with other epidemiological shreds of evidence that breastfeeding might protect against obesity and diabetes [20]. Likewise, breastfeeding increases *CDKN2A* gene expression via epigenetic changes, as a result, it has the potential to protect against cancer [21]. These findings provide the following insights for future research: the potential role of epigenetics in the associations of breastfeeding with long-term benefits on cognition is worth elucidating.

Much research on the benefits of breastfeeding has been mostly restricted to short-term outcomes that reduce mortality and morbidity due to infectious diseases such as lower respiratory tract infections, otitis media, and gastroenteritis in setting where poverty, poor sanitation, and malnutrition are prevalent [22, 23]. In the longer term, the risk of developing inflammatory bowel disease, childhood leukemia/lymphoma, hypertension, cardiovascular disease, hyperlipidemia, obesity, and diabetes (type I and II) is reduced by breastfeeding [24, 25].

Breastfeeding confers early skin-to-skin contact between mothers and newborns and has some neurobehavioral advantages, which may help to adopt extrauterine life [26]. Breastfeeding seems to have an analgesic effect during a painful procedure, and this effect is due to the enhanced maternal-infant bond. Higher salivary cortisol levels found in breastfed infants affirmed this analgesic effect compared to formula-fed infants [27]. Exclusive breastfeeding and a longer duration of breastfeeding render the greatest protection against sudden infant death syndrome [28]. This section presents the findings of the recent research, meta-analysis, and review that intended to raise awareness of this growing body of research, by focusing on the key themes of the influence of breastfeeding on intelligence and social-language development in the developing brain.

2   Breastfeeding and Intelligence

The cognitive development of an infant consists of erratic evolutionary drives formed by genetic and environmental factors that interact mutually. Breastfeeding mothers are engaged in behaviors that stimulate their children's development. This might contribute to the observed differences in cognitive performance between breastfed children and others. Breastfeeding promotes reaching developmental milestones like language, cognition, and fine motor skills earlier. A large and growing body of literature has investigated the beneficial effect on intelligence with higher results on measures of cognitive development among children and adults who have been breastfed [29–32]. In light of the consensus of many reports on breastfed infants, it is recognized that IQ scores increased by 3–5 points in a dose-dependent manner [33, 34]. Bernard et al. [35] showed that prolonged duration of exclusive breastfeeding improved problem-solving abilities besides improved cognitive and motor development in 2- and 3-year-old children. Some of the current literature on these cognitive benefits of breastfeeding pays particular attention to its enduring effect on childhood and adolescence.

A small proportion of the studies presented thus far provide evidence that breastfeeding does not influence on enhancement of the child's intelligence [36–38]. However, the problem with these inferences is the deprived capacity to consider all the astonishing variables of social factors in the determination of cognitive development into account. While presenting the current findings, it is important to consider how different methodologies for evaluating children's intelligence and how those differ between studies in terms of how well they correlate with objective measurements of human milk consumption. Additionally, earlier research has noted the conflicting impacts of elements like maternal IQ and obesity on children's cognition [33, 39].

Regarding the comparison between human milk and other formulas' effect on intelligence, Bellando et al. [40] showed favorable scores in breastfed children on tests of language and cognition with differences in performance notes, versus cow's milk formula and soy formula in groups aged 5 years. Researchers have aspired to conduct these studies in such a convenient group of 'Preschoolers' in order to exclude the potential impact of school education and social stimuli on cognitive development. However, many analyze have a number of serious drawbacks. To distinguish whether the breastfeeding benefits on cognitive development reflect a real nutritional advantage derived from breast milk as indicated previously or from the socioeconomic advantage is complicated. The most surprising observation from the studies to emerge from the data comparison is mostly no significant differences have been revealed after adjusting for confounders such as socioeconomic status, home environment, and maternal verbal ability [30, 36, 41, 42].

Maternal sensitivity is a mother's ability to perceive and capacity to understand her infant's signs and the meaning behind her infant's behavioral signals and to respond to them promptly and appropriately [43]. Mothers' display of sensitive caregiving with their infants is shown to be related to breastfeeding. For this reason, breastfeeding is frequently encouraged in order to increase maternal sensitivity during the postpartum period [44]. Breastfeeding has been linked to the production of oxytocin, a vital hormone connected to social competence and effective caregiving behaviors, as well as to the activation of brain regions associated with caregiving [45, 46]. Gibbs et al. [47] advocated that maternal frequency of reading and maternal sensitivity is a primary component of the relationship between breastfeeding and early cognitive development. They suggested the assessment of other parenting habits beyond infant feeding practices in order to promote early children's cognitive development.

Prior studies have shown that the longer duration of breastfeeding promotes brain development, especially of the white matter, and is associated with improved intelligence [33, 48, 49]. Mortensen et al. [50] reported that the duration of breastfeeding was significantly associated with higher IQ scores of the Wechsler adult intelligence scores positively [99.4, 101.7, 102.3, 106.0, and 104.0 for breastfeeding durations of ≤ 1 month, 2–3 months, 4–6 months, 7–9 months, and >9 months, respectively ($P = 0.003$)]. Jedrychowski et al. [51] reported persisting cognitive benefits across ages from 1 to 7 years as a result of prolonged exclusive breastfeeding duration by using the Wechsler Intelligence Scale for Children [51]. In a population-based cohort study, Leventakou et al. [52] showed the positive association of breastfeeding duration with increased scores in the scales of cognitive, language, and fine motor scales development at 18 months of age by using the Bayley scales of infant toddler development. The long-term outcomes of the prospective birth cohort trial conducted with a three decades follow-up found strong associations between breastfeeding with a duration of 12 months and cognitive development. It was shown that breastfeeding with a duration of 12 months has improved performance in intelligence tests, educational attainment, and monthly income [53].

A broader perspective has been adopted by studies that focused on the potential impact of breastfeeding on the cognitive development of the developing brain has expanded using methodologies such as electroencephalography (EEG) and magnetic resonance imaging (MRI) [3]. Correlations with structural and functional neurodevelopment of breastfeeding showed that optimal evoked response potentials within visual and auditory areas, diminished ventricular volumes, increased head circumferences, and early brain maturation by myelination and white matter development were obtained [54–56].

Mother-infant affectionate touch patterns influence both breastfeeding and the infant's positive temperament and result in neuroprotective benefits for newborns. Infant EEG patterns have been linked by several studies to variations in the child-rearing environment. A relationship exists between an infant's differential brain activation patterns (EEG asymmetry and power) and their differences in the trajectory of neuroplasticity across development [57, 58]. One such study compared breastfed and formula-fed infants by measuring EEG spectral power longitudinally throughout the course of the first year of life in a cohort of healthy infants. This study revealed that formula-fed infants showed an earlier peak in EEG power than breast-fed infants (at 6 months) in the frequency range known to be most affected by myelination (0.1–3 Hz) [59]. These different patterns may reflect the early neurodevelopment, which may lead to differential trajectories in brain and cognitive development between breastfed and formula-fed infants.

Over the first 24 months of life, maturational variations in newborn EEG power are linked to positive mother affect [60]. In babies of depressed mothers, patterns of right frontal EEG asymmetry (a dysregulated physiological pattern linked to depressive disorders) have been found [61]. While in infants with stable breastfeeding, the interaction with the left frontal asymmetry was detected. It is not surprising to inform that left frontal activity in EEG has been associated with advancing maturation and higher-order processing skills [58, 62–64]. In a recent study, Hardin et al. [58] found an interaction between the 'left frontal asymmetry' in infants to stable breastfeeding.

Breastfeeding mothers exhibit more interactive behaviors toward their infants, like touching and gazing, besides more affectionate reactions while feeding compared to formula-feeding mothers. Brain imaging studies have shown an association between the structural composition of the human brain and breastfeeding. For instance, increased white matter volume, total gray matter volume, and regional cortical thickness were correlated to increased breastfeeding duration and the percentage of breast milk in an infant's diet [65]. Furthermore, neuroimaging finds have been associated with improved cognitive function as measured by IQ [13, 66–68]. Kim et al. [45] examined the relationship between breastfeeding, the maternal brain response to infant stimuli, and maternal sensitivity toward their infants with functional magnetic resonance imaging (fMRI). Their results proved that several limbic and cortical brain regions previously known to be important for caregiving behaviors and empathy were more active among breastfeeding mothers in comparison with formula-feeding mothers while listening to their own baby cry versus a control baby cry [45]. Using fMRI scanning, Olsavsky et al. [69] concluded that increased amygdala activation to own infant's cry and higher amygdala-supplementary motor area functional connectivity suggest motor responses to their baby's distress.

Breastfeeding positively impacts 'affectionate touch behaviors' for both mothers and their offspring and is affiliated with an infant's temperament positively, which results in better neuroprotective outcomes [58, 70]. The outbreak of coronavirus disease 2019 (COVID-19) which was caused by the severe acute respiratory syndrome coronavirus-2 was declared a pandemic by WHO in March 2020. A retrospective analysis of COVID-19 in pregnancy showed that none of the women had detectable viral loads of SARS-CoV-2 in breast milk, but the close proximity between mother and child arouse the concern of droplet transmission and cause disadvantage of some hesitancy in breastfeeding [71]. In a multinational study, Ceulemans et al. [72] found high levels of depressive symptoms and generalized anxiety among pregnant and breastfeeding women during the COVID-19 outbreak. These findings emphasized the importance of monitoring perinatal mental health during pandemics in order to maintain maternal and infant mental health. So far, there is not enough data to identify the consequences of this hesitancy and to distinguish the long-term risks of COVID-19 for ASD and cognitive disabilities in children [73].

The current data highlight the importance of breastfeeding, which has a positive impact on a child's and adolescent's IQ scores. The causal role of breastfeeding in improving cognition has been demonstrated by the fact that mothers who breastfeed their children are more likely to give them a stimulating environment. The positive effect of breastfeeding on cognition could be due to the family environment besides breast milk's nutritional facts. According to several reports, breastfeeding may be a sign of good parenting strategies that foster a child's development. Depending on the methodological design, the impact of confounding factors should be taken into account in order to evaluate the validity of these reports. The methodology ought to be less prone to misclassification, self-selection bias, and residual confounding. Moreover, rapid improvements in neuroimaging techniques have opened the door to a more comprehensive assessment of the relationship between breastfeeding and brain development, including higher white matter volume and larger cortical thickness in white matter as well as differential brain activation patterns.

3 Breastfeeding and Social Development

Infants and toddlers need secure attachments to develop the social competency required to successfully cruise peer relationships [74]. Children's nutrition in the first 1000 days (from conception to 2 years of age) is an essential factor in their neurodevelopment and lifelong mental health [75]. Children's early years are critically important for socioemotional development, and their benefits extend far beyond the first 1000 days. In animal studies, monkey neonates exposed to increased tactile stimulation had advanced motor, social, and cognitive skills in the first 3 months of life [76]. However, there are contradictory results among studies. For instance, Belfort et al. [77] suggested that a longer duration of exclusive or nonexclusive breastfeeding was not associated with better social-emotional development in mid-childhood. In the systematic review, Turner et al. [78] advocated that several studies showed a positive association between breastfeeding and socio-emotional competencies. However, they also emphasized there is a lack of satisfying evidence to confirm such an association. The contradictory results of the studies could be attributed to the difference in defining the socio-emotional competencies and the variability of the instruments preferred to use in assessing them.

Sensitive responding to emotions in others is a basic social skill that aids to predict the actions of others and coordinate our behaviors while interacting with them. Autism spectrum disorder (ASD) is a neurodevelopmental disorder characterized by deficits in social communication and interaction and restricted, repetitive patterns of behaviors, interests, or activities. Studies on autism spectrum disorder provide us with some evidence to suggest that attending to the eyes plays an important role in early social development. Krol et al. [79] demonstrated that infants pay attention to the emotional cues in their mother's eye, as a vital social skill during infancy. Their findings associated this skill with genetic variations related to the oxytocin system and exclusive breastfeeding experience. In the literature on the etiology of ASD, the relative importance of breastfeeding is debated. The etiology of ASD is likely to involve genetic and nongenetic factors (sociodemographic features, pregnancy complications, breastfeeding, exposure to chemicals, maternal infections, and diet) [80, 81]. The association between the duration of breastfeeding in newborns and the pathogenesis of autism spectrum disorder is controversial. In light of a recent nationwide cross-sectional study by Huang et al. [82], toddlers who had partly or never breastfed for the first 6 months of life had a higher odds ratio (OR) of receiving a diagnosis of ASD versus those exclusively breastfed [OR: 2.34, 95% confidence interval (CI):1.10–4.82; OR: 1.55, CI:0.90–2.74]. Similarly, Ghozy et al. [83] reported that breastfeeding was associated with a lower risk of being diagnosed with ASD in children in their meta-analysis (combined OR, 0.24; 95% CI, 0.18–0.32). Moreover, they suggested that breastfeeding for 12–24 months was associated with the most significant reduction in the risk of autism spectrum disorder. This concept has been challenged by the study of Dodds et al. [84] among 129,733 children, which argued that breastfeeding at discharge was not associated with an increased risk of ASD. Likewise, Husk et al. [85] carried out a large, nationally representative survey of US children ($n = 37,901$, 2–5 years) and found no association between breastfeeding and ASD.

According to studies conducted to date, there is no conclusive evidence that the difficulties of breastfeeding are related to early developmental disturbances, such as emotion regulation problems, motor development, and sleep disturbances, in children with ASD [86, 87]. To develop a full picture of breastfeeding affiliation to cognitive and social development, additional studies will be needed.

4 Breastfeeding and Language Development

Language is one of the key elements of cognitive development, which maintains communication between parents and their offspring, and envisions subsequent academic achievement. Children make rapid advancements in all aspects of development during the first 3 years of life, including the development of communication and language skills. Children's expressive gestures and vocalizations to caregivers are a part of their developing communication skills, which start in early infancy. It has been suggested that early communicative actions of toddlers served as the inspiration for the development of more conventional oral language, which typically starts to emerge with children's first expressive vocabulary at around 1 year of age.

The neurological system consists of a vast network organized throughout pregnancy, infancy, and toddlerhood. The fundamental building blocks of the system can vary with the early dietary status leading to diversities in brain structure. Infants must develop new connections between brain cells, reshape the brain's architecture, and build a wall that is selectively permeable to the outside environment in addition to developing new brain cells. The raw resources needed for these tasks are provided by their diet [88]. There are some potential explanations put up to explain how infants' diet affects their speech-language development. First, the fatty acid content of human milk is the essential ingredient of cell membranes that influence gene expression within those cells. Second, the variable constituents of human milk might promote optimal neurodevelopment. The third idea is that the positive impact of breastfeeding on immune regulation of neural inflammation, which becomes ineffective in neurodegenerative diseases, has a possible influence on learning and memory. A fourth potential mechanism involves the consequences of lactation on mothers, which in turn customizes their children's learning and language. All of these possible mechanisms should be acknowledged together to provide a partially sufficient explanation for such a complex procedure as neurodevelopment.

Early examples of research into whether breastfeeding might influence speech-language outcomes found that formula-fed children, particularly boys, were more prone to have slower communicative development [88]. It has also been suggested that starting breastfeeding as soon as possible after birth will help lower children's risk of developing cognitive impairment. In order to determine this, a clinical study compared the breastfeeding histories of 4- to 11-year-old children with specific language impairment (SLI) to those of healthy children. Children with language impairment were found to be considerably less likely than healthy children to have been breastfed immediately after birth [89]. The evidence suggests that high maternal education is one of the other crucial factors for fostering children's cognitive development and language. On the other hand, the evidence on the role of paternal education is more limited [90, 91]. According to Pancsofar et al. [92], children of more educated fathers showed advanced language and cognitive development, which persisted after adjustment for family income and mothers' education.

Trends in this topic have led to an increment of studies that concern the duration of breastfeeding. The dose-related effect of breastfeeding is more potently observed with more exclusivity and duration. Vestergaard et al. [93] pointed out that 73.4% of the infants exclusively breastfed for 6 months were engaging in various babbling, compared to 34.0% of the formula-fed infants. Shorter breastfeeding duration was associated with lower scores on the Peabody picture vocabulary test among 6-year-old children and 10-year-old children [42, 94]. Quinn et al. [95] found dose-dependent assistance of breastfeeding duration on verbal intelligence abilities with the revised Peabody picture vocabulary test in a cohort from infancy to 5 years of age. According to this study, at age 5, children who had been breastfed for at least six months scored the best in verbal intelligence, while children who had never been breastfed scored the lowest. Guzzardi et al. [96] found that exclusive breastfeeding ensures improved hearing and language scores in girls aged 5 years, independent of parents' age, maternal weight, and IQ, or children's weight and weight gain. Existing research recognized the critical role played by a longer duration of breastfeeding on communication development, which appears to improve communication development at 18 months [52]. A recent randomized trial on children at 16 years of age found that prolonged exclusive breastfeeding had a sustained effect on linguistic skills but not on any other neurocognitive measures [97].

5 Conclusion

Breastfeeding provides a bond between mothers and their offspring besides supplying an optimal way of adequate nutrition. In addition to being an essential source of nutrition for the infant, studies indicate that breastfeeding has profound implications on children's cognition, behavior, and mental health. Furnishing a stimulating habitat for the infant is the essence of promoting cognitive development. In light of the literature, the recompense of improving public health efforts to increase exclusive breastfeeding is far beyond short-term outcomes. Numerous studies from various nations have shown a connection between breastfeeding and later cognitive development, including better memory retention, increased language skills, and IQ scores. These motivations should provide stronger arguments in public health for promoting not only initiating but also continuing a longer duration of breastfeeding.

References

1. Black RE, Victora CG, Walker SP, et al. Maternal and child undernutrition and overweight in low-income and middle-income countries. Lancet. 2013;382:427–51.
2. Satar M, Engin Arısoy A, Çelik İH. Turkish Neonatal Society guideline on neonatal infections-diagnosis and treatment. Turk Pediatr Ars. 2018;53:88–100.
3. Krol KM, Grossmann T. Psychological effects of breastfeeding on children and mothers. Bundesgesundheitsblatt Gesundheitsforschung Gesundheitsschutz. 2018;61:977–85.
4. UNICEF Innocenti Research Centre. 1990–2005 Celebrating the Innocenti Declaration on the Protection, Promotion and Support of Breastfeeding: past achievements, present challenges and the way forward for infant and young child feeding. Italy: Innocenti Publications; 2005.
5. Binns CW, Lee MK. Exclusive breastfeeding for six months: the WHO six months recommendation in the Asia Pacific Region. Asia Pac J Clin Nutr. 2014;23:344–50.
6. Scott JA, Binns CW, Oddy WH, Graham KI. Predictors of breastfeeding duration: evidence from a cohort study. Pediatrics. 2006;117:e646–55.
7. Odom EC, Li R, Scanlon KS, et al. Reasons for earlier than desired cessation of breastfeeding. Pediatrics. 2013;131:e726–32.
8. Rollins NC, Bhandari N, Hajeebhoy N, et al. Why invest, and what it will take to improve breastfeeding practices? Lancet. 2016;387:491–504.
9. Ballard O, Morrow AL. Human milk composition: nutrients and bioactive factors. Pediatr Clin N Am. 2013;60:49–74.
10. Andreas NJ, Kampmann B, Mehring L-DK. Human breast milk: a review on its composition and bioactivity. Early Hum Dev. 2015;91:629–35.
11. Eriksen KG, Christensen SH, Lind MV, Michaelsen KF. Human milk composition and infant growth. Curr Opin Clin Nutr Metab Care. 2018;21:200–6.
12. Guesnet P, Alessandri JM. Docosahexaenoic acid (DHA) and the developing central nervous system (CNS) - Implications for dietary recommendations. Biochimie. 2011;93:7–12.
13. Kafouri S, Kramer M, Leonard G, et al. Breastfeeding and brain structure in adolescence. Int J Epidemiol. 2013;42:150–9.
14. Caspi A, Williams B, Kim-Cohen J, et al. Moderation of breastfeeding effects on the IQ by genetic variation in fatty acid metabolism. Proc Natl Acad Sci U S A. 2007;104:18860–5.
15. Zeisel SH. Choline: critical role during fetal development and dietary requirements in adults. Annu Rev Nutr. 2006;26:229–50.
16. Zeisel SH, Niculescu MD. Perinatal choline influences brain structure and function. Nutr Rev. 2006;64:197–203.
17. Hartwig FP, De Mola CL, Davies NM, et al. Breastfeeding effects on DNA methylation in the offspring: a systematic literature review. PLoS One. 2017;12:e0173070.
18. Alsaweed M, Hartmann PE, Geddes DT, Kakulas F. MicroRNAs in breastmilk and the lactating breast: potential immunoprotectors and developmental regulators for the infant and the mother. Int J Environ Res Public Health. 2015;12:13981–4020.
19. Karlsson O, Rodosthenous RS, Jara C, et al. Detection of long non-coding RNAs in human breastmilk extracellular vesicles: implications for early child development. Epigenetics. 2016;11:721–9.
20. Victora CG, Bahl R, Barros AJD, et al. Breastfeeding in the 21st century: epidemiology, mechanisms, and lifelong effect. Lancet. 2016;387:475–90.
21. Deng Y, Chan SS, Chang S. Telomere dysfunction and tumour suppression: the senescence connection. Nat Rev Cancer. 2008;8:450–8.
22. Horta BL, Victora CG, World Health Organization. Short-term effects of breastfeeding: a systematic review on the benefits of breastfeeding on diarrhoea and pneumonia mortality. Geneva: World Health Organization; 2013. p. 1–49.
23. Yu C, Binns CW, Lee AH. Comparison of breastfeeding rates and health outcomes for infants receiving care from hospital outpatient clinic and community health centres in China. J Child Health Care. 2016;20:286–93.

24. Bar S, Milanaik R, Adesman A. Long-term neurodevelopmental benefits of breastfeeding. Curr Opin Pediatr. 2016;28:559–66.
25. Binns C, Lee M, Low WY. The long-term public health benefits of breastfeeding. Asia Pac J Public Health. 2016;28:7–14.
26. Bergman NJ. Birth practices: maternal-neonate separation as a source of toxic stress. Birth Defects Res. 2019;111:1087–109.
27. Cao Y, Rao SD, Phillips TM, et al. Are breast-fed infants more resilient? Feeding method and cortisol in infants. J Pediatr. 2009;154:452–4.
28. Thompson JMD, Tanabe K, Moon RY, et al. Duration of breastfeeding and risk of SIDS: an individual participant data meta-analysis. Pediatrics. 2017;140:e20171324.
29. Anderson JW, Johnstone BM, Remley DT. Breast-feeding and cognitive development: a meta-analysis. Am J Clin Nutr. 1999;70:525–35.
30. Kramer MS, Aboud F, Mironova E, et al. Breastfeeding and child cognitive development: new evidence from a large randomized trial. Arch Gen Psychiatry. 2008;65:578–84.
31. Jenkins JM, Foster EM. The effects of breastfeeding exclusivity on early childhood outcomes. Am J Public Health. 2014;104(Suppl 1):S128–35.
32. Banerjee PN, McFadden KE, Shannon JD, Davidson LL. Does breastfeeding account for the association between maternal sensitivity and infant cognitive development in a large, nationally representative cohort? BMC Pediatr. 2022;22:61.
33. Horta BL. Loret De Mola C, Victora CG. Breastfeeding and intelligence: a systematic review and meta-analysis. Acta Paediatr. 2015;104:14–9.
34. Strøm M, Mortensen EL, Kesmodel US, et al. Is breast feeding associated with offspring IQ at age 5? Findings from prospective cohort: Lifestyle During Pregnancy Study. BMJ Open. 2019;9:e023134.
35. Bernard JY, De Agostini M, Forhan A, et al. Breastfeeding duration and cognitive development at 2 and 3 years of age in the EDEN mother-child cohort. J Pediatr. 2013;163:36–42.
36. Der G, Batty GD, Deary IJ. Effect of breast feeding on intelligence in children: prospective study, sibling pairs analysis, and meta-analysis. BMJ. 2006;333:945–8.
37. Veena SR, Krishnaveni GV, Srinivasan K, et al. Infant feeding practice and childhood cognitive performance in South India. Arch Dis Child. 2010;95:347–54.
38. Lind JN, Li R, Perrine CG, Schieve LA. Breastfeeding and later psychosocial development of children at 6 years of age. Pediatrics. 2014;134(Suppl 1):S36–41.
39. Hinkle SN, Schieve LA, Stein AD, et al. Associations between maternal prepregnancy body mass index and child neurodevelopment at 2 years of age. Int J Obes. 2012;36:1312–9.
40. Bellando J, McCorkle G, Spray B, et al. Developmental assessments during the first 5 years of life in infants fed breast milk, cow's milk formula, or soy formula. Food Sci Nutr. 2020;8:3469–78.
41. Zhou SJ, Baghurst P, Gibson RA, Makrides M. Home environment, not duration of breastfeeding, predicts intelligence quotient of children at four years. Nutrition. 2007;23:236–41.
42. Oddy WH, Kendall GE, Blair E, et al. Breast feeding and cognitive development in childhood: a prospective birth cohort study. Paediatr Perinat Epidemiol. 2003;17:81–90.
43. Mateus V, Osório A, Miguel HO, et al. Maternal sensitivity and infant neural response to touch: an fNIRS study. Soc Cogn Affect Neurosci. 2021;16:1256–63.
44. Weaver JM, Schofield TJ, Papp LM. Breastfeeding duration predicts greater maternal sensitivity over the next decade. Dev Psychol. 2018;54:220–7.
45. Kim P, Feldman R, Mayes LC, et al. Breastfeeding, brain activation to own infant cry, and maternal sensitivity. J Child Psychol Psychiatry. 2011;52:907–15.
46. Whitley J, Wouk K, Bauer AE, et al. Oxytocin during breastfeeding and maternal mood symptoms. Psychoneuroendocrinology. 2020;113:104581.
47. Gibbs BG, Forste R. Breastfeeding, parenting, and early cognitive development. J Pediatr. 2014;164:487–93.
48. Victora CG, Barros AJD. Effect of breastfeeding on infant and child mortality due to infectious diseases in less developed countries: a pooled analysis. Lancet. 2000;355:451–5.

49. Rouw E, von Gartzen A, Weißenborn A. The importance of breastfeeding for the infant. Bundesgesundheitsblatt Gesundheitsforschung Gesundheitsschutz. 2018;61:945–51.
50. Mortensen EL, Michaelsen KF, Sanders SA, Reinisch JM. The association between duration of breastfeeding and adult intelligence. JAMA. 2002;287:2365–71.
51. Jedrychowski W, Perera F, Jankowski J, et al. Effect of exclusive breastfeeding on the development of children's cognitive function in the Krakow prospective birth cohort study. Eur J Pediatr. 2012;171:151–8.
52. Leventakou V, Roumeliotaki T, Koutra K, et al. Breastfeeding duration and cognitive, language and motor development at 18 months of age: Rhea mother-child cohort in Crete, Greece. J Epidemiol Comm Health. 2015;69:232–9.
53. Victora CG, Horta BL, de Mola CL, et al. Association between breastfeeding and intelligence, educational attainment, and income at 30 years of age: a prospective birth cohort study from Brazil. Lancet Glob Health. 2015;3:e199–205.
54. Khedr E, Farghaly W, Amry SE-D, Osman A. Neural maturation of breastfed and formula-fed infants. Acta Paediatr. 2004;93:734–8.
55. Herba CM, Roza S, Govaert P, et al. Breastfeeding and early brain development: the Generation R study. Matern Child Nutr. 2013;9:332–49.
56. Deoni SCL, Dean DC, Piryatinsky I, et al. Breastfeeding and early white matter development: a cross-sectional study. NeuroImage. 2013;82:77–86.
57. Gartstein MA, Hancock GR, Potapova NV, et al. Modeling development of frontal electroencephalogram (EEG) asymmetry: sex differences and links with temperament. Dev Sci. 2020;23:e12891.
58. Hardin JS, Jones NA, Mize KD, Platt M. Affectionate touch in the context of breastfeeding and maternal depression influences infant neurodevelopmental and temperamental substrates. Neuropsychobiology. 2021;80:158–75.
59. Jing H, Gilchrist JM, Badger TM, Pivik RT. A longitudinal study of differences in electroencephalographic activity among breastfed, milk formula-fed, and soy formula-fed infants during the first year of life. Early Hum Dev. 2010;86:119–25.
60. Bernier A, Calkins SD, Bell MA. Longitudinal associations between the quality of mother-infant interactions and brain development across infancy. Child Dev. 2016;87:1159–74.
61. Goodman SH, Liu R, Lusby CM, et al. Consistency of EEG asymmetry patterns in infants of depressed mothers. Dev Psychobiol. 2021;63:768–81.
62. Poole BD, Gable PA. Affective motivational direction drives asymmetric frontal hemisphere activation. Exp Brain Res. 2014;232:2121–30.
63. Zhu C, Guo X, Jin Z, et al. Influences of brain development and ageing on cortical interactive networks. Clin Neurophysiol. 2011;122:278–83.
64. Harmon-Jones E, Gable PA, Peterson CK. The role of asymmetric frontal cortical activity in emotion-related phenomena: a review and update. Biol Psychol. 2010;84:451–62.
65. Deoni S, Dean D, Joelson S, et al. Early nutrition influences developmental myelination and cognition in infants and young children. NeuroImage. 2018;178:649–59.
66. Ou X, Andres A, Pivik RT, et al. Voxel-based morphometry and fMRI revealed differences in brain gray matter in breastfed and milk formula-fed children. AJNR Am J Neuroradiol. 2016;37:713–9.
67. Isaacs EB, Fischl BR, Quinn BT, et al. Impact of breast milk on intelligence quotient, brain size, and white matter development. Pediatr Res. 2010;67:357–62.
68. Luby JL, Belden AC, Whalen D, et al. Breastfeeding and childhood IQ: the mediating role of gray matter volume. J Am Acad Child Adolesc Psychiatry. 2016;55:367–75.
69. Olsavsky AK, Stoddard J, Erhart A, et al. Reported maternal childhood maltreatment experiences, amygdala activation and functional connectivity to infant cry. Soc Cogn Affect Neurosci. 2021;16:418–27.
70. Ferber SG, Feldman R, Makhoul IR. The development of maternal touch across the first year of life. Early Hum Dev. 2008;84:363–70.

71. Dashraath P, Wong JLJ, Lim MXK, et al. Coronavirus disease 2019 (COVID-19) pandemic and pregnancy. Am J Obstet Gynecol. 2020;222:521–31.
72. Ceulemans M, Foulon V, Ngo E, et al. Mental health status of pregnant and breastfeeding women during the COVID-19 pandemic- A multinational cross-sectional study. Acta Obstet Gynecol Scand. 2021;100:1219–29.
73. Kara B. Could Maternal COVID-19 Disease be a Risk Factor for Neurodevelopmental Disorders in the Child? Turk Arch Pediatr. 2021;56:542–4.
74. Gibbs BG, Forste R, Lybbert E. Breastfeeding, parenting, and infant attachment behaviors. Matern Child Health J. 2018;22:579–88.
75. Schwarzenberg SJ, Georgieff MK. Advocacy for improving nutrition in the first 1000 days to support childhood development and adult health. Pediatrics. 2018;141:e20173716.
76. Simpson EA, Sclafani V, Paukner A, et al. Handling newborn monkeys alters later exploratory, cognitive, and social behaviors. Dev Cogn Neurosci. 2019;35:12–9.
77. Belfort MB, Rifas-Shiman SL, Kleinman KP, et al. Infant breastfeeding duration and mid-childhood executive function, behavior, and social-emotional development. J Dev Behav Pediatr. 2016;37:43–52.
78. Turner S, Mayumi Maruyama J, Matijasevich A, Pastor-Valero M. Breastfeeding and the development of socio-emotional competencies: a systematic review. Breastfeed Med. 2019;14:691–704.
79. Krol KM, Monakhov M, Lai PS, et al. Genetic variation in CD38 and breastfeeding experience interact to impact infants' attention to social eye cues. Proc Natl Acad Sci U S A. 2015;112:E5434–42.
80. Fujiwara T, Morisaki N, Honda Y, et al. Chemicals, nutrition, and autism spectrum disorder: a mini-review. Front Neurosci. 2016;10:174.
81. Ng M, de Montigny JG, Ofner M, Do MT. Environmental factors associated with autism spectrum disorder: a scoping review for the years 2003-2013. Health Promot Chronic Dis Prev Can. 2017;37:1–23.
82. Huang S, Wang X, Sun T, et al. Association of breastfeeding for the first six months of life and autism spectrum disorders: a national multi-center study in China. Nutrients. 2021;14:45.
83. Ghozy S, Tran L, Naveed S, et al. Association of breastfeeding status with risk of autism spectrum disorder: a systematic review, dose-response analysis and meta-analysis. Asian J Psychiatr. 2020;48:101916.
84. Dodds L, Fell DB, Shea S, et al. The role of prenatal, obstetric and neonatal factors in the development of autism. J Autism Dev Disord. 2011;41:891–902.
85. Husk JS, Keim SA. Breastfeeding and autism spectrum disorder in the national survey of children's health. Epidemiology. 2015;26:451–7.
86. Lemcke S, Parner ET, Bjerrum M, et al. Early regulation in children who are later diagnosed with autism spectrum disorder. A longitudinal study within the Danish National Birth Cohort. Infant Ment Health J. 2018;39:170–82.
87. Stadler DD, Musser ED, Holton KF, et al. Recalled initiation and duration of maternal breastfeeding among children with and without ADHD in a well characterized case-control sample. J Abnorm Child Psychol. 2016;44:347–55.
88. Mahurin SJ. Breastfeeding and language outcomes: a review of the literature. J Commun Disord. 2015;57:29–40.
89. Diepeveen FB, van Dommelen P, Oudesluys-Murphy AM, Verkerk PH. Specific language impairment is associated with maternal and family factors. Child Care Health Dev. 2017;43:401–5.
90. Patra K, Greene MM, Patel AL, Meier P. Maternal education level predicts cognitive, language, and motor outcome in preterm infants in the second year of life. Am J Perinatol. 2016;33:738–44.
91. Vollmer S, Bommer C, Krishna A, et al. The association of parental education with childhood undernutrition in low- and middle-income countries: comparing the role of paternal and maternal education. Int J Epidemiol. 2017;46:312–23.

92. Pancsofar N, Vernon-Feagans L. Fathers' early contributions to children's language development in families from low-income rural communities. Early Child Res Q. 2010;25:450–63.
93. Vestergaard M, Obel C, Henriksen T, et al. Duration of breastfeeding and developmental milestones during the latter half of infancy. Acta Paediatr. 1999;88:1327–32.
94. Whitehouse AJO, Robinson M, Li J, Oddy WH. Duration of breast feeding and language ability in middle childhood. Paediatr Perinat Epidemiol. 2011;25:44–52.
95. Quinn PJ, O'Callaghan M, Williams GM, et al. The effect of breastfeeding on child development at 5 years: a cohort study. J Paediatr Child Health. 2001;37:465–9.
96. Guzzardi MA, Granziera F, Sanguinetti E, et al. Exclusive breastfeeding predicts higher hearing-language development in girls of preschool age. Nutrients. 2020;12:1–12.
97. Yang S, Martin RM, Oken E, et al. Breastfeeding during infancy and neurocognitive function in adolescence: 16-year follow-up of the PROBIT cluster-randomized trial. PLoS Med. 2018;15(4):e1002554.
98. Cerdó T, Diéguez E, Campoy C. Infant growth, neurodevelopment and gut microbiota during infancy: which nutrients are crucial? Curr Opin Clin Nutr Metab Care. 2019;22:434–41.
99. Dror DK, Allen LH. Overview of nutrients in human milk. Adv Nutr. 2018;9(Suppl 1):278S–94S.
100. Hampel D, Dror DK, Allen LH. Micronutrients in human milk: analytical methods. Adv Nutr. 2018;9(Suppl 1):313S–31S.
101. Hampel D, Allen LH. Analyzing B-vitamins in human milk: methodological approaches. Crit Rev Food Sci Nutr. 2016;56:494–511.
102. Allen LH. B vitamins in breast milk: relative importance of maternal status and intake, and effects on infant status and function. Adv Nutr. 2012;3:362–9.
103. Salem N, Van Dael P. Arachidonic acid in human milk. Nutrients. 2020;12:626.

Breastfeeding in Immune-Mediated Demyelinating Disorders of the Central Nervous System

Tuğçe Damla Dilek, Sema Saltık, and Bülent Kara

1 Introduction

Neuroinflammation refers to the process by which the brain's innate immune system is triggered following an inflammatory challenge such as those caused by injury, infection, exposure to a toxin, neurodegenerative disease, or aging [1].

Neuroinflammatory diseases (NDs) are mainly immune-mediated and present with a wide variety of symptoms such as encephalopathy, seizures, and movement disorders [2]. NDs can be classified as acquired demyelinating diseases, immune-mediated epilepsies, primary rheumatologic conditions with central nervous system (CNS) manifestations, CNS vasculitis, and neurodegenerative/genetic conditions according to the clinical presentation, the pathophysiologic mechanism (antibody-mediated, innate immunity-mediated, etc.) or imaging and laboratory findings [3].

Demyelination refers to the loss of myelin that occurs due to various conditions targeting oligodendroglia or myelin membranes [4]. The immune-mediated demyelinating syndromes of the CNS are a group of acquired diseases and can be roughly divided into two groups, monophasic and multiphasic [5]. Monophasic diseases consist of acute disseminated encephalomyelitis (ADEM) and clinically isolated syndromes (CIS). Multiphasic diseases consist of multiple sclerosis (MS), neuromyelitis optica spectrum disorder (NMO-SD), and diseases associated with myelin-oligodendrocyte glycoprotein antibody (MOGAD) [6].

T. D. Dilek (✉) · S. Saltık
Cerrahpasa Medical Faculty, Division of Pediatric Neurology, Department of Pediatrics, Istanbul University, Istanbul, Türkiye

B. Kara
Faculty of Medicine, Division of Pediatric Neurology, Department of Pediatrics, Kocaeli University, Kocaeli, Türkiye
e-mail: bulent.kara@kocaeli.edu.tr

Ö. N. Şahin et al. (eds.), *Breastfeeding and Metabolic Programming*, https://doi.org/10.1007/978-3-031-33278-4_25

In this section, breastfeeding will be discussed in children whose mothers suffer from immune-mediated demyelinating disorders of the central nervous system. In monophasic diseases, only breastfeeding during acute treatment will be described. Since prophylactic treatment will not be required for these diseases, breastfeeding will not be an issue. In multiphasic diseases, the prophylactic treatment options will be discussed and breastfeeding during these treatments will be mentioned.

2 Monophasic Demyelinating Diseases

2.1 Acute Disseminated Encephalomyelitis (ADEM)

ADEM is a monophasic inflammatory demyelinating disease characterized by encephalopathy and multifocal brain lesions. Neurologic deficits can include ataxia, dysarthria, focal weakness, vision loss due to optic neuritis, and weakness or sensory changes due to spinal cord syndrome [7].

2.2 Clinically Isolated Syndromes (CIS)

Clinically isolated syndromes are another monophasic demyelinating event of CNS. It is usually considered the first presentation of MS. The typical patient with CIS is a young adult with a single episode of central nervous system dysfunction such as unilateral optic neuritis, a focal brain syndrome, a focal brainstem or cerebellar syndrome, or partial myelopathy [8]. Although CIS is limited to only a single attack, multifocal abnormalities can be seen. CIS is clinically indistinguishable from MS but does not fully meet the diagnostic criteria for MS. So, CIS is considered a potential precursor of MS. As the diagnostic criteria for MS have expanded, fewer patients meet the strict criteria for CIS [9].

3 Multiphasic Demyelinating Diseases

3.1 Neuromyelitis Optica Spectrum Disorder (NMO-SD)

NMO-SD is a spectrum of demyelinating diseases with prominent features of optic neuritis (ON) and longitudinally extensive transverse myelitis (LETM) [10]. NMO-SD is often associated with serum aquaporin-4 immunoglobulin G antibodies (AQP4-IgG), which differs from MS. The core findings of patients with NMO-SD include clinical symptoms of the spinal cord, optic nerve, brainstem, diencephalon, area postrema, and other cerebral localizations, and brain and/or spinal cord MRI findings consistent with these symptoms [11]. NMO-SD has a relapsing course. The relapses can lead to vision loss due to ON, weakness, sensory changes, bowel/bladder issues due to LETM, and intractable nausea/vomiting due to area postrema syndrome [12].

Due to the high rate of relapses, prevention therapy should begin as soon as possible. Corticosteroids, azathioprine, mycophenolate mofetil, eculizumab, and rituximab are first-line immunomodulatory drugs [13]. Methotrexate, mitoxantrone, and cyclophosphamide are second-line immunomodulatory drugs [14].

3.2 Myelin-Oligodendrocyte Glycoprotein Antibody-Associated Disease

Myelin-oligodendrocyte glycoprotein antibody-associated disease (MOGAD) is a recently identified autoimmune disorder that leads to CNS demyelination in both adults and children [15]. Although there are clinical phenotypic overlaps between MOGAD, MS, and NMO-SD, discrimination among them is based on neuropathological evidence [16].

Approximately 50% of patients with positive MOG antibodies have relapsing courses and these relapses can occur within a few months or years after the first attack. Long-term treatment regimens including monthly intravenous Immunoglobulin (IVIG), monthly high-dose steroids, mycophenolate mofetil, azathioprine, and rituximab are used in relapsing cases [17].

3.3 Multiple Sclerosis (MS)

MS is the most common chronic autoimmune disorder of the CNS characterized by recurrent inflammation with demyelination and progressive neurodegeneration [18]. MS mostly affects young women of childbearing age and often occurs as a relapsing-remitting disease. In relapses, optic nerve dysfunction, diplopia, dizziness, and weakness or numbness in one extremity are common but may present with the involvement of any part of the central nervous system [19]. MS can also present with slowly progressive symptoms such as gait disorder, bladder/bowel dysfunction, and blindness. Diagnosis is based on the 2017- Mc Donald Criteria [20]. The etiology of MS is unknown. It is believed that genetic and environmental factors may play a role in the etiopathogenesis of MS. Family history, smoking, low vitamin D level, and Epstein-Barr virus exposure can be counted among these factors [21].

Many treatment options have been developed for long-term therapy of MS. These treatment options are broadly subdivided into three categories—injectables, oral medications, and infusions [18]. Interferon-b (IFN-b) and glatiramer acetate are injectable treatment options. Oral treatment options include fingolimod, dimethyl fumarate, and teriflunomide. Monoclonal antibodies such as natalizumab, rituximab, alemtuzumab, ocrelizumab, and ofatumumab are used as infusions in the treatment [22].

MS commonly affects young women of childbearing age, so effect of pregnancy on MS is an important clinical issue. It is observed that the attack rate during pregnancy decreases in women with MS. The underlying mechanism is based on the transition from Th1 to Th2 responses during pregnancy. As a result, the transition from cellular immunity to humoral immunity occurs, and it is known that it returns to its original state after birth. On the other hand, clinical observations showed that the relapse rate in the postpartum period is increased. In the study where 227 patients with MS were followed prospectively, an approximately 70% reduction in relapse rates during the third trimester of pregnancy was shown, and the postpartum relapse rate was found higher than pre-pregnancy [23]. However, it was observed that this temporary increase in relapses subsided over the following postpartum year, and rates returned to baseline pre-pregnancy levels [23]. It is thought that estrogens and other sex hormones activate immunological transformation during pregnancy by shifting T helper cells to mostly Th2 (anti-inflammatory effect), instead of Th 1 (pro-inflammatory effect), while after the delivery immunomodulation is reversed.

In animal studies, neuroprotective effects of sex hormones such as estrogens (17-estradiol (E2) and estriol (E3)), progesterone, and testosterone have been demonstrated in experimental allergic encephalomyelitis (EAE). These results may explain the course of MS during pregnancy [24]. It is thought that delivery may have a proinflammatory impact and this may be valid on also CNS. Recent studies conducted on women with NMO-SD support this idea. It was found that NMO-SD symptoms occur in the first year after pregnancy and the rate of relapse has been shown to increase in the first 6 months [25].

The number of studies investigating the risk of MS relapse in the postdelivery period is very limited, so the information on relapse risk factors in this period is very limited. The effects of factors such as breastfeeding, starting treatment after pregnancy, diet, and vitamin D deficiency are not clear [26]. Luteinizing hormone (LH) levels are low, while prolactin levels are high during breastfeeding. The ovaries are suppressed and lactational amenorrhea occurs [27]. As long as breastfeeding continues at intense and frequent intervals, this hormonal balance is maintained in this way. During the transition to supplementary food, the absorption times will be shortened and the durations will be shortened, and prolactin levels will decrease. Ovarian activity will return to pre-pregnancy and menses will soon resume [28]. It has also been observed that the proinflammatory molecule (TNF)-alpha, which is important in MS, fluctuates during the menstrual period [29]. Not breastfeeding or breastfeeding less frequently may cause earlier periods to return, which may mean returning to a period of more intense pro-inflammatory effects [26].

Studies have shown that relapses decrease in the third trimester of pregnancy, whereas increased relapses occur in the postpartum period [30]. Another study showed that the most important predictor of postpartum relapse risk was the frequency of relapse before pregnancy [31]. The effect of breastfeeding on postpartum relapses has not been demonstrated.

There is no clear information on when to start treatment or when breastfeeding should be interrupted in the postpartum period in MS patients. The patients who have the active disease before pregnancy, restarting disease-modifying treatments (DMTs) could be considered earlier [32]. However, patients with milder MS may also have postpartum relapses. Individual patients and their clinicians must weigh their decision to breastfeed on a case-by-case basis.

4 Breastfeeding in Acute Attack Treatment of Immune-Mediated Demyelinating Disorders of the Central Nervous System

Acute attack treatment modalities include high-dose intravenous corticosteroids, therapeutic plasma exchange, and intravenous immunoglobulin.

4.1 Corticosteroids

Corticosteroids are approved by the United States Food and Drug Administration (FDA) for the treatment of acute exacerbations of MS and other immune-mediated demyelinating disorders [33]. Commonly, high-dose methylprednisolone, which has powerful anti-inflammatory and immunosuppressive activities, is administered. There is limited data about transferring corticosteroids to human milk. Generally, it has been recommended that a breastfeeding mother should discontinue breastfeeding during corticosteroid treatment [34].

The methylprednisolone reaches its maximum level in the first hour after administration and then decreases rapidly in the milk of a mother with MS receiving intravenous methylprednisolone therapy [23]. Similar results have been observed in previous studies and the authors concluded that mothers who received intravenous corticosteroids could breastfeed 2–4 hours after administration [23].

4.2 Intravenous Immunoglobulin (IVIG)

IVIG is another treatment option for MS relapses. In a retrospective study of 108 women with relapsing-remitting MS, 69 of these patients received IVIG in the postpartum period, and no adverse effects were observed in any of these mothers' babies

[35]. Another study designed on 168 mothers with MS who received IVIG treatment in the postpartum period showed no adverse effect in breastfed infants [36]. These studies suggest that IVIG can be used safely in the pregnant and/or breastfeeding mother for MS relapses [37, 38].

5 Breastfeeding in Disease-Modifying Treatments of Immune-Mediated Demyelinating Disorders of the Central Nervous System

There is limited information about disease-modifying treatments (DMTs) in immune-mediated demyelinating disorders regarding the transition to human milk and its effects on the breastfed infant. Very limited numbers of DMTs are licensed for the use during breastfeeding [39]. It is suggested that decisions should be made on an individual basis [39].

The first-line of injectable medications such as interferons and glatiramer acetate is thought as safe during breastfeeding.

5.1 *Interferons*

Interferons are molecules with immunomodulatory, antiviral, and antiproliferative properties that have been used in the first-line therapy of MS for many years [40]. They have large protein sizes and are bound to plasma proteins in the mother's body. It is considered that IFNs are not generally excreted in breast milk. Additionally, IFNs are not orally bioavailable. It is thought that although IFNs pass into breast milk, they will break down and be inactivated in the gastrointestinal tract of the baby. In a study of six women receiving IFN therapy, no significant adverse events occurred in the infants of these mothers [41]. Another study evaluated 39 women using IFNs and breastfeeding their babies [42]. In this study, infants who were exposed to IFNs (median duration 8.5months) were followed in the first year of life and no adverse outcomes were observed. Therefore, breastfeeding of patients with MS receiving IFN therapy is considered to be theoretically safe [42].

According to the European Medicines Agency (EMA) Summaries of Product Characteristics of IFN beta-1a and beta-1b, both can be used during breastfeeding [43]. However, according to the FDA, interferon beta-1a can be used with caution in lactating women, but the use of IFN-1b should be decided by considering how necessary it is for the mother [44, 45].

5.2 Glatiramer Acetate (GA)

GA is a synthetic polypeptide agent used to treat relapsing-remitting MS [18]. It directs the proinflammatory Th1 T cell response to the noninflammatory, regulatory Th2 T cell response. GA is administered as a subcutaneous injection like IFNs. Its molecular weight is also similar to IFNs. In a study conducted on 34 breastfeeding women who received glatiramer acetate, no side effect associated with potential infant exposure to glatiramer acetate was observed [42]. Though GA is considered safe by most experts, studies conducted on large groups are needed [42]. According to FDA, due to a lack of the knowledge about excretion of glatiramer acetate in human milk, caution should be exercised when GA is administered to a breastfeeding woman [46].

5.3 Teriflunomide

Teriflunomide is a small molecule with a molecular weight of 270 Da and is received orally [47]. It shows its effect by selectively and reversibly blocking dihydro-orotate dehydrogenase, which is involved in de novo pyrimidine synthesis, and consequently reduces the proliferation of activated T and B lymphocytes. In animal studies, teriflunomide was found teratogenic and embryotoxic [48]. So, teriflunomide is contraindicated for MS patients planning to conceive. Despite the various guidelines recommending efficient contraception, pregnancies exposed to teriflunomide have been recorded. In a study that analyzed the outcomes of 222 pregnancies occurring during treatment with teriflunomide, maternal death, stillbirth, spontaneous abortions, and birth defects were reported. Since teriflunomide is of small molecular weight, it is considered to have a high potential to pass into the milk, and according to the FDA, the use of teriflunomide in breastfed mothers is contraindicated [48].

5.4 Dimethyl Fumarate

Dimethyl fumarate is a fumaric ester derivative. It is thought to exert its anti-inflammatory effects by reducing CD4+ and CD8+ T cells and adhesion molecules [49]. Its metabolites also have antioxidant effects. In animal studies, high-dose dimethyl fumarate has been shown to cause fetal growth retardation [50]. According to the information at the 2013 Annual Meeting of the American Academy of Neurology, there was no increase in the rates of spontaneous abortion or fetal malformation in the infants of mothers who took dimethyl fumarate during pregnancy. However, due to limited data, it is still not recommended to use dimethyl fumarate during pregnancy. The data on the use of dimethyl fumarate during breastfeeding is also limited. However, monomethyl fumarate, which is the active metabolite of dimethyl fumarate, is thought to be low in breast milk. According to the FDA, caution should be exercised when dimethyl fumarate is administered to a breastfeeding mother [51].

5.5 Fingolimod

Fingolimod is a sphingosine-1-phosphate receptor agonist. It prevents the egress of lymphocytes from lymphoid tissues, thus preventing lymphocyte infiltration into the brain. In July 2019, the EMA updated restrictions for fingolimod use in pregnancy and recommended stopping fingolimod at least 2 months before conception. These updated restrictions were based on previous reports of birth defects (heart, muscles, bone abnormalities, etc.) being twice as high for infants exposed to fingolimod in pregnancy.

It is shown that some women experience severe MS relapses as early as 1–4 months after cessation of fingolimod [52]. To avoid disease reactivation in women desiring pregnancy, switching to natalizumab is recommended before pregnancy [53]. Fingolimod is also concentrated in the breast milk of animals, relative to the blood. Therefore, breastfeeding is not recommended [54].

5.6 Natalizumab

Natalizumab is a large molecular weight IgG4 humanized monoclonal antibody and shows its effect by binding to $\alpha_4\beta_1$-integrin and blocking its interaction with VCAM-1 [55]. Natalizumab is thought to be unable to cross the placental barrier [55]. It is administered as an intravenous infusion once a month. In the studies on pregnant women taking natalizumab, no association was found in terms of major malformations, low birth weight, and premature birth [56]. In a recent study investigating pregnancy outcomes of women with MS using natalizumab in the third trimester, hematological alterations such as anemia and thrombocytopenia were observed in newborns [57]. The British Association of Neurologists' updated 2019 guidance on pregnancy management in MS recommends continuing natalizumab therapy up to 34 weeks of pregnancy for women with high MS activity. In the postpartum period, it is recommended that it is necessary to wait 8–12 weeks to return to treatment. To reduce the exposure, instead of 4-weekly infusions, natalizumab infusions can be reduced to 8-weekly [58]. In terms of breastfeeding, the latest studies show that the concentration of natalizumab in the serum of newborns and breast milk is low. Therefore, breastfeeding under natalizumab is likely to be safe [42]. FDA has suggested no contraindication about natalizumab during breastfeeding [59]. However, it was reported that natalizumab can be detected in human milk and the exact effect of exposure is unknown [60].

5.7 Cladribine

Cladribine is a chlorinated analog of deoxyadenosine. Although it is deactivated in many cell types, it remains active in lymphocytes and induces apoptosis by inhibiting DNA synthesis and repair. As a result, it depletes T and B lymphocytes, while other cell types are protected from the toxic effect [61]. Previous studies showed no congenital malformations in pregnancies that occurred during cladribine treatment or within 6 months after the last dose [62]. Furthermore, a noninterventional post-authorization safety study has been initiated to obtain more information [62]. In a recent case study, the transition of cladribine into human milk was shown in a patient who experienced a relapse 4 months after birth and began cladribine treatment [63]. Although cladribine levels were measured as 281.2 ng/mL at 1 h following a 20-mg dose, it was not detected in the milk samples at 48, 72, and 96 h. According to the FDA breastfeeding during cladribine treatment and until 10 days after the last dose is contraindicated [63].

5.8 Ocrelizumab

Ocrelizumab is a recombinant humanized anti-CD20 monoclonal antibody [62]. It has a large molecular weight and is expected to be in low concentrations in breast milk. There is no data on the presence of ocrelizumab in human milk. There are limited studies about breastfeeding under ocrelizumab treatment. In a recent study, conducted on 6 patients who received anti-CD 20 therapies such as rituximab and ocrelizumab during lactation, the amount of these molecules in breast milk has been determined to be very low [64]. The effect of low breast milk levels of these molecules on the infant is unknown. The FDA reported that the developmental benefits of breastfeeding on the infant should be considered along with the mother's clinical need for ocrelizumab [65].

5.9 Rituximab

Rituximab is a human monoclonal antibody that targets CD20, a B-cell-specific surface antigen [66]. In some studies, the amount of rituximab in the milk was found very low [64]. It is thought to be the result of its high molecular weight. In a study, breast milk samples were collected from 9 women with multiple sclerosis who received rituximab, and it was shown that rituximab had a peak milk concentration 1–7 days after infusion. Rituximab concentration in milk was virtually undetectable by 90 days postinfusion in all women. Breastfed infants experienced no adverse effects during maternal use of rituximab in this study. However, there is insufficient information on the effects of the low amount of rituximab excreted in breast milk on the infant. FDA advises women not to breastfeed during treatment with rituximab and for 6 months after the last dose due to the potential serious adverse reactions of rituximab in breastfed children [67].

5.10 Ofatumumab

Ofatumumab is another anti-CD20 monoclonal antibody used in MS [68]. There is no data about the effect of ofatumumab on breastfed infants. FDA suggests that the developmental and health benefits of breastfeeding should be considered along with the mother's clinical need for ofatumumab treatment [69].

5.11 Alemtuzumab

Alemtuzumab is a humanized IgG1 monoclonal antibody specific for CD52 and is recommended for adults with highly active relapsing-remitting MS [70]. In animal studies, alemtuzumab is detected in milk but there is no clear data in humans [71]. It is thought to be unlikely transferred to breast milk owing to its large molecular weight. FDA suggests that the decision of whether continue or discontinue alemtuzumab should be based according to the mother's need to use this drug [72].

5.12 Methotrexate

Methotrexate is an antagonist of folic acid, which plays an important role in DNA synthesis and cell proliferation [73]. In animal studies, it has been shown to cause many malformations such as the cleft palate and spina bifida. It is contraindicated during pregnancy due to its teratogenic effects [74]. Information on the use of methotrexate during breastfeeding is limited. No information is available on the effects of methotrexate on a breastfed infant or milk production. Due to potentially serious side effects, including myelosuppression, the FDA recommends that women not breastfeed during methotrexate therapy [75].

5.13 Mitoxantrone

Mitoxantrone is an antineoplastic antibiotic that is used in the treatment of leukemia, lymphoma, and prostate and breast cancer, but also for late-stage, severe multiple sclerosis [76]. The FDA reports that it can cause fetal harm when administered to a pregnant woman [77]. Mitoxantrone is excreted in human milk. Breastfeeding is not recommended during mitoxantrone treatment due to its potential serious adverse reactions [77].

5.14   Cyclophosphamide

Cyclophosphamide is another antineoplastic drug that can be used in demyelinating diseases [78]. It appears to be high in human milk and is considered that it has highly toxic active metabolites for the infant [79]. In some studies, neutropenia, thrombocytopenia, low hemoglobin, and diarrhea are observed in infants breastfed by women treated with cyclophosphamide. It may take 6 weeks for milk levels to drop to a safe level after a dose of cyclophosphamide [80, 81]. FDA recommends discontinuing breastfeeding during cyclophosphamide therapy [80, 81].

5.15   Mycophenolate Mofetil (MM)

MM is an anti-inflammatory agent that can be used in many inflammatory diseases [79]. It is the precursor of mycophenolic acid and inhibits the proliferation of T and B lymphocytes by inhibiting inosine-5′-monophosphate dehydrogenase, preferentially by depleting guanosine nucleosides in T and B lymphocytes. Animal studies showed that MM was excreted in the milk [82]. A few infants have been reported being breastfed during MM treatment, and no adverse effect was observed [80]. Nevertheless, due to limited data on using MM treatment during breastfeeding, FDA recommends discontinuing breastfeeding during MM treatment [83].

5.16   Azathioprine

Azathioprine is a purine analog that can be used as an immunosuppressive agent in autoimmune diseases [84]. It is a purine metabolism antagonist, and it is thought to inhibit DNA, RNA, and protein synthesis, thereby inhibiting T and B cells. In some studies, azathioprine is found in breast milk. Due to its potential side effects such as tumorigenicity, FDA does not recommend continuing azathioprine during breastfeeding [85, 86].

6   Conclusion

The drugs used in the treatment of acute attacks in acquired demyelinating diseases have not been shown to have a toxic effect on the mother or infant in the pregnancy and lactation periods; therefore, it is thought that there is no harm in their use. There is not enough information about plasmapheresis. Recommendations for the use of DMTs in acquired demyelinating diseases requiring long-term, preventive treatment during pregnancy, and lactation vary according to the drug.

Although there is a significant decrease in the frequency of relapses during pregnancy, it is known that the frequency of relapses in the lactation period is more common than in the pre-pregnancy period in women with MS. Therefore, it is important to prevent attacks during lactation with high disease activity of MS. The possible toxic effects of DMTs used in the treatment of MS in breastfeeding women on the infant play a role in determining the drugs to be chosen for treatment. Drugs that are safe for use in breastfeeding women with MS are limited to interferons and natalizumab. Oral disease-modifying drugs are not recommended for use during pregnancy and lactation. Although the effects of CD20 and CD52-targeted monoclonal antibody treatments on infants in breastfeeding mothers are not well-known, it is suggested that they can be used by considering the benefits and harms for the mother and infant. In conclusion, the balance between not depriving the infant of the potential benefits of breastfeeding and keeping the mother under control with safe DMTs due to the increased risk of relapse during lactation needs to be well discussed.

References

1. Heneka MT, Kummer MP, Latz E. Innate immune activation in neurodegenerative disease. Nat Rev Immunol. 2014;14:463–77.
2. Walker AK, Kavelaars A, Heijnen CJ, Dantzer R. Neuroinflammation and comorbidity of pain and depression. Pharmacol Rev. 2014;66:80–101.
3. Malani SN, Lotze TE, Muscal E. Inflammatory diseases of the central nervous system. Neurol Clin. 2021;39:811–28.
4. Höftberger R, Lassmann H. Inflammatory demyelinating diseases of the central nervous system. Handb Clin Neurol. 2017;145:263–83.
5. Longoni G, Deborah ML, Ann EY. The changing landscape of childhood inflammatory central nervous system disorders. J Pediatr. 2016;179:24–32.
6. Popescu BF, Lucchinetti CF. Pathology of demyelinating diseases. Annu Rev Pathol. 2012;7:185–217.
7. Wang CX. Assessment and management of acute disseminated encephalomyelitis (ADEM) in the pediatric patient. Paediatr Drugs. 2021;23:213–21.
8. Miller DH, Chard DT, Ciccarelli O. Clinically isolated syndromes. Lancet Neurol. 2012;11:157–69.
9. Thompson AJ, Banwell BL, Barkhof F, et al. Diagnosis of multiple sclerosis: 2017 revisions of the McDonald criteria. Lancet Neurol. 2018;17:162–73.
10. Waliszewska-Prosół M, Chojdak-Łukasiewicz J, Budrewicz S, Pokryszko-Dragan A. Neuromyelitis optica spectrum disorder treatment- Current and future prospects. Int J Mol Sci. 2021;22:2801.
11. Malani Shukla N, Lotze TE, Muscal E. Inflammatory diseases of the central nervous system. Neurol Clin. 2021;39:811–28.
12. Wingerchuk DM, Banwell B, Bennett JL, et al. International consensus diagnostic criteria for neuromyelitis optica spectrum disorders. Neurology. 2015;85:177–89.
13. Trebst C, Jarius S, Berthele A, et al. Update on the diagnosis and treatment of neuromyelitis optica: recommendations of the Neuromyelitis Optica Study Group (NEMOS). J Neurol. 2014;261:1–16.
14. Chan KH, Lee CY. Treatment of neuromyelitis optica spectrum disorders. Int J Mol Sci. 2021;22:8638.

15. Huda S, Whittam D, Bhojak M, Chamberlain J, Noonan C, Jacob A. Neuromyelitis optica spectrum disorders. Clin Med (Lond). 2019;19:169–76.
16. Marignier R, Hacohen Y, Cobo-Calvo A, et al. Myelin-oligodendrocyte glycoprotein antibody-associated disease. Lancet Neurol. 2021;20:762–72.
17. Hacohen Y, Banwell B. Treatment approaches for MOG-Ab-associated demyelination in children. Curr Treat Options Neurol. 2019;21:2.
18. Doshi A, Chataway J. Multiple sclerosis, a treatable disease. Clin Med (Lond). 2016;16(Suppl 6):s53–9.
19. Filippi M, Bar-Or A, Piehl F, et al. Multiple sclerosis. Nat Rev Dis Primers. 2018;4:43.
20. Yamout BI, Alroughani R. Multiple sclerosis. Semin Neurol. 2018;38:212–25.
21. Amato MP, Derfuss T, Hemmer B, et al. Environmental modifiable risk factors for multiple sclerosis: report from the 2016 ECTRIMS focused workshop. Mult Scler. 2018;24:590–603.
22. Scolding N, Barnes D, Cader S, et al. Association of British Neurologists: revised (2015) guidelines for prescribing disease-modifying treatments in multiple sclerosis. Pract Neurol. 2015;15:273–9.
23. Voskuhl R, Momtazee C. Pregnancy: Effect on multiple sclerosis, treatment considerations, and breastfeeding. Neurotherapeutics. 2017;14:974–84.
24. Mendibe Bilbao M, Boyero Durán S, Bárcena Llona J, Rodriguez-Antigüedad A. Multiple sclerosis: Pregnancy and women's health issues. Neurologia (Engl Ed). 2019;34:259–69.
25. Langer-Gould A, Beaber BE. Effects of pregnancy and breastfeeding on the multiple sclerosis disease course. Clin Immunol. 2013;149:244–50.
26. Langer-Gould AM. Pregnancy and family planning in multiple sclerosis. Continuum (Minneap Minn). 2019;25:773–92.
27. Zhang F, Xia H, Shen M, et al. Are prolactin levels linked to suction pressure? Breastfeed Med. 2016;11:461–8.
28. Vieira Borba V, Shoenfeld Y. Prolactin, autoimmunity, and motherhood: when should women avoid breastfeeding? Clin Rheumatol. 2019;38:1263–70.
29. Chakravarty EF, Murray ER, Kelman A, Farmer P. Pregnancy outcomes after maternal exposure to rituximab. Blood. 2011;117:1499–506.
30. Confavreux C, Hutchinson M, Hours MM, Cortinovis-Tourniaire P, Moreau T. Rate of pregnancy-related relapse in multiple sclerosis. Pregnancy in multiple sclerosis group. N Engl J Med. 1998;339:285–91.
31. Vukusic S, Michel L, Leguy S, Lebrun-Frenay C. Pregnancy with multiple sclerosis. Rev Neurol (Paris). 2021;177:180–94.
32. Miller DH, Fazekas F, Montalban X, Reingold SC, Trojano M. Pregnancy, sex and hormonal factors in multiple sclerosis. Mult Scler. 2014;20:527–36.
33. Le Page E, Veillard D, Laplaud DA, et al. Oral versus intravenous high-dose methylprednisolone for treatment of relapses in patients with multiple sclerosis (COPOUSEP): a randomised, controlled, double-blind, non-inferiority trial. Lancet. 2015;386:974–81.
34. Cooper SD, Felkins K, Baker TE, Hale TW. Transfer of methylprednisolone into breast milk in a mother with multiple sclerosis. J Hum Lact. 2015;31:237–9.
35. Achiron A, Kishner I, Dolev M, et al. Effect of intravenous immunoglobulin treatment on pregnancy and postpartum-related relapses in multiple sclerosis. J Neurol. 2004;251:1133–7.
36. Haas J, Hommes OR. A dose comparison study of IVIG in postpartum relapsing-remitting multiple sclerosis. Mult Scler. 2007;13:900–8.
37. Argyriou AA, Makris N. Multiple sclerosis and reproductive risks in women. Reprod Sci. 2008;15:755–64.
38. United States Food and Drug Administration. Octagam 10% liquid solution for intravenous administration. https://www.fda.gov/media/70911/download. Accessed Mar 2022.
39. Portaccio E, Amato MP. Breastfeeding and post-partum relapses in multiple sclerosis patients. Mult Scler. 2019;25:1211–6.

40. Chiang J, Gloff CA, Yoshizawa CN, Williams GJ. Pharmacokinetics of recombinant human interferon-beta ser in healthy volunteers and its effect on serum neopterin. Pharm Res. 1993;10:567–72.

41. Hale TW, Siddiqui AA, Baker TE. Transfer of interferon β-1a into human breastmilk. Breastfeed Med. 2012;7:123–5.

42. Ciplea AI, Langer-Gould A, Stahl A, et al. Safety of potential breast milk exposure to IFN-B or glatiramer acetate: one-year infant outcomes. Neurol Neuroimmunol Neuroinflamm. 2020;7:e757.

43. United States Food and Drug Administration. Interferon beta-1a: Summary of product characteristics. March 2009, https://www.Ema.Europa.Eu/En/Documents/Product-Information/Avonex-Epar-Product-Information_En.Pdf. Accessed 19 Dec 2019.

44. United States Food and Drug Administration. REBIF: Prescribing information. July 2019, https://www.accessdata.fda.gov/drugsatfda_docs/label/2019/103780s5204lbl.pdf. Accessed July 2019.

45. United States Food and Drug Administration. Interferon beta-1b, Betaseron. March 2003, https://www.accessdata.fda.gov/drugsatfda_docs/label/2003/ifnbchi031403lb.pdf. Accessed Nov 2005.

46. United States Food and Drug Administration. COPAXONE: Prescribing information. January 2018, https://www.accessdata.fda.gov/drugsatfda_docs/label/2018/020622s102lbl.pdf. Accessed Jan 2018.

47. Varytė G, Arlauskienė A, Ramašauskaitė D. Pregnancy and multiple sclerosis: an update. Curr Opin Obstet Gynecol. 2021;33:378–83.

48. US Food and Drug Administration. Aubagio: Prescribing information. June 2016, https://www.accessdata.fda.gov/drugsatfda_docs/label/2016/202992s003lbl.pdf. Accessed June 2016.

49. Hart FM, Bainbridge J. Current and emerging treatment of multiple sclerosis. Am J Manag Care. 2016:159–70.

50. Gold R, Phillips JT, Havrdova E, et al. Delayed-release dimethyl fumarate and pregnancy: preclinical studies and pregnancy outcomes from clinical trials and postmarketing experience. Neurol Ther. 2015;4(2):93–104.

51. United States Food and Drug Administration. TECFIDERA (Dimethyl fumarate): Prescribing information. March 2013, https://www.accessdata.fda.gov/drugsatfda_docs/label/2013/204063lbl.pdf. Accessed Mar 2013.

52. Meinl I, Havla J, Hohlfeld R, Kümpfel T. Recurrence of disease activity during pregnancy after cessation of fingolimod in multiple sclerosis. Mult Scler. 2018;24:991–4.

53. Alroughani R, Inshasi J, Al-Asmi A, et al. Disease-modifying drugs and family planning in people with multiple sclerosis: a consensus narrative review from the Gulf Region. Neurol Ther. 2020;9:265–80.

54. Alroughani R, Altintas A, Jumah MA, et al. Pregnancy and the use disease-modifying therapies in patients with multiple sclerosis: benefits versus risks. Mult Scler Int. 2016;2016:1034912.

55. European Summary of Product Characteristics Publishing: Tysabri (natalizumab). 2019, https://www.medicines.org.uk/emc/product/222. Accessed 14 Mar 2021.

56. Ebrahimi N, Herbstritt S, Gold R, Amezcua L, Koren G, Hellwig K. Pregnancy and fetal outcomes following natalizumab exposure in pregnancy. A prospective, controlled observational study. Mult Scler. 2015;21:198–205.

57. Triplett JD, Vijayan S, Rajanayagam S, Tuch P, Kermode AG. Pregnancy outcomes amongst multiple sclerosis females with third trimester natalizumab use. Mult Scler Relat Disord. 2020;40:101961.

58. Dobson R, Dassan P, Roberts M, Giovannoni G, Nelson-Piercy C, Brex PA. UK consensus on pregnancy in multiple sclerosis: 'Association of British Neurologists' guidelines. Pract Neurol. 2019;19:106–14.

59. National Institute of Child Health and Human Development. Drugs and Lactation Database (LactMed®). Natalizumab. 2006, https://www.ncbi.nlm.nih.gov/sites/books/NBK501613. Accessed May 2022.

60. United States Food and Drug Administration. Tysabri: Prescribing information. January 2012, https://www.accessdata.fda.gov/drugsatfda_docs/label/2012/125104s0576lbl.pdf. Accessed Jan 2012.
61. United States Food and Drug Administration. Cladribine: Prescribing information. 2019, https://www.accessdata.fda.gov/drugsatfda_docs/label/2019/022561s000lbl.pdf. Accessed Mar 2021.
62. Giovannoni G, Galazka A, Schick R, et al. Pregnancy outcomes during the clinical development program of cladribine in multiple sclerosis: an integrated analysis of safety. Drug Saf. 2020;43:635–43.
63. United States Food and Drug Administration. MAVENCLAD: Prescribing information. April 2019, https://www.accessdata.fda.gov/drugsatfda_docs/label/2019/022561s000lbl.pdf. Accessed April 2019
64. Varytė G, Zakarevičienė J, Ramašauskaitė D, et al. Pregnancy and multiple sclerosis: An update on the disease modifying treatment strategy and a review of pregnancy's impact on disease activity. Medicina (Kaunas). 2020;56:49.
65. United States Food and Drug Administration. OKREVUS: Prescribing information. March 2017, https://www.accessdata.fda.gov/drugsatfda_docs/label/2017/761053lbl.pdf. Accessed March 2017.
66. RITUXAN (Rituximab) injection for intravenous use. Full prescribing information. September 2019, www.gene.com/download/pdf/rituxan_prescribing.pd. Accessed Sept 2019.
67. United States Food and Drug Administration. RITUXAN: Prescribing information. June 2021, https://www.accessdata.fda.gov/drugsatfda_docs/label/2021/103705s5464lbl.pdf. Accessed June 2021.
68. Hauser SL, Bar-Or A, Cohen JA, et al. ASCLEPIOS I and ASCLEPIOS II Trial Groups. Ofatumumab versus Teriflunomide in Multiple Sclerosis. N Engl J Med. 2020;383:546–57.
69. United States Food and Drug Administration. KESIMPTA: Prescribing information. August 2020, https://www.accessdata.fda.gov/drugsatfda_docs/label/2020/125326s070lbl.pdf. Accessed August 2020.
70. Syed YY. Alemtuzumab: A review in relapsing remitting multiple sclerosis. Drugs. 2021;81:157–68.
71. National Institute of Child Health and Human Development. Drugs and Lactation Database (LactMed®). Alemtuzumab. 2006, https://www.ncbi.nlm.nih.gov/books/NBK501803/. Accessed 15 Feb 2023.
72. United States Food and Drug Administration. LEMTRADA: Prescribing information November 2017, https://www.accessdata.fda.gov/drugsatfda_docs/label/2017/103948s5158lbl.pdf. Accessed 2017.
73. Gray OM, McDonnell GV, Forbes RB. A systematic review of oral methotrexate for multiple sclerosis. Mult Scler. 2006;12:507–10.
74. Milunsky A, Graef JW, Gaynor MF. Methotrexate induced congenital malformations. J Pediatr. 1968;72:790–5.
75. United States Food and Drug Administration. REDITREX: Prescribing information. December 2019, https://www.accessdata.fda.gov/drugsatfda_docs/label/2019/210737s000lbl.pdf. Accessed Dec 2019.
76. Evison BJ, Sleebs BE, Watson KG, Phillips DR, Cutts SM. Mitoxantrone, more than just another topoisomerase II poison. Med Res Rev. 2016;36:248–99.
77. United States Food and Drug Administration. NOVANTRONE: Prescribing information. June 2010, https://www.accessdata.fda.gov/drugsatfda_docs/label/2010/019297s033s034lbl.pdf. Accessed June 2019.
78. Patti F, Lo FS. Lights and shadows of cyclophosphamide in the treatment of multiple sclerosis. Autoimmune Dis. 2011;2011:961702.
79. Murthy RK, Theriault RL, Barnett CM, et al. Outcomes of children exposed in utero to chemotherapy for breast cancer. Breast Cancer Res. 2014;16:500.

80. Codacci-Pisanelli G, Honeywell RJ, Asselin N, et al. Breastfeeding during R-CHOP chemotherapy: Please abstain! Eur J Cancer. 2019;119:107–11.
81. United States Food and Drug Administration. CYCLOPHOSPHAMIDE: Prescribing information. May 2013, https://www.accessdata.fda.gov/drugsatfda_docs/label/2013/012141s09 0,012142s112lbl.pdf. Accessed May 2013.
82. Allison AC. Mechanisms of action of mycophenolate mofetil. Lupus. 2005;14(Suppl 1):s2–8.
83. National Institute of Child Health and Human Development. Drugs and Lactation Database (LactMed®). Mycophenolate. 2006, https://www.ncbi.nlm.nih.gov/books/NBK501638/. Accessed 30 Nov 2022.
84. United States Food and Drug Administration. CellCept: Prescribing information. June 2009, https://www.accessdata.fda.gov/drugsatfda_docs/label/2009/050722s021,050723s019,05075 8s019,050759s024lbl.pdf. Accessed June 2009.
85. Casetta I, Iuliano G, Filippini G. Azathioprine for multiple sclerosis. Cochrane Database Syst Rev. 2007;2007:CD003982.
86. United States Food and Drug Administration. IMURAN (azathioprine): Prescribing information. May 2011, https://www.accessdata.fda.gov/drugsatfda_docs/label/2011/016324s034s035lbl.pdf. Accessed May 2011.

Part IV
Breastfeeding and Infections

Role of Breastfeeding in the Prevention of Infectious Diseases

Funda Çipe, Ayşe Engin Arısoy, Emin Sami Arısoy, and Sheldon L. Kaplan

1 Introduction

Neonates live in a protected area in intrauterine life; passing through the birth channel, they are exposed to a broad spectrum of maternal microflora, most of which are harmless, even if they could be defensive. The babies will have resistance against these microflora organisms with the aid of breastfeeding [1, 2].

The newborn's immune system is naïve to extrauterine life and is trained to give responses after the exposure of variable antigens by contact via the respiratory and gastrointestinal tracts [2]. The lymphocytes in human milk are available in limited numbers and specificity. Expansion of T cell functions starts during delivery and continues with exposure to microorganisms in mucosal membranes. Increased T cell numbers after birth migrate over the vast gastrointestinal surface and continue to spread and become more specified [3].

F. Çipe (✉)
Department of Pediatric Allergy-Immunology, Al Qassimi Women's and Children's Hospital, Sharjah, United Arab Emirates

A. E. Arısoy
Division of Neonatology, Department of Pediatrics, Faculty of Medicine, Kocaeli University (Emeritus), Kocaeli, Türkiye

E. S. Arısoy
Division of Pediatric Infectious Diseases, Department of Pediatrics, Faculty of Medicine, Kocaeli University (Emeritus), Kocaeli, Türkiye

S. L. Kaplan
Division of Infectious Diseases, Department of Pediatrics, Baylor College of Medicine, and Infectious Disease Service, Texas Children's Hospital, Houston, TX, USA
e-mail: slkaplan@texaschildrens.org

Ö. N. Şahin et al. (eds.), *Breastfeeding and Metabolic Programming*,
https://doi.org/10.1007/978-3-031-33278-4_26

Studies from high-income countries reported that exclusive breastfeeding for the first 6 months of life and starting other food decrease the risk of common childhood infections [4–8]. While some studies have revealed that breastfeeding protects babies against gastroenteritis and respiratory infections such as acute otitis media, breastfeeding is not as protective for urinary infections and oral thrush [9, 10].

The protective features of breastfeeding have been attributed to the multiple components of human milk, including antibodies and nutritional, immunoregulatory, and immunomodulatory factors regarding defense mechanisms. A World Health Organization (WHO) collaborative study from Ghana showed that infant mortality decreased by 22% in babies who started breastfeeding within the first hour after birth, compared to starting after 3 days [11, 12]. An analysis concluded that promoting breastfeeding could prevent approximately 720 postneonatal deaths annually in the United States of America (USA) [13].

Among the death causes in infancy, gastroenteritis is one of the most common. Exclusive breastfeeding for 6 months is associated with less gastroenteritis than for 3 months of breastfeeding [14]. It was also reported that the death rate due to diarrhea could be decreased to 14–24 times less if the babies were exclusively breastfeeding compared to the infants receiving supplementary foods [15]. The protective feature of breast milk against recurrent wheezing, upper respiratory tract infections, otitis media, pneumonia, and measles has been demonstrated in various studies when babies were exclusively breastfed for the first 4–6 months compared to those who were not [5, 16, 17]. A Spanish study reported that exclusive breastfeeding in the first 4 months reduced hospitalizations by 56% in infancy [7].

The frequency of allergic diseases and upper and lower respiratory tract infections decreases in babies exclusively breastfed for the first 6 months [18, 19]. In two large population-based studies, breastfeeding was found protective against common childhood infections; however, this effect was the greatest when exclusive breastfeeding was given for the first 6 months [20, 21]. Shorter durations could be less protective, and combined breastfeeding with formula had no significant protective effect. It was also concluded that breastfeeding is still very valuable in reducing the frequency of doctor visits and hospitalizations, even though disorders are present such as gastroenteritis and pneumonia.

It is unclear how much breast milk is required to see the anti-infective effects. Giving at least 50 mL of breast milk per kg of body weight per day through the first 4 weeks has been proposed as a threshold amount needed to reduce the sepsis rate in very-low-birth-weight (VLBW; <1500 g) babies [22]. However, giving this volume to extremely premature infants generally may be challenging.

2 The Components of Breast Milk

Breast milk contains several immunological molecules that help the baby's immune system development with the actions of microbiota, antibodies, and immune cells. It also comprises micro-RNAs, oligosaccharides, hormones, bioactive compounds such as growth factors, and antimicrobial peptides like lactoferrin. Breastfeeding helps to develop and differentiate the infant's immune system over the early months of life [23, 24]. Owing to all these immune components, an infant's immune system is educated to tolerate nonharmful antigens, such as in foods and commensal microbes, and develop a strong immune defense against pathogenic microorganisms [25].

Besides these immunological factors, some other features of breast milk also affect the immune system. For instance, fatty acids produced by triglyceride degradation in breast milk have been identified as a primary energy source and significant regulators of immune function and metabolism. This feature is important because 93–97% of breast milk lipids are triglycerides [26].

The breast milk composition depends on the time after delivery. Colostrum is secreted in the first few days, called "gold liquid," and is rich in proteins such as immunoglobulins (Igs). However, breast milk has the highest antibody content by 6 weeks of lactation. Between 3 and 12 months, breast milk contains more calories with fats and carbohydrates to support the infant's growth. By 2 years of age, it becomes again like colostrum rich in proteins and immunological molecules like a boost [23].

2.1 Protein Components

2.1.1 Lactoferrin

Lactoferrin and secretory immunoglobulin A (sIgA) account for 26% of the protein content of breast milk. Lactoferrin, an essential glycoprotein encompassing 690 amino acid residues, is contained in colostrum at about 5–7 g/L, while more than 1–3 g/L in mature milk [27]. However, over time, higher lactoferrin levels are maintained in the mothers' breast milk of premature newborns [28, 29].

Lactoferrin belongs to the transferrin protein family and has two subunits binding iron (Fe). Lactoferrin binds ferric iron (Fe^{+3}) with high affinity. Human lactoferrin is released from neutrophils (15 $\mu g/10^6$ neutrophils) at the site of infection and all exocrine glands and functions as a part of innate immunity [30]. A particular receptor is present on the intestinal surfaces for lactoferrin and its derivatives [31]. Lactoferricin, produced after gastric digestion from the N-terminus of lactoferrin, also has an antipathogenic effect [32]. Lactoferrin and lactoferricin function to increase the number of *Bifidobacteria* and *Lactobacillus* species in breast milk [33].

Lactoferrin has immunomodulatory and anti-inflammatory functions and antibacterial, antiviral, and antifungal features. Lactoferrin also increases the release of inflammatory cytokines such as interleukin (IL)-1 beta (IL-1β), tumor necrosis factor-alpha (TNFα), IL-6, and IL-8; however, it blocks transcription of the *nuclear factor kappa-light-chain-enhancer of activated B cells* (NF-ƙB). It seems beneficial in preventing infections and suppressing the inflammatory response [34]. Its anti-inflammatory effects also occur by entering the host cell via endocytosis and migrating to the nucleus to cause decreased proinflammatory cytokine gene expression [35, 36].

2.1.2 Immunoglobulins

Antibodies against numerous microorganisms exist in breast milk, representing the mother's immunological memory [25]. Breastfeeding provides passive immunity to infants by the transfer of Igs. Although only IgG can cross the placenta, all different Ig groups (IgA, IgG, IgM, IgE) are present in breast milk, with the predominancy of sIgA (80–90%); the secretory IgM concentration is the second highest after IgA [37].

Secretory IgA is the most substantial Ig found in breast milk regarding its highest concentration and biological functions [27]. Secretory IgA, found in approximately 12 g/L in colostrum, 0.5–1 g/L in the milk of later days, blocks the binding of microorganisms to the mucosal surfaces by binding itself to them without consuming energy during this reaction [38]. After exposure to microflora and pathogenic microorganisms, the mother's lymphoid cells in the Peyer's patches in the gut move to different mucosal surfaces and produce the sIgA antibodies against these microorganisms. Thus, breast milk contains sIgA antibodies against the mother's gastrointestinal microflora, a process named the "enteromammarian link" [9]. The existing commensal bacteria in breast milk also might promote plasma cells to produce sIgA and thus resistance against colonization by pathogens [39].

Secretory IgA of breast milk remains stable after digestion in the newborn's gastrointestinal tract; its effects continue, such as the capability to bind microbes, toxins, and other antigenic molecules like lipopolysaccharide [25]. Secretory IgA can also inhibit the activation of the other Igs, such as IgM and IgG; therefore, it blocks the complement system from being activated and the production of the proinflammatory cytokines indirectly [40].

Breastfeeding immediately after delivery provides the newborn sIgA-mediated immunity [12]. Correlation between the IgA levels and IL-6, IL-10, and transforming growth factor-beta (TGF-β) concentrations in breast milk has been reported. Increased IgA is also protective against the development of allergic diseases, especially milk allergy [41]. Exclusive breastfeeding may be required to acquire significant protection against infectious illnesses because findings suggest that a threshold level may exist for the passive immunity provided by maternal sIgA and other protective compounds in breast milk to the infant [42].

In addition to sIgA and IgA, IgM is the second-highest immunoglobulin in breast milk at a concentration of up to 2.5 mg/mL in colostrum. Both have elevated binding capacity to viruses and bacteria to protect mucosal surfaces and have roles in pathogen agglutination. This function helps the development of the baby's adaptive immunity after B cell activation [43, 44]. Selective IgA-deficient patients show higher concentrations of secretory IgM (sIgM) antibodies in breast milk and compensate for the absence of sIgA at mucosal surfaces [45].

Immunoglobulin G is found in breast milk at a concentration of about 0.1 ± 0.03 g/L, approximately 1% of serum values. Compared to other immunoglobulins, this percentage is low. Immunoglobulin G has many roles in opsonization, complement activation, antibody-dependent cytotoxicity, and neutralizing antibody function [44]. Immunoglobulin G antibodies in breast milk do not inhibit vaccine responses, unlike the transplacentally transferred IgG antibodies; on the contrary, breast milk supports the immune response to vaccines [17, 46].

2.1.3 Other Protein Components

Whey proteins and casein are among the essential components of breast milk. While the whey protein part is more liquid and easier to digest, casein is thicker and can make some lumps in the baby's stomach. Protein varieties containing at least 20 different free amino acids, which have effects on the growth of the immune system, have been defined in breast milk. In addition, breast milk comprises elastase carboxypeptidase B2, kallikrein, thrombin, cathepsin D, and plasmin members of innate proteases and their inhibitors. These are usually active molecules and cause the degradation of milk proteins [23, 47].

Osteoprotegerin, a product of epithelial cells of mammary tissue, is found in breast milk almost 1000 times more than in blood. Osteoprotegerin shows features binding to TNF-related apoptosis-inducing ligand, afterward stimulating caspase-dependent apoptosis; the immunologic reaction is essential in balancing T helper (Th) 1/Th 2 cell response [48].

2.2 Carbohydrate Components

2.2.1 Oligosaccharides

Breast milk also contains glycoproteins, oligosaccharides, and glycolipids in varying amounts. Oligosaccharides are present highly in terms of amount in breast milk after lactose and fats. Mammarian glands produce 90 different types of oligosaccharides. It appears the baby's intestinal microbiota is also affected by these oligosaccharides [49].

Most microbes bind to carbohydrate structures on the mucosal cell membranes to infect the host. The oligosaccharides in breast milk function as receptor agonists, block microbial attachment to mucosal surfaces, and cover the sites to which microorganisms could bind [40, 50]. With this critical function, oligosaccharides prevent the infant's intestinal mucosa from disease-triggering organisms in the gastrointestinal tract [51].

The oligosaccharides have also been described as containing tolerogenic factors that affect human dendritic cells and modulate the augmentation of the immune system in the newborn [52].

Prebiotics are essential for infant intestinal microbiota development. Recently breast milk oligosaccharides have been shown to function as prebiotics by using the metabolism of resident microflora in the gut to produce short-chain fatty acids [53].

2.3   Lipid Components

In stored milk, until at least after the first two days at 4 °C, antiviral activity does not happen; in contrast, in the stomach, the enzymatic process of fatty acid release by lipases is more rapid [54]. Lipoprotein lipase function is high, especially in stored milk triglycerides. Fragmentation of cellular and viral membranes by fatty acids makes breast milk to have antimicrobial effects against enveloped viruses. Linoleic acid is another milk lipid content that contributes to cell lysis [54]. The membrane destabilizing effect of free fatty acids makes breast milk antimicrobial; therefore, viral spread from mother to baby via breastfeeding and the vertical spread of pathogens during delivery is reduced. Breast milk lipids could also be modified in the gastrointestinal tract to be used on mucosal surfaces [54, 55].

2.4   Immune Cells

Lactocytes, mammary stem cells, epithelial cells, and leukocytes are significant residents of breast milk, which differs from other body fluids [56]. Most leukocytes are neutrophils and macrophages, around 80%, and are found in higher numbers in colostrum and then decrease. Thus, mature milk contains only 2% of the number of leukocytes found in colostrum [57]. Besides epithelial cells, macrophages, and neutrophils, different lymphocytes subsets have also been studied, mainly showing CD3+ T cells, CD4+ and CD8+ cells in equal amounts, natural killer (NK) cells, Tγδ + cells, and B cells are in lower numbers [38].

Regarding lymphocyte subsets, T cells (~85%) are predominant cells when compared to B cells in breast milk obtained 0–45 days after birth (~4%) [57]. Breast milk CD4+ T cells show CD45RO expression related to T cell memory and are found in a stimulated situation [25]. Similar to T cells, B cells of breast milk are mainly CD27+ IgD- switched memory cells responsible for releasing immunoglobulins after stimulation of plasma cells [58]. The proportion could differ according to the time breast milk is collected. Probiotic supplementation to pregnant women increases IL-6 release by stimulating IgG and IgA, indirectly contributing to the development of the immune system [57, 59].

Scurfin, also known as forkhead box P3 (FOXP3), is a protein involved in immune system responses as a member of the FOX protein family. FOXP3 appears to function as a master regulator of the regulatory pathway in the development and function of regulatory T (Treg) cells. *The* FOXP3+ *Treg cells, naturally expressing the transcription factor* FOXP3, *are critical in maintaining immune tolerance and homeostasis of the immune system.* Exosomes have been reported to inhibit the release of IL-2 and interferon-γ induced by T cells [60]. The FOXP3+ CD4+ CD25+ Treg cells were reported as high after the stimulation of milk-derived exosomes in infants [61]. So, breast milk exosomes and FOXP3+ T cells act together to maintain immunologic balance in the baby. Shaping the thymus and helping T-cell development can also be performed by breast milk to contribute to adaptive immunity [62, 63]. A decrease in CD4 and CD8 levels was detected in infants after ceasing breastfeeding [62].

2.5 Cytokines, Soluble Receptors, and Anti-Inflammatory Factors

Breast milk also includes immunomodulatory factors such as growth factors (epidermal growth factor [EGF], insulin-like growth factor [IGF] 1 and II), cytokines, soluble receptors, vitamins, and CXC chemokines (CXCL8, CCL2, CCL5, and CXCL10). All have significant roles in expanding an infant's gastrointestinal immune system [64]. Many of these molecules are produced by immune cells in breast milk and cells in the mammary glands, while others come from the mother's bloodstream. Interleukin-6, transforming growth factor-beta (TGF-β), soluble CD14 (sCD14), and IL-10 were reported to be helpful in the tolerance mechanisms against foods [65]. CXC chemokines are small proteins; CXC refers to the location of the two cysteine residues near the N-terminal, with the X representing any amino acid. Levels of CXC chemokines are also high in breast milk; they act as initiators of neutrophil functions and the chemotaxis of intraepithelial lymphocytes [66].

Essential cytokines in human milk, TGF-β1, TGF-β2, and IL-10, downregulate the inflammation [67]. While TGF-β1 is more predominant in the serum, TGF-β2 is more in breast milk; however, both are rare in infant formulas. Transforming growth factor-β is found in breast milk in nonactivated form and is activated by the acidic ingredients of the baby's stomach [68]. Moreover, CD103+ dendritic cells can activate TGF-β and induce Tregs, vital in tolerance development [69]. A report investigating the outcome of cytokines showed that high IgA levels, but not IgM, increased TGF levels in colostrum [70].

Interleukin-10 has an anti-inflammatory effect in breast milk. It shows its effects by blocking Th1 responses, reducing major histocompatibility complex (MHC)-class II expression on monocytes to limit antigen presentation and increase B cells [63]. Interleukin-6 has an anti-inflammatory effect by inducing the production of IgA and follicular T helper cells in the newborn intestine, although it is a well-known pro-inflammatory cytokine [71]. Interleukin-7, related to the thymus, is another cytokine in breast milk. A study showed that the thymus was 2 times larger in breastfed infants than in nonbreastfed infants [72]. Interleukin-7 has been defined as having effects on thymus size and the production of Tγδ lymphocytes from the thymus accumulated in the crypts of intestinal mucosa [73].

Soluble receptors are known as having immunoregulatory effects in breast milk. Breast milk contains numerous soluble innate immune receptors, like soluble Toll-like 2 receptors (sTLR2s), sCD14, receptor antagonists such as IL-1 receptor antagonist protein (IL-1RA), and soluble cytokine receptors such as sTNF-R1, sTNF-R2, sIL-6R. These molecules have a regulatory role in signaling parts of immune response via membrane-bound receptors in newborns [64]. These receptor antagonists might act as competitive antagonists of cytokines, inhibiting them from binding and showing their inflammatory effects [74].

There are also many molecules acting as an anti-inflammatory in breast milk. For instance, the complement system can be blocked by lactoferrin, lysozyme, or α-lactalbumin; prostaglandins inhibit the release of neutrophilic enzymes; some anti-proteases such as α1-antichymotrypsin and α1-antitrypsin inhibit tissue-damaging enzymes [75, 76]. Lysozyme is another enzyme that can bind to the residues of *N*-acetylglucosamine and *N*-acetylmuramic acid of the wall of Gram-positive bacteria and hydrolyses their β-1,4 bonds. Additionally, lysozyme could kill Gram-negative bacteria by acting with lactoferrin and attaching lipopolysaccharide in the bacterial wall [77].

Soluble CD14 levels also are around 20 times serum levels in colostrum and mature milk. Soluble CD14 acts as a coreceptor for TLR2 and TLR4 and facilitates the recognition of their ligands. Soluble CD14 activates phagocytes in the gut via binding to TLR4 of Gram-negative and TLR2 of Gram-positive bacteria wall [78, 79]. It may be concluded that sCD14 modulates intestinal innate and adaptive immunity during the growth of beneficial bacteria in the neonatal intestine [78].

Breast milk contains additional hormones, chemokines, cytokines, and complement-inhibiting, maturation, and growth factors. Most are little in amount, and knowledge about their functions has not been established well [39]. Studies differ with regard to functions and amounts of the cytokines and soluble receptors in breast milk [64].

Breast milk also includes antioxidant molecules because significant oxidative stress emerges from delivery. These molecules abolish free radicals and consequently restrict the harm of oxidative stress. Neutrophils naturally produce hydrogen peroxide as they have catalase, and breast milk works as an antioxidant [80].

Endogenous antioxidants may be defined as either nonenzymatic molecules such as catalase, L-histidine, glutathione, α-tocopherol, β-carotene, ascorbic acid, and lactoferrin, or enzymatic molecules such as catalase superoxide dismutase and glutathione peroxidase or hormones like melatonin. Colostrum has a higher antioxidant capacity compared to mature milk. Antioxidants, immunological, and nutritional properties can be decreased after some processes, such as pasteurization or storage. Carotenoids, vitamins, and polyphenols are antioxidants derived from food and are found in certain amounts in breast milk [81].

Granulocyte colony-stimulating factor (G-CSF), granulocyte-macrophage colony-stimulating factor (GM-CSF), and macrophage colony-stimulating factor (M-CSF) are also detectable in breast milk. They act on milk macrophages and neutrophils in terms of their diversity, expansion, and survival. Their concentrations are much higher in milk than in serum levels [82, 83].

Nucleotides are one of the nonprotein contents in human milk. They might have roles in the immune response by increasing IL-2 production, NK cell activity, iron absorption, bifidobacterium expansion, and gastrointestinal mucosa repair [84].

2.6 Microbiome

Breast milk includes a variety of microorganisms; if a baby receives 800 mL of breast milk in a day, he/she will ingest approximately 1×10^5–1×10^7 bacteria [85]. Lactobacilli, streptococci, staphylococci, *Bifidobacterium*, and *Propionibacterium* are the majority of these microbes. Bacteriophages infect bacteria and cause bacterial cell death, comprising 95% of viruses in infant stool and breast milk [86]. The viruses in breast milk have been reported mainly as deoxyribonucleic acid (DNA) viruses with the family of bacteriophages such as Myoviridae, Siphoviridae, and Podoviridae, followed by eucaryotic viruses such as Herpesviridae [87, 88].

Even before pregnancy and lactation, bacteria are found in the mammary tissue; however, during breastfeeding, infants continue to take some other microbes orally to their gastrointestinal system, which have an essential role in the healthy immune response. On the other hand, infants will also ingest maternal skin and oral cavity microbiome by breastfeeding. So, breastfeeding is a critical source of infant microbiota [87, 88].

The microbiota has been defined as having 2–18 taxa in main breast milk, though it varies regarding the methodologies and the population of the studies; it is likely to be affected by geographic and lifestyle factors such as health condition, mother's diet, weight, lactation stage, way of delivery, and antibiotic usage [23, 89]. Breast milk of mothers living in rural areas seems more diverse than that in urban sites [90]. However, studies have shown that *Bifidobacterium* has the highest level among all species in breastfed baby's intestines, as the oligosaccharides in breast milk are nutrients for this bacterium [91]. In contrast, formula-fed infants show *more Bacteroides*, *Firmicutes*, *Eubacterium, and Veillonella* in their gut [92].

All previous reports propose that microbiota in breast milk colonize infants' gastrointestinal microbiomes. The human gastrointestinal microbiota plays an essential part in nutrition, immunity against pathogens, metabolism, and as a hypothesis, even in human behavior and emotion. The transmission of these beneficial microbes to the infant gastrointestinal system contributes to immune tolerance and development by improving intestinal epithelial blockade of the intestine [93, 94].

The diverse composition of breast milk microbiota has not been fully understood yet regarding portions of prokaryotes (archaea) and eukaryotes (fungi). A few studies have reported *Saccharomyces*, *Candida*, and *Malassezia* as the significant fungi found in breast milk [23, 95]. Two species of methanogenic archaea, *Methanobrevibacter oralis* and *Methanobrevibacter smithii,* have been identified in breast milk by genome sequencing [96].

2.7 *Microribonucleic Acids (MicroRNAs)*

Microribonucleic acids (microRNAs, miRNAs), small RNA molecules bundled inside exosomes, have regulatory functions in several gene expressions. Kosaka et al. [97] showed miRNA expression in breast milk in 2010, and subsequent studies identified it as rich [97, 98]. Their expression levels were also high in the first 6 months of lactation. Additionally, these miRNA molecules are not affected by gastric acidity, are absorbed easily by the gastrointestinal system of infants, and have a regulatory role on the immune system in the gut. Breast milk's freeze and thawing processes do not cause denaturation of the miRNAs [97].

High levels of some miRNAs, such as miR-155 and miR-181, have a role in B cell development. Other defined miRNAs have been shown as acting on the activation or proliferation of different immune cells, such as miR-92 and miR-17 on the differentiation of B and T cells and the monocytic cell development, miR-223 on granulocytes proliferation, miR-150, and miR-30b-5p on suppression of B cells and stimulation of some other immune cells, and miR-182-5p on adaptive immunity mediated by T cell [99–103].

Sources and function mechanisms of major breast milk components are summarized in Table 1.

Table 1 Sources and function mechanisms of major breast milk components

Name	Source	Function	Reference
Protein component			
Lactoferrin	Exocrine glands and neutrophils	Blocks transcription of NF-ƙB Induces the production of the pro-inflammatory cytokines IL-1β, TNFα, IL-6, and IL-8 Enters the host cell through receptor-mediated endocytosis and translocates into the nucleus causing down-regulation of proinflammatory cytokine gene expression	[34] [36]
Immunoglobulins Secretory IgA	Entero-mammary link Plasma cells	Blocks binding of microorganisms, toxins, viruses, and other antigens to the mucosal surfaces by binding to them Inhibit the activation of IgM and IgG; therefore, it blocks the complement system from being activated High avidity to viruses and bacteria to Protect mucosal surfaces	[34, 45]
IgM	Plasma cells, mammary blood flow	Have roles in the pathogen agglutination resulting in B cell activation	[40]
IgG	Plasma cells, mammary blood flow		
	Mammary gland epithelial cells	Opsonization, complement activation, and antibody-dependent cytotoxicity Neutralizing antibody function	[40, 43] [40]
Osteoprotegerin		Binding to TNF-related apoptosis-inducing ligand stimulate caspase-dependent apoptosis Balancing of Th1/Th2 cell response	[48]
HAMLET (human alpha-lactalbumin made lethal to tumor cells)		HAMLET	[118]
Carbohydrate components Oligosaccharides	Mammary gland	Act as receptor agonists and prevent microbial adhesion Affect human dendritic cells with its tolerogenic factors	[43, 49] [52]
Lipid Components	Mammary gland	Fragmentation of cellular and viral membranes by fatty acids	[52]

(continued)

Table 1 (continued)

Name	Source	Function	Reference
Immune cells			
CD45RO memory T cells Switched memory B cells	Mammary blood flow mammary blood flow	Adaptive immunity related to T cell memory Secrete antibodies	[25] [58]
Cytokines, soluble (s) receptors, and anti-inflammatory factors	Mammary gland cells, mammary blood flow, immune cells		
TGF-β, IL-10		Tolerance mechanisms to foods Blocking Th1 responses, increasing B cells, and reducing MHC-II expression Regulatory role in signaling parts of immune response via membrane-bound receptors	[66]
IL-6		Inducing the production of IgA and follicular Th cells	[72]
IL-7		Effects on thymus size	[74]
		Stimulate Tγδ lymphocytes output off the thymus	
CXC chemokines		Initiators of neutrophil functions	[67]
		Chemotaxis of intraepithelial lymphocytes	
sIL-6R, sTNF-RI-RII, IL-1RA,		Receptor antagonists act as competitive antagonist inhibits their inflammatory effects	[65, 75]
sCD14, sTLR2		Coreceptor for TLR2 and TLR4	[76]
Prostaglandins		Inhibit the release of neutrophilic enzymes	[76]
α1- antitrypsin, α1-antichymotrypsin		Block tissue-damaging enzymes	[77]
Lysozyme		Bind to the wall of Gram-negative and Gram-positive bacteria	[77]
Antioxidant molecules		Restrict the harm of oxidative stress due to delivery	[80]
Colony-stimulating factors (CSFs)		Functions in the proliferation, differentiation, and survival of milk neutrophils and macrophages	[82, 83]
Nucleotides		Increase iron absorption, NK cell activity, and IL-2 production; expansion of *Bifidobacterium* and repair of the gastrointestinal mucosa	[84]

Table 1   (continued)

Name	Source	Function	Reference
Microbiome	Mammary gland, maternal skin, and gut	Infect bacteria and cause bacterial cell death Colonization of the infant's gastrointestinal microbiome Immune tolerance and maturation by improving intestinal epithelial barrier function	[93, 94]
MicroRNAs (miRNAs)	Maternal mammary	Acts as a regulatory on immune system gene expression	
miR-17 and miR-92 miR-223 miR-150 and miR-30b-5p miR-182-5p miR-181 and miR-155	cells	Regulation of monocyte development and the maturation of B and T cells Granulocytes proliferation Suppression of B cells and activation of several immune cells T cell-mediated immune responses Which have a role in the B cell development	[100] [101] [102, 103] [103] [98]

Ig immunoglobulin, *IL* interleukin, *MHC* major histocompatibility complex, *NF-kB nuclear factor kappa-light-chain-enhancer of activated B cells, NK* natural killer, *TGF-β* transforming growth factor-beta, *Th* T helper, *TLR* Toll-like receptor, *TNF* tumor necrosing factor

3   Antimicrobial Effects

3.1   *Antibacterial Effects*

Almost all molecules in breast milk have been described as having antibacterial effects. Lactoferrin can have bacteriostatic or bactericidal effects on different bacteria with separate mechanisms, which can be iron dependent or independent. Free iron is one of the vital nutrients required for bacteria; iron binding by lactoferrin has a bacteriostatic effect of preventing bacterial growth. Besides, in a low-iron status environment, only beneficial bacteria that need low iron can grow, and lactoferrin indirectly promotes the growth of *Lactobacillus* and *Bifidobacterium* [104]. Lactoferrin also blocks the adherence of *Haemophilus influenzae* and enteropathogenic *Escherichia coli* [105]. Lactoferrin stimulates the secretion of lipopolysaccharide (LPS) by binding to the lipid A of LPS [105]. Regardless of the binding iron, both lactoferrin and its fragments destabilize the wall of many Gram-negative and Gram-positive bacteria. With this action, lysozyme, also found in breast milk, makes bacteria more sensitive to lysis [106]. Lactoferricin, the cationic peptide derivative located in the N-terminal region of lactoferrin, is responsible for bactericidal activity. Lactoferricin is more effective than the whole protein, which has a bacteriostatic effect [107, 108]. In mice with tuberculosis, oral administration of lactoferrin decreased *Mycobacterium tuberculosis* levels and inflammation in the lungs and was associated with a higher percentage of CD8+ and CD4+ cells, NK cells found in regional lymph nodes, and peripheral blood monocytes [109, 110].

Antimicrobial and antibiofilm features of some oligosaccharides in breast milk against *Streptococcus agalactiae* (group B streptococcus; GBS) have been reported; as well known, GBS is one of the most commonly seen bacteria in neonatal infections [111]. Casein in breast milk reduces the mucosal binding of *Actinomyces, Helicobacter pylori,* and streptococci [40, 50].

Because of the immunomodulatory features, lactoferrin supplementation in preterm infants was investigated; however, conflicting results have been reported. In some studies, lactoferrin supplementation reduced late-onset neonatal sepsis and necrotizing enterocolitis (NEC) rates [110, 112]. In contrast, no decrease was noted in others, especially in the incidence of late-onset neonatal sepsis [113, 114]. Secretory IgA in breast milk protects against infections caused by *Giardia lamblia, Vibrio cholerae,* enterotoxigenic *E. coli, Shigella,* and *Campylobacter* [40]. Secretory IgA also helps form a thin biofilm on the intestinal epithelial cells, which can induce microflora placement [115]. It has been shown that IgG2 antibodies in breast milk have long-lasting effects against *H. influenzae* type b, *S. pneumoniae,* live poliovirus vaccination, tetanus, and diphtheria [17, 46].

"Human alpha-lactalbumin made lethal to tumor cells" (HAMLET), a protein–lipid complex in breast milk, has bactericidal activity against some bacteria, including *M. tuberculosis*, *H. influenzae*, and *Streptococcus pneumoniae*. This complex binds to bacterial membranes and causes membrane depolarization [116, 117]. The bactericidal activity is enhanced when it acts together with kinase activity; kinase inhibition can block bacterial death. A recent study showed that HAMLET could kill three diverse types of streptococci by increasing the effects of lincosamides and macrolides more than beta-lactams [118]. These promising results suggest that using HAMLET in combination with antibiotic treatment has a potential role in the treatment.

Breast milk has the effect of decreasing the function of NF-ƙB via IƙBα-related signaling. Therefore, these possible mechanisms in newborns can prevent inflammatory bowel diseases such as NEC [119].

Compared to boys, exclusive breastfeeding in girls can also reduce urinary tract infections (UTIs) [120]. A hypothesis is that the placement of the urinary system in girls is close to the intestinal bacterial flora, which may explain why it is more beneficial in female babies by affecting the gut flora. This protective effect remains beyond 2 years old [121]. Protection from UTIs by breastfeeding has been described as associated with antiadhesive oligosaccharides [121, 122]. Lactoferrin and sIgA antibodies in breast milk contribute to the protective effect in breastfed babies with nonspecific antibacterial effects [120, 122].

A study reported that lactoperoxidase, a glycoprotein, catalyzes the oxidation of thiocyanate in the infant's saliva, triggers hydrogen peroxide production, and forms hypothiocyanate that can kill Gram-negative and Gram-positive bacteria [123]. Lytic forms of bacteriophages in breast milk have also been defined as having a part in the immune defense against bacterial pathogens. Moreover, these phages control the natural bacterial composition of the infant's gastrointestinal microbiota by the active interaction between bifidobacteria and bifidophages [124].

A small subunit of casein, ƙ-casein, inhibits the binding of *H. pylori* to gastric surfaces by showing a receptor-like effect with sialic acid residues [125]. Haptocorrin is another protein found in breast milk in a small amount with the capability to bind to vitamin B12, so bacteria cannot access it to grow [126]. It has also been shown that digested and undigested forms could inhibit enteropathogenic *E. coli* at similar levels.

3.2 Antiviral Features

Innate immunity components of breast milk have a primary role in host defenses, like a barrier against viral damage. Lactoferrin has a substantial role with its anti-inflammatory effects on mucosal surfaces and binding iron. Oligosaccharides also are likely to have effects as imitators of viral receptors and inhibit their attachment to host cells [127]. Additionally, free fatty acids show antiviral activity through their lytic effect [54].

Lactoferrin prevents the entry of viruses into cells, thus preventing the early stages of infection. However, it has been shown that by adding lactoferrin during infections such as rotavirus and human immunodeficiency virus (HIV) infections, antiviral activity continues, suggesting that lactoferrin affects the intracellular steps of virus infection [37, 128]. Whey protein supplementation decreases the clinical manifestations of rotavirus gastroenteritis by modulating immunity to rotavirus [129]. Lactoferrin also has antiviral activity toward both bare and enveloped viruses such as human papillomavirus, HIV, cytomegalovirus (CMV), herpes simplex virus (HSV), calicivirus, hepatitis C virus (HCV), rotavirus, Picornaviridae (poliovirus, enterovirus 71, echovirus 6), adenovirus, parainfluenza virus, respiratory syncytial virus (RSV), influenza A virus, and hepatitis B virus (HBV) [37, 107, 130]. Blockage of the viral entrance into epithelial cells through competition with the negative compounds such as glycosaminoglycans (GAGs) of heparan sulfate and chondroitin sulfate for attaching to receptors on the cell membrane has been reported in several studies [130–132]. The binding of lactoferrin to specific particles of some viruses such as HCV (heparan sulfate, E1, and E2 proteins), RSV (F protein), and HIV (gp120 protein), as well as host epithelial cells also contributes to the antiviral activity of lactoferrin. Valenti et al. [128] described this glycoprotein as "an important brick in the mucosal wall, effective against viral attacks." In one study, lactoferrin showed a dose-dependent inhibitory activity against adenovirus, while α-lactalbumin, mucin, and β-lactoglobulin were ineffective [133]. Other metal ions, besides iron $Fe^{3+,}$ are also bound by lactoferrin and inhibit competitive metal ion saturation. In one experimental study, breast milk fully saturated with ions of zinc, ferric, and manganese had an antiviral effect of inhibiting adenovirus infections via lactoferrin [134].

In the era of the *coronavirus disease 2019 (COVID-19)* pandemic *caused by the* severe acute respiratory syndrome coronavirus 2 (SARS-CoV-2), Lang et al. [135] revealed that lactoferrin could inhibit attachment of the viral spike protein to the host cells at the early viral adhesion phase. Although it did not block the viral entry by binding to spike protein directly, it interacts with heparan sulfate proteoglycans of the virus responsible for transporting extracellular viral particles into the cell. In brief, lactoferrin can defend the host against SARS-CoV-2 infection by inhibiting the early steps of viral pathogenesis [37, 135].

Lactoferrin can exert negative regulatory effects on cell migration by inhibiting plasminogen, which controls the viral-induced coagulation cascade [136]. Positively charged forms of lactoferrin and lactoferricin were also demonstrated to have anti-viral activity against CMV infection in vitro [137].

Regarding rotavirus infections, breastfed infants may have an asymptomatic infection or show the delayed appearance of rotavirus antigen in their stools due to high sIgA levels [138–140]. Lactadherin, a mucin-bound glycoprotein, has also been described as blocking rotavirus replication [40, 57].

Whereas lactoferrin and oligosaccharides have antiviral roles in inhibiting viral entrance by either blocking viral adherence to the mucosa or mimicking viral receptors, breast milk also provides a wide variety of antibodies against different viruses [23]. This passive immunity by maternal IgG antibodies gives antiviral protection to the infant until it starts to diminish after the first 6 to 12 months of life [141].

3.3 Antifungal and Antiprotozoal Features

Despite *Candida albicans* on the mother's nipple, factors in breast milk have protective effects against *Candida* infections in oral cavities; moreover, partially breastfed infants are more susceptible to the oral carriage of different *Candida* strains [20, 142].

Lactoferrin also has a fungistatic effect by iron binding, similar to its bacteriostatic property. It has also shown that lactoferrin and fungal cell surface interaction has a more direct fungicidal effect regardless of the iron presence [143, 144].

In preterm babies, the antifungal property of lactoferrin is essential. In a study, bovine lactoferrin was added to standard formulas and compared to a regular formula containing cow's milk. The authors did not report differences in growth rates among infants fed both formulas; however, the infants fed formulas with lactoferrin supplementation showed smoother stool viscosity compared to standard-formula-fed infants [145].

Free fatty acids have been reported to have antiprotozoal effects shown on *Giardia* [54].

4 Conclusion

Breast milk has a complex composition that provides newborns with unique essentials for optimal growth and education of their immune system. The oligosaccharides promote the expansion of commensal enteric bacteria and impact mucosal immunity along with the immunoglobulin fraction of breast milk. All the remaining molecules related to the immune system play roles in cell development and signaling multidirectional interaction. Additional studies are required to comprehend how immune components of breast milk induce the engagement of beneficial microflora in the gut so that they can compete with enteric pathogens. Breastfeeding probably has many valuable influences on growth, development, anti-infective resistance, and chronic diseases in adulthood, such as diabetes, leukemia, ulcerative colitis, and asthma.

References

1. Hanson LA, Korotkova M, Telemo E. Breast-feeding, infant formulas, and the immune system. Ann Allergy Asthma Immunol. 2003;90(6 Suppl 3):59–63.
2. Carr LE, Virmani MD, Rosa F, et al. Role of human milk bioactives on infants' gut and immune health. Front Immunol. 2021;12:604080.
3. Johansen FE, Baekkevold ES, Carlsen HS, Farstad IN, Soler D, Brandtzaeg P. Regional induction of adhesion molecules and chemokine receptors explains disparate homing of human B cells to systemic and mucosal effector sites: dispersion from tonsils. Blood. 2005;15:593–600.
4. Bachrach VR, Schwarz E, Bachrach LR. Breastfeeding and the risk of hospitalization for respiratory disease in infancy: a meta-analysis. Arch Pediatr Adolesc Med. 2003;157:237–43.
5. Oddy WH, Sly PD, de Klerk NH, et al. Breast feeding and respiratory morbidity in infancy: a birth cohort study. Arch Dis Child. 2003;88:224–8.
6. Pettigrew MM, Khodaee M, Gillespie B, Schwartz K, Bobo J, Foxman B. Duration of breast-feeding, daycare, and physician visits among infants 6 months and younger. Ann Epidemiol. 2003;13:431–5.
7. Talayero JMP, Lizan-Garcia M, Puime AO, et al. Full breastfeeding and hospitalization as a result of infections in the first year of life. Pediatrics. 2006;118:e92–9.
8. Duijts L, Jaddoe VW, Hofman A, Moll HA. Prolonged and exclusive breastfeeding reduces the risk of infectious diseases in infancy. Pediatrics. 2010;126:e18–25.
9. Hanson LA. Protective effects of breastfeeding against urinary tract infection. Acta Paediatr. 2004;93:154–6.
10. Darwazeh AM, al-Bashir A. Oral candidal flora in healthy infants. J Oral Pathol Med. 1995;24:361–4.
11. Bahl R, Frost C, Kirkwood BR, et al. Infant feeding patterns and risks of death and hospitalization in the first half of infancy: multicentre cohort study. Bull World Health Organ. 2005;83:418–26.
12. Edmond K, Zandoh C, Quigley M, Amenga-Etego S, Owusu-Agyei S, Kirkwood BR. Delayed breastfeeding initiation increases risk of neonatal mortality. Pediatrics. 2006;117:e380–6.
13. Chen A, Rogan WJ. Breastfeeding and the risk of postneonatal death in the United States. Pediatrics. 2004;113:e435–9.

14. Kramer MS, Guo T, Platt RW, et al. Infant growth and health outcomes associated with 3 compared with 6 mo of exclusive breastfeeding. Am J Clin Nutr. 2003;78:291–5.
15. Kaiser AM. A warm chain for breastfeeding. Lancet. 1994;344:1239–41.
16. Chantry CJ, Howard CR, Auinger P. Full breastfeeding duration and associated decrease in respiratory tract infection in US children. Pediatrics. 2006;117:425–32.
17. Duijts L, Ramadhani MK, Moll HA. Breastfeeding protects against infectious diseases during infancy in industrialized countries. a systematic review. Matern Child Nutr. 2009;5:199–210.
18. Tromp I, Jong JK-D, Raat H, et al. Breastfeeding and the risk of respiratory tract infections after infancy: the generation R study. PLoS One. 2017;12:e0172763.
19. Bowatte G, Tham R, Allen KJ, et al. Breastfeeding and childhood acute otitis media: a systematic review and meta-analysis. Acta Paediatr. 2015;104:85–95.
20. Ladomenou F, Moschandreas J, Kafatos A, Tselentis Y, Galanakis E. Protective effect of exclusive breastfeeding against infections during infancy: a prospective study. Arch Dis Child. 2010;95:1004–8.
21. Payne S, Quigley MA. Breastfeeding and infant hospitalisation: analysis of the UK 2010 infant feeding survey. Matern Child Nutr. 2017;13:e12263.
22. Furman L, Taylor G, Minich N, Hack M. The effect of maternal milk on neonatal morbidity of very low-birth-weight infants. Arch Pediatr Adolesc Med. 2003;157:66–71.
23. Duale A, Singh P, Al KS. Breast milk: a meal worth having. Front Nutr. 2022;26:800927.
24. Agostoni C, Braegger C, Decsi T, et al. Breastfeeding: a commentary by the ESPGHAN Committee on Nutrition. J Pediatr Gastroenterol Nutr. 2009;49:112–25.
25. Palmeira P, Carneiro-Sampaio M. Immunology of breast milk. Rev Assoc Med Bras. 2016;62:584–93.
26. Ramiro-Cortijo D, Singh P, Liu Y, et al. Breast milk lipids and fatty acids in regulating neonatal intestinal development and protecting against intestinal injury. Nutrients. 2020;12:534.
27. Goldman AS, Thorpe LW, Goldblum RM, Hanson LA. Anti-inflammatory properties of human milk. Acta Paediatr Scand. 1986;75:689–95.
28. Hirai Y, Kawakata N, Satoh K, et al. Concentrations of lactoferrin and iron in human milk at different stages of lactation. J Nutr Sci Vitaminol (Tokyo). 1990;36:531–44.
29. Hsu YC, Chen CH, Lin MC, Tsai CR, Liang JT, Wang TM. Changes in preterm breast milk nutrient content in the first month. Pediatr Neonatol. 2014;55:449–54.
30. Actor JK, Hwang SA, Kruzel ML. Lactoferrin as a natural immune modulator. Curr Pharm Des. 2009;15:1956–73.
31. Kawakami H, Lönnerdal B. Isolation and function of a receptor for human lactoferrin in human fetal intestinal brush-border membranes. Am J Phys. 1991;261:g841–6.
32. Park YW, Nam MS. Bioactive peptides in milk and dairy products: a review. Korean J Food Sci Anim Resour. 2015;35:831–40.
33. Vega-Bautista A, de la Garza M, Carrero JC, Campos-Rodríguez R, Godínez-Victoria M, Drago-Serrano ME. The impact of lactoferrin on the growth of intestinal inhabitant bacteria. Int J Mol Sci. 2019;20:4707.
34. Togawa JI, Nagase H, Tanaka K, et al. Lactoferrin reduces colitis in rats via modulation of the immune system and correction of cytokine imbalance. Am J Physiol Gastrointest Liver Pathol. 2002;283:g187–95.
35. Frioni A, Conte MP, Cutone A, et al. Lactoferrin differently modulates the inflammatory response in epithelial models mimicking human inflammatory and infectious diseases. Biometals. 2014;27:843–56.
36. Liao Y, Jiang R, Lönnerdal B. Biochemical and molecular impacts of lactoferrin on small intestinal growth and development during early life. Biochem Cell Biol. 2012;90:476–84.
37. Demers-Mathieu V, Underwood MA, Beverly RL, Nielsen SD, Dallas DC. Comparison of human milk immunoglobulin survival during gastric digestion between preterm and term infants. Nutrients. 2018;10:631.
38. Lepage P, Van de Perre P. The immune system of breast milk: antimicrobial and anti-inflammatory properties. Adv Exp Med Biol. 2012;743:121–37.

39. Vorbach C, Capecchi MR, Penninger JM. Evolution of the mammary gland from the innate immune system? BioEssays. 2006;28:606–16.

40. Hanson LA. Feeding and infant development breastfeeding and immune function. Proc Nutr Soc. 2007;66:384–96.

41. Böttcher MF, Jenmalm MC, Garofalo RP, Björkstén B. Cytokines in breast milk from allergic and nonallergic mothers. Pediatr Res. 2000;47:157–62.

42. Raisler J, Alexander C, O'Campo P. Breastfeeding and infant illness: a dose response relationship? Am J Public Health. 1999;89:25–30.

43. Cacho NT, Lawrence RM. Innate immunity and breast milk. Front Immunol. 2017;8:584.

44. Hanson LA, Korotkova M, Lundin S, et al. The transfer of immunity from mother to child. Ann N Y Acad Sci. 2003;987:199–206.

45. Palmeira P, Costa-Carvalho BT, Arslanian C, Pontes GN, Nagao AT, Carneiro-Sampaio MM. Transfer of antibodies across the placenta and in breast milk from mothers on intravenous immunoglobulin. Pediatr Allergy Immunol. 2009;20:528–35.

46. Silfverdal SA, Bodin L, Ulanova M, Hahn-Zoric M, Hanson LA, Olcen P. Long term enhancement of the IgG2 antibody response to *Haemophilus influenzae* type b by breastfeeding. Pediatr Infect Dis J. 2002;21:816–21.

47. Dallas DC, German JB. Enzymes in human milk. Intest Microb. 2017;88:129–36.

48. Vidal K, van den Broek P, Lorget F, Donnet-Hughes A. Osteoprotegerin in human milk: a potential role in the regulation of bone metabolism and immune development. Pediatr Res. 2004;55:1001–8.

49. Rudloff S, Pohlentz G, Diekmann L, Egge H, Kunz C. Urinary excretion of lactose and oligosaccharides in preterm infants fed human milk or infant formula. Acta Paediatr. 1996;85:598–603.

50. Newburg DS, Ruiz-Palacios GM, Morrow AL. Human milk glycans protect infants against enteric pathogens. Annu Rev Nutr. 2005;25:37–58.

51. Plaza-Díaz J, Fontana L, Gil A. Human milk oligosaccharides and immune system development. Nutrients. 2018;10:1038.

52. Xiao L, van De Worp WR, Stassen R, et al. Human milk oligosaccharides promote immune tolerance via direct interactions with human dendritic cells. Eur J Immunol. 2019;49:1001–14.

53. Hu M, Li M, Li C, Miao M, Zhang T. Effects of human milk oligosaccharides in infant health based on gut microbiota alteration. J Agric Food Chem. 2023;71:994–1001.

54. Isaacs CE, Thormar H, Pessolano T. Membrane-disruptive effect of human milk: inactivation of enveloped viruses. J Infect Dis. 1986;154:966–71.

55. Isaacs CE, Thormar H. The role of milk-derived antimicrobial lipids as antiviral and antibacterial agents. Adv Exp Med Biol. 1991;310:159–65.

56. Ballard O, Morrow AL. Human milk composition: nutrients and bioactive factors. Pediatr Clin N Am. 2013;60:49–74.

57. Wirt DP, Adkins LT, Palkowetz KH, Schmalstieg FC, Goldman AS. Activated and memory T lymphocytes in human milk. Cytometry. 1992;13:282–90.

58. Tuaillon E, Valea D, Becquart P, et al. Human milk-derived B cells: a highly activated switched memory cell population primed to secrete antibodies. J Immunol. 2009;182:7155–62.

59. Demers-Mathieu V, Mathijssen GB, DaPra C, Medo E. The effects of probiotic supplementation on the gene expressions of immune cell surface markers and levels of antibodies and pro-inflammatory cytokines in human milk. J Perinatol. 2021;41:1083–91.

60. Melnik BC, John SM, Schmitz G. Milk: an exosomal microRNA transmitter promoting thymic regulatory T cell maturation preventing the development of atopy? J Transl Med. 2014;12:43.

61. Admyre C, Johansson SM, Qazi KR, et al. Exosomes with immune modulatory features are present in human breast milk. J Immunol. 2007;179:1969–78.

62. Hsu PS, Nanan R. Does breast milk nurture T lymphocytes in their cradle? Front Pediatr. 2018;6:268.

63. Hasselbalch H, Jeppesen DL, Engelmann MD, Michaelsen KF, Nielsen MB. Decreased thymus size in formula-fed infants compared with breastfed infants. Acta Paediatr. 1996;85:1029–32.

64. Dawod B, Marshall JS. Cytokines and soluble receptors in breast milk as enhancers of oral tolerance development. Front Immunol. 2019;10:16.

65. Hawkes JS, Bryan DL, Gibson RA. Cytokine production by human milk cells and peripheral blood mononuclear cells from the same mothers. J Clin Immunol. 2002;22:338–44.

66. Cocchi F, DeVico AL, Garzino-Demo A, Arya SK, Gallo RC, Lusso P. Identification of RANTES, MIP-1 alpha, and MIP-1 beta as the major HIV suppressive factors produced by CD8+ T cells. Science. 1995;270:1811–5.

67. Hvas CL, Kelsen J, Agnholt J, et al. Crohn' disease intestinal CD4 + T cells have impaired interleukin-10 production which is not restored by probiotic bacteria. Scand J Gastroenterol. 2007;42:592–601.

68. Nakamura Y, Miyata M, Ando T, et al. The latent form of transforming growth factor-β administered orally is activated by gastric acid in mice. J Nutr. 2009;139:1463–8.

69. Worthington JJ, Czajkowska BI, Melton AC, Travis MA. Intestinal dendritic cells specialize to activate transforming growth factor-β and induce Foxp3+ regulatory T cells via integrin αvβ8. Gastroenterology. 2011;141:1802–12.

70. Ogawa J, Sasahara A, Yoshida T, et al. Role of transforming growth factor-beta in breast milk for initiation of IgA production in newborn infants. Early Hum Dev. 2004;77:67–75.

71. Xing Z, Gauldie J, Cox G, et al. IL-6 is an anti-inflammatory cytokine required for controlling local or systemic acute inflammatory responses. J Clin Invest. 1998;101:311–20.

72. Ngom PT, Collinson A, Pido-Lopez J, Henson SM, Prentice AM, Aspinall R. Improved thymic function in exclusively breastfed babies is associated with higher breast milk IL-7 concentrations in their mothers' breast milk. Am J Clin Nutr. 2004;80:722–8.

73. Laky K, Lewis JM, Tigelaar RE, Puddington L. Distinct requirements for IL-7 in development of TCR gamma delta cells during fetal and adult life. J Immunol. 2003;170:4087–94.

74. Buescher ES, Malinowska I. Soluble receptors and cytokine antagonists in human milk. Pediatr Res. 1996;40:839–44.

75. Ogundele MO. Inhibitors of complement activity in human breast-milk: a proposed hypothesis of their physiological significance. Mediat Inflamm. 1999;8:69–75.

76. Garofalo RP, Goldman AS. Expression of functional immunomodulatory and anti-inflammatory factors in human milk. Clin Perinatol. 1999;26:361–77.

77. Ellison RTJ, Giehl TJ. Killing of Gram-negative bacteria by lactoferrin and lysozyme. J Clin Invest. 1991;88:1080–91.

78. Labeta MO, Vidal K, Nores JE, et al. Innate recognition of bacteria in human milk is mediated by a milk-derived highly expressed pattern recognition receptor, soluble CD14. J Exp Med. 2000;191:1807–12.

79. Vidal K, Labeta MO, Schiffrin EJ, Donnet-Hughes A. Soluble CD14 in human breast milk and its role in innate immune responses. Acta Odontol Scand. 2001;59:330–4.

80. Friel JK, Martin SM, Langdon M, Herzberg GR, Buettner GR. Milk from mothers of both premature and full-term infants provides better antioxidant protection than does infant formula. Pediatr Res. 2002;51:612–8.

81. Gila-Diaz A, Arribas SM, Algara A, et al. A review of bioactive factors in human breastmilk: a focus on prematurity. Nutrients. 2019;11:1307.

82. Hara T, Irie K, Saito S, et al. Identification of macrophage colony-stimulating factor in human milk and mammary epithelial cells. Pediatr Res. 1995;37:437–43.

83. Gilmore WS, McKelvey-Martin VJ, Rutherford S, et al. Human milk contains granulocyte colony stimulating factor. Eur J Clin Nutr. 1994;48:222–4.

84. Pickering LK, Granoff DM, Erickson JR, et al. Modulation of the immune system by human milk and infant formula containing nucleotides. Pediatrics. 1998;101:242–9.

85. Heikkilä MP, Saris PE. Inhibition of *Staphylococcus aureus* by the commensal bacteria of human milk. J Appl Microbiol. 2003;95:471–8.

86. Pannaraj PS, Ly M, Cerini C, et al. Shared and distinct features of human milk and infant stool viromes. Front Microbiol. 2018;9:1162.
87. Stinson LF, Sindi ASM, Cheema AS, et al. The human milk microbiome: who, what, when, where, why, and how? Nutr Rev. 2021;79:529–43.
88. Fitzstevens JL, Smith KC, Hagadorn JI, Caimano MJ, Matson AP, Brownell EA. Systematic review of the human milk microbiota. Nutr Clin Pract. 2017;32:354–64.
89. Murphy K, Curley D, O'Callaghan TF, et al. The composition of human milk and infant faecal microbiota over the first three months of life: a pilot study. Sci Rep. 2017;7:40597.
90. Lackey KA, Williams JE, Meehan CL, et al. What's normal? microbiomes in human milk and infant feces are related to each other but vary geographically: the INSPIRE study. Front Nutr. 2019;6:45.
91. Thomson P, Medina DA, Garrido D. Human milk oligosaccharides and infant gut bifidobacteria: molecular strategies for their utilization. Food Microbiol. 2018;75:37–46.
92. Fallani M, Amarri S, Uusijarvi A, et al. Determinants of the human infant intestinal microbiota after the introduction of first complementary foods in infant samples from five European centres. Microbiology. 2011;157:1385–92.
93. Toscano M, De Grandi R, Grossi E, Drago L. Role of the human breast milk-associated microbiota on the newborns' immune system: a mini review. Front Microbiol. 2017;8:2100.
94. Belkaid Y, Hand TW. Role of the microbiota in immunity and inflammation. Cell. 2014;157:121–41.
95. Boix-Amorós A, Martinez-Costa C, Querol A, Collado MC, Mira A. Multiple approaches detect the presence of fungi in human breastmilk samples from healthy mothers. Sci Rep. 2017;7:1–13.
96. Togo AH, Grine G, Khelaifia S, et al. Culture of methanogenic archaea from human colostrum and milk. Sci Rep. 2019;9:18653.
97. Kosaka N, Izumi H, Sekine KO. MicroRNA as a new immune-regulatory agent in breast milk. Silence. 2010;1:7.
98. Carrillo-Lozano E, Sebastián-Valles F, Knott-Torcal C. Circulating microRNAs in breast milk and their potential impact on the infant. Nutrients. 2020;12:3066.
99. Ventura A, Young AG, Winslow MM, et al. Targeted deletion reveals essential and overlapping functions of the miR-17~92 family of miRNA clusters. Cell. 2008;132:875–86.
100. Johnnidis JB, Harris MH, Wheeler RT, et al. Regulation of progenitor cell proliferation and granulocyte function by microRNA-223. Nature. 2008;451:1125–9.
101. Zhou B, Wang S, Mayr C, Bartel DP, Lodish HF. miR-150, a microRNA expressed in mature B and T cells, blocks early B cell development when expressed prematurely. Proc Natl Acad Sci U S A. 2007;104:7080–5.
102. Gaziel-Sovran A, Segura MF, Di Micco R, et al. miR-30b/30d regulation of GalNAc transferases enhances invasion and immunosuppression during metastasis. Cancer Cell. 2011;20:104–18.
103. Stittrich AB, Haftmann C, Sgouroudis E, et al. The microRNA miR-182 is induced by IL-2 and promotes clonal expansion of activated helper T lymphocytes. Nat Immunol. 2010;11:1057–62.
104. Anghel L, Radulescu A, Erhan RV. Structural aspects of human lactoferrin in the iron-binding process studied by molecular dynamics and small-angle neutron scattering. Eur Phys J E Soft Matter. 2018;41:109.
105. Hendrixson DR, Qii J, Shewry SC, et al. Human milk lactoferrin is a serine protease that cleaves *Haemophilus* surface proteins at arginine-rich sites. Mol Microbiol. 2003;47:607–17.
106. Leitch EC, Willcox MD. Synergic antistaphylococcal properties of lactoferrin and lysozyme. J Med Microbiol. 1998;47:837–42.
107. Berlutti F, Pantanella F, Natalizi T, et al. Antiviral properties of lactoferrin - a natural immunity molecule. Molecules. 2011;16:6992–7018.

108. Bellamy W, Takase M, Wakabayashi H, Kavase K, Tomita M. Antibacterial spectrum of lactoferricin B, a potent bactericide peptide derived from the N-terminal region of bovine lactoferrin. J Appl Bacteriol. 1992;73:472–9.
109. Welsh KJ, Hwang SA, Boyd S, Kruzel ML, Hunter RL, Actor JK. Influence of oral lactoferrin on *Mycobacterium tuberculosis* induced immunopathology. Tuberculosis. 2011;91:s105–13.
110. Liu KY, Comstock SS, Shunk JM, Monaco MH, Donovan SM. Natural killer cell populations and cytotoxic activity in pigs fed mother's milk, formula, or formula supplemented with bovine lactoferrin. Pediatr Res. 2013;74:402–7.
111. Ackerman DL, Doster RS, Weitkamp JH, Aronoff DM, Gaddy JA, Townsend SD. Human milk oligosaccharides exhibit antimicrobial and antibiofilm properties against group B streptococcus. ACS Infect Dis. 2017;3:595–605.
112. Welsh KJ, Hwang SA, Hunter RL, Kruzel ML, Actor JK. Lactoferrin modulation of mycobacterial cord factor trehalose 6-6'-dimycolate induced granulomatous response. Transl Res. 2010;156:207–15.
113. ELFIN trial investigators group. Enteral lactoferrin supplementation for very preterm infants: a randomised placebo-controlled trial. Lancet. 2019;393:423–33.
114. Asztalos EV, Barrington K, Lodha A, Tarnow-Mordi W, Martin A. Lactoferrin infant feeding trial Canada (LIFT Canada): protocol for a randomized trial of adding lactoferrin to feeds of very-low-birth-weight preterm infants. BMC Pediatr. 2020;20:40.
115. Bollinger RR, Everett ML, Palestrant D, Love SD, Lin SS, Parker W. Human secretory immunoglobulin A may contribute to biofilm formation in the gut. Immunology. 2003;109:580–7.
116. Meikle V, Mossberg AK, Mitra A, Hakansson AP, Niederweis M. A protein complex from human milk enhances the activity of antibiotics and drugs against *Mycobacterium tuberculosis*. Antimicrob Agents Chemother. 2018;63:e01846–18.
117. Marks LR, Clementi EA, Hakansson AP. The human milk protein-lipid complex HAMLET sensitizes bacterial pathogens to traditional antimicrobial agents. PLoS One. 2012;7(8):e43514.
118. Alamiri F, Riesbeck K, Hakansson AP. HAMLET, a protein complex from human milk has bactericidal activity and enhances the activity of antibiotics against pathogenic *streptococci*. Antimicrob Agents Chemother. 2019;63:e01193–19.
119. Minekawa R, Takeda T, Sakata M, et al. Human breast milk suppresses the transcriptional regulation of IL-1beta-induced NF-kappaB signaling in human intestinal cells. Am J Physiol Cell Physiol. 2004;287:c1404–11.
120. Mårild S, Hansson S, Jodal U, Odén A, Svedberg K. Protective effect of breastfeeding against urinary tract infection. Acta Paediatr. 2004;93:164–8.
121. Jakaitis BM, Denning PW. Human breast milk and the gastrointestinal innate immune system. Clin Perinatol. 2014;41:423–35.
122. Levy I, Comarsca J, Davidovits M, et al. Urinary tract infection in preterm infants: the protective role of breastfeeding. Pediatr Nephrol. 2009;24(3):527–31.
123. Björck L, Rosén CG, Marshall V, Reiter B. Antibacterial activity of lactoperoxidase system in milk against pseudomonas and other Gram negative bacteria. Appl Microbiol. 1975;30:199–204.
124. Lugli GA, Milani C, Turroni F, et al. Prophages of the genus *Bifidobacterium* as modulating agents of the infant gut microbiota. Environ Microbiol. 2016;18:2196–213.
125. Lönnerdal B. Nutritional and physiologic significance of human milk proteins. Am J Clin Nutr. 2003;77:s1537–43.
126. Adkins Y, Lönnerdal B. Potential host-defense role of a human milk vitamin B-12-binding protein, haptocorrin, in the gastrointestinal tract of breastfed infants, as assessed with porcine haptocorrin in vitro. Am J Clin Nutr. 2003;77:1234–40.
127. Morozov V, Hansman G, Hanisch FG, Schroten H, Kunz C. Human milk oligosaccharides as promising antivirals. Mol Nutr Food Res. 2018;62:e1700679.
128. Valenti P, Marchetti M, Superti F, et al. Antiviral activity of lactoferrin. Adv Exp Med Biol. 1998;443:199–203.

129. Perez-Cano FJ, Marin-Gallen S, Castell M, et al. Supplementing suckling rats with whey protein concentrate modulates the immune response and ameliorates rat rotavirus-induced diarrhea. J Nutr. 2008;138:2392–8.
130. Wakabayashi H, Oda H, Yamauchi K, Abe F. Lactoferrin for prevention of common viral infections. J Infect Chemother. 2014;20:666–71.
131. El Yazidi-Belkoura I, Legrand D, Nuijens J, Slomianny MC, van Berkel P, Spik G. The binding of lactoferrin to glycosaminoglycans on enterocyte-like HT29-18-C1 cells is mediated through basic residues located in the N-terminus. Biochim Biophys Acta. 2001;1568:197–204.
132. Shukla D, Spear PG. Herpesviruses and heparan sulfate: an intimate relationship in aid of viral entry. J Clin Invest. 2001;108:503–10.
133. Ng TB, Cheung RCF, Wong JH, et al. Antiviral activities of whey proteins. Appl Microbiol Biotechnol. 2015;99:6997–7008.
134. Arnold D, Di Biase AM, Marchetti M, et al. Antiadenovirus activity of milk proteins: lactoferrin prevents viral infection. Antivir Res. 2002;53:153–8.
135. Lang J, Yang N, Deng J, et al. Inhibition of SARS pseudovirus cell entry by lactoferrin binding to heparan sulfate proteoglycans. PLoS One. 2011;6:e23710.
136. Zwirzitz A, Reiter M, Skrabana R, et al. Lactoferrin is a natural inhibitor of plasminogen activation. J Biol Chem. 2018;293:8600–13.
137. Andersen JH, Osbakk SA, Vorland LH, Traavik T, Gutteberg TJ. Lactoferrin and cyclic lactoferricin inhibit the entry of human cytomegalovirus into human fibroblasts. Antivir Res. 2001;51:141–9.
138. Espinoza F, Paniagua M, Hallander H, Svensson L, Strannegard O. Rotavirus infections in young Nicaraguan children. Pediatr Infect Dis J. 1997;16:564–71.
139. Gianino P, Mastretta E, Longo P, et al. Incidence of nosocomial rotavirus infections, symptomatic and asymptomatic, in breastfed and non-breast-fed infants. J Hospital Infect. 2002;50:13–7.
140. Clemens J, Rao M, Ahmed F, et al. Breast-feeding and the risk of life-threatening rotavirus diarrhea: prevention or postponement? Pediatrics. 1993;92:680–5.
141. Henrick BM, Yao XD, Nasser L, Roozrogousheh A, Rosenthal KL. Breastfeeding behaviours and the innate immune system of human milk: working together to protect infants against inflammation, HIV-1, and other infections. Front Immunol. 2017;8:1631.
142. Kadir T, Uygun B, Akyüz S. Prevalence of *Candida* species in Turkish children: relationship between dietary intake and carriage. Arch Oral Biol. 2005;50:33–7.
143. Al-Sheikh H. Effect of lactoferrin and iron on the growth of human pathogenic *Candida* species. Pak J Biol Sci. 2009;12:91–4.
144. Kondori N, Baltzer L, Dolphin GT, Mattsby-Baltzer I. Fungicidal activity of human lactoferrin-derived peptides based on the antimicrobial alphabeta region. Int J Antimicrob Agents. 2011;37:51–7.
145. Johnston WH, Ashley C, Yeiser M, et al. Growth and tolerance of formula with lactoferrin in infants through one year of age: double-blind, randomized, controlled trial. BMC Pediatr. 2015;15:173.

Vaccination and Breastfeeding

Gonca Keskindemirci and Gülbin Gökçay

1 Introduction

Vaccines enable the immune system of the organism to recognize and destroy pathogens. Vaccination is one of the most effective public health initiatives [1, 2]. Vaccines protect the vaccinated individuals and through "herd immunity" or "indirect effects" reduce the disease among unimmunized individuals in the community [3]. There are several types of vaccines such as attenuated live vaccines, inactivated vaccines, polysaccharide vaccines, and toxoid vaccines. Every country has national vaccination programs. While this program is being formed by the epidemiological data on the burden of disease in that country, the efficacy and effectiveness of the vaccine related to the disease, the cost, and the sustainability of the vaccine supply are evaluated [4].

2 Breastfeeding and Vaccination Practices

In addition to being a great source of nutrition for the baby, breast milk also strengthens the baby's defense mechanism against infections with its immunological and anti-infective properties. Immunoglobulins of IgA, IgG, and IgM are found in breast

G. Keskindemirci (✉) · G. Gökçay
Division of Social Pediatrics, Department of Pediatrics, İstanbul Faculty of Medicine, İstanbul University, İstanbul, Türkiye

Department of Social Pediatrics, Institute of Child Health, Istanbul University, İstanbul, Türkiye

Ö. N. Şahin et al. (eds.), *Breastfeeding and Metabolic Programming*, https://doi.org/10.1007/978-3-031-33278-4_27

milk. Breast milk plays a critical role in the transmission of immunity from mother to child, and the number of antibodies may increase during breastfeeding in response to the infant's needs [5]. Colostrum is the most powerful natural immune booster known to science. Breast milk has antibodies to many pathogens that the mother has come into contact with during her lifetime. Secretory IgA (SIgA) constitutes the largest proportion, followed by IgM and IgG antibodies in colostrum [6–8]. One of the mechanisms underlying such a potent effect of breastfeeding is the transfer of maternal SIgA specific for some pathogens through breast milk [8]. Although there are some reservations about vaccination during breastfeeding, routinely recommended vaccines can be safely applied to nursing mothers in general. In a few situations, vaccination during breastfeeding is contraindicated. In addition, it has been observed that the immune responses of breastfed babies after their own vaccinations are higher than those of who are not breastfed [9, 10].

2.1   BCG Vaccine

First introduced in the 1920s, the Bacillus Calmette-Guerin (BCG) vaccine is still the only approved vaccine against tuberculosis. BCG vaccine was derived from Mycobacterium Bovis live attenuated strain [11]. Over the years, after the first BCG vaccine, a wide variety of strains were produced by various laboratories around the world as a result of passages under different conditions. There are genetic differences between these strains. BCG vaccines used today were obtained by the passage from the first BCG strain. World Health Organisation supports the production of vaccine lots using strains Denmark 1331, Tokyo 172-1, Russia BCG-I, and Moreau RDJ, which have been shown to be effective and safe in humans [12]. There is no contraindication for BCG vaccination of nursing mothers if it is required [13]. On the other hand, infants who are breastfed and given BCG vaccine at birth have a good cellular immune response to vaccine [14]. There is no need to discontinue breastfeeding after tuberculin skin testing or to avoid skin testing in nursing mothers [15].

2.2   COVID-19 Vaccine

Coronavirus Disease 2019 (COVID-19) is the disease that is caused by a new coronavirus called severe acute respiratory syndrome coronavirus 2. Current evidence suggests that the virus mainly spreads between people who are in close contact with one another [16]. Four different types of vaccines are available all over the world; these are mRNA, viral vector, inactivated virus, and recombinant vaccines [17]. World Health Organization recommends vaccination of mothers during breastfeeding [18]. Breastfed babies who are not vaccinated due to their age can be protected by SIgA and IgG antibodies against COVID-19 that appear in breast milk after maternal vaccination [17, 19–21]. Studies demonstrated that administering the

COVID-19 vaccines is safe and poses no risk for the nursing mother and for her baby [17–22]. Therefore, health authorities and professional organizations recommend offering the COVID-19 vaccines to nursing mothers in terms of the potential advantages of maternal vaccination during breastfeeding [18, 23, 24].

2.3 Diphtheria Tetanus Pertussis Vaccine

The diphtheria vaccine is produced by mixing *Corynebacterium diphtheria* exotoxin with formaldehyde and turning it into a "toxoid" after inactivation. Diphtheria toxoid vaccines are shown in two different ways, according to the amount of antigen in their content, as "D" for those containing high-dose toxoids and as "d" for those containing low doses. Low-dose vaccines are administered to those over 7 years of age [25]. Acellular pertussis vaccines used today contain two or more immunogens in the structure of *Bordetella pertussis* bacteria. Acellular pertussis vaccines have begun to replace previously administered whole-cell pertussis vaccines [26–28]. Tetanus vaccine is a toxoid vaccine obtained by inactivating the neurotoxin called tetanospasmin of *Clostridium tetani* bacteria with formaldehyde. The same type of tetanus vaccine is used for all ages. There is no obstacle to the vaccination of the nursing mother with the adult-type Tetanus-adult-type diphtheria and acellular pertussis (Tdap) vaccine. Tdap contains tetanus, a reduced dose of diphtheria toxoids, and a reduced dose of acellular pertussis antigens. Centers for Disease Control and Prevention recommends maternal vaccination with the Tdap vaccine during pregnancy [29, 30]. Studies have shown that women with maternal Tdap vaccine have significantly higher concentrations of anti-pertussis toxin antibodies in their colostrum compared to women who gave birth at term and were not vaccinated. These antibodies of vaccinated mothers persist in the breast milk up to 12 weeks after delivery [31]. Vaccination of mothers will provide additional protection for infants during the most vulnerable period when the vaccination of their children has not been completed. "Cocoon strategy" is an immunization strategy [32]. In this strategy, influenza and pertussis vaccines are given to household members around infants, who cannot be vaccinated, and are susceptible to illness [33]. This strategy is designed for people who have close contact with their babies. Mothers are recommended to receive the vaccine as soon as possible after delivery if not vaccinated during pregnancy. Rowe et al. reported that pertussis infection was reduced by 77% in infants after vaccinating both parents [34]. Breastfeeding also reduces the adverse effects of routine childhood vaccines on the infant [32].

2.4 Hemophilus Influenza Type B Vaccine

There are polysaccharide and conjugate vaccines against *Hemophilus Influenza Type B* (Hib). With the introduction of the conjugated Hib vaccine, the interest in the efficacy and safety of the polysaccharide vaccine has decreased. Four conjugated

Hib vaccines have been developed. These are PRP-D, HbOC, PRP-OMP, and PRP-T [35]. Vaccines differ in carrier protein, size of the PRP portion, and chemical bonds. Conjugated Hib vaccines are also used in combination with DaBT-Hib, DaBT-Hib-inactivated polio vaccine (IPV) or DaBTHib-IPV-Hepatitis B vaccines [36]. In addition, when the immune responses of breastfed and not breastfed infants vaccinated with conjugated Hib vaccine at 2, 4, and 6 months were compared, there was no significant difference between feeding methods in antibody levels in the early period. On the other hand, antibody levels were significantly higher at 7 months and 12 months of age in breastfed infants. These findings were seen as strong evidence of the importance of breastfeeding in the development of the immune response during the first year of life [37]. Silfverdal et al. stated that exclusively breastfed infants for at least 90 days have better post-vaccination protection against Haemophilus influenza type B and pneumococcal serotypes 6B and 14 [38]. There is no risk for the mother to be vaccinated during breastfeeding. The immune responses of breastfed babies to the vaccination are much better [39].

2.5   *Hepatitis A Vaccine*

Hepatitis A vaccine is an inactivated virus vaccine containing antigens obtained from viruses produced in human fibroblast cell cultures and inactivated with formalin. Although there is an attenuated hepatitis A vaccine produced and licensed in China, inactivated hepatitis A vaccine is widely used all over the world. There is no known contraindication for immunization of breastfeeding mothers if vaccination against hepatitis A is necessary [40, 41].

2.6   *Hepatitis B Vaccine*

There are different types of hepatitis B vaccines, depending on the source from which they are obtained. Plasma-derived hepatitis B vaccine is prepared from the HBsAg particle derivative obtained from individuals who are chronic hepatitis B carriers. Recombinant hepatitis B vaccine derived from yeast is obtained by cloning the hepatitis B virus S gene produced by recombinant DNA technology from yeast cells and is the most commonly used vaccine. Recombinant hepatitis B vaccines produced in mammalian cells contain antigens of the pre-S regions. Heplisav-B is a recombinant vaccine produced from yeast containing HBsAg [42, 43]. There are monovalent or combined forms of the hepatitis B vaccine. Combined forms include diphtheria–tetanus–pertussis (DTP), Haemophilus influenza type b (Hib), and inactivated polio vaccine (IPV) [36]. Additionally, there is a combined hepatitis B and hepatitis A vaccine. There is no harm to mothers in getting vaccinated with the hepatitis B vaccine and continuing to breastfeed their infants [44].

2.7 Herpes Zoster Vaccine

Varicella zoster virus causes Herpes zoster, and the same virus also causes chicken-pox (varicella). After a person heals from chickenpox, the virus remains inactive (dormant) in the body and can reactivate years later, causing shingles. Anyone recovering from chickenpox can develop shingles, and the risk of shingles increases when persons get older. The shingles can't be transmitted to the baby through breast milk [45]. The attenuated live vaccine is available in many countries. Currently, recombinant zoster vaccine replaced attenuated live vaccine. In many countries, vaccination of the inactive zoster is recommended for adults aged 50 years and older in terms of preventing shingles and related complications, and also for adults aged 19 and over who have weakened immune systems due to an illness or treatment [46, 47]. Recombinant zoster vaccination has no known risks to nursing mothers or their infants [46]. So, there is no contraindication for zoster vaccination of nursing moth-ers if there is a need for protection against herpes zoster.

2.8 Human Papillomavirus (HPV) Vaccine

There are three different types of HPV vaccines. A purified bivalent vaccine of HPV contains types 16 and 18, quadrivalent vaccines of HPV contain types 6, 11, 16, and 18), and nonvalent vaccines of HPV contain types 6, 11, 16, 18, 31, 33, 45, 52, and 58 viral L1 proteins [48]. There is no evidence that the risk of vaccine-related adverse events in mothers or their infants is increased after administration of the HPV vaccine to breastfeeding women. There is no need for the cessation of breast-feeding after HPV vaccination. So, there is no contraindication for administering the HPV vaccine to breastfeeding mothers [49–51].

2.9 Influenza Vaccine

The influenza vaccine is available in two forms, inactivated and attenuated live vac-cines. Both vaccines have trivalent forms containing two subtypes of influenza A and one subtype of influenza B2, and quadrivalent forms of influenza A containing two subtypes of influenza B. The attenuated live vaccine is administered intrana-sally, while the inactivated vaccine is administered by injection [52]. Brady et al. reported that levels of influenza antibodies were higher in breast milk after inacti-vated vaccine than in attenuated live vaccine, and no influenza virus was detected in the milk of mothers who were given attenuated live vaccine [53]. Presence of anti-influenza IgA antibodies at least 6 months after vaccination was reported in the milk of mothers who were vaccinated in the third trimester [54]. According to the find-ings of another study, postnatal influenza vaccination of the nursing mother has been associated with a significant decrease in infants' influenza-related morbidity during the influenza season, and there is a significant decrease not only in disease-related morbidity but also in healthcare seeking and antibiotic use [55]. Authorities recommend that nursing mothers should be vaccinated with the influenza vaccine if the mother is not vaccinated during the pregnancy period [56, 57].

2.10 Measles-Rubella-Mumps Vaccine

Measles-rubella-mumps vaccine (MMR) is a combined vaccine contains attenuated live strains of measles, mumps, and rubella viruses. In addition, there is a vaccine in the form of measles-rubella-mumps-chickenpox, including the varicella vaccine. Although the weakened virus was detected in breast milk after rubella vaccination, no infant was infected during the observation period [58, 59]. In addition, it was determined that children with rubella virus detected in breast milk later responded normally to the rubella-containing vaccine. No studies reported that measles or mumps virus was detected in breast milk after MMR vaccination. There is no contraindication for the administration of the measles vaccine or the measles-rubella-mumps vaccine to nursing mothers if the vaccination of the mother is necessary [60, 61].

2.11 Meningococcal Vaccines

Meningococcal encapsulated, nonspore, Gram (−), aerobic diplococci microorganisms cannot survive for a long time in the external environment. There are inactivated vaccines such as polysaccharide meningococcal vaccines and conjugated meningococcal vaccines. Conjugated vaccines are: Serogroup C conjugate vaccine, Serogroup A conjugate vaccine, Hib-meningococcal serogroup CY conjugate vaccine, Serogroup A/C/W/Y conjugate vaccines, and Serogroup B vaccines [62]. Lakshman et al. showed that with the administration of quadrivalent polysaccharide meningococcal vaccine to three nursing mothers, serogroup A and C specific secretory IgA's were found in breast milk, serum, and saliva samples collected 2 weeks after the vaccine. It has been shown that antibody levels rise to very high levels after vaccination [63]. Breastfeeding has not been reported as a barrier to meningococcal vaccine administration in nursing mothers [63].

2.12 Monkeypox Vaccine

The disease is caused by the monkeypox virus (Monkeypox), a member of the genus Orthopoxvirus in the family of Poxviridae [64]. An orthopoxvirus infection or an orthopoxvirus vaccine immunization leads to immunologic cross-protection against other viruses in the genus. Orthopoxviruses which are large, double-stranded DNA viruses (Family Poxviridae, Genus Orthopoxvirus), include multiple species, such as the Vaccinia virus, Variola virus, Cowpox virus, Monkeypox virus, and newly discovered viruses [65]. Monkeypox virus is usually transmitted from wild animals to humans, such as primates and rodents, but it can also be transmitted through human to human. The lesions are transmitted from one person to another through contact with contaminated materials such as body fluids, respiratory droplets, and bedding. Eating undercooked meat and other animal products of infected animals is a possible risk factor. Based on the experiences in Africa, the World Health Organization (WHO) reports that the smallpox vaccine will provide 85% protection from monkeypox [64]. However, the smallpox vaccine has not been applied since 1980.

For this reason, people who have been vaccinated against smallpox today are those aged 40–50 years and over. Today, smallpox vaccines are no longer available for widespread use. Only people at risk (for example, someone who has had close contact with someone with monkeypox) should be considered for vaccination. Mass vaccination is not recommended at this time [65]. There are two types of vaccines. ACAM2000 vaccine contains replication-competent vaccinia viruses, and JYNNEOS vaccine contains replication-deficient modified vaccinia viruses Ankara [66–69]. In November 2021, for primary and booster vaccinations, the ACIP voted in favor of JYNNEOS as an alternative to ACAM2000 without opposition [65]. However, the efficacy and safety of JYNNEOS have not been assessed in nursing mothers. It is unknown if JYNNEOS is excreted in mothers' milk, and data is not available to evaluate the JYNNEOS vaccine for effect on milk production or the safety in breastfed infants. However, the attenuated virus in the JYNNEOS vaccine lacks replication. This characteristic of the vaccine may decrease the transmission risk to breastfed infants. On the other hand, there is no clear recommendation about the use of monkeypox among nursing mothers due to a lack of evidence.

2.13 Pneumococcal Vaccine

The pneumococcal vaccine is available in two forms: polysaccharide and conjugate. The polysaccharide vaccine is recommended for those over 65 and in special circumstances [70]. Deubzer et al. determined in their study that adhesion of *Streptococcus pneumoniae* 6B and 14 serotypes to pharyngeal epithelial cells was reduced with the colostrum of a mother who received a pneumococcal vaccine during pregnancy. The authors of this study suggested that the breast milk of vaccinated mothers can also prevent pneumococcal disease in infants [71]. Finn et al. reported that after vaccinating three lactating mothers with a 23-valent polysaccharide vaccine, specific SIgA increased >twofold in breast milk and postulated that capsule-specific SIgA could initiate the killing of *S. pneumoniae* and that vaccine-induced mucosal SIgA could support functional bactericidal activity [72]. It has also been shown that children who were exclusively breastfed for 90 days or more may achieve better post-vaccination serological protection against the 6B and 14 serotypes of pneumococcus and Hib [38]. There is no contraindication for the administration of pneumococcal vaccines to nursing mothers.

2.14   Poliomyelitis Vaccine

The polioviruses include three serotypes. Humans are the only natural reservoir for poliovirus. There are two types of polio vaccine: attenuated live oral and inactive parenteral vaccine. Only inactive polio vaccine (IPV) takes place in the national immunization schedules of high-income countries. IPV includes the three serotypes, which are inactivated with formaldehyde and grown in human diploid cells or Vero cells. IPV exists in combination with other childhood vaccines (such as pertussis, Haemophilus influenzae, diphtheria tetanus and hepatitis B) [29, 32]. The oral polio vaccine (OPV) is mainly used in low- and middle-income countries. Since the withdrawal of trivalent OPV, which contains poliovirus serotypes 1, 2, and 3, from routine immunization in 2016, bivalent OPV (bOPV), which contains poliovirus serotypes 1 and 3, has become the primary vaccine used in routine immunization of low and middle-income countries and supplementary immunization activities [73, 74]. Breastfeeding is not a contraindication to IPV or OPV administration [73]. Breastfed infants must be vaccinated according to the national immunization schedules of their countries. Some studies reported that breastfeeding might improve infant response to the oral polio vaccine [75, 76].

2.15   Rabies Vaccine

The rabies virus is an RNA virus from the Rhabdoviridae family. Rabies is almost always fatal in unvaccinated persons. WHO recommends concentrated and embryonated egg-based rabies vaccines, which are purified cell cultures (CCEEVs). CEEVs contain inactivated rabies virus that has been grown in cell culture (e.g., Vero cells, primary chick embryo cells, or human diploid cells) or embryonated eggs (e.g., embryonated chicken or duck eggs) [77, 78]. Nguyen et al. reported pregnant and lactating mothers who were not vaccinated due to unfounded concerns about the vaccination, according to the information received from their families, died due to rabies after exposure [79]. Vaccinations given to a nursing mother do not affect the safety of breastfeeding for mothers or infants. Breastfeeding can continue after rabies vaccination. There is no contraindication [41].

2.16   Smallpox Vaccine

The smallpox vaccine is an attenuated live vaccine. It has been reported that smallpox rashes were seen in the infant whose mother had a smallpox lesion in her areola 10 days after her husband was vaccinated with the smallpox vaccine [80]. The smallpox vaccine is no longer in use, and it is contraindicated to administer to lactating mothers [81].

2.17   Varicella Zoster Vaccine

Varicella zoster virus (VZV), the causative agent of chickenpox infection and shingles, is a double-stranded DNA virus belonging to the alpha herpesvirus family. Transmission of this virus occurs after direct contact with patients' vesicular fluids or zoster lesions, or after the spread of respiratory secretions. Vaccination is the most effective way to prevent chickenpox infection. The vaccine is a live attenuated lyophilized vaccine produced by serial passages in different cell cultures of the virus isolated from a child naturally infected with a wild virus, reducing its virulence. Bohlke et al. reported that no varicella DNA was detected in the milk of any mother by PCR after varicella vaccination of lactating mothers at 1-month postpartum interval. No seropositivity was found in their babies either [82]. There is no evidence that the virus passes into breast milk after vaccination. Breastfeeding mothers who have been vaccinated against chickenpox can continue to breastfeed [83].

2.18   Yellow Fever Vaccine

The yellow fever vaccine is a live, attenuated virus. Cases of transmission of yellow fever vaccine virus by breastfeeding have been reported. Yellow fever-specific immunoglobulin M and yellow fever-specific antigens were detected in the serum and cerebrospinal fluid of the infants [84–86]. If yellow fever vaccination is planned, the vaccination should be postponed if possible, but if the travel of breastfeeding mothers to yellow fever endemic areas cannot be avoided or postponed, this mother should be vaccinated and breastfeeding should be interrupted [87]. There is no data on how long breastfeeding should be interrupted if a nursing mother is vaccinated against yellow fever. It is recommended that she should not breastfeed for at least 2 weeks and should express and discard her milk. On the other hand, in a recent study in Brazil, it was reported that no virus was detected in breast milk samples taken on the 8th, 10th, and 15th days after yellow fever vaccination of nursing mothers. In this study, it was recommended that the mother should not breastfeed for 10 days instead of 2 weeks [88].

3 Conclusion

The benefits of breastfeeding for both mother and baby are well known. There are also many advantages for vaccination of nursing mothers. These advantages are for the infants of nursing mothers in addition to mothers themselves. In the light of the information obtained so far, there is no contraindication for vaccinating the nursing mothers, except for two vaccines. These two vaccines are yellow fever and smallpox vaccine [89]. In case of insufficient data on the vaccination of nursing mothers, the epidemiology of the disease and the risks and benefits of breastfeeding should be evaluated.

References

1. Greenwood B. The contribution of vaccination to global health: past, present, and future. Phil Trans R Soc B. 2014;369:20130433.
2. World Health Organization. Vaccines, https://www.who.int/topics/vaccines/en/. Accessed 5 July 2022.
3. John TJ, Samuel R. Herd immunity and herd effect: new insights and definitions. Eur J Epidemiol. 2000;16:601–6.
4. World Health Organization. Principles and considerations for adding a vaccine to a national immunization program: from the decision to implementation and monitoring, https://www.who.int/immunization/programmes_systems/policies_strategies/vaccine_intro_resources/nvi_guidelines/en/. Accessed 5 July 2022.
5. Lyons KE, Ryan CA, Dempsey EM, Ross RP, Stanton C. Breast Milk, a source of beneficial microbes and associated benefits for infant health. Nutrients. 2020;12:1039.
6. Palmeira P, Carneiro-Sampaio M. Immunology of breast milk. Rev Assoc Med Bras (1992). 2016;62:584–93.
7. Lawrence RM. Host-resistance factors and immunologic significance of human milk. In: Lawrence RA, Lawrence RM, editors. Breastfeeding: a guide for the medical profession. 9th ed. Philadelphia, PA: Elsevier; 2022. p. 145–92.
8. Verhasselt V. Is Infant immunization by breastfeeding possible? Philos Trans R Soc Lond Ser B Biol Sci. 2015;370:20140139.
9. Center for Disease Control and Prevention. Vaccinations, https://www.cdc.gov/breastfeeding/breastfeeding-special-circumstances/vaccinations-medications-drugs/vaccinations.html. Accessed 5 July 2022.
10. Dórea JG. Breast-feeding and responses to infant vaccines: constitutional and environmental factors. Am J Perinatol. 2012;29:759–75.
11. World Health Organization. 2019 Global tuberculosis report 2019, https://www.who.int/publications/i/item/9789241565714. Accessed 6 July 2022.
12. Hanekom WA, Hawn TR, Ginsberg AM. Tuberculosis Vaccines. In: Plotkin SA, Orenstein WA, Offit PA, Edwards KM, editors. Plotkin's vaccines. 7th ed. Philadelphia, PA: Elsevier; 2018. p. 1095–13.
13. World Health Organization. BCG vaccine: WHO position paper, February 2018–recommendations. Vaccine. 2018;36:3408–10.
14. Pabst HF, Godel J, Grace M, Cho H, Spady DW. Effect of breastfeeding on the immune response to BCG vaccination. Lancet. 1989;1(8633):295–7.
15. Drugs and Lactation Database (LactMed) Bethesda (MD): National Library of Medicine (US); 2006-. Tuberculin. https://www.ncbi.nlm.nih.gov/books/NBK501131. Accessed 6 July 2022.

16. Centers for Disease Control and Prevention. SARS-CoV-2 transmission. https://www.cdc.gov/coronavirus/2019-ncov/science/science-briefs/sars-cov-2-transmission.html#:~:text=References-,SARS%2DCoV%2D2%20is%20transmitted%20by%20exposure%20to%20infectious%20respiratory,respiratory%20fluids%20carrying%20infectious%20virus. Accessed 1 Aug 2022.

17. Juncker HG, Mulleners SJ, Coenen ERM, van Goudoever JB, van Gils MJ, van Keulen BJ. Comparing human milk antibody response after 4 different vaccines for COVID-19. JAMA Pediatr. 2022;176:611–2.

18. World Health Organisation. Coronavirus disease (COVID-19): Vaccines. https://www.who.int/news-room/questions-and-answers/item/coronavirus-disease-(covid-19)-vaccines. Accessed 1 Aug 2022.

19. Valcarce V, Stafford LS, Neu J, et al. Detection of SARS-CoV-2-specific IgA in the human milk of COVID-19 vaccinated lactating health care workers. Breastfeed Med. 2021;16:1004–9.

20. Selma-Royo M, Bäuerl C, Mena-Tudela D, Aguilar-Camprubí L, et al. Anti-SARS-CoV-2 IgA and IgG in human milk after vaccination is dependent on vaccine type and previous SARS-CoV-2 exposure: a longitudinal study. Genome Med. 2022;14:42.

21. Fox A, DeCarlo C, Yang X, Norris C, Powell RL. Comparative profiles of SARS-CoV-2 spike-specific milk antibodies elicited by COVID-19 vaccines currently authorized in the USA. medRxiv. Pre-print 2021:2021.07.19.21260794.

22. McLaurin-Jiang S, Garner CD, Krutsch K, Hale TW. Maternal and child symptoms following COVID-19 vaccination among breastfeeding mothers. Breastfeed Med. 2021;16:702–9.

23. American College of Obstetricians and Gynecologists. Vaccinating pregnant and lactating patients against COVID-19:Practice advisory. https://www.acog.org/clinical/clinicalguidance/practice-advisory/articles/2020/12/vaccinating-pregnantand-lactating-patients-against-covid-19. Accessed 1 Aug 2022.

24. Royal College of Obstetricians and Gynaecologists. COVID-19 vaccines, pregnancy and breastfeeding. https://www.rcog.org.uk/en/guidelines-research-services/guidelines/coronavirus. Accessed 1 Aug 1, 2022.

25. World Health Organization. The Global Vaccine Action Plan 2011-2020. Strategic Advisory Group of Experts on Immunization review and lessons learned 2019.

26. American Academy of Pediatrics. Pertussis. In: Kimberlin DW, Brady MT, Jackson MA, Long SS, editors. Red Book: 2018 Report of the Committee on Infectious Diseases, vol. 2018. 31st ed. Itasca, IL: American Academy of Pediatrics. p. 620–34.

27. Cherry JD, Heininger U. Pertussis and other Bordetella infections. In: Feigin RD, Cherry JD, Demmler-Harrison GJ, Kaplan SL, editors. Textbook of pediatric infectious diseases. 7th ed. Philadelphia, PA: Saunders Elsevier; 2014. p. çp.1616–39.

28. Long SS, Edwards KM. Bordetella pertussis (pertussis) and other species. In: Long SS, Pickering LK, Prober CG, editors. Principles and practice of pediatric infectious diseases. 4th ed. Churchill Livingstone, Elsevier: Philadelphia, PA; 2012. p. 865–73.

29. Drugs and Lactation Database (LactMed). Bethesda (MD): National Library of Medicine (US); 2006-. Diphtheria-Tetanus-Pertussis Vaccines, https://www.ncbi.nlm.nih.gov/books/NBK500572. Accessed 7 July 2022.

30. Centers for Disease Control and Prevention. Pertussis Vaccination. https://www.cdc.gov/pertussis/vaccines.html. Accessed 1 Aug 2022.

31. Orije MRP, Larivière Y, Herzog SA, et al. Breast milk antibody levels in tdap-vaccinated women after preterm delivery. Clin Infect Dis. 2021;73:e1305–13.

32. Centers for Disease Control and Prevention. Prevention of pertussis, tetanus, and diphtheria with vaccines in the United States: recommendations of the advisory committee oniImmunization practices (ACIP). MMWR. 2018;67:1–44.

33. Nitsch-Osuch A. Cocoon strategy of vaccination: Benefits and limitations. In: Afrin F, Hemek H, Ozbak H, editors. Vaccines. London: IntechOpen; 2017. p. 3–20.

34. Rowe SL, Tay EL, Franklin LJ, et al. Effectiveness of parental cocooning as a vaccination strategy to prevent pertussis infection in infants: a case-control study. Vaccine. 2018;36:2012–9.

35. Nanduri SA, Sutherland AR, Gordon LK, Santosham M. Haemophilus influenza type b vaccines. In: Plotkin SA, Orenstein WA, Offit PA, Edwards CM, editors. Plotkin's vaccines. 7th ed. Amsterdam: Elsevier; 2018. p. 301–18.
36. Centers for Disease Control and Prevention. Vaccines and Preventable Disease. https://www.cdc.gov/vaccines/vpd/hib/public/index.html Accessed 8 July 2022.
37. Pabst HF, Spady DW. Effect of breastfeeding on antibody response to conjugat the e vaccine. Lancet. 1990;4:269–70.
38. Silfverdal SA, Ekholm L, Bodin L. Breastfeeding enhances the antibody response to Hib and pneumococcal serotype 6B and 14 after vaccination with conjugate vaccines. Vaccine. 2007;9:1497–502.
39. Dòrea JG. Breastfeeding is an essential complement to vaccination. Acta Paediatr. 2009;98:1244–50.
40. World Health Organization. WHO position paper on hepatitis A vaccines – June 2012. https://apps.who.int/iris/bitstream/handle/10665/241938/WER8728_29_261-276.PDF?sequence=1. Accessed 8 July 2022.
41. Kroger A, Bahta L, Hunter P. General Best Practice Guidelines for Immunization. Best Practices Guidance of the Advisory Committee on Immunization Practices (ACIP). https://www.cdc.gov/vaccines/hcp/acip-recs/general-recs/index.html , Accessed 10 July 2022.
42. Centers for Disease Control and Prevention. Heplisav-B® (HepB-CpG) Vaccin, https://www.cdc.gov/vaccines/schedules/vacc-updates/heplisav-b.pdf. Accessed 15 July 2022.
43. Food and Drug Administration. HEPLISAV-B [package insert]. Emeryville, CA: Dynavax Technologies Corporation; 2017–2019. US https://www.fda.gov/media/108745/download. Accessed 15 July 2022.
44. World Health Organization. Hepatitis B vaccines: WHO position paper, July 2017 - recommendations. Vaccine. 2019;37:223–5.
45. Centers for Disease Control and Prevention. Shingles. https://www.cdc.gov/breastfeeding/breastfeeding-special-circumstances/maternal-or-infant-illnesses/shingles.html. Accessed 15 July 2022.
46. Centers for Disease Control and Prevention. Shingles (Herpes Zoster) vaccination. https://www.cdc.gov/shingles/vaccination.html. Accessed 15 July 2022.
47. Anderson TC, Masters NB, Guo A, et al. Use of recombinant zoster vaccine in immunocompromised adults aged ≥19 years: recommendations of the advisory committee on immunization practices - United States, 2022. MMWR Morb Mortal Wkly Rep. 2022;71:80–4.
48. World Health Organization. Human papillomavirus vaccines: WHO position paper, May 2017–Recommendations. Vaccine. 2017;35:5753–5.
49. Markowitz LE, Dunne EF, Saraiya M, et al. Centers for Disease Control and Prevention (CDC). Human papillomavirus vaccination: recommendations of the Advisory Committee on Immunization Practices (ACIP). MMWR Recomm Rep. 2014;63:1–30.
50. American College of Obstetricians and Gynecologists' Committee on Adolescent Health Care, American College of Obstetricians and Gynecologists' Immunization, Infectious Disease, and Public Health Preparedness Expert Work Group. Human papillomavirus vaccination: ACOG committee opinion, Number 809. Obstet Gynecol. 2020;136:e15–21.
51. Drugs and Lactation Database (LactMed) Bethesda (MD): National Library of Medicine (US); 2006-. Human Papillomavirus Vaccines. https://www.ncbi.nlm.nih.gov/books/NBK501705/?report=classic). Accessed 14 July 2022.
52. World Health Organization. Vaccines against influenza:WHO position paper –May 2022. https://www.who.int/publications/i/item/who-wer9719. Accessed 1 Aug 2022.
53. Brady RC, Jackson LA, Frey SE, et al. Randomized trial comparing the safety and antibody responses to live attenuated versus inactivated influenza vaccine when administered to breast-feeding women. Vaccine. 2018;36:4663–71.
54. Schlaudecker EP, Steinhoff MC, Omer SB, et al. IgA and neutralizing antibodies to influenza a virus in human milk: a randomized trial of antenatal influenza immunization. PLoS One. 2013;8:e70867.

55. Maltezou HC, Fotiou A, Antonakopoulos N, et al. Impact of postpartum influenza vaccination of mothers and household contacts in preventing febrile episodes, influenza-like illness, healthcare seeking, and administration of antibiotics in young infants during the 2012-2013 influenza season. Clin Infect Dis. 2013;57:1520–6.
56. World Health Organization. Tailoring immunization programmes for seasonal influenza (TIP FLU): A guide for promoting uptake of maternal influenza vaccination. https://apps.who.int/iris/handle/10665/351329. Accessed 1 Aug 2022.
57. Drugs and Lactation Database (LactMed). Bethesda (MD): National Library of Medicine (US); 2006-. Influenza vaccines. https://www.ncbi.nlm.nih.gov/books/NBK500990/#). Accessed 14 July 2022.
58. Buimovici-Klein E, Hite RL, Byrne T, Cooper LZ. Isolation of rubella virus in milk after postpartum immunization. J Pediatr. 1977;9:939–41.
59. Losonsky GA. FishautJM, Strussenberg J, Ogra PL. Effect of immunization against rubella on lactation products II. Maternal-neonatal interactions. J Infect Dis. 1982;145:661–6.
60. Alain S, Dommergues MA, Jacquard AC, Caulin E, Launay O. State of the art: Could nursing mothers be vaccinated with attenuated live virus vaccine? Vaccine. 2012;30:4921–6.
61. Centers for Disease Control and Prevention. Vaccines and Preventable Diseases https://www.cdc.gov/vaccines/vpd/mmr/public/index.html. Accessed 1 Aug 2022.
62. World Health Organization. Meningococcal vaccines: WHO position paper, November 2011. Weekly Epidemiological Record= Relevé épidémiologique hebdomadaire. 2011;86:521–539.
63. Lakshman R, Seymour L, Akhtar S, et al. Secretory antibody responses to quadrivalent meningococcal vaccine in lactating mothers. Clin Infect Dis. 2000;31:321. Abstract 629
64. World Health Organization. Clinical management and infection prevention and control for monkeypox interim rapid response guidance 10 June 2022.
65. Rao AK, Petersen BW, Whitehill F, et al. Use of JYNNEOS (Smallpox and Monkeypox Vaccine, Live, Nonreplicating) for preexposure vaccination of persons at risk for occupational exposure to orthopoxviruses: recommendations of the advisory committee on immunization practices - United States. MMWR Morb Mortal Wkly Rep. 2022;71:734–42.
66. Centers for Disease Control and Prenevtion. Considerations for monkeypox vaccination. https://www.cdc.gov/poxvirus/monkeypox/considerations-for-monkeypox-vaccination.html. Accessed 4 Aug 2022.
67. World Health Organization. Monceypox. https://www.who.int/news-room/questions-and-answers/item/monkeypox?gclid=Cj0KCQjw8uOWBhDXARIsA OxKJ2HIO44Esm0QW-goB7I30nakNcOBBWLpHREYNuOWBhDXARIsAOxKJ2HIO44Esm0QWgo-B7I30nakNcOBBWLWYrArNcqm9wCHFALYK7I30nakNcObLWyr. Accessed 15 July 2022.
68. Food and Drug Administration. ACAM2000 (Smallpox Vaccine) Questions and Answers, https://www.fda.gov/vaccines-blood-biologics/vaccines/acam2000-smallpox-vaccine-questions-and-answers. Accessed 15 July 2022.
69. United Kingdom. Health SEurity Acency. Monkeypox: waiting for your vaccination. https://www.gov.uk/government/publications/monkeypox-vaccination-resources/monkeypox-waiting-for-your-vaccination. Accessed 15 July 2022.
70. Center for Disease Control and Prevention. Vaccines and Preventable Diseases. Pnuemococcal. https://www.cdc.gov/vaccines/vpd/pneumo/index.html. Accessed 8 July 2022.
71. Deubzer HE, Obaro SK, Newman VO, Adegbola RA, Greenwood BM, Henderson DC. Colostrum obtained from women vaccinated with pneumococcal vaccine during pregnancy inhibits epithelial adhesion of Streptococcus pneumoniae. J Infect Dis. 2004;190:1758–61.
72. Finn A, Zhang Q, Seymour L, Fasching C, Pettitt E, Janoff EN. Induction of functional secretory IgA responses in breast milk, by pneumococcal capsular polysaccharides. J Infect Dis. 2002;15(186):1422–9.
73. American Academy of Pediatrics. Poliovirus infections. In: Kimberlin DW, Brady MT, Jackson MA, Long SS, editors. Red Book: 2018 Report of the Committee on Infectious Diseases. 31st ed. Itasca, IL: American Academy of Pediatrics; 2018. p. 601–7.

74. World Health Organization. Poliomyelitis. https://www.who.int/teams/health-product-policy-and-standards/standards-and-specifications/vaccines-quality/poliomyelitis. Accessed 29 July 2022.

75. Brickley EB, Wieland-Alter W, Connor RI, et al. Intestinal immunity to poliovirus following sequential trivalent inactivated polio vaccine/bivalent oral polio vaccine and trivalent inactivated polio vaccine-only immunization schedules: analysis of an open-label, randomized, controlled trial in chilean infants. Clin Infect Dis. 2018;67(Suppl 1):S42–50.

76. Haque R, Snider C, Liu Y, et al. Oral polio vaccine response in breast fed infants with malnutrition and diarrhea. Vaccine. 2014;32:478–82.

77. World Health Organization. Expert Consultation on Rabies, third report: WHO Technical Series Report No. 1012, Geneva, 2018.

78. World Health Organization. Rabies vaccines: WHO position paper, April 2018–Recommendations. Vaccine. 2018;36:5500–3.

79. Nguyen HT, Tran CH, Dang AD, et al. Rabies Vaccine Hesitancy and Deaths Among Pregnant and Breastfeeding Women — Vietnam, 2015–2016. MMWR Morb Mortal Wkly Rep. 2018;67:250–2.

80. Garde V, Harper D, Fairchok MP. Tertiary contact vaccinia in a breastfeeding infant. JAMA. 2004;291:725–7.

81. Centers for Disease Control and Prevention. Smallpox. Smallpox Vaccine Basis. Available at: https://www.cdc.gov/smallpox/vaccine-basics/index.html. Last accessed 15 July 2022.

82. Bohlke K, Galil K, Jackson LA, Schmid DS, Starkovich P, Loparev VN, Seward JF. Postpartum varicella vaccination: is the vaccine virus excreted in breast milk? Obstet Gynecol. 2003;102:970–7.

83. Centers for Disease Control and Prevention. Varicella vaccination. Available at: https://www.cdc.gov/vaccines/vpd/varicella/hcp/recommendations.html#:~:text=There%20is%20no%20need%20to,vaccine%20may%20continue%20to%20breastfeed. Last accessed 15 July 2022.

84. Traiber C, Coelho-Amaral P, Ritter VR, Winge A. Infant meningoencephalitis caused by yellow fever vaccine virus transmitted via breastmilk. J Pediatr (Rio J). 2011;87:269–72.

85. Kuhn S, Twele-Montecinos L, MacDonald J, et al. Case report: Probable transmission of vaccine strain of yellow fever virus to an infant via breast milk. CMAJ. 2011;183:E243–5.

86. Centers for Disease Control and Prevention. Transmission of yellow fever vaccine virus through breast-feeding: Brazil: 2009. MMWR Morb Mortal Wkly Rep. 2010;59:130–2.

87. Centers for Disease Control and Prevention. Travelers' health. chapter 4 travel-related infectious diseases- yellow fever. Available at: https://www.nc.cdc.gov/travel/yellowbook/2020/travel-related-infectious-diseases/yellow-fever. July 15, 2022.

88. Fernandes EG, Nogueira JS, Porto VBG, Sato HK. The search for yellow fever virus vaccine in breast milk of inadvertently vaccinated women in Brazil. Rev Inst Med Trop Sao Paulo. 2020;62:e33.

89. Centers for Disease Control and Prevention. Vaccinations. https://www.cdc.gov/breastfeeding/breastfeeding-special-circumstances/vaccinations-medications-drugs/vaccinations.html. Accessed 1 Aug 2022.

Breastfeeding and Maternal Bacterial Infections

Özge Kaba, Ayşe Engin Arısoy, Emin Sami Arısoy, and Sheldon L. Kaplan

1 Introduction

Breast milk is a miraculous nutrient specially produced for each baby. Breast milk, the essential source of infant nutrition, provides different benefits with every component it contains. Skin-to-skin contact with the mother during breastfeeding reduces the baby's stress, eases the baby's adaptation to the world, and contributes to neurobehavioral development [1]. Breast milk has many more benefits further than growth and development. The formation of the gastrointestinal microbiota, reduction in the risk of necrotizing enterocolitis (NEC), protection against various diseases such as oral candidiasis, otitis media, and respiratory, gastrointestinal, and urinary tract infections, and a reduction in the mortality risk in the first months of life for any reason are some of the short-term benefits provided by breast milk [1–5].

In addition to its immunoglobulin (Ig) content, breast milk plays a role in structuring an infant's immune system by providing a balance between tissue macrophage profile, thymus development, and T helper cells [6]. Moreover, long-term studies also demonstrated with different evidence levels that breast milk can

Ö. Kaba (✉)
İstanbul Çam and Sakura Hospital, Section of Pediatric Infectious Diseases, University of Health Science, İstanbul, Türkiye

A. E. Arısoy
Faculty of Medicine, Division of Neonatology (Emeritus), Department of Pediatrics, Kocaeli University, Kocaeli, Türkiye

E. S. Arısoy
Faculty of Medicine, Division of Pediatric Infectious Diseases (Emeritus), Department of Pediatrics, Kocaeli University, Kocaeli, Türkiye

S. L. Kaplan
Division of Infectious Diseases, Department of Pediatrics, Baylor College of Medicine, and Infectious Disease Service, Texas Children's Hospital, Houston, TX, USA

Ö. N. Şahin et al. (eds.), *Breastfeeding and Metabolic Programming*, https://doi.org/10.1007/978-3-031-33278-4_28

effectively prevent some diseases, including autoimmune, allergic, and cardiovascular diseases, obesity, type 1 and 2 diabetes mellitus, and some types of malignancies such as leukemia and breast cancer [7–11]. The World Health Organization (WHO), the United Nations International Children's Emergency Fund (UNICEF), the American Academy of Pediatrics (AAP), and many other organizations recommend that infants should be exclusively breastfed for the first 6 months, starting within the first hour of birth [11, 12].

2   Protective Elements of Breast Milk

Breast milk, mainly composed of water, is comprised of nutritional compounds, electrolytes, vitamins, minerals, enzymes, carrier molecules, hormones, growth factors, cytokines, Igs, and other molecules involved in various functions [13]. Many breast milk constituents, including secretory IgA (sIgA) and other Igs, lactoferrin, lysozyme, free fatty acids, bile-salt stimulated lipase, stem cells, white blood cells, haptocorrin, alpha-lactalbumin, casein, lactoperoxidase, mucins, and oligosaccharides with prebiotic activity are the main substances effective in preventing infections.

2.1   *Immunoglobulins*

It was first shown in 1961 that the predominant immunoglobulin in breast milk is IgA [14]. Secretory IgA, synthesized by plasma cells on the basal surface of the mammary epithelium, is involved in pathogen neutralization with its stable and resistant structure [15]. Secretory IgA in breast milk protects against enteric and systemic pathogens [16, 17]. Its dynamic structure changes due to factors such as gestational age, nutrition, vaccination, maternal diseases, and smoking. Antibodies specific to intestinal and respiratory pathogens are present in breast milk even when not in the mother's circulation [13].

Secretory IgA is produced by stimulation of T and B lymphocytes as a result of encountering any pathogen of the mother's respiratory and gastrointestinal mucosal barrier. This system, known as the bronchomammarian and enteromammarian axes, helps protect the baby from infections [18–20]. These antibodies protect against bacteria such as *Haemophilus influenzae, Streptococcus pneumoniae, Escherichia coli, Vibrio cholerae, Clostridium difficile,* and *Salmonella* spp. and many types of viruses and fungi [21].

Immunoglobulin A, which accounts for 88% of colostrum content with an amount of 7500 mg/L in the colostrum secreted in the first days of life, continues to be the most dominant Ig; however, its contribution decreases to 68–81% in the following days [22]. Although the main Ig is 11S sIgA, Igs G, M, D, and E also are present in breast milk. The IgM amount increases with breast milk maturation and reaches 22%; the IgG concentration is lower than IgA and IgM in breast milk [23].

The highest IgG subtypes are IgG1 and IgG2 in colostrum and mature milk. A study with mice by Zheng et al. [24] showed that IgG in breast milk provides protection against mucosal and systemic infections induced by enterotoxigenic *E. coli*. Immunoglobulins found at lower levels in breast milk are IgE, dominant in allergic processes, and IgD, which functions similarly to IgM and plays a role in the local immune response of the breast tissue [25–28].

2.2 *Lysozyme*

Fleming first detected the lytic activity of lysozyme in 1921, and its presence in breast milk was demonstrated by Bordet in 1924 [29]. Lysozyme, also called N-acetyl muramidase, an enzyme consisting of a 130 amino acid polypeptide chain, is also found in body fluids such as saliva and tears [30]. Lysozyme destroys gram-positive bacteria by hydrolyzing peptidoglycan polymers in the bacterial cell wall [8, 31] and gram-negative bacteria in vitro synergistically with lactoferrin [32]. In addition to the broad antimicrobial spectrum, lysozyme also contributes to the enrichment of beneficial microbiota and reduction in harmful microbiota in the intestines [33]. With heating, lysozyme amount and thus its activity decrease by 50–80% [34]. Unlike other protective elements, lysozyme concentration increases proportionally with the duration of lactation [30, 35].

2.3 *Lactoferrin*

A Danish chemist described lactoferrin in 1939 as a red protein in cow's milk [29]. A similar protein was identified in human milk in 1951 and isolated in 1960 [29]. Lactoferrin is a glycosylated protein consisting of 691 amino acids belonging to the transferrin family [35]. Lactoferrin has an antibacterial effect by binding iron, and it can destroy the bacteria via damage to the membrane with a direct effect [36]. Together with lysozyme, sIgA, and lactoperoxidase, lactoferrin provides a bacteriostatic state on mucosal surfaces [16, 37]. Lactoferrin, also known to support the antibacterial activity of lysozyme [34], exhibits bacteriostatic activity against *E. coli* and bactericidal activity against pathogens such as *V. cholerae* and *Streptococcus mutans* [35, 38]. Lactoferrin also inactivates colonization factors synthesized by *H. influenzae* [39], and shows anti-inflammatory properties by preventing the synthesis of many pro-inflammatory cytokines [40].

The lactoferrin amount is reduced in mature milk, but its glycosylation properties vary; it is suggested that the process contributes to microbiota development [34, 41]. Lactoferrin can cause stimulation, differentiation, and cell activity through its receptors in other immune system elements [42]. Animal and human studies showed lactoferrin prevents urinary tract infection and colitis and reduces the rates of late-onset sepsis and lower respiratory tract infections [40, 43, 44].

2.4 Alpha-Lactalbumin

Alpha (α)-lactalbumin, the main whey protein, comprises 25–35% of human milk and consists of 123 amino acids [13]. Cysteine and tryptophan in the α-lactalbumin content affect the immune system [45]. Alpha-lactalbumin has a very high nutritional value and prevents the attachment of pathogens to the intestinal mucosa [35]. Pellegrini et al. [46] demonstrated in monkeys the antibacterial activity of polypeptides obtained by the degradation of α-lactalbumin against *E. coli, Klebsiella pneumoniae, Staphylococcus aureus, Staphylococcus epidermidis*, and *Streptococcus* spp. They concluded that similar antibacterial activity might be observed through the similarity of human and monkey α-lactalbumin molecules [47]. Some of these polypeptides show bifidogenic activity [13, 48]. Brück et al. [49] showed that α-lactalbumin could inhibit the growth of various potential pathogens such as enteropathogenic *E. coli* (EPEC), *Salmonella typhimurium, Bacteroides,* and *Clostridium* spp. Another study reported that α-lactalbumin provides resistance to *EPEC* diarrhea in monkeys [34]. In addition to its nutritional and antimicrobial properties, the antitumoral activity of α-lactalbumin is currently under investigation [50].

2.5 Human Milk Oligosaccharides

Human milk oligosaccharides (HMOs), carbohydrates resistant to digestion found in breast milk, are known for their contribution to immunity rather than growth [51]. Although there are more than 200 HMOs, only half have been understood in detail. The HMOs found up to 20–23 g/L in colostrum and 5–15 g/L in mature milk [52] help beneficial intestinal bacteria such as *Bifidobacterium* and *Lactobacillus* colonize and support the shaping of the intestinal microbiota [53]. The HMOs act as a receptor, preventing mucosal adhesion and colonization of enteric pathogens [16, 54]. *Campylobacter jejuni, H. influenzae, S. pneumoniae,* and EPEC are some pathogens whose adhesion is prevented by HMOs [13]. The HMOs strengthen the intestine's barrier by increasing mucus secretion [55]. Some data suggest that excreted HMOs in the urine also reduce the incidence of urinary tract infections [13]. The HMOs can change cytokine responses by interacting with various molecules of immune system elements [56].

2.6 Milk Fat Globule Membrane

Milk fat globule membrane (MFGM), the complex compounds, a mixture of carbohydrates, lipids, and proteins surrounded by a triple membrane system show an antibacterial effect by preventing the adhesion of pathogens to the intestinal mucosa. Mucins, lactadherin, butyrophilin, and adipophilin are some of the glycoproteins identified as MFGM [34, 35]. Mucins show pathogen-specific activity; for example, mucin-1 functions against *S. typhimurium,* and mucins are also involved in protection [34, 57]. Bhinder et al. [58] showed that MFGM-containing nutrition protects against *C. difficile* infections. Studies in humans and animals have demonstrated the positive effects of MFGM-enriched nutrition on the neurological, immunological, and gastrointestinal systems [35]. However, in addition to the studies reporting a decrease in acute otitis media, respiratory tract infections, and diarrhea, studies also exist, documenting no difference or even increases in these infections [59].

2.7   Cells

The cells in breast milk were first described as Donne particles in an atlas published in 1845 [29]. The number of live and active cells in newly expressed breast milk may vary between 10,000 and 13,000,000/mL [13]. Cell count is particularly high in colostrum [60]. The primary cells in breast milk are epithelial cells, leukocytes, and stem cells. Approximately 10^8 maternal leukocytes daily are delivered to infants by breast milk produced during the early lactation period [57]. The cell number in breast milk increases during the infectious processes of the mother or the baby.

Leukocytes go to immune stations such as the spleen and lymph nodes of newborns via the gastrointestinal tract [61]. Although the distribution of leukocytes varies according to the milk stage, macrophages, polymorphonuclear neutrophils, and lymphocytes, especially T lymphocytes, are dominant. Stem cells at rest in breast tissue are activated during breastfeeding. Stem cells in breast milk can differentiate into adipose tissue cells, chondrocytes, neurons, osteoblast, cardiac muscle cells, hepatocytes, and pancreatic cells, which can occur from all 3 germ layers [62].

2.8   Cytokines

Cytokines, first shown in breast milk in the 1990s, are suggested to be secreted by immune cells in the mammary glands; however, the exact sources are still unknown. Cytokines have various immunomodulatory functions such as growth stimulation, differentiated immunoglobulin production, thymocyte proliferation, and suppression of interleukin (IL) -2 and IgE production [13]. Interleukin-1 beta (IL-1β) and tumor necrosis factor-alpha (TNF-α) were the first to be quantified [63]. Some cytokines, such as transforming growth factor-beta 2 (TGF-β2), IL-2, IL-6, IL-10, epidermal growth factor (EGF), insulin-like growth factor (IGF), and TNF-α, perform well-defined tasks such as sIgA production, mucin production in the airways and intestines, intestinal maturation, prevention of resistant pathogen colonization and control of inflammatory responses [61–65]. In addition to cytokines whose function has been understood more clearly, such as IL-7, which supports thymus growth, the presence of cytokines whose function has not yet been determined, such as interferon-gamma (IFN-γ), has also been reported [64]. Interleukin-6 and IL-8 are found at higher rates in mothers with mastitis breast milk [57].

2.9 Lactoperoxidase

The lactoperoxidase enzyme supports the immune system by forming hypothiocyanate by oxidation of thiocyanate in the presence of hydrogen peroxide [66]. Hypothiocyanate is a powerful antimicrobial that kills gram-positive and gram-negative bacteria [67]. Thiocyanate is also found in saliva, where it contributes to oral mucosal immunity. The hydrogen peroxide molecule required for the lactoperoxidase enzyme's function is formed due to xanthine oxidoreductase activity. The lactoperoxidase enzyme inhibits the growth of *E. coli* and *Salmonella enteritidis* in vitro [34].

2.10 Bacteriocins

Bacteriocins, frequently used in food preservation, are antibacterial peptides produced against other bacteria. Some bacteriocins undergo modification after being synthesized; this activity is observed in *Lactobacillus, Enterococcus, Streptococcus,* and many other gram-positive and gram-negative bacteria. Bacteriocins continued to be studied for their antibacterial properties for developing new antibiotics and discovering new cancer treatments [68].

2.11 Kappa-Casein

Kappa (κ) casein is a glycoprotein, one of the 3 casein types found in breast milk. Peptides formed by proteolysis show many bioactive properties, especially antimicrobial and immunomodulatory activities [69]. They prevent attaching pathogens such as EPEC, *S. typhimurium,* and *Shigella flexneri* to the intestinal mucosa [13]. The degraded glycomacropeptide (GMP) inhibits the adhesion of *Helicobacter pylori* to the gastric mucosa [70]. The contribution of glycomacropeptide to the microbiota has been proven by its bifidogenic effect on *Bifidobacterium infantis* and *Bifidobacterium bifidum* [71].

2.12 Haptocorrin

Haptocorrin, a heavily glycosylated protein, contributes to vitamin B_{12} absorption as well as protection from pathogens [34]. Although its mechanism has not been fully elucidated, in vitro studies demonstrate that haptocorrin provides protection against EPEC [72].

2.13   Breast Milk Microbiota

Breast milk microbiota, much richer than intestinal microbiota [73], plays an essential role in shaping the intestinal microbiota and, thus, in the maturation of the immune system. Zimmermann and Curtis [5] reviewed 44 studies in terms of breast milk microbiota; the most commonly detected generas were *Staphylococcus, Streptococcus Lactobacillus, Pseudomonas, Bifidobacterium, Corynebacterium, Enterococcus, Acinetobacter, Rothia, Cutibacterium, Veillonella,* and *Bacteroides.* Breastfed infants have a *Bifidobacterium*-predominant intestinal microbiota [74]. Despite the diversity in breast milk microbiota, antibacterial products synthesized by lactic acid-producing bacteria and *Parabacteroides* prevent other bacteria from showing pathogenicity [5, 75]. In addition, lactic acid-producing bacteria prevent the proliferation of some types of bacteria, such as *Pseudomonas, Salmonella, Shigella, and Listeria,* not found in the breast milk microbiota [76]. Many factors such as gestational age, delivery mode, sex, parity, intrapartum antibiotics, presence of human immunodeficiency virus (HIV) infection, lactation stage, diet, body mass index (BMI), probiotic use during pregnancy, and smoking have been studied with respect to the formation of breast milk microbiota. These studies, conducted with a relatively limited number of participants, did not have consistent results, and investigators concluded that large-scale studies with more participants were needed [5]. The effects of different practices, such as the mother's use of probiotics and the addition of probiotics to breast milk, on the infant's microbiota are among the most intriguing future studies.

3   Breastfeeding and Maternal Infections

Although breast milk is protective against infections, it can also cause the transmission of some infectious diseases. Although rare, transmission can occur by ingesting breast milk or by contact, droplet, or airborne during breastfeeding. Excessive fear of contagion will prevent the baby from getting breast milk, providing growth and development and protecting it from infections. For this reason, knowing the absolute contraindications and avoiding incorrect contraindications is important for breastfeeding.

3.1   Anthrax

Anthrax is a zoonotic disease caused by *Bacillus anthracis.* It is transmitted to humans by contact with infected animals and animal products. Clinically, it may cause mostly cutaneous, less frequently inhalational, and/or gastrointestinal involvement [77]. Direct human-to-human transmission occurs by contact of non-intact skin or mucosa with the infected lesion. No data exist on transmission through breast milk [78].

To continue breastfeeding, the mother's general health status, the presence of a cutaneous lesion, and the location of the lesion, if any, should be considered. Depending on the mother's condition, treatment or prophylaxis should be started, and the agents to be used should be chosen among agents that are safe for breast-feeding, such as penicillin, amoxicillin, ampicillin, clindamycin, meropenem, and imipenem [79]. If there are cutaneous lesions, they should be covered, and hands should be washed before touching the baby. When these conditions are met, breast-feeding is continued [80].

The baby should be evaluated in terms of the necessity of prophylaxis. If the mother's general condition is poor and a lesion exists -on the breast/s- in an area that may contaminate the milk, breastfeeding status and method should be reconsidered [81]. After 24–48 h of effective antibacterial therapy, breastfeeding should be resumed as the contagion is considered over [81].

3.2 Brucellosis

Brucellosis is a worldwide zoonosis, and the primary source is sheep, goats, and cattle. *Brucella* species, gram-negative coccobacillus bacteria, are mainly transmit-ted from animal to human through infected animal tissues and the consumption of raw meat [82]. Although rare, *Brucella* species may be transmitted from person to person through transfusion, bone marrow or organ transplant, sexual contact, trans-placental, and breastfeeding [83]. Three case reports suggest the possibility of trans-mission through breast milk based on the growth in breast milk cultures [84–86]. Treatment should be started as soon as the diagnosis is made because the conse-quences may lead to mortality. Gentamicin, streptomycin, trimethoprim-sulfamethoxazole, and rifampin for 4 to 6 weeks are acceptable medications for mothers breastfeeding [80]. For this extended period, doxycycline should be used cautiously in the lactating woman [80]. If a breast abscess has occurred, it should be drained [87]. Babies whose mothers have brucellosis should not be breastfed until the infection clears and should be closely monitored for evidence of infection [82].

3.3 Chlamydial Infections

Chlamydia pneumoniae and *Chlamydia trachomatis* are gram-negative bacteria transmitted by droplets and sexually, respectively. *Chlamydia* species can cause pneumonia, trachoma, and genitourinary infections such as vaginitis, urethritis, cervicitis, endometritis, and pelvic inflammatory disease in adults. In infants, *C. trachomatis* can cause pneumonia and conjunctivitis with perinatal transmission [88]. No evidence exists of transmission through breast milk [78]. Since a prolonged infection may result in adhesions and infertility, the mother must be treated with agents suitable for breastfeeding. The infant should also be evaluated for the need for treatment. The significance of antibodies in the breast milk of seropositive mothers in terms of protection is not yet known [89]. The general recommendation is to treat the mother-infant dyad, if necessary, and to continue breastfeeding [80].

3.4 Diarrheal Infections

Bacillus cereus, a gram-positive bacillus that causes food poisoning with a short incubation period, is transmitted by improperly prepared food intake. Since heat-resistant *B. cereus* spores can cause disease despite pasteurization, breast milk from a milk bank or donor should be used cautiously [90].

Clostridium difficile is a gram-positive spore-forming bacillus. Asymptomatic intestinal colonization is common, especially in infants under 2 years of age [91]. Contact precautions should be applied in addition to standard precautions for infants of hospitalized mothers for *C. difficile* infection. If the mother's general condition is good, breastfeeding may be continued during treatment [80]. Vancomycin and metronidazole may be used safely in both mother and baby.

In diarrheal infections caused by other agents, including *Campylobacter fetus, Campylobacter jejuni, E. coli* O157:H7, *Salmonella enteritidis, Shigella* spp., *V. cholerae, Vibrio parahaemolyticus, Yersinia enterocolitica,* and *Yersinia pseudo-tuberculosis*, standard and contact precautions should be followed [92]. Many animal and human studies have proven the protective effect of breast milk, especially against *E. coli, Shigella spp.,* and *V. cholerae* [13]. For this reason, it is recommended to continue breastfeeding with adequate hydration support to be provided to the mother during diarrhea.

3.5 Diphtheria

Diphtheria, an infectious disease of the respiratory tract or skin, is caused by *Corynebacterium diphtheriae* transmitted by droplet route or contact with infected material. It can also affect the nervous system, heart, and kidneys, with the distribution of toxins into the systemic circulation [93]. Diphtheria, a significant mortality cause before the vaccine era, has been reduced to almost non-existence after global immunization, but it continues to be a threat for some countries. The transmission of *C. diphtheriae* to breast milk has not yet been demonstrated. It is recommended to continue breastfeeding if there is no lesion caused by *C. diphtheriae* on the breast skin that could contaminate the breast milk [80].

3.6 **Haemophilus influenzae** *Infections*

Haemophilus influenzae type b (Hib) was a significant cause of severe invasive diseases and related mortality, especially in children. As a result of effective and widespread vaccination, a significant decrease was achieved in the incidence and mortality of Hib diseases [94]. *Haemophilus influenzae* type b, transmitted via droplet or contact with respiratory secretions, can cause bacteremia and affects many systems, primarily the respiratory tract and central nervous system. No data exists on its transmission into breast milk. Furthermore, breast milk limits throat colonization of *H. influenzae* [95]. After the 24th hour of the mother's treatment for *H. influenzae* infection, breastfeeding may be continued if the mother's general condition is good [92]. Since infants are not yet immunized with the Hib vaccine, chemoprophylaxis with rifampin should be provided [96].

3.7 *Listeria Infections*

Listeria monocytogenes often cause self-limited foodborne infections. More serious diseases caused by *L. monocytogenes,* such as bacteremia, sepsis, meningitis, and brain abscess, may occur in pregnant and immunocompromised patient groups [97]. Perinatal *L. monocytogenes* infection may result in intrauterine death, preterm birth, early and late neonatal sepsis, meningitis, and even mortality [98]. Although many articles exist about mastitis in animals, the transmission of *L. monocytogenes* to breast milk has not been shown in humans [78, 99]. Continuity of breastfeeding should be ensured as soon as the general health status of the mother-baby dyad allows.

3.8 *Mastitis*

Lactational mastitis occurs in 3–33% of lactating women, which starts with poor milk flow but can develop into bacterial mastitis within 12–24 h [100]. The most common causative agent of mastitis is *S. aureus*; less frequently, other bacteria such as *Streptococcus, Bacteroides, Corynebacterium, Pseudomonas, and Klebsiella* may also be seen [101]. Antistaphylococcal antibiotics, such as cephalexin, and clindamycin, suitable for breastfeeding, should be used for the mother. If an abscess is formed, it should be drained, and the breast should be emptied by breastfeeding or expressing [102].

3.9 Mycobacterial Infections

3.9.1 Mycobacterium leprae

Mycobacterium leprae is an obligate intracellular bacterium that can infect the skin, as in anthrax and diphtheria. The peripheral nervous system and mucous membranes may also be involved. *Mycobacterium leprae* may be transmitted by prolonged close contact or droplets [103]. No transmission of *M. leprae* via breastfeeding has been reported. Data show that the immune response changes caused by leprae negatively affect the growth and development of infants [80]. Although *M. leprae* is not transmitted by breastfeeding, the safety of dapsone and clofazimine used in the treatment is unclear. However, some experts advocate the continuation of breastfeeding; the decision should be made by considering the risk-benefit ratio [104].

3.9.2 Mycobacterium tuberculosis

Mycobacterium tuberculosis, an obligate intracellular bacterium, can infect all organs in the body. The 2022 WHO report shows tuberculosis still has a severe disease burden [105]. Wars, uncontrolled immigration, and the increasing number of newly diagnosed HIV-infected cases make tuberculosis challenging to control. *Mycobacterium tuberculosis* is transmitted by inhalation of droplet nuclei scattered from a person with laryngeal, pulmonary, or endobronchial tuberculosis disease, considered contagious. *Mycobacterium tuberculosis* may be transmitted from mother to baby by the hematogenous route during pregnancy, ingesting amniotic fluid or secretions during delivery for mothers with genitourinary tuberculosis, and by airway during postpartum breastfeeding [106]. When transmitted during pregnancy, tuberculosis can cause miscarriage, perinatal death, preterm birth, low birth weight, and congenital disease. Therefore, antituberculous treatment should be started as soon as possible after the mother is diagnosed [107]. The placenta must be examined histologically and microbiologically. Every mother diagnosed with tuberculosis should be evaluated for HIV infection and antituberculous drug susceptibility. Treatment and follow-up processes should be continued according to national and international guidelines. Pyridoxine support should not be forgotten for pregnant and lactating mothers.

Although congenital tuberculosis is rare, its mortality is quite high [108]. Congenital tuberculosis may manifest nonspecific signs of a sepsis-like syndrome, such as fever, hepatomegaly, respiratory distress, decreased suction and weight gain, lethargy, and convulsions [109–111]. The diagnostic process is complex as these findings may also be seen in any congenital infection. Rapid clinical and laboratory evaluation with the tuberculin skin test (TST), interferon-gamma release assay (IGRAs), chest radiography, and lumbar puncture should be performed in infants whose mothers were diagnosed with tuberculosis.

If tuberculosis is detected, the baby should be treated and isolated from other babies. If tuberculosis is undetected in the infant, breastfeeding should be delayed until the mother appropriately completes the first 2 weeks of treatment [111]. After the second week of the antituberculous treatment, breastfeeding may be started if the disappearance of contagiousness is microbiologically proven with smear-negative sputum [111, 112]. Meanwhile, breast milk may be expressed according to the appropriate guidelines, provided no tuberculosis involvement exists on the breast skin or tuberculosis mastitis. Another -uninfected- person can feed the baby with the mother's breast milk through a bottle or spoon. Chemoprophylaxis also should be started for the undiseased baby of the mother with tuberculosis.

3.10 Neisseria Infections.

3.10.1 Gonococcal Infections

Asymptomatic carriage and genitourinary involvement, such as urethritis, vaginitis, vulvitis, cervicitis, and disseminated disease, may be caused by *Neisseria gonorrhoeae*, a gram-negative diplococcus. Extragenital skin involvement with *N. gonorrhoeae* is often associated with trauma and its presence in the fingers [113]. No evidence of breast milk-mediated transmission of *N. gonorrhoeae* exists [78].

Neisseria gonorrhoeae can be transmitted to the baby in the birth canal or by contact with an infected person during the postpartum period. In infants, *N. gonorrhoeae* disseminated disease, ophthalmia neonatorum, or scalp abscesses due to scalp monitoring may be seen [114]. As soon as the gonococcal infection is diagnosed in the mother, treatment should be started, and the mother should be screened for other sexually transmitted infections (STIs). Empirical preventive treatment should also be started in babies whose mothers have proven gonococcal infection, and babies should be followed closely for disease status. After the 24th hour of treatment, the patient with gonococcal infection is considered non-infectious. It would be appropriate to isolate the mother-baby dyad from other mother-baby pairs for 24 h without separating from each other [80].

3.10.2 Meningococcal Infections

Neisseria meningitidis, a gram-negative diplococcus transmitted through droplets, causes severe invasive infections that can result in mortality. It is essential to follow the droplet precautions as the infectiousness continues in the first 24 h of the treatment [115]. Prophylaxis with appropriate agents such as rifampin or ceftriaxone should be started as soon as possible in infants at risk of exposure, whether breastfed or not [116]. After the 24th hour of the treatment, the mother's general health will determine the breastfeeding continuity. Separating the mother-infant couple or interrupting breastfeeding is not required for the baby has already been exposed [80].

3.11 Pertussis

Bordetella pertussis, the causative agent of pertussis, is transmitted by close exposure to large respiratory droplets of infected individuals. Pertussis has a milder course in adults; however, it often infects infants and small children and can lead to serious complications such as severe apnea and paroxysmal coughing attacks, pneumonia, pulmonary hypertension, seizures, and encephalopathy [117].

Since the baby is unprotected until the first dose of the pertussis vaccine, only maternal antibodies may protect a baby until pertussis vaccine administration. It is recommended that the mother be vaccinated between 27–36 weeks of gestation to produce antibodies against *B. pertussis* [118, 119]. Although the cost-effectiveness data are controversial, the cocoon strategy can also be done [118].

Chemoprophylaxis is recommended for all household contacts of the patient since the contagiousness of pertussis is high, and complications are challenging [118]. Azithromycin or cotrimoxazole (if >8 weeks) is suitable for infants [120]. Additionally, the vaccine series can be started if the baby is older than 6 weeks. However, no permanent immunity is provided by vaccines in the long term. Droplet and standard precautions should be followed during the first 5 days of the mother's treatment [80]. In cases where treatment is impossible, precautions should be extended to 21 days.

3.12 Staphylococcal Infections

Staphylococcus aureus causes local infections such as cellulitis, impetigo, soft tissue infections, and invasive diseases such as pneumonia, meningitis, osteomyelitis, septic arthritis, and endocarditis [121]. *Staphylococcus aureus* is also the most common bacterial cause of mastitis. *Staphylococcus aureus* frequently colonizes the nasal mucosa and umbilicus and can be transmitted from person to person by direct contact. Data showed that maternal and parental colonizations play a principal role in *S. aureus* colonization in infants and young children, respectively [122, 123].

Community-acquired methicillin-resistant *S. aureus* (CA-MRSA) transmission to infants via breast milk has been reported; however, *S. aureus* was not detected in expressed breast milk samples after pasteurization [80]. Nguyen et al. [80] reported breastfeeding was not a risk factor for MRSA infection in well-infant nursery outbreaks.

When a mild or moderate staphylococcal infection, such as impetigo, pustulosis, cellulitis, abscess, mastitis, and breast abscess, develops in the mother and/or **term** infant, treatment should be initiated by following standard and contact precautions without dividing the two and breastfeeding should be continued [80]. However, when a staphylococcal infection develops in the mother and/or her **preterm** baby, it should be treated appropriately, and the breast milk should be cultured and monitored. The breast milk culture result should be negative before resuming breastfeeding [80].

Staphylococcus aureus can also cause a toxin-mediated disease. In the literature, only one case, a breastfed infant with staphylococcal scalded skin syndrome, has been reported [124]. Starting treatment and continuing breastfeeding is recommended if the mother's health condition is good.

Staphylococcus epidermidis is a frequently detected microorganism in breast milk, especially in preterm infants. In addition to standard and contact precautions, training of mothers with preterm infants on the expression, collection, transportation, and storage of breast milk should also be supported [124].

3.13   Group B Streptococcal Infections

Streptococcus agalactiae (group B streptococcus; GBS) frequently colonizes the genital and gastrointestinal tracts of women [125]. A meta-analysis showed that the GBS colonization rate ranged from 1.4% to 48.4% [126]. Group B streptococcus may cause asymptomatic bacteriuria, urinary system infection, chorioamnionitis, endometritis, bacteremia, and rarely meningitis, sepsis, and endocarditis during pregnancy and the postpartum period in mothers, and bacteremia, sepsis, meningitis and other invasive infections in neonates.

Although a relationship between GBS colonization and pregnancy loss, stillbirth, and preterm birth has been established, the linkage between preterm birth and the mother's colonization status is quite complex [126, 127]. Maternal GBS colonization status is a significant risk factor for early-onset and late-onset neonatal sepsis. All pregnant women should be screened first in the early pregnancy stage and between the $36^{0/7}$ and $37^{6/7}$ weeks of pregnancy [128]. If colonization with GBS, cystitis, pyelonephritis, asymptomatic bacteriuria, or a previous history of GBS-infected newborn exists, intrapartum antibiotic prophylaxis (IAP) should be provided [128]. However, studies have shown that anti-GBS sIgA antibodies in breast milk reduce the risk of colonization, which supports the continuation of breastfeeding [129].

For high-risk preterm newborns in the neonatal intensive care unit (NICU) and term newborns, whose mothers are positive for GBS, IAP should be administered to the mother, breastfeeding should be supported, and the baby should be followed up for clinical findings. For high-risk preterm newborns whose mothers have mastitis and are followed up in the NICU, breast milk should be cultured, the mother should be treated with appropriate antibiotics, and the baby should be monitored clinically. If the culture result is positive, interrupting breastfeeding should be considered until pasteurization, or the culture result is negative [130].

For newborns with early-onset GBS sepsis, feeding with breast milk should be continued if possible. For newborns with late-onset GBS sepsis, the mother's urine, vaginal, rectal, and breast milk cultures should be obtained, and the mother should be treated if the breast milk culture is positive [131].

4 Conclusion

Breast milk is a unique source of nutrition with each ingredient's flawless and personalized composition. Breast milk contributes to growth and development, disease protection, and survival. Contraindications that require interruption or termination of breastfeeding due to maternal bacterial infections are limited in numbers. Physicians must be aware of these contraindications and avoid incorrect contraindications to ensure infants' access to breast milk, which is their right.

References

1. Prentice AM. Breastfeeding in the modern world. Ann Nutr Metab. 2022;78(Suppl 2):29–38.
2. American Academy of Pediatrics Committee on Drugs. Transfer of drugs and other chemicals into human milk. Pediatrics. 2001;108:776–89.
3. Kawalec A, Zwolińska D. Emerging role of microbiome in the prevention of urinary tract infections in children. Int J Mol Sci. 2022;23(2):870.
4. Altobelli E, Angeletti PM, Verrotti A, Petrocelli R. The impact of human milk on necrotizing enterocolitis: a systematic review and meta-analysis. Nutrients. 2020;12(5):1322.
5. Zimmermann P, Curtis N. Breast milk microbiota: a review of the factors that influence composition. J Infect. 2020;81:17–47.
6. Röszer T. Mother-to-child signaling through breast milk biomolecules. Biomol Ther. 2021;11(12):1743.
7. Eidelman AI, Schanler RJ, Johnston M, et al. Section on breastfeeding, Breastfeeding and the use of human milk. Pediatrics. 2012;129:e827–41.
8. Lönnerdal B. Bioactive proteins in human milk-potential benefits for preterm infants. Clin Perinatol. 2017;44:179–91.
9. Pai UA, Chandrasekhar P, Carvalho RS, Kumar S. The role of nutrition in immunity in infants and toddlers: an expert panel opinion. Clin Epidemiol Glob Health. 2018;7:155–9.
10. Horta BL, de Lima NP. Breastfeeding and type 2 diabetes: systematic review and meta-analysis. Curr Diab Rep. 2019;19(1):1.
11. Meek JY, Noble L. Policy statement: Breastfeeding and the use of human milk. Pediatrics. 2022;150(1):e2022057988.
12. World Health Organization. Guideline: protecting, promoting and supporting breastfeeding in facilities providing maternity and newborn services. Geneva: World Health Organization; 2017. p. 1–120. https://www.who.int/publications/i/item/9789241550086. Accessed 3 Mar 2023).
13. Kim JH, Bode L, Ogra PL. Human milk. In: Wilson CB, Nizet V, Maldonado YA, Remington JS, Klein JO, editors. Remington and Klein's infectious diseases of the fetus and newborn infant. 8th ed. Philadelphia, PA: Elsevier; 2016. p. 189–213.
14. Hanson LA. Comparative immunological studies of the immune globulins of human milk and of blood serum. Int Arch Allergy Appl Immunol. 1961;18:241–67.

15. Johansen FE, Braathen R, Brandtzaeg P. The J chain is essential for polymeric Ig receptor-mediated epithelial transport of IgA. J Immunol. 2001;167:5185–92.
16. Kleist SA, Knoop KA. Understanding the elements of maternal protection from systemic bacterial infections during early life. Nutrients. 2020;12(4):1045.
17. Capasso L, Borrelli A, Cerullo J, et al. Role of immunoglobulins in neonatal sepsis. Transl Med UniSa. 2014;11:28–33.
18. Fishaut M, Murphy D, Neifert M, McIntosh K, Ogra PL. Bronchomammary axis in the immune response to respiratory syncytial virus. J Pediatr. 1981;99:186–91.
19. Guarner F, Malagelada JR. Gut flora in health and disease. Lancet. 2003;361(9356):512–9.
20. Lamounier JA, Moulin ZS, Xavier CC. Recomendações quanto à amamentação na vigência de infecção materna [Recommendations for breastfeeding during maternal infections]. J Pediatr (Rio J). 2004;80(5 Suppl):s181–188. [article in Portuguese, abstract in English].
21. Sharma N, Devi B, Sharma M. Impressive antimicrobial potential of human milk: a blessing for nascent life. In: Cole JI, editor. Human milk nutritional content and role in health and disease. 1st ed. New York: Nova Science Publishers; 2021. p. 1–69.
22. Rio-Aige K, Azagra-Boronat I, Castell M, et al. The breast milk immunoglobulinome. Nutrients. 2021;13(6):1810.
23. Reddy V, Bhaskaram C, Raghuramulu N, Jagadeesan V. Antimicrobial factors in human milk. Acta Paediatr Scand. 1977;66:229–32.
24. Zheng W, Zhao W, Wu M, et al. Microbiota-targeted maternal antibodies protect neonates from enteric infection. Nature. 2020;577(7791):543–8.
25. Nguyen TG. The therapeutic implications of activated immune responses via the enigmatic immunoglobulin D. Int Rev Immunol. 2022;41:107–22.
26. Litwin SD, Zehr BD, Insel RA. Selective concentration of IgD class-specific antibodies in human milk. Clin Exp Immunol. 1990;80:263–7.
27. Meng X, Dunsmore G, Koleva P, et al. The profile of human milk metabolome, cytokines, and antibodies in inflammatory bowel diseases versus healthy mothers, and potential impact on the newborn. J Crohns Colitis. 2019;13:431–41.
28. Bahna SL, Keller MA, Heiner DC. IgE and IgD in human colostrum and plasma. Pediatr Res. 1982;16:604–7.
29. Goldman AS, Chheda S. The immune system in human milk: a historic perspective. Ann Nutr Metab. 2021;77:189–96.
30. Hendricks GM. Bioactive components in human milk. In: Guo M, editor. Human milk biochemistry and infant formula manufacturing technology. 1st ed. Philadelphia, PA: Elsevier; 2014. p. 33–54.
31. Benkerroum N. Antimicrobial activity of lysozyme with special relevance to milk. Afr J Biotechnol. 2009;725(25):4856–67.
32. Chang R, Ng TB, Sun WZ. Lactoferrin as potential preventative and adjunct treatment for COVID-19. Int J Antimicrob Agents. 2020;56(3):106118.
33. Maga EA, Desai PT, Weimer BC, Dao N, Kültz D, Murray JD. Consumption of lysozyme-rich milk can alter microbial fecal populations. Appl Environ Microbiol. 2012;78(17):6153–60.
34. Demmelmair H, Prell C, Timby N, Lönnerdal B. Benefits of lactoferrin, osteopontin and milk fat globule membranes for infants. Nutrients. 2017;9(8):817.
35. Almeida CC, Mendonça Pereira BF, Leandro KC, Costa MP, Spisso BF, Conte-Junior CA. Bioactive compounds in infant formula and their effects on infant nutrition and health: a systematic literature review. Int J Food Sci. 2021;2021:8850080.
36. Brandenburg K, Jürgens G, Müller M, Fukuoka S, Koch MH. Biophysical characterization of lipopolysaccharide and lipid A inactivation by lactoferrin. Biol Chem. 2001;382:1215–25.
37. Alexander DB, Iigo M, Yamauchi K, Suzui M, Tsuda H. Lactoferrin: an alternative view of its role in human biological fluids. Biochem Cell Biol. 2012;90:279–306.
38. Lönnerdal B. Infant formula and infant nutrition: bioactive proteins of human milk and implications for composition of infant formulas. Am J Clin Nutr. 2014;99:s712–7.

39. Qiu J, Hendrixson DR, Baker EN, Murphy TF, St Geme JW 3rd, Plaut AG. Human milk lactoferrin inactivates two putative colonization factors expressed by *Haemophilus influenzae*. Proc Natl Acad Sci U S A. 1998;95(21):12641–6.

40. Hanson LA, Korotkova M. The role of breastfeeding in prevention of neonatal infection. Semin Neonatol. 2002;7:275–81.

41. Barboza M, Pinzon J, Wickramasinghe S, et al. Glycosylation of human milk lactoferrin exhibits dynamic changes during early lactation enhancing its role in pathogenic bacteria-host interactions. Mol Cell Proteomics. 2012;11(6):M111.015248.

42. Suzuki YA, Lopez V, Lönnerdal B. Mammalian lactoferrin receptors: structure and function. Cell Mol Life Sci. 2005;62:2560–75.

43. Håversen LA, Engberg I, Baltzer L, Dolphin G, Hanson LA, Mattsby-Baltzer I. Human lactoferrin and peptides derived from a surface-exposed helical region reduce experimental Escherichia coli urinary tract infection in mice. Infect Immun. 2000;68:5816–23.

44. Manzoni P, Rinaldi M, Cattani S, et al. Italian Task Force for the Study and Prevention of Neonatal Fungal Infections, Italian Society of Neonatology Bovine lactoferrin supplementation for prevention of late-onset sepsis in very low-birth-weight neonates: a randomized trial. JAMA. 2009;302:1421–8.

45. Layman DK, Lönnerdal B, Fernstrom JD. Applications for α-lactalbumin in human nutrition. Nutr Rev. 2018;76:444–60.

46. Pellegrini A, Thomas U, Bramaz N, Hunziker P, von Fellenberg R. Isolation and identification of three bactericidal domains in the bovine alpha-lactalbumin molecule. Biochim Biophys Acta. 1999;1426:439–48.

47. Golinelli LP, Del Aguila EM, Paschoalin VF, Silva JT, Conte-Junior CA. Functional aspect of colostrum and whey proteins in human milk. J Hum Nutr Food Sci. 2014;2(3):1035.

48. Lönnerdal B, Erdmann P, Thakkar SK, Sauser J, Destaillats F. Longitudinal evolution of true protein, amino acids and bioactive proteins in breast milk: a developmental perspective. J Nutr Biochem. 2017;41:1–11.

49. Brück WM, Graverholt G, Gibson GR. A two-stage continuous culture system to study the effect of supplemental alpha-lactalbumin and glycomacropeptide on mixed cultures of human gut bacteria challenged with enteropathogenic *Escherichia coli* and *Salmonella* serotype *Typhimurium*. J Appl Microbiol. 2003;95:44–53.

50. Gustafsson L, Hallgren O, Mossberg AK, et al. HAMLET kills tumor cells by apoptosis: structure, cellular mechanisms, and therapy. J Nutr. 2005;135:1299–303.

51. Kulinich A, Liu L. Human milk oligosaccharides: the role in the fine-tuning of innate immune responses. Carbohydr Res. 2016;432:62–70.

52. Wang Y, Zhou X, Gong P, et al. Comparative majör oligosaccharides and lactose between Chinese human and animal milk. Int Dairy J. 2020;108:104727.

53. Thongaram T, Hoeflinger JL, Chow J, Miller MJ. Human milk oligosaccharide consumption by probiotic and human-associated bifidobacteria and lactobacilli. J Dairy Sci. 2017;100:7825–33.

54. Moossavi S, Atakora F, Miliku K, et al. Integrated analysis of human milk microbiota with oligosaccharides and fatty acids in the CHILD cohort. Front Nutr. 2019;6:58.

55. Wu RY, Li B, Koike Y, et al. Human milk oligosaccharides increase mucin expression in experimental necrotizing enterocolitis. Mol Nutr Food Res. 2019;63(3):e1800658.

56. Triantis V, Bode L, van Neerven RJJ. Immunological effects of human milk oligosaccharides. Front Pediatr. 2018;6:190.

57. Kim YJ. Immunomodulatory effects of human colostrum and milk. Pediatr Gastroenterol Hepatol Nutr. 2021;24:337–45.

58. Bhinder G, Allaire JM, Garcia C, et al. Milk fat globule membrane supplementation in formula modulates the neonatal gut microbiome and normalizes intestinal development. Sci Rep. 2017;7:45274.

59. Ambrożej D, Dumycz K, Dziechciarz P, Ruszczyński M. Milk fat globule membrane supplementation in children: systematic review with meta-analysis. Nutrients. 2021;13(3):714.

60. Brooker BE. The epithelial cells and cell fragments in human milk. Cell Tissue Res. 1980;210:321–32.

61. Bardanzellu F, Peroni DG, Fanos V. Human breast milk: bioactive components, from stem cells to health outcomes. Curr Nutr Rep. 2020;9:1–13.

62. Hassiotou F, Beltran A, Chetwynd E, et al. Breastmilk is a novel source of stem cells with multilineage differentiation potential. Stem Cells. 2012;30:2164–74.

63. Rudloff HE, Schmalstieg FC Jr, Mushtaha AA, Palkowetz KH, Liu SK, Goldman AS. Tumor necrosis factor-alpha in human milk. Pediatr Res. 1992;31:29–33.

64. Ngom PT, Collinson AC, Pido-Lopez J, Henson SM, Prentice AM, Aspinall R. Improved thymic function in exclusively breastfed infants is associated with higher interleukin 7 concentrations in their mothers' breast milk. Am J Clin Nutr. 2004;80:722–8.

65. Saso A, Blyuss O, Munblit D, Faal A, Moore SE, Le Doare K. Breast milk cytokines and early growth in Gambian infants. Front Pediatr. 2019;6:414.

66. Zou Z, Bauland J, Hewavitharana AK, et al. A sensitive, high-throughput fluorescent method for the determination of lactoperoxidase activities in milk and comparison in human, bovine, goat, and camel milk. Food Chem. 2021;339:128090.

67. Sousa SG, Delgadillo I, Saraiva JA. Effect of thermal pasteurisation and high-pressure processing on immunoglobulin content and lysozyme and lactoperoxidase activity in human colostrum. Food Chem. 2014;151:79–85.

68. Chikindas ML, Weeks R, Drider D, Chistyakov VA, Dicks LM. Functions and emerging applications of bacteriocins. Curr Opin Biotechnol. 2018;49:23–8.

69. Gridneva Z, Tie WJ, Rea A, et al. Human milk casein and whey protein and infant body composition over the first 12 months of lactation. Nutrients. 2018;10(9):1332.

70. Strömqvist M, Falk P, Bergström S, et al. Human milk kappa-casein and inhibition of *Helicobacter pylori* adhesion to human gastric mucosa. J Pediatr Gastroenterol Nutr. 1995;21:288–96.

71. Wada Y, Lönnerdal B. Bioactive peptides derived from human milk proteins--mechanisms of action. J Nutr Biochem. 2014;25:503–14.

72. Adkins Y, Lönnerdal B. Potential host-defense role of a human milk vitamin B-12-binding protein, haptocorrin, in the gastrointestinal tract of breastfed infants, as assessed with porcine haptocorrin in vitro. Am J Clin Nutr. 2003;77:1234–40.

73. Biagi E, Quercia S, Aceti A, et al. The bacterial ecosystem of mother's milk and infant's mouth and gut. Front Microbiol. 2017;8:1214.

74. Zimmermann P, Curtis N. Factors influencing the intestinal microbiome during the first year of life. Pediatr Infect Dis J. 2018;37:e315–35.

75. Nakano V, Ignacio A, Fernandes MR, Fukugaiti MH, Avila-Campos MJ. Intestinal *Bacteroides* and *Parabacteroides* species producing antagonistic substances. Microbiology. 2006;1:61–4.

76. Jiang M, Zhang F, Wan C, et al. Evaluation of probiotic properties of *Lactobacillus plantarum* WLPL04 isolated from human breast milk. J Dairy Sci. 2016;99:1736–46.

77. Swartz MN. Recognition and management of anthrax - an update. N Engl J Med. 2001;345:1621–6.

78. Lawrence RM, Lawrence RA. Breast milk and infection. Clin Perinatol. 2004;31:501–28.

79. Meaney-Delman D, Zotti ME, Creanga AA, et al. Special considerations for prophylaxis for and treatment of anthrax in pregnant and postpartum women. Emerg Infect Dis. 2014;20(2):e130611.

80. Lawrence RM. Tranmission of infectious diseases through breast milk and breastfeeding. In: Lawrence RA, Lawrence RM, Noble L, Rosen-Carole C, Stuebe AM, editors. Breastfeeding: a guide for the medical profession. 9th ed. Philadelphia, PA: Elsevier; 2021. p. 393–456.

81. Bradley JS, Peacock G, Krug SE, et al. AAP Committee on Infectious Diseases and Disaster Preparedness Advisory Council. Pediatric anthrax clinical management. Pediatrics. 2014;133:e1411–36.

82. American Academy of Pediatrics. Brucellosis. In: Kimberlin DW, Barnett ED, Lynfield R, Sawyer MH, editors. Red Book: 2021-2024 Report of the Committee on Infectious Diseases. 32nd ed. Itasca, IL: American Academy of Pediatrics; 2021. p. 238–40.

83. Dadar M, Shahali Y, Alamian S. Isolation of *Brucella melitensis* biovar 1 from human milk confirms breastfeeding as a possible route for infant infection. Microb Pathog. 2021;157:104958.

84. Celebi G, Külah C, Kiliç S, Ustündağ G. Asymptomatic *Brucella* bacteraemia and isolation of *Brucella melitensis* biovar 3 from human breast milk. Scand J Infect Dis. 2007;39:205–8.

85. Al-Mafada SM, Al-Eissa YA, Saeed ES, Kambal AM. Isolation of *Brucella melitensis* from human milk. J Infect. 1993;26:346–8.

86. Tikare NV, Mantur BG, Bidari LH. Brucellar meningitis in an infant - evidence for human breast milk transmission. J Trop Pediatr. 2008;54:272–4.

87. Nemenqani D, Yaqoob N, Khoja H. Breast brucellosis in Taif, Saudi Arabia: cluster of six cases with emphasis on FNA evaluation. J Infect Dev Ctries. 2009;3:255–9.

88. Hammerschlag MR, Kohlhoff SA. Chlamydia infections. In: Feigin RD, Cherry JD, Harrison GJ, Kaplan SL, Steinbach WJ, Hotez PJ, editors. Feigin and Cherry's textbook of pediatric infectious diseases. 8th ed. Philadelphia, PA: Elsevier; 2019. p. 1952–62.

89. Skaug K, Otnaess AB, Orstavik I, Jerve F. Chlamydial secretory IgA antibodies in human milk. Acta Pathol Microbiol Immunol Scand C. 1982;90:21–5.

90. Jandová M, Měřička P, Fišerová M, et al. Quantitative risk assessment of *Bacillus cereus* growth during the warming of thawed pasteurized human banked milk using a predictive mathematical model. Foods. 2022;11(7):1037.

91. Lees EA, Miyajima F, Pirmohamed M, Carrol ED. The role of *Clostridium difficile* in the paediatric and neonatal gut - a narrative review. Eur J Clin Microbiol Infect Dis. 2016;35:1047.

92. Lawrence RM. Precautions and breastfeeding recommendations for selected maternal infections. In: Lawrence RA, Lawrence RM, Noble L, Rosen-Carole C, Stuebe AM, editors. Breastfeeding: a guide for the medical profession. 9th ed. Philadelphia, PA: Elsevier; 2021. p. 738–53.

93. Stechenberg BW. Diphtheria. In: Feigin RD, Cherry JD, Harrison GJ, Kaplan SL, Steinbach WJ, Hotez PJ, editors. Feigin and Cherry's textbook of pediatric infectious diseases. 8th ed. Philadelphia, PA: Elsevier; 2019. p. 931–8.

94. Wahl B, O'Brien KL, Greenbaum A, et al. Burden of *Streptococcus pneumoniae* and *Haemophilus influenzae* type b disease in children in the era of conjugate vaccines: global, regional, and national estimates for 2000-15. Lancet Glob Health. 2018;6:e744.

95. Hokama T, Sakamoto R, Yara A, Asato Y, Takamine F, Itokazu K. Incidence of *Haemophilus influenzae* in the throats of healthy infants with different feeding methods. Pediatr Int. 1999;41:277–80.

96. American Academy of Pediatrics. *Haemophilus influenzae* infections. In: Kimberlin DW, Barnett ED, Lynfield R, Sawyer MH, editors. Red Book: 2021-2024 Report of the Committee on Infectious Diseases. 32nd ed. Itasca, IL: American Academy of Pediatrics; 2021. p. 345–54.

97. Xing F, Lo SKF, Lau SKP, Woo PCY. Listeriosis in a metropolitan hospital: is targeted therapy a risk factor for infection? Front Med (Lausanne). 2022;9:888038.

98. Charlier C, Perrodeau É, Leclercq A, et al. Clinical features and prognostic factors of listeriosis: the MONALISA national prospective cohort study. Lancet Infect Dis. 2017;17:510.

99. Malik SV, Barbuddhe SB, Chaudhari SP. Listeria infections in humans and animals in the Indian subcontinent: a review. Trop Anim Health Prod. 2002;34:359–81.

100. Lai BY, Yu BW, Chu AJ, et al. Risk factors for lactation mastitis in China: a systematic review and meta-analysis. PLoS One. 2021;16(5):e0251182.

101. Angelopoulou A, Field D, Ryan CA, Stanton C, Hill C, Ross RP. The microbiology and treatment of human mastitis. Med Microbiol Immunol. 2018;207:83–94.

102. Crepinsek MA, Taylor EA, Michener K, Stewart F. Interventions for preventing mastitis after childbirth. Cochrane Database Syst Rev. 2020;9(9):CD007239.

103. Cruz AT. Leprosy and Buruli ulcer: the major cutaneous mycobacterioses. In: Feigin RD, Cherry JD, Harrison GJ, Kaplan SL, Steinbach WJ, Hotez PJ, editors. Feigin and Cherry's textbook of pediatric infectious diseases. 8th ed. Philadelphia, PA: Elsevier; 2019. p. 995–1012.
104. Ozturk Z, Tatliparmak A. Leprosy treatment during pregnancy and breastfeeding: a case report and brief review of literature. Dermatol Ther. 2017;30(1) https://doi.org/10.1111/dth.12414.
105. World Health Organisation. Global tuberculosis report 2022. Geneva: World Health Organisation. 2022:1–51. https://www.who.int/teams/global-tuberculosis-programme/tb-reports. Accessed 3 Mar 2023.
106. Li C, Liu L, Tao Y. Diagnosis and treatment of congenital tuberculosis: a systematic review of 92 cases. Orphanet J Rare Dis. 2019;14(1):131.
107. Miele K, Bamrah Morris S, Tepper NK. Tuberculosis in pregnancy. Obstet Gynecol. 2020;135:1444–53.
108. Gould JM, Aronoff SC. Tuberculosis and pregnancy - maternal, fetal, and neonatal considerations. Microbiol Spectr. 2016;4:1–6.
109. Pop LG, Bacalbasa N, Suciu ID, Ionescu P, Toader OD. Tuberculosis in pregnancy. J Med Life. 2021;14:165–9.
110. Lee LH, Le Vea CM, Graman PS. Congenital tuberculosis in a neonatal intensive care unit: case report, epidemiologic investigation and management of exposures. Clin Infect Dis. 1998;27:474–7.
111. American Academy of Pediatrics. Tuberculosis. In: Kimberlin DW, Barnett ED, Lynfield R, Sawyer MH, editors. Red Book: 2021-2024 Report of the Committee on Infectious Diseases. 32nd ed. Itasca, IL: American Academy of Pediatrics; 2021. p. 786–814.
112. Snider DE Jr, Powell KE. Should women taking antituberculosis drugs breastfeed? Arch Intern Med. 1984;144:589–90.
113. Scott MJ Jr, Scott MJ Sr. Primary cutaneous *Neisseria gonorrhoeae* infections. Arch Dermatol. 1982;118:351.
114. American Academy of Pediatrics. Gonococcal infections. In: Kimberlin DW, Barnett ED, Lynfield R, Sawyer MH, editors. Red Book: 2021-2024 Report of the Committee on Infectious Diseases. 32nd ed. Itasca, IL: American Academy of Pediatrics; 2021. p. 338–44.
115. Gardner P. Clinical practice. Prevention of meningococcal disease. N Engl J Med. 2006;355:1466–73.
116. Cohn AC, MacNeil JR, Clark TA, et al. Prevention and control of meningococcal disease: recommendations of the Advisory Committee on Immunization Practices (ACIP). MMWR Recomm Rep 2013; 62:RR-2:1–28.
117. Cherry JD, Heininger U. Pertussis and other *Bordetella* infections. In: Feigin RD, Cherry JD, Harrison GJ, Kaplan SL, Steinbach WJ, Hotez PJ, editors. Feigin and Cherry's textbook of pediatric infectious diseases. 8th ed. Philadelphia, PA: Elsevier; 2019. p. 1159–77.
118. American Academy of Pediatrics. Pertussis. In: Kimberlin DW, Barnett ED, Lynfield R, Sawyer MH, editors. Red Book: 2021-2024 Report of the Committee on Infectious Diseases. 32nd ed. Itasca, IL: American Academy of Pediatrics; 2021. p. 578–89.
119. Havers FP, Moro PL, Hunter P, Hariri S, Bernstein H. Use of tetanus toxoid, reduced diphtheria toxoid, and acellular pertussis vaccines: updated recommendations of the Advisory Committee on Immunization Practices - United States, 2019. MMWR Morb Mortal Wkly Rep. 2020;69(3):77–83.
120. Long SS, Edwards KM, Mertsola J. *Bordotella pertussis* (pertussis) and other *Bordotella* species. In: Long SS, Prober CG, Fischer M, Kimberlin DW, editors. Principles and practice of pediatric infectious diseases. 6th ed. Philadelphia, PA: Elsevier; 2023. p. 909–18.
121. Thomsen I, Creech CB. Staphylococcus aureus. In: Long SS, Prober CG, Fischer M, Kimberlin DW, editors. Principles and practice of pediatric infectious diseases. 6th ed. Philadelphia, PA: Elsevier; 2023. p. 710–23.

122. Chatzakis E, Scoulica E, Papageorgiou N, Maraki S, Samonis G, Galanakis E. Infant colonization by *Staphylococcus aureus*: role of maternal carriage. Eur J Clin Microbiol Infect Dis. 2011;30:1111–7.
123. Regev-Yochay G, Raz M, Carmeli Y, et al. Parental *Staphylococcus aureus* carriage is associated with staphylococcal carriage in young children. Pediatr Infect Dis J. 2009;28:960–5.
124. Katzman DK, Wald ER. Staphylococcal scalded skin syndrome in a breastfed infant. Pediatr Infect Dis J. 1987;6:295–6.
125. Karimi M, Eslami Z, Shamsi F, Moradi J, Ahmadi AY, Baghianimoghadam B. The effect of educational intervention on decreasing mothers' expressed breast milk bacterial contamination whose infants are admitted to neonatal intensive care unit. J Res Health Sci. 2012;13:43–7.
126. Edwards MS, Nizet V, Baker CJ. Group B Streptococcal Infections. In: Wilson CB, Nizet V, Maldonado YA, Remington JS, Klein JO, editors. Remington and Klein's infectious diseases of the fetus and newborn infant. 8th ed. Philadelphia, PA: Elsevier; 2016. p. 411–56.
127. Bianchi-Jassir F, Seale AC, Kohli-Lynch M, et al. Preterm birth associated with Group B streptococcus maternal colonization worldwide: systematic review and meta-analyses. Clin Infect Dis. 2017;65(suppl_2):s133–42.
128. Seale AC, Bianchi-Jassir F, Russell NJ, et al. Estimates of the burden of Group B streptococcal disease worldwide for pregnant women, stillbirths, and children. Clin Infect Dis. 2017;65(suppl_2):s200–19.
129. Prevention of Group B streptococcal early-onset disease in newborns: ACOG Committee Opinion, Number 797. Obstet Gynecol. 2020;135:e51–72. [erratum: Obstet Gynecol. 2020;135:978–979].
130. Le Doare K, Bellis K, Faal A, et al. SIgA, TGF-β1, IL-10, and TNFα in colostrum are associated with infant Group B *Streptococcus* colonization. Front Immunol. 2017;8:1269.
131. Davanzo R, De Cunto A, Travan L, Bacolla G, Creti R, Demarini S. To feed or not to feed? case presentation and best practice guidance for human milk feeding and group B streptococcus in developed countries. J Hum Lact. 2013;29:452–7.

Breastfeeding and Maternal Viral Infections

Murat Sütçü, Funda Yıldız, and Fatma Levent

1 Introduction

Breast milk is uniquely suitable for the infant in its nutritional composition and bioactive molecules that support survival and development. Breast milk contains macro and micronutrients, bioactive molecules, growth factors, and immunoprotective factors.

Exclusive breastfeeding is recommended for approximately the first 6 months of life and continuing until age two, with the transition to appropriate complementary foods.

However, some maternal and infant diseases may limit breastfeeding. In such cases, the healthcare professional should have sufficient knowledge and communication skills to assess the appropriateness of breastfeeding. Breast milk is not sterile; it can be a source of maternally provided commensal and pathogenic microorganisms. Most maternal infections are not contraindicated for breastfeeding; in most cases, breast milk supplies antibodies and protection for the infant. Infected breastfeeding mothers can contaminate pathogenic agents in their infants. Some bacterial, viral, fungal, or parasitic diseases can be transmitted from mother to infant by breast milk.

M. Sütçü (✉)
Division of Pediatric Infectious Diseases, Department of Pediatrics, Faculty of Medicine, Istinye University İstanbul, İstanbul, Türkiye

F. Yıldız
Department of Pediatrics, Faculty of Medicine, Istinye University İstanbul, İstanbul, Türkiye

F. Levent
Division of Pediatric Infectious Diseases, Department of Pediatrics, School of Medicine, Texas Tech University, Lubbock, TX, USA
e-mail: fatma.levent@ttuhsc.edu

© The Author(s), under exclusive license to Springer Nature Switzerland AG 2023
Ö. N. Şahin et al. (eds.), *Breastfeeding and Metabolic Programming*,
https://doi.org/10.1007/978-3-031-33278-4_29

Breastfeeding is recommended for most maternal viral infections except for very few, like HIV infection. Breast milk is also not suggested for infants of human T-lymphotropic virus type 1 or 2 infected mothers. Current evidence for emerging pathogens such as severe acute respiratory syndrome-2 (SARS-CoV-2) is available in the policy statement by the American Academy of Pediatrics (AAP). As contact between the mother and other infected family members expose the infant to respiratory secretions, hand hygiene, and covering the nose and mouth with a mask are recommended while the infected mother is breastfeeding [1].

2   Cytomegalovirus Infection

Cytomegalovirus (CMV) is a DNA virus that is a member of Herpesviridae and is highly prevalent. Most people infected with CMV are asymptomatic and have a lifelong latency [2, 3]. Studies have estimated that the seroprevalence of CMV is 83% globally and 66% in Europe [4].

Cytomegalovirus can be transmitted from mother to child in utero, intrapartum, and postnatal ways. In utero transmission may cause congenital CMV infection. Intrapartum and postnatal transmission occur by contact with infected body fluids (saliva, urine, blood, human milk) [5]. Postnatal infection is not typically related to clinical signs in healthy-term infants. There is no evidence to prohibit breastfeeding of healthy full-term infants whose mothers are CMV infected [1, 6].

Postnatal CMV infection in preterm low-birth-weight infants may be symptomatic and present with a sepsis-like syndrome and multi-organ involvement, particularly respiratory distress and hepatosplenomegaly. However, these symptoms do not cause long-term sequelae [7]. Therefore, the benefits of breastfeeding preterm infants outweigh the risk of postpartum symptomatic CMV infection, and it is recommended to continue breastfeeding [1].

It is beneficial to mention that CMV can also be transmitted to infants from asymptomatic seropositive mothers. Up to 95% of healthy seropositive women experience CMV reactivation by shedding viral DNA into breast milk during breastfeeding. This is especially important for preterm infants with a high risk of symptomatic infection. The CMV reactivation occurs in cases of low immunological status, stress, and DNA damage and in healthy mothers during lactation [2, 8].

According to the Centers for Disease Control and Prevention (CDC), breastfeeding is appropriate for CMV seropositive mothers. However, breastfed infants born <30 weeks gestational age and <1500 g whose mothers are CMV seropositive may risk a late-onset sepsis-like syndrome. When deciding to breastfeed the premature infants of CMV seropositive mothers, the risk of CMV transmission should be considered against the unique benefits of breast milk. Freezing and pasteurizing breast milk can reduce the risk of CMV transmission, but freezing does not eliminate the risk [9]. Freezing or pasteurization of breast milk may be beneficial to reduce neonatal CMV infection in preterm infants. Pasteurization reduces the nutritional and immunological substances in breast milk, but CMV viral load can be abolished by pasteurizing breast milk. Freezing does not alter the beneficial components of breast milk, but current studies show that freezing breast milk does not eliminate CMV but only lowers viral load [2, 8, 10].

3 Herpes Simplex Virus Infection

Herpes simplex virus (HSV) is a member of the Herpesviridae family and a DNA virus. HSV is divided into two types, HSV-1 and HSV-2. HSV-1 is commonly spread through oral-to-oral contact. HSV-1 is the primary cause of oral herpes and can lead to genital herpes. HSV-2 leads to genital herpes and is transmitted sexually. Most HSV infections are asymptomatic. Painful blisters or ulcers that recur over time are the symptoms of HSV infection.

Herpes simplex virus is quite common worldwide. The estimation of the World Health Organization (WHO) is that 3.7 billion people (67%) under the age of 50 have HSV-1 infection, and 491 million people (13%) between the ages of 15 and 49 have HSV-2 infection worldwide [11].

Both types of HSV can infect newborns and infants, and painful blisters from herpes can appear anywhere on the body. HSV frequently causes severe infections in newborn infants with high mortality and morbidity rates. All precautions should be taken to protect the baby from contact with the herpes virus, and proper hand hygiene should be practiced before handling the baby [12].

Herpes simplex virus can be transmitted from mother to infant in utero, intrapartum, or postpartum. Intrapartum transmission is usually by contact with genital lesions during delivery, and postpartum transmission occurs by direct contact. Mothers with active herpetic lesions can transmit the virus to their babies by direct or indirect contact. Breastfeeding is recommended if the mother has no herpetic lesions on her breasts and all active lesions on her body are completely and adequately placed under cover. It is not recommended for the mother to breastfeed her baby from the breast with a herpetic lesion or feed the baby with expressed milk from this breast. Breast milk may be contaminated with HSV if an active herpetic lesion is touched while expressed by hand or pump. Therefore, mothers with active herpetic lesions on the breast should discard the milk expressed from the affected breast until all lesions heal. To prevent mother-to-child transmission, lesions on the affected breast should be totally and appropriately covered, and breast milk expressed from the unaffected breast should be used. For the continuity of breast milk production, expressing milk from the breast with the lesion will be beneficial, even if it is not used to feed the infant. Mothers should practice hand hygiene very well and be very careful about cleaning pump parts. Breastfeeding directly from the breast with an active herpetic lesion is not recommended by the AAP; however, unlike the CDC, which states that it would be appropriate to feed with breast milk expressed from the affected breast [12].

4 Shingles

Shingles is caused by the varicella-zoster virus (VZV) that causes chickenpox (varicella) and is also called herpes zoster. After chickenpox is cured, the virus remains inactive and can reactivate, causing shingles.

Shingles is not transmitted from person to person or the infant by breast milk. However, VZV may be transmitted from someone with active shingles to someone who has never had chickenpox or has not had the vaccine. In this case, VZV leads to chickenpox. The virus is transmitted directly through the blisters' liquid [13].

If the mother with shingles does not have a breast lesion, she can continue breastfeeding. If a shingles lesion exists on or near the areola where the baby's mouth touches while feeding, breastfeeding should be discontinued from that affected breast. However, milking should be continued to ensure the continuity of breast milk and prevent mastitis. During this period, breastfeeding can continue on the unaffected breast. All lesions should be covered with a clean, dry cloth until healed to avoid contact with the infant. Mothers should practice proper hand hygiene until all lesions have crusted over [13].

5 Human Immunodeficiency Virus Infection

Human immunodeficiency virus (HIV) is one of the retroviruses. It attacks to CD4+ T cells and gradually reduces their number during infection. Human immunodeficiency virus may be transmitted from mother to infant in utero, peripartum, and postnatal periods. When HIV infection is treated, the risk of perinatal transmission is significantly reduced; however, if left untreated, the risk of transmission is between 20 and 40% [14, 15].

Breastfeeding is one of the postnatal ways of transmission. Evidence of HIV transmission from breast milk to infants has been obtained from studies showing that HIV detection in breast milk and infants of HIV-infected mothers who continue to be breastfed are more likely to be infected. In addition, the fact that mothers infected with HIV in the postnatal period and continuing to breastfeed transmit the infection to their infants supports this evidence. There are also cases that the disease was transmitted to infants born to HIV-free surrogate mothers and breastfed by HIV-infected mothers. The best option to prevent HIV transmission by breast milk is not to breastfeed. The CDC and the American Academy of Pediatrics recommend that mothers with HIV infection with access to clean water and affordable infant formula in the United States should not breastfeed their infants, regardless of anti-retroviral therapy (ART) and viral load. Infant formula and pasteurized donor human milk are safe feeding alternatives for infants of mothers with HIV infection [1, 16]. In resource-limited environments, such as parts of Africa, the World Health Organization (WHO) recommends breastfeeding. Infants should be exclusively breastfed for the first 6 months and continue to be breastfed for at least one more year after starting appropriate complementary foods. Mainly these mothers should be supported to reduce the risk of HIV transmission to the baby through breastfeeding and to comply with ART for their health [17]. Previous studies have suggested that shortening the duration of breastfeeding may reduce the risk of HIV transmission. Previous guidelines from WHO have also included this recommendation to limit the risk of HIV transmission. However, subsequent studies have shown that short-term breastfed infants have higher morbidity and mortality than long-term breastfed infants. It was hypothesized that the infant's mixed feeding would reduce viral load and lower the risk of disease for less exposure to HIV-infected breast milk. However, studies have not supported this idea [18–20]. Breast milk is the best nutrition for very low birth weight (VLBW) infants because it prevents the significant complications of prematurity, including the risk of necrotizing enterocolitis. Pasteurized donor human milk is recommended for VLBW infants when the mother's milk is unavailable or is contraindicated, such as for mothers with HIV infection [16].

6 Hepatitis B Virus Infection

Hepatitis B is a life-threatening liver infection caused by the hepatitis B virus (HBV) that can lead to cirrhosis and hepatocellular carcinoma. Hepatitis B virus is a DNA virus and can cause acute or chronic infection of the liver [21]. Hepatitis B virus is transmitted from mother to child during birth via vertical and horizontal transmission in early childhood. According to the WHO report, 296 million people with chronic hepatitis B infection in 2019, and 1.5 million more are added annually [22].

Hepatitis B is a vaccine-preventable infectious disease, and vaccines are safe, available, and effective. All newborns whose mothers have HBV should be practiced both hepatitis B immune globulin (HBIG) and the first dose of the hepatitis B vaccine within the first 12 h after birth. The second dose of the vaccine should be given when the infant is 1–2 months old, and the third dose at 6 months. At 9–12 months of age, after completion of the vaccine series, the infant should be tested to determine if the vaccine is working and whether HBV has been transmitted to the baby by contact with the mother's blood during delivery.

It is not recommended to delay breastfeeding until the infant is fully immunized. If babies whose mothers are HBsAg positive are administered the hepatitis B vaccine and hepatitis B immunoglobulin (HBIG) at birth, the risk of HBV transmission through breast milk in these cases is very low. However, mothers should not be asked to donate breast milk carriers of HBV [23]. The safety of the drugs used by mothers with chronic HBV infection who continued HBV antiviral therapy after birth is uncertain for infants. In these cases, whether there is an alternative to breastfeeding and the benefits of breastfeeding should be discussed. The decision to breastfeed should be made according to the mother's preference. Since nucleoside and nucleotide analogs are excreted into breast milk, it is mentioned in the drug package inserts to avoid using these drugs while breastfeeding.

7 Hepatitis C Virus Infection

Hepatitis C virus (HCV) infection causes acute or chronic liver inflammation. Acute HCV hepatitis can be cured or lead to chronic hepatitis, progressive hepatic fibrosis, and liver cancer. Infected blood can transmit HCV from mother to child in utero, intrapartum, and postnatally [24, 25]. Currently, there is no effective HCV vaccine worldwide. According to the WHO report, almost 290,000 people died from hepatitis C in 2019, mainly caused by cirrhosis and hepatocellular carcinoma. An estimated 58 million people worldwide have chronic HCV infection, and about 1.5 million new infections are added yearly. The WHO also estimates that 3.2 million children and adolescents have chronic HCV infection [26].

Hepatitis C virus DNA has been detected in maternal colostrum, but transmission by breastfeeding has not been reported. Since there is no evidence of HCV transmission through breastfeeding, maternal HCV infection is not contraindicated for breastfeeding [1].

8 Human T-Lymphotropic Virus (HTLV) Infection

Human T-Lymphotropic Virus is a member of the Retroviridae family and has subtypes. The virus can cause adult T-cell leukemia/lymphoma. The HTLV is transmitted through infected bodily fluids, including breast milk. It can be transmitted by breastfeeding; the longer the breastfeeding period and the higher the mother's viral load, the more contagious it is. The risk of mother-to-child transmission through breastfeeding is approximately 16–30%. A difference exists in transmission between HTLV and HIV because HTLV is primarily transmitted by breastfeeding, not in utero or birth [27]. HTLV-positive mother is contraindicated from breastfeeding and expressing human milk [1].

9 Influenza

Influenza is an RNA virus with four types: A, B, C, and D. Influenza A and B viruses cause seasonal diseases, also called flu and may cause epidemics. Influenza is an acute, contagious viral infection that attacks the respiratory system. Nose, throat, bronchi, and sometimes the lungs are affected [28]. Influenza can cause mild to severe symptoms and serious complications and rarely can lead to death. The flu is not transmitted from mother to baby by breastfeeding. Flu is transmitted from person to person by tiny droplets while infected people sneeze, cough, or talk. In addition, if the hands are rubbed into the mouth or nose after touching an object with influenza, the flu is transmitted. Breastfeeding is also recommended when the mother has the flu, as breast milk contains immunological factors and antibodies that protect the infant from influenza. If the mother is too ill to breastfeed her baby from the breast, it is recommended that the mother expresses her milk and the caregiver feed the baby with breast milk. However, before expressing, mothers should wash their hands thoroughly with soap and water [29].

The flu vaccine can be safely administered to infants older than 6 months and breastfeeding mothers. In addition, antibodies formed in mothers who received the flu vaccine while pregnant or breastfeeding are passed to the baby through breast milk. Breastfeeding also protects against the flu in infants younger than 6 months old who cannot get the flu vaccine. With current information, an annual flu shot is recommended for anyone over 6 months of age. In addition, it is necessary and recommended that caregivers and household members be vaccinated against influenza to protect children under 6 months of age [29].

10 Ebola Virus Infection

Ebola virus disease (EVD), also known as Ebola hemorrhagic fever, is a rare but severe and mortal disease caused by Ebola (EBOV). Ebola virus disease is an RNA virus and occasionally causes deadly outbreaks. The Ebola virus is transmitted by direct contact with body fluids such as blood, urine, saliva, sweat, feces, vomit, and breast milk of a person who is sick or who has died from the Ebola virus. There is no current information about when the Ebola virus passes into breast milk during the disease and when it is cleared [30]. Therefore, breastfeeding is not recommended for mothers with proven or suspected Ebola virus disease [1]. The virus can also be transmitted from mother to child through close contact. Breastfeeding should be discontinued in mothers with suspected or confirmed Ebola disease, and the baby and mother should be separated. The mother and baby should remain separate if the baby is also diagnosed with the Ebola virus. Alternative nutritional diets should continue to be used instead of breast milk. However, in environments with limited resources, continued breastfeeding should be considered if the baby is under 6 months old, not well cared for, and has no alternative food to breast milk. Mothers who wish to continue breastfeeding after treatment for the Ebola virus require testing for Ebola virus RNA in breast milk to determine when they can start breastfeeding. Vaccination with recombinant vesicular stomatitis virus—Zaire Ebola vaccine (rVSV-ZEBOV) is recommended for mothers without Ebola disease living in areas with the Zaire Ebola virus outbreak. However, data on vaccine effects during breastfeeding are limited. Guidelines recommend not initiating breastfeeding until two consecutive negative test results are 24 h apart [31].

11   Coronavirus Disease-2019 (COVID-19)

Coronavirus disease 2019 (COVID-19) is an infectious disease caused by the severe acute respiratory syndrome coronavirus 2 (SARS-CoV-2), ranging from mild illness to fatal conditions. There is no evidence of SARS-CoV-2 transmission through breast milk from mother to child [32]. Centers for Disease Control and Prevention recommends taking precautions for breastfeeding mothers who have suspected or confirmed COVID-19 and mothers who have been in close contact with someone who has COVID-19 and is not fully vaccinated. Washing hands using soap and water before touching the child and wearing a mask when less than 6 ft. from the child are recommended. Mothers in this situation should carefully follow the recommendations while breastfeeding or expressing the milk [33]. Breastfeeding does not affect the time of vaccination. In addition, SARS-CoV-2 antibodies generated by vaccination can pass into breast milk and provide passive protection to the baby. Vaccines do not contain infectious viruses, and very few vaccines will likely pass into breast milk. The infant's gastrointestinal tract probably inactivates this amount. Therefore, current vaccines are unlikely to pose a risk to the infant [34].

12   Zika Virus Infection

Zika virus is a member of Flaviviridae and an RNA virus. Zika virus is transmitted to humans by biting an infected Aedes mosquito. Most people infected with the Zika virus have no symptoms. People with symptoms develop fever, conjunctivitis, muscle and joint pain, weakness, and headache. There is no vaccine or treatment for Zika virus infection. Zika virus has been detected in breast milk, but it has not been proven whether it is transmitted to an infected infant. Breast milk is a possible tool for transmitting the Zika virus, but knowledge remains limited. Since the benefits of breastfeeding outweigh the risk of transmission of the Zika virus through breast milk, it is recommended that mothers with Zika virus infection, living in or traveling to risk areas continue breastfeeding. No complications have been reported in infants with postnatal Zika virus infection or exposure [35, 36].

13   West Nile Virus Infection

West Nile is a member of Flaviviridea and an RNA virus. West Nile virus is transmitted to people by infected mosquitoes. Cases occur in the summer, when mosquitoes are plentiful, and continue during autumn. The disease is asymptomatic in most people. Symptoms occur in one out of every five infected people, and about one out of hundred and fifty infected people have severe disease. Serious disease symptoms are high fever, headache, disorientation, neck stiffness, tremors, convulsions, and coma. Currently, there is no vaccine or treatment for the West Nile virus. According to the CDC, West Nile virus may be transmitted from mother to child through breast milk. No evidence of the mother's West Nile infection harming the baby exists. Therefore, the possibility of an infection that can be transmitted through breast milk theoretically harming the baby is less than the benefits of breast milk, and breastfeeding is recommended [37, 38].

14 Conclusion

Breast milk is a unique source of nutrients for infants. Thanks to the immunological factors and antibodies in breast milk, it is protective against many infectious diseases. There are very few infections that are considered to be contraindications to breastfeeding. According to current evidence, breastfeeding is not recommended for infants of mothers with HIV, HTLV, and Ebola viruses. Standard precautions should be followed in cases other than these infections. Mothers should always use hand hygiene to protect their infants from infectious diseases. Mothers with infectious blisters should ensure that they completely cover the lesions while breastfeeding and that their babies do not come into contact with them. To protect the infant from respiratory diseases, mothers with flu-like illnesses should wear a mask to prevent the spread of droplets.

References

1. Meek JY, Noble L. Section on breastfeeding. Policy statement: breastfeeding and the use of human milk. Pediatrics. 2022;150(1):e2022057988.
2. Bardanzellu F, Fanos V, Reali A. Human breast milk acquired cytomegalovirus infection: certainties, doubts and perspectives. Curr Pediatr Rev. 2019;15:30–41.
3. Fakhreddine AY, Frenette CT, Konijeti GG. A practical review of cytomegalovirus in gastroenterology and hepatology. Gastroenterol Res Pract. 2019;2019:6156581.
4. Zuhair M, Smit GSA, Wallis G, et al. Estimation of the worldwide seroprevalence of cytomegalovirus: a systematic review and meta-analysis. Rev Med Virol. 2019;29(3):e2034.
5. Davis NL, King CC, Kourtis AP. Cytomegalovirus infection in pregnancy. Birth Defects Res. 2017;109:336–46.
6. Cattaneo A, Yngve A, Koletzko B, Guzman LR. Protection, promotion and support of breastfeeding in Europe: current situation. Public Health Nutr. 2005;8:39–46.
7. Jim WT, Chiu NC, Ho CS, et al. Outcome of preterm infants with postnatal cytomegalovirus infection via breast milk: a two-year prospective follow-up study. Medicine (Baltimore). 2015;94(43):e1835.
8. Hamprecht K, Goelz R. Postnatal cytomegalovirus infection through human milk in preterm infants: transmission, clinical presentation, and prevention. Clin Perinatol. 2017;44:121–30.
9. Centers for Disease Control and Prevention. Cytomegalovirus (CMV) and congenital CMV infection. https://www.cdc.gov/cmv/clinical/overview.html. Accessed 21 Feb 2023.
10. Hamprecht K, Maschmann J, Müller D, et al. Cytomegalovirus (CMV) inactivation in breast milk: reassessment of pasteurization and freeze-thawing. Pediatr Res. 2004;56:529–35.

11. World Health Organization. Herpes simplex virus. https://www.who.int/news-room/fact-sheets/detail/herpes-simplex-virus. Accessed 21 Feb 2023.
12. Centers for Disease Control and Prevention. Herpes simplex virus (HSV). https://www.cdc.gov/breastfeeding/breastfeeding-special-circumstances/maternal-or-infant-illnesses/herpes.html. Accessed 21 Feb 2023.
13. Centers for Disease Control and Prevention. Shingles. https://www.cdc.gov/breastfeeding/breastfeeding-special-circumstances/maternal-or-infant-illnesses/shingles.html. Accessed 21 Feb 2023.
14. Capriotti T. HIV/AIDS: An update for home healthcare clinicians. Home Healthc Now. 2018;36:348–55.
15. John GC, Kreiss J. Mother-to-child transmission of human immunodeficiency virus type 1. Epidemiol Rev. 1996;18:149.
16. Centers for Disease Control and Prevention. Human immunodeficiency virus (HIV). https://www.cdc.gov/breastfeeding/breastfeeding-special-circumstances/maternal-or-infant-illnesses/hiv.html. Accessed 21 Feb 2023.
17. World Health Organization. Guideline updates on HIV and infant feeding. Geneva: World Health Organization. 2016:1–58. https://apps.who.int/iris/bitstream/handle/10665/246260/9789241549707-eng.pdf. Accessed 21 Feb 2023.
18. Kafulafula G, Hoover DR, Taha TE, et al. Frequency of gastroenteritis and gastroenteritis-associated mortality with early weaning in HIV-1-uninfected children born to HIV-infected women in Malawi. J Acquir Immune Defic Syndr. 2010;53:6.
19. Onyango-Makumbi C, Bagenda D, Mwatha A, et al. Early weaning of HIV-exposed uninfected infants and risk of serious gastroenteritis: findings from two perinatal HIV prevention trials in Kampala, Uganda. J Acquir Immune Defic Syndr. 2010;53:20.
20. Arpadi S, Fawzy A, Aldrovandi GM, et al. Growth faltering due to breastfeeding cessation in uninfected children born to HIV-infected mothers in Zambia. Am J Clin Nutr. 2009;90:344.
21. Society for Maternal-Fetal Medicine, Dionne-Odom J, Tita ATN, Silverman NS. Hepatitis B in pregnancy screening, treatment, and prevention of vertical transmission. Am J Obstet Gynecol. 2016;214(1):6–14.
22. World Health Organization. Hepatitis B. https://www.who.int/news-room/fact-sheets/detail/hepatitis-b. Accessed 21 Feb 2023.
23. Centers for Disease Control and Prevention. Hepatitis B. https://www.cdc.gov/breastfeeding/breastfeeding-special-circumstances/maternal-or-infant-illnesses/hepatitis.html. Accessed 21 Feb 2023.
24. Society for Maternal-Fetal Medicine, Hughes BL, Page CM, Kuller JA. Hepatitis C in pregnancy: screening, treatment, and management. Am J Obstet Gynecol. 2017;217(5):b2–12.
25. Mok J, Pembrey L, Tovo PA, Newell ML, European Paediatric Hepatitis C Virus Network. When does mother to child transmission of hepatitis C virus occur? Arch Dis Child Fetal Neonatal Ed. 2005;90:f156–60.
26. World Health Organization. Hepatitis B or C infections. https://www.cdc.gov/breastfeeding/breastfeeding-special-circumstances/maternal-or-infant-illnesses/hepatitis.html. Accessed 21 Feb 2023.
27. Carneiro-Proietti AB, Amaranto-Damasio MS, Leal-Horiguchi CF, et al. Mother-to-child transmission of human t-cell lymphotropic viruses-1/2: what we know, and what are the gaps in understanding and preventing this route of infection. J Pediatr Infect Dis Soc. 2014;3(Suppl 1):s24–9.
28. Hutchinson EC. Influenza virus. Trends Microbiol. 2018;26:809–10.
29. Centers for Disease Control and Prevention. Influenza (flu).. https://www.cdc.gov/breastfeeding/breastfeeding-special-circumstances/maternal-or-infant-illnesses/influenza.html. Accessed 21 Feb 2023.
30. Centers for Disease Control and Prevention. Ebola virus disease. https://www.cdc.gov/breastfeeding/breastfeeding-special-circumstances/maternal-or-infant-illnesses/ebola.html. Accessed 21 Feb 2023.

31. Chertow DS, Bray M, Palmore TN. Treatment and prevention of Ebola virus disease. In: Hirsch MS, editor. UpToDate 2022. www.uptodate.com. Accessed 21 Feb 2023.
32. Centeno-Tablante E, Medina-Rivera M, Finkelstein JL, et al. Transmission of SARS-CoV-2 through breast milk and breastfeeding: a living systematic review. Ann N Y Acad Sci. 2021;1484(1):32–54.
33. Centers for Disease Control and Prevention. Care for breastfeeding people. https://www.cdc.gov/coronavirus/2019-ncov/hcp/care-for-breastfeeding-women.html. Accessed 21 Feb 2023.
34. Berghella V, Hughes BL. COVID-19: intrapartum and postpartum issues. In: Lockwood CJ, ed. UpToDate 2022. www.uptodate.com. Accessed 21 Feb 2023.
35. Blohm GM, Lednicky JA, Márquez M, et al. Evidence for mother-to-child transmission of Zika virus through breast milk. Clin Infect Dis. 2018;55:1120–1.
36. Colt S, Garcia-Casal MN, Peña-Rosas JP, et al. Transmission of Zika virus through breast milk and other breastfeeding-related bodily fluids: a systematic review. PLoS Negl Trop Dis. 2017;11:e0005528.
37. World Health Organization. West Nile virus. https://www.who.int/news-room/fact-sheets/detail/west-nile-virus. Accessed 21 Feb 2023.
38. Centers for Disease Control and Prevention. Breastfeeding and special circumstances. https://www.cdc.gov/breastfeeding/breastfeeding-special-circumstances/maternal-or-infant-illnesses/west-nile-virus.html. Accessed 21 Feb 2023.

Breastfeeding and Maternal Fungal Infections

Derin Oygar and Despina D. Briana

1 Introduction

Breast milk is the ideal source of nutrition for infants in the first 6 months of life [1]. All major health organizations like The World Health Organization (WHO), the American Academy of Pediatrics (AAP), and American Academy of Family Physicians (AAFP) recommend exclusive breastfeeding for the first 6 months of life and after 6 months with the introduction of complementary foods, continuation of breastfeeding until at least 24 months of age [2–4].

Breast milk consists of water (87%), fat (3.8%), proteins (1.0%), and lactose (7%), lactose, and fat providing 40 and 50% of the total energy provided by human milk, respectively [5]. Nutrient contents may change through lactation, over the course of a day, and within a feeding and differ among women. Aside from nutrients required by the newborn infant for energy and metabolism, breast milk contains non-nutritional components like microRNAs, hormones, and bioactive components that promote infant health, growth, and development [6]. The main bioactive components include cytokines, chemokines, immunoglobulins, hormones, growth factors, oligosaccharides, and antimicrobial peptides such as bacteriocin and lactoferrin [7]. Although the physiological significance of all these substances is not fully determined, non-nutrient factors are important for neonates, in the transition of intrauterine to extrauterine life as their digestive systems and barrier function host defenses are still immature and susceptible to infections.

D. Oygar (✉)
Department of Pediatric Infectious Diseases, Neurology Department, Dr. Burhan Nalbantoğlu State Hospital, Nicosia, Northern Cyprus

D. D. Briana
NICU, Third Department of Pediatrics, National and Kapodistrian University of Athens, University General Hospital "ATTIKON", Athens, Greece

© The Author(s), under exclusive license to Springer Nature Switzerland AG 2023

Ö. N. Şahin et al. (eds.), *Breastfeeding and Metabolic Programming*, https://doi.org/10.1007/978-3-031-33278-4_30

Once considered as sterile, breast milk is known to contain a microbiome of its own [8–10]. It contains up to 109 microbes/L, the most common groups being staphylococci, streptococci, corynebacteria, lactobacilli, micrococci, propionibacteria, and bifidobacteria [11, 12]. Although the origin of breast milk bacteria is not definitely known, it is believed to originate from the perinatal period which starts during the third trimester of pregnancy and continue through lactation [13]. While in certain reports, the human milk microbiota was proposed that it could have been derived from colonization from the mother's skin, the infant's oral cavity during suckling, or the mother's gut via the entero-mammary pathway [14–16]. Others proposed the existence of a commensal microbiota in human breast tissue, suggesting that specific microbes inhabit the breast tissue and potentially colonize the milk ducts and colostrum already contains bacteria before suckling [17, 18]. With the advancement of polymerase chain reaction techniques and next-generation sequencing platforms the existence of a diverse breast-milk microbial community has been confirmed [19, 20].

While breast milk is established as a source of diverse and viable bacteria [21] only a few studies have assessed fungi in human milk [22–27]. The gastrointestinal tract is sterile at birth and is subsequently colonized by microbes acquired from the mother and the surrounding environment [28].

Fungi constitute an important component of the human microbiome [29, 30] and fungal and bacterial colonization occur in parallel during early life [31], hence the presence of fungi in breast milk is not surprising. Although all determinants of milk fungi are not fully understood it was reported that fungi in breast milk were significantly associated with environmental characteristics, human milk oligosaccharides, and milk bacterial composition [32]. In the same study the most prevalent fungi were reported to be Candida species.

Apart from being the best nutrient for the newborn and young children breast milk also protects them from diarrhea [33, 34], necrotizing enterocolitis [35, 36], respiratory infections [34, 37–40], acute otitis media [37, 38], oral candiadiasis [37], enterovirus infection [41] as well as atopic dermatitis [33], obesity [42, 43], allergic disease [44]. Breastfeeding can reduce risk for sudden infant death syndrome (SIDS) by up to 64% and overall infant death risk by as much as 40% [45].

Breastfeeding has also significant and long-term effects on cognition, behavior, and mental health for children [46]. For nursing women, breastfeeding gives protection against breast cancer, and it might also protect against ovarian cancer and type 2 diabetes [47].

Although breast milk is unique and breastfeeding is physiologic, not everyone can breastfeed or continue breastfeeding for as long as desired. Many factors including lack or insufficient prenatal, perinatal, and postnatal encouragement and education as well as emotional and financial support of families during breast feeding, unavailability of workplace break time with a clean, private location for expressing milk or provision of lactation rooms as well as living in an unsupportive breastfeeding society are proposed as factors responsible for attaining breastfeeding. Persistent pain associated with breastfeeding is another common cause for early breastfeeding cessation [48].

Pain and discomfort experienced during breastfeeding are common especially in the first few weeks postpartum [49] while persistent pain which is described as pain beyond 2 weeks should be evaluated. The differential diagnosis of persistent nipple and/or breast pain is extensive. Several etiologies including abnormal latch/suck dynamic, breast pump trauma, dermatoses, postpartum depression as well as infections could lead to persistent nipple/breast pain.

Several studies were conducted in order to identify which, if any, microbes may cause persistent nipple/breast pain during lactation, but the roles of bacteria and yeast could not be determined: Both *Staphylococcus* and *Candida* species were found on nipples and in breast milk of women having no symptoms [25, 50, 51]. The individuality of breastfeeding, the complex physiology, and dynamic microbiomes of lactating breast together with biofilm forming *Staphylococcus* and *Candida* species challenge the diagnosis of infections during breastfeeding.

Breastfeeding is not considered as a predisposing factor for fungal infections. Furthermore, recent reports accumulate on absence of scientific proofs on yeasts being responsible of (particularly *Candida* spp.) nipple and breast pain [52, 53].

The use of medication by the nursing mother is another common reason for the cessation of breastfeeding. Especially antifungal therapy is challenging during breastfeeding due to limited data on efficacy and safety of antifungal agents in breastfeeding women. Although the Food and Drug Administration (FDA) pregnancy category provides guidance regarding a drug's potential fetal risks, a specific toxic dose or predisposing pregnancy trimester is not mentioned limiting its applicability. Furthermore, antifungal recommendations during lactation are only available for a few fungal infections in accepted guidelines [54].

2 Breastfeeding and Candida

Candida species are part of the normal microbial flora of the human gut and *Candida albicans* is by far the most prevalent of the *Candida* species found in humans [55]. When opportunity arises, the organism can overgrow and result in an infectious process particularly in immunodeficient individuals. Breastfeeding practitioners commonly suggest *Candida albicans* as the cause of deep breast pain during lactation while pediatricians diagnose oral thrush in neonates frequently.

Candida species are diploid polymorphic yeasts that reproduce by budding. They are common fungal commensal in the human body, which are present on the skin and in the mouth, intestinal tract, and vagina of immunocompetent people. Newborn infants are often colonized from the mother's genital tract. *Candida* can adhere to epidermal keratinocytes and exists on the nipple-areolar complex as part of healthy human skin's network of protective and interacting microbiota and biofilms.

Candida albicans can grow hyphae and may penetrate through epithelium in favorable circumstances like friction, heat, moisture, reduced pH but the infection usually remains superficial due to skin barrier defenses and host immunity. *C.*

albicans invades systemically only in immunocompromised patients, for example, who have HIV or are undergoing chemotherapy as well as very low birth weight premature neonates [56, 57].

2.1 Oral Candidiasis (Thrush)

Oral thrush is an opportunistic infection of buccal mucosa, palate, tongue, and oropharynx by commensal *Candida* species and is a frequent diagnosis in infants. Colonization by *Candida* yeast is thought to occur at an early age, with the organism being acquired vertically during passage through the birth canal or horizontally from the environment, mainly from colonized hands, skin or improperly cleaned bottle nipples. There are approximately 200 *Candida* species, and *C. albicans* accounts for the majority of oral thrush cases. Thrush occurs, when innate and acquired host-defense mechanisms do not act in concert with the resident bacterial flora. This leads to an imbalance within the system, providing an ecological advantage for overgrowth of *C. albicans*. In most cases, thrush is limited to the neonatal and infant periods of life but is also observed in immunocompromised patients as well as those with polyendocrine disorders and due to use of antibiotics or steroids. Thrush affects both males and females equally and it is reported to be rare during the first week of life. Its incidence peaks around fourth to sixth weeks of life and is relatively uncommon between 6 and 9 months of age. Oral thrush beyond 6 months of age in the absence of risk factors should raise the suspicion of immunodeficiency including HIV infection. Undernourishment is proposed as a risk factor for development of thrush.

Oral candidiasis can be classified into a number of distinct clinical forms: acute pseudomembranous candidiasis, acute atrophic candidiasis, chronic atrophic candidiasis, chronic hyperplastic candidiasis, and chronic mucocutaneous candidiasis. Acute pseudomembranous form tends to occur in infants. Acute pseudomembranous candidiasis usually presents as white raised patches observed on buccal mucosa, gums, or tongue. If untreated, patches can develop to form confluent plaques. They are usually painless and do not lead to symptoms. They may spread to oropharynx and esophagus and can present with difficulty in feeding. The pseudomembranes in thrush easily dislodge revealing an erythematous bleeding surface beneath. The diagnosis of oral thrush is primarily based on history and physical examination. Laboratory confirmation is rarely conducted. Since it is not uncommon for infants to have a white coating due to milk on their tongues, misdiagnosis of thrush is common. *Candida* can spread to gastrointestinal tract and can cause rash in the diaper area as well. Diaper rash due to *Candida* presents with papules and plaques with sharp edges and scales as well as surrounding satellite lesions. Presence of Candida diaper dermatitis is suggestive of oral thrush.

In addition to the inconsistent and subjective clinical signs and symptoms, diagnosis is complicated by the fact that *C. albicans* is a normal inhabitant of mucous membranes. Even if laboratory confirmation is performed, it is difficult to interpret the results, as the presence of *C. albicans* may indicate colonization rather than infection. Hence diagnosis of oral thrush is not straightforward. Oral nystatin and oral fluconazole are the preferred treatments for thrush in infants [58] while topical nystatin, miconazole, and clotrimazole are preferred agents for the treatment of candida diaper dermatitis.

2.2 *Nipple/Breast Pain and Candida*

The association of *Candida* with nipple/breast pain remains controversial. It has been shown that human milk does not inhibit growth of *Candida* in fungal cultures [59]. While some authors did not find a correlation between symptoms and the presence of *Candida* [59, 60] others demonstrated candida as a causative agent of nipple/breast pain. Prolonged nipple/breast pain is one of the reasons of early cessation of breastfeeding.

Symptoms due to candida in mothers are described as sharp, burning pain deep in the breast during and especially after feedings, acute nipple pain, itching of the breast with or without rash as well as total lack of maternal symptoms in the presence of infantile oral thrush [61]. These symptoms are not specific to thrush and can also be observed in physical trauma from incorrect latch-on/or positioning, bacterial mastitis, or chronic dermatoses unrelated to breastfeeding. In candida infection the nipples or areolas are described as shiny pink or flaky in appearance [25, 62] but nipples which are subject to repetitive micro-trauma due to breastfeeding may appear pink and shiny, with fine scaling and itch, hence the appearance and symptoms are not diagnostic of candidiasis. Thrush in infant's mouth or in the diaper area and recent use of antibiotics in mother or child are predisposing factors for women to develop Candida infection [63]. Hence some authors emphasized on overdiagnosis of candida infections as a cause of breast/nipple pain during breastfeeding and extended or improper use of antifungals [52, 64]. Although there are controversies on *Candida* species being responsible for nipple and breast pain topical nystatin and oral fluconazole are agents commonly used as treatment.

3   Breastfeeding and Antifungals

Prescribing drugs to the nursing mother is challenging. The drugs should have no effect on milk supply or milk composition and offer effective pharmacologic treatment to the nursing mother.

Drugs are secreted into breast milk by passive diffusion. The milk-to-plasma (M:P) ratio is an index that determines the extent of drug secretion into breast milk [65, 66]. The M:P ratio is not known for most agents. Thus, relative infant dose (RID) is calculated to estimate the amount of drug exposure in the breastfeeding infant. It is estimated by evaluating the predicted amount secreted into breast milk, the daily volume of milk ingested by the infant, and the predicted or measured plasma concentration of the mother. In general, RID value less than 10% is considered acceptable in a healthy postnatal infant and a value greater than 25% may have a therapeutic effect on the infant if absorbed through the gastrointestinal tract [67].

Antifungal medications used during breastfeeding are prescribed mainly for yeast infections.

Nystatin, the most frequently prescribed antifungal during breastfeeding is not absorbed through gastrointestinal system hence nystatin use is compatible with breastfeeding [68]. Another frequently administered antifungal *Fluconazole* is widely distributed in tissues, but the highest concentrations in breast milk are less than the recommended neonatal dosages [69], hence fluconazole is rated compatible with breastfeeding by the American Academy of Pediatrics [70]. Like fluconazole, *Itraconazole* is secreted into breast milk. A pharmacokinetic study conducted by the manufacturer revealed that doses in human milk seems insignificant [71] however, itraconazole has an active metabolite and tends to accumulate in tissues; thus, with continued daily dosing, milk levels are likely to increase over time. Hence, the use of itraconazole by lactating women are not usually recommended unless it has a definite indication. *In preclinical animal studies Posaconazole* distribution was observed [72]. There are no studies available on distribution of *Posaconazole* into breast milk. However, it is very likely that it is distributed to breast milk as well. The manufacturer recommends against its use in breastfeeding women unless clearly indicated. The distribution of *voriconazole* into breast milk is unknown [67]. In animal studies, voriconazole was found to be teratogenic and embryotoxic hence it is recommended to avoid voriconazole during breastfeeding by the manufacturer [73].

Amphotericin B has a large molecular size, poor absorption, and high protein binding capacity. Hence it is estimated breast milk levels are likely to be none to very low [74]. Based on these data, amphotericin is considered safe for use during lactation.

Echinocandins (Caspofungin, micafungin, and anidulafungin) were found to be secreted in breast milk in rats, but their distribution in human breast milk is not known [67]. The manufacturers caution against the use of these agents during breastfeeding.

Oral *terbinafine* is distributed in human milk with an M:P ratio of 7:1 hence it is not recommended for breastfeeding women [75] while due to its minimal systemic absorption it can be used topically during breastfeeding. The distribution of *flucytosine* in human breast milk is unknown [76]. *Griseofulvin* is an antifungal well known for its teratogenicity and embryotoxicity [77]. The distribution of griseofulvin in human breast milk is unknown. There are no recent publications concerning the use of griseofulvin or flucytosine in pregnancy, and these agents are typically avoided, as safer options are available.

Antifungal therapy during lactation is challenging because of the limited available data on breast milk distribution of most antifungal agents. In general, topical azoles are favored for superficial fungal infections during lactation, whereas amphotericin B is preferred for invasive fungal infections. Nystatin and fluconazole are preferred oral agents during breastfeeding.

4 Conclusion

The benefits of breastfeeding to the health of children in terms of nutrition, gastro-intestinal function, host defenses, neurodevelopment and chronic diseases of childhood as well as to maternal health are well established. Breastfeeding not only provides complete nutrition for the infant, but it is also associated with lower rates of infectious illness during infancy. Fungal infections during breastfeeding can be challenging in terms of diagnosis and treatment. Correct diagnosis is critical to promote the continuation of breastfeeding as well as to avoid the unnecessary prescription of antifungals.

References

1. Nutrition EC, Agostoni C, Braegger C, Decsi T, Kolacek S, Koletzko B, et al. Breast-feeding: a commentary by the ESPGHAN committee on nutrition. J Pediatr Gastroenterol Nutr. 2009;49:112–25. https://doi.org/10.1097/MPG.0b013e31819f1e05.
2. American Academy of Family Physicians. Breastfeeding, family physicians supporting (position paper). https://www.aafp.org/about/policies/all/breastfeeding-support.html. Accessed 22 Apr 2017.
3. Johnston M, Landers S, Noble L, Szucs K, Viehmann L. Breastfeeding and the use of human milk. Pediatrics. 2012;129(3):e827–41.
4. World Health Organization. Infant and young child nutrition. Global strategy on infant and young child feeding. Report by the secretariat. April 16, 2002. http://apps.who.int/gb/archive/pdf_files/WHA55/ea5515.pdf?ua=1. Accessed 1 May 2017.
5. Guo M. Human milk biochemistry and infant formula manufacturing technology. 1st ed. Sawston: Woodhead Publishing; 2014.
6. Zimmermann P, Curtis N. Breast milk microbiota: a review of the factors that influence composition. J Infect. 2020;81:17–47.
7. Gura T. Nature's first functional food. Science. 2014;345:747–9.
8. Cacho NT, Lawrence RM. Innate immunity and breast milk. Front Immunol. 2017;8:584.
9. Hill DR, Newburg DS. Clinical applications of bioactive milk components. Nutr Rev. 2015;73:463–76.
10. Gila-Diaz A, Arribas SM, Algara A, Martín-Cabrejas MA, López de Pablo ÁL, Sáenz de Pipaón M, et al. A review of bioactive factors in human breastmilk: a focus on prematurity. Nutrients. 2019;11:1307.
11. Asquith MT, Harrod JR. Reduction in bacterial contamination in banked human milk. J Pediatr. 1979;95:993–4.
12. West PA, Hewitt JH, Murphy OM. The infl uence of methods of collection and storage on the bacteriology of human milk. J Appl Bacteriol. 1979;46:269–77.
13. Jost T, Lacroix C, Braegger C, Chassard C. Impact of human milk bacteria and oligosaccharides on neonatal gut microbiota establishment and gut health. Nutr Rev. 2015;73(7):426e37.
14. Rautava S, Luoto R, Salminen S, Isolauri E. Microbial contact during pregnancy, intestinal colonization and human disease. Nat Rev Gastroenterol Hepatol. 2012;9(10):565e76.

15. Fernández L, Langa S, Martin V, Maldonado A, Jiménez E, Martín R, et al. The human milk microbiota: origin and potential roles in health and disease. Pharmacol Res. 2013;69(1):1–10.
16. Rodriguez JM. The origin of human milk bacteria:is there a bacterial enteromammary pathway during late pregnancy and lactation? Adv Nutr. 2014;5(6):779e84.
17. Urbaniak C, Cummins J, Brackstone M, Macklaim JM, Gloor GB, Baban CK, et al. Microbiota of human breast tissue. Appl Environ Microbiol. 2014;80(10):3007e14.
18. Xuan C, Shamonki JM, Chung A, Dinome ML, Chung M, Sieling PA, et al. Microbial dysbiosis is associated with human breast cancer. PLoS One. 2014;9(1):e83744.
19. Jeurink PV, van Bergenhenegouwen J, Jimenez E, Knippels LM, Fernandez L, Garssen J, et al. Human milk: a source of more life than we imagine. Benef Microbes. 2013;4(1):17e30.
20. McGuire MK, McGuire MA. Human milk: mother nature's prototypical probiotic food? Adv Nutr. 2015;6(1):112e23.
21. McGuire MK, McGuire MA. Got bacteria? The astounding, yet not-sosurprising, microbiome of human milk. Curr Opin Biotechnol. 2017;44:63–8.
22. Boix-Amoros A, Martinez-Costa C, Querol A, Collado MC, Mira A. Multiple approaches detect the presence of Fungi in human Breastmilk samples from healthy mothers. Sci Rep. 2017;7(1):13016.
23. Jimenez E, de Andres J, Manrique M, Pareja-Tobes P, Tobes R, Martinez-Blanch JF, et al. Metagenomic analysis of Milk of healthy and mastitis-suffering women. J Hum Lact. 2015;31(3):406–15.
24. Boix-Amoros A, Puente-Sanchez F, du Toit E, Linderborg KM, Zhang Y, Yang B, et al. Mycobiome profiles in milk from healthy women depend on mode of delivery, geographic location and interaction with bacteria. Appl Environ Microbiol. 2019;85(9):e02994–18.
25. Amir LH, Donath SM, Garland SM, Tabrizi SN, Bennett CM, Cullinane M, et al. Does Candida and/or Staphylococcus play a role in nipple and breast pain in lactation? A cohort study in Melbourne, Australia. BMJ Open. 2013;3(3):e002351.
26. Heisel T, Nyaribo L, Sadowsky MJ, Gale CA. Breastmilk and NICU surfaces are potential sources of fungi for infant mycobiomes. Fungal Genet Biol. 2019;128:29–35.
27. Morrill JF, Pappagianis D, Heinig MJ, Lonnerdal B, Dewey KG. Detecting *Candida albicans* in human milk. J Clin Microbiol. 2003;41(1):475–8.
28. Mackie RI, Sghir A, Gaskins HR. Developmental microbial ecology of the neonatal gastrointestinal tract. Am J Clin Nutr. 1999;69(Suppl):s1035–45.
29. Huseyin CE, O'Toole PW, Cotter PD, Scanlan PD. Forgotten fungi-the gut mycobiome in human health and disease. FEMS Microbiol Rev. 2017;41(4):479–511.
30. Laforest-Lapointe I, Arrieta MC. Microbial Eukaryotes: a missing link in gut microbiome studies. mSystems. 2018;3(2):e00201–17.
31. Ward TL, Dominguez-Bello MG, Heisel T, Al-Ghalith G, Knights D, Gale CA. Development of the human mycobiome over the first month of life and across body sites. mSystems. 2018;3(3):e00140–17.
32. Moossavi S, Fehr K, Derakhshani H, Sbihi H, Robertson B, Bode L, et al. Human milk fungi: environmental determinants and inter-kingdom associations with milk bacteria in the CHILD Cohort Study. BMC Microbiol. 2020;20(1):146.
33. Kramer MS, Chalmers B, Hodnett ED, Sevkovskaya Z, Dzikovich I, Shapiro S, et al. PROBIT Study Group (Promotion of Breastfeeding Intervention Trial). Promotion of Breastfeeding Intervention Trial (PROBIT): a randomized trial in the Republic of Belarus. JAMA. 2001;285(4):413–20.
34. Duijts L, Jaddoe VW, Hofman A, Moll HA. Prolonged and exclusive breastfeeding reduces the risk of infectious diseases in infancy. Pediatrics. 2010;126(1):e18–25.
35. Meinzen-Derr J, Poindexter B, Wrage L, Morrow AL, Stoll B, Donovan EF. Role of human milk in extremely low birth weight infants' risk of necrotizing enterocolitis or death. J Perinatol. 2009;29(1):57–62.
36. Herrmann K, Carroll K. An exclusively human milk diet reduces necrotizing enterocolitis. Breastfeed Med. 2014;9(4):184–90.

37. Ladomenou F, Moschandreas J, Kafatos A, Tselentis Y, Galanakis E. Protective effect of exclusive breastfeeding against infections during infancy: a prospective study. Arch Dis Child. 2010;95(12):1004–8.
38. López-Alarcón M, Villalpando S, Fajardo A. Breast-feeding lowers the frequency and duration of acute respiratory infection and diarrhea in infants under six months of age. J Nutr. 1997;127(3):436–43.
39. Tromp I, Kiefte-de Jong J, Raat H, Jaddoe V, Franco O, Hofman A, et al. Breastfeeding and the risk of respiratory tract infections after infancy: The Generation R Study. PLoS One. 2017;12(2):e0172763.
40. Lanari M, Prinelli F, Adorni F, Di Santo S, Vandini S, Silvestri M, et al. Study Group of Italian Society of Neonatology on Risk Factors for RSV Hospitalization. Risk factors for bronchiolitis hospitalization during the first year of life in a multicenter Italian birth cohort. Ital J Pediatr. 2015;41:40.
41. Sadeharju K, Knip M, Virtanen SM, Savilahti E, Tauriainen S, Koskela P, et al. Finnish TRIGR Study Group. Maternal antibodies in breast milk protect the child from enterovirus infections. Pediatrics. 2007;119(5):941–6.
42. von Kries R, Koletzko B, Sauerwald T, von Mutius E, Barnert D, Grunert V, et al. Breast feeding and obesity: cross sectional study. BMJ. 1999;319(7203):147–50.
43. Gillman MW, Rifas-Shiman SL, Camargo CA Jr, Berkey CS, Frazier AL, Rockett HR, et al. Risk of overweight among adolescents who were breastfed as infants. JAMA. 2001;285(19):2461–7.
44. Munblit D, Verhasselt V. Allergy prevention by breastfeeding: possible mechanisms and evidence from human cohorts. Curr Opin Allergy Clin Immunol. 2016;16(5):427–33.
45. Hauck FR, Thompson J, Tanabe KO, Moon RY, Vennemann M. Breastfeeding and reduced risk of sudden infant death syndrome: a meta- analysis. Pediatrics. 2011;128(1):103–110.46.
46. Raju TN. Breastfeeding is a dynamic biological process—not simply a meal at the breast. Breastfeed Med. 2011;6:257–9.
47. Victora CG, Bahl R, Barros AJ, França GV, Horton S, Krasevec J, et al. Breastfeeding in the 21st century: Epidemiology, mechanisms, and lifelong effect. Lancet. 2016;387:475–90.
48. Odom E, Li R, Scanlon K, Perrine CG, Grummer-Strawn L. Reasons for earlier than desired cessation of breastfeeding. Pediatrics. 2013;131:e726–32.
49. Division of Nutrition Physical Activity and Obesity. National Center for Chronic Disease Prevention and Health Promotion. Infant Feeding Practices Survey II: Results. Centers for Disease Control and Prevention. 2009. Available at www.cdc.gov/ifps/results/ch2/table2–37.htm. Accessed 11 Nov 2015.
50. von Eiff C, Proctor RA, Peters G. Coagulase-negative staphylococci. Pathogens have major role in nosocomial infections. Postgrad Med 2001;110:63–64, 69–70, 73–66.
51. Melchior MB, Vaarkamp H, Fink-Gremmels J. Biofilms: A role in recurrent mastitis infections? Vet J. 2006;171:398–407.
52. Jiménez E, Arroyo R, Cárdenas N, Marín M, Serrano P, Fernández L, et al. Mammary candidiasis: a medical condition without scientific evidence? PLoS One. 2017;12(7):e0181071.
53. Kaski K, Kvist LJ. Deep breast pain during lactation: a case-control study in Sweden investigating the role of Candida albicans. Int Breastfeed J. 2018;13:21. https://doi.org/10.1186/s13006-018-0167-8. Published 2018 Jun 7
54. Kauffman CA, Bustamante B, Chapman SW, Pappas PG. Clinical practice guidelines for the management of sporotrichosis: 2007 update by the Infectious Diseases Society of America. Clin Infect Dis. 2007;45(10):1255–65.
55. McManus BA, Coleman DC. Molecular epidemiology, phylogeny and evolution of Candida albicans. Infect Genet Evol. 2014;21:166–8.
56. Kuhbacher A, Burger-Kentischer A, Rupp S. Interaction of *Candida* species with the skin. Microorganisms. 2017;5:32.
57. Dadar M, Tiwari R, Karthik K, Chakraborty S, Shahali Y, Dhama K. *Candida albicans* – biology, molecular characterization, pathogencitiy, and advances in diagnosis and control - an update. Microb Pathog. 2018;117:128–38.

58. Brent NB. Thrush in the breastfeeding dyad: results of a survey on diagnosis and treatment. Clin Pediatr (Phila). 2001;40(9):503–6.
59. Hale TW, Bateman TL, Finkelman MA, Berens PD. The absence of Candida albicans in milk samples of women with clinical symptoms of ductal candidiasis. Breastfeed Med. 2009;4:57–63.
60. Graves S, Wright W, Harman R, et al. Painful nipples in nursing mothers: Fungal or staphylococcal? Aust Fam Physician. 2003;32:570–1.
61. Andrews JI, Fleener D, Messer S, Hansen WF, Pfaller MA, Diekema DJ. The yeast connection: is Candida linked to breastfeeding associated pain? Am J Obstet Gynecol. 2007;197:e421–4.
62. Barrett ME, Heller MM, Fullerton Stone H, Murase JE. Dermatoses of the breast in lactation. Dermatol Ther. 2013;26:331–6.
63. Berens P, Eglash A, Malloy M, Steube AM. ABM clinical protocol #26: persistent pain with breastfeeding. Breastfeed Med. 2016;11(2):46–53.
64. Douglas P. Overdiagnosis and overtreatment of nipple and breast candidiasis: a review of the relationship between diagnoses of mammary candidiasis and *Candida albicans* in breastfeeding women. Womens Health (Lond). 2021;17:17455065211031480.
65. Anderson GD. Using pharmacokinetics to predict the effects of pregnancy and maternal-infant transfer of drugs during lactation. Expert Opin Drug Metab Toxicol. 2006;2(6):947–60.
66. Atkinson HC, Begg EJ, Darlow BA. Drugs in human milk. Clinical pharmacokinetic considerations. Clin Pharmacokinet. 1988;14(4):217–40.
67. Njoku JC, Gumeel D, Hermsen ED. Antifungal therapy in pregnancy and breastfeeding. Curr Fungal Infect Rep. 2010;4:62–9.
68. Datta P, Baker T, Hale TW. Balancing the use of medications while maintaining breastfeeding. Clin Perinatol. 2019;46(2):367–82.
69. Samaranayake LP, Keung Leung W, Jin L. Oral mucosal fungal infections. Periodontol 2000. 2009;49:39–59.
70. American Academy of Pediatrics: Committee on Drugs. Transfer of drugs and other chemicals into human milk. Pediatrics. 2001;108(3):776–89.
71. Force RW. Fluconazole concentrations in breast milk. Pediatr Infect Dis J. 1995;14(3):235–6.
72. Briggs GG, Freeman RK, Yaffe SJ. A reference guide to fetal andneonatal risk. In: Drugs in pregnancy and lactation. 6th ed. Baltimore: Lippincott Williams & Wilkins; 2002.
73. Moore JN, Healy JR, Kraft WK. Pharmacologic and clinical evaluation of posaconazole. Expert Rev Clin Pharmacol. 2015;8(3):321–34.
74. Vfend (voriconazole) tablets and injection [package insert]. NewYork: Pfizer; 2005.
75. Ilett KF, Kristensen JH. Drug use and breastfeeding. Expert Opin Drug Saf. 2005;4(4):745–68.
76. Khaled A, Chtourou O, Zeglaoui F, Fazaa B, Jones M, Kamoun MR. Tinea faciei: a report on four cases. Acta Dermatovenerol Alp Panonica Adriat. 2007;16(4):170–3.
77. Ancobon (Flucytosine) [package insert]. Costa Mesa, CA: Valeant Pharmaceuticals; 2002.

Breastfeeding and Maternal Parasitic Infections

Yıldız Ekemen Keleş, Ayşe Engin Arısoy, Emin Sami Arısoy, and Armando G. Correa

1 Introduction

Breast milk is the ideal nutritional source for almost all infants. Breast milk meets the infant's needs for macro- and micronutrients, functioning immune cells, enhanced growth of nonpathogenic flora and growth factors, and immunoprotective substances beyond nutrition [1]. Breast milk contains many biologically active constituents with antimicrobial and immunomodulatory properties supporting the development of gastrointestinal system function [2, 3]. Immunoglobulins (Igs), mainly secretory IgA (sIgA), in breast milk protect infants from many pathogenic microorganisms by several mechanisms, such as immobilizing pathogens, preventing attachment to epithelial cell surfaces, neutralizing toxins and virulence factors, and reducing colonization [2–4].

Several microorganisms causing severe infections in infants may be detected in breast milk [5, 6]. Nursing mothers with acute infections are concerned about the

Y. E. Keleş (✉)
Section of Pediatric Infectious Diseases, Tepecik Training and Research Hospital, University of Health Sciences, İzmir, Türkiye

A. E. Arısoy
Division of Neonatology, Department of Pediatrics, Faculty of Medicine, Kocaeli University (Emeritus), Kocaeli, Türkiye

E. S. Arısoy
Division of Pediatric Infectious Diseases, Department of Pediatrics, Faculty of Medicine, Kocaeli University (Emeritus), Kocaeli, Türkiye

A. G. Correa
Division of Academic General Pediatrics, Department of Pediatrics, Baylor College of Medicine, and Section of International and Destination Medicine, Texas Children's Hospital, Houston, TX, USA
e-mail: acorrea@bcm.edu

Ö. N. Şahin et al. (eds.), *Breastfeeding and Metabolic Programming*, https://doi.org/10.1007/978-3-031-33278-4_31

399

transmission risk of microorganisms to their infants via breastfeeding. In deciding whether a mother with an infection breastfeeds, the potential benefits and harms should be weighed against the known or estimated risk of the infant acquiring a clinically significant infection through breastfeeding and the potential severity of the illness. Multiple factors should be considered to demonstrate whether breast milk is the primary transmission route for a clinically significant infection in the infant [6]. However, excluding other likely transmission routes of infectious disease may be challenging because the organisms in question may be commonly transmitted prenatally, perinatally, and postnatally in different ways.

Parasitic diseases, as old as human history, were first mentioned in ancient Egypt inscriptions [7]. Parasitic infections are caused by endo- and ectoparasites. Endoparasites are mostly transmitted via the fecal-oral route, usually through contaminated food or water. Endoparasites are divided into two major groups: Protozoa, one-celled parasites, and helminths, parasitic worms. The helminths include the Nematoda, named roundworms, and the Platyhelminthes, flatworms. Platyhelminthes are further composed of two groups, cestodes (tapeworms) and trematodes (flukes) [7]. This chapter discusses some possible parasitoses that can be transmitted through breast milk.

2 Protozoa Infections

2.1 Chagas Disease (American Tripanosomiasis): Trypanosoma cruzi

Trypanosoma cruzi, the causative agent of American trypanosomiasis, also called Chagas disease, is one of the protozoan parasites transmitted by Triatominae bugs [8]. All triatomine species are potential vectors of *T. cruzi*, only those well adapted to living with humans, such as *Triatoma infestans,* are considered medically important. Triatominae vectors can infect humans when they defecate during feeding with human blood, spread feces containing parasites through the bite site, or come into contact with mucous membranes [9]. In addition, *T. cruzi* may be transmitted through blood products, transplantation from an infected donor, ingesting contaminated food or beverages, and transmission under laboratory conditions [10–12]. Congenital infection from mother to infant has also been reported [13]. When *T. cruzi* infection is transmitted orally, a more severe disease appears to be associated with a higher mortality rate [14].

Trypanosoma cruzi infection presents in acute and chronic phases. The acute phase lasts 8–12 weeks and, if not successfully treated, progresses to the chronic phase, which can be lifelong [15]. Although acute Chagas disease may occur at any age, most cases are detected before the age of 15 years [16]. During the acute phase of Chagas disease, patients may be asymptomatic or have constitutional symptoms and signs such as malaise, fever, anorexia, hepatosplenomegaly, and generalized lymphadenopathy [9, 15]. Within 2–3 weeks, a chagoma, an indurated lesion, may appear at the site of parasite entry [17]. Severe acute Chagas disease rarely occurs and may cause acute myocarditis, pericardial effusion, and meningoencephalitis, leading to fatal cardiac or gastrointestinal involvement [14, 15].

Symptoms experienced during the acute phase usually resolve, and the chronic phase begins [17]. Most Chagas disease patients are asymptomatic during the first years to decades of chronic infection; generally, antibodies to various *T. cruzi* antigens may be detected [18, 19]. Cardiac and gastrointestinal involvements occur in 20 to 40% [17]. Cardiac involvement is Chagas disease's most common chronic complication [20]. Mural thrombi are common, and the apical aneurysm is pathognomonic for progressive cardiac involvement [21].

Chagas disease should be suspected in persons who have historically lived in or traveled to rural areas of the southern half of the United States of America (USA) and Latin America, where *T. cruzi* is endemic [22]. However, diagnosis of Chagas disease is challenging during the relatively brief acute phase, in which trypomastigotes can be detected by microscopy of fresh blood preparations [23]. Another diagnostic tool is the polymerase chain reaction (PCR) more sensitive during the acute phase of Chagas disease [24]. Currently, a test with good sensitivity and specificity to diagnose the chronic phase of *T. cruzi* infection is unavailable; a positive result from a single test is insufficient to confirm the diagnosis [25]. Therefore, additional samples may be needed to increase the sensitivity of the tests. Most helpful tests are based on enzyme-linked immunosorbent assay (ELISA) or indirect-immunofluorescence assay (IFA) [15, 26].

Transmission of *T. cruzi* during breastfeeding has been reported [27–30]. Interruption of breastfeeding in a mother with Chagas disease is not recommended unless the risk of possible infection to the infant outweighs the benefits of breastfeeding [27, 31]. In one study, 97 breastfed infants whose mothers had been diagnosed with chronic Chagas disease and born free of infection were tested for IgG antibodies to *T. cruzi* by IFA test, and no infection was detected [28]. However, the authors concluded that mothers with chronic Chagas disease have intermittent parasitemia and should avoid breastfeeding if nipple bleeding is present. If transmission does occur, treatment of acute infections in infants and children is more successful, and adverse drug reactions occur less frequently [32].

Animal models on the potential transmission of acute *T. cruzi* infections during breastfeeding have been inconclusive [33–35]. A few studies have not been able to demonstrate the transmission of *T. cruzi* during breastfeeding [33, 34]. Some authors have postulated that maternal antibodies transmitted by breast milk protect against the spread of infection [28, 33]. In contrast, experimental oral and peritoneal administration of unpasteurized human breast milk samples contaminated with *T. cruzi* resulted in infection, but not if the breast milk was first pasteurized [29]. The authors concluded that pasteurization of human milk inactivates trypomastigotes of *T. cruzi*. Others have recommended microwave treatment of human milk to prevent Chagas disease transmission [30]. In yet another study, direct observation, culture, and inoculation failed to demonstrate the presence of *T. cruzi* in the colostrum and breast milk of 40 women with Chagas disease [36].

2.2 *Toxoplasmosis:* **Toxoplasma gondii**

Toxoplasma gondii is a protozoan that causes toxoplasmosis and has a worldwide distribution [37]. At least 60% of some populations are seropositive for toxoplasmosis [38]. The prevalence varies worldwide because of variations in the foods consumed, preparation methods, personal hygiene, and handling of animals [37]. Water provides an important route for toxoplasmosis transmission, particularly in regions with low socioeconomic levels [39].

The reproductive cycle of *T. gondii* is completed in cats and kittens which play an essential role in the animal-to-human transmission and spread of the parasites; the oocyst form is found in cat feces [40, 41]. These infected feces with oocysts are contagious to the environment [42]. In humans, *T. gondii* infection can be transmitted by contaminated water, food, and soil, consuming infected meat with tissue cysts, and organ transplants from an infected donor [42, 43].

Following human ingestion, the parasites are released from ingested oocysts or tissue cysts and invade the epithelial cells of the gastrointestinal tract to transform into tachyzoites [40]. Because of the immune response, the tachyzoites may either be destroyed or transformed into slowly proliferating bradyzoites that form persistent intracellular cysts [40]. These cysts may contain many parasites and occur preferentially in neurons of the brain, retina, and muscle cells [44]. In the chronic phase of infection, the immune system plays a critical role in combating the parasites but may also contribute to disease, particularly in the eye [44, 45].

Primary *T. gondii* infection is usually asymptomatic; however, in some individuals, it can lead to an acute systemic and/or ocular disease [46]. The initial *T. gondii* infection lasts a few weeks, after which the latent infection persists for life [47]. If the immune defenses are weakened, reactivation may occur; such patients typically present with multiple abscess-like formations of the central nervous system (CNS) [48]. Primary infection during pregnancy can result in severe or even fatal disease of the fetus [43, 49, 50]. The typical symptoms of acute toxoplasmosis are mild fever, chills, sweats, and sometimes a mononucleosis-like illness [51]. The fever generally lasts for several days [51]. Other rare symptoms include headache, myalgias, pharyngitis, hepatosplenomegaly, and maculopapular skin eruptions [49, 52]. Lymphadenopathy usually occurs bilaterally, is symmetrical, is not painful, and usually involves the cervical region [52]. Reactivated *T. gondii* infection may cause symptoms such as fever, headache, nausea, confusion, incoordination, and seizures [49].

Toxoplasma gondii may be found in the bloodstream of humans and animals, especially in the acute stage [53–56]. Studies have shown that *T. gondii* can be transmitted by the transmammary route [54, 57, 58]. Transmission of toxoplasmosis from goats to humans has been reported via the consumption of unpasteurized goat milk [54, 57, 59]. In humans, the transmission of *T. gondii* from mother to child may occur if the mother is infected during the third trimester of pregnancy or breastfeeding [60, 61]. During the first or second trimester of pregnancy, the transmission of toxoplasmosis to the fetus is unlikely but frequently leads to severe disease when it occurs [62]. Oral transmission via breastfeeding during acute infection is not expected because the tachyzoites are too sensitive to the proteolytic activity of the oral and gastric secretions [58, 63]. However, satiety may decrease pepsin digestion, leading to the invasion of tachyzoites into the gastric mucosa [64].

Transmission of *T. gondii* through breast milk has been reported [65, 66]. A 2-month-old exclusively-breastfed infant was diagnosed with toxoplasmosis simultaneously with his mother; she was one of 17 individuals who contracted toxoplasmosis by eating raw sheep meat [65]. Khamsian et al. [66] extracted *T. gondii* deoxyribonucleic acid (DNA) in 300 randomly collected human milk samples. In contrast to these reports, some claim that *T. gondii* could have been transmitted by infected water or other body fluids rather than breast milk [67–69]. An animal study reported trophozoites could survive for days in human tears, saliva, and urine [69]. The authors postulated that these body fluids might represent another route of human-to-human transmission.

The often asymptomatic nature of postnatal infection and the lack of data demonstrating transmission of *T. gondii* via breast milk are reasons enough to continue breastfeeding even if the mother has acute toxoplasmosis. Other possible routes of *T. gondii* transmission rather than breastfeeding should be excluded, such as congenital disease, infected water, and other contaminated foods [56, 67].

3   Platyhelminth Infections

3.1   *Schistosomiasis:* Schistosoma *Species*

Schistosomiasis is one of the most important human parasitic diseases in terms of socioeconomic impact, primarily causing significant morbidity and mortality. Schistosomiasis is mainly caused by *Schistosoma haematobium, Schistosoma japonicum*, and *Schistosoma mansoni* species, infecting humans, of the *Schistosoma* genus blood trematodes [70, 71]. S*chistosoma mansoni* and *S. japonicum* mainly infect the gastrointestinal tract, whereas *S. haematobium* the genitourinary tract [72]. *Schistosoma* species live in freshwater snails which can lead to water contamination. Humans are infected when the skin comes into contact with contaminated water [73–75].

Schistosomiasis is common in low-income tropical and subtropical countries without safe drinking water and adequate sanitation [76, 77]. Schistosomiasis primarily affects farmers, fishermen, and children; poor hygiene and contact with infected water make them particularly vulnerable to infection [70, 75, 76]. The World Health Organization (WHO) estimates more than 236 million people have been infected with *Schistosoma* spp. worldwide, and at least 90% of those needing treatment for schistosomiasis live in Africa [70]. In children, worm burden increases with age, and recurrent infections may occur [74, 78]. Most patients have mild-to-moderate disease with limited morbidity; relatively few develop severe infections and death [79, 80].

The clinical manifestations of schistosomiasis are caused by the immune response to the parasites [75, 81]. The chronic stage occurs months to years after the initial infection and results from the immune response leading to the formation of granulomas around the infected tissue [75].

The initial stage of schistosomiasis, called cercarial dermatitis or swimmer's itch, starts 24 h after the cercariae enter the dermis, and lasts 3–8 weeks [75]. In cercarial dermatitis, an itchy maculopapular rash confined to the areas immersed in water develops within a few hours of contaminated water contact [82]. After the first hours to several days of infection, the itching becomes more intense, and the rash typically develops into papules and vesicles. Cercarial dermatitis is self-limiting within several weeks [83]. Diagnosis during the cercarial dermatitis stage is challenging; serologic test results may be negative, and no eggs are found in the urine or stool [81]. The cercariae remain in the bloodstream until they reach the liver. The circulating parasites become adults and may embolize in the liver, lungs, spleen, brain, or spinal cord, causing inflammation and subsequent fibrosis [81].

Another form of acute schistosomiasis, called Katayama syndrome, is an immune reaction against parasitic antigen-antibody complexes that occurs 3–8 weeks after infection [84]. Katayama syndrome usually occurs in nonimmune travelers and may appear in more than half of infected persons [83–85]. Acute schistosomiasis syndrome clinical manifestations include fever, urticaria, angioedema, myalgia, chills, arthralgia, dry cough, diarrhea, abdominal pain, and headache [86]. Symptoms are usually mild and resolve spontaneously within a few days to weeks. In rare cases, weight loss, diarrhea, and neurologic symptoms may occur [86–88].

Chronic schistosomiasis primarily affects persons with childhood-acquired reinfection in poor rural areas [88]. The severity of the disease depends on the density and location of the parasite in the infected tissue, the immune response, and the duration and severity of the infection [89]. Chronic schistosome disease primarily affects the liver, spleen, urogenital tract, gastrointestinal tract, lungs, and CNS. In chronic schistosomiasis, hepatosplenomegaly with hepatic granulomas may be present. In the later stages of the disease, the granulomas gradually progress to periportal fibrosis, leading to portal hypertension and even death due to esophageal variceal bleeding [90]. Severe morbidity associated with genitourinary system involvement and bladder squamous cell carcinoma in schistosomiasis has also been reported [91, 92].

Schistosoma species that enter the bloodstream and multiply in tissue vessels can theoretically also become established in breast tissue and disrupt the vascular structure. In one of the studies on breastfeeding and *Schistosoma* antigens, the effect of breastfeeding on the transfer of lymphocyte response to *S. mansoni* antigens from infected mothers to 50 breastfed infants was examined [93]. Fifty-six percent of infants breastfed had positive delayed-type hypersensitivity reactions. The authors concluded that cellular hypersensitivity to *S. mansoni* antigens in the colostrum of infected mothers might be transmitted to their infants. Another study supported the association between gastrointestinal allergic manifestations in breastfed infants and the presence of immunoglobulin E against the *S. mansoni* antigens [94]. The authors concluded that gastrointestinal allergy in breastfed infants of mothers infected with *S. mansoni* might be due to hypersensitivity to *S. mansoni* antigens in breast milk [94].

4 Nematode Infections

4.1 *Toxocariasis:* **Toxocara canis** *and* **Toxocara cati**

Toxocara, the cause of visceral and ocular larval migrans syndromes, is a common nematode, especially in low-income countries. Toxocariasis results from the accidental infection of humans with the larvae of *Toxocara canis* or *Toxocara cati*, which cannot develop into adult forms in the human body [95, 96]. Humans become infected by ingesting embryonated eggs in contaminated food or *Toxocara* larvae encapsulated in the tissues of transport (paratenic) hosts due to improper cooking of their meat [95].

After ingesting the embryonated eggs, the larvae open in the intestine and enter the bloodstream, spreading throughout the body, causing a marked inflammatory reaction and various clinical symptoms, depending on the organs affected [95, 97]. Toxocariasis is usually asymptomatic; in symptomatic patients, clinical manifestations depend on the density of migrating larvae, the organs they invade, and the inflammatory reaction developed in response to them. Visceral toxocariasis is characterized by the invasion of tissues by numerous larvae migrating through the body and causing inflammation and disease symptoms. In rare cases, the larvae may migrate to the CNS and cause eosinophilic meningoencephalitis or granuloma. The systemic reaction may present as fever, cough, wheezing, abdominal pain, and hepatomegaly [98].

The medical and public health implications may be underestimated because toxocariasis is often asymptomatic [97]. The diagnosis of toxocariasis is based on clinical symptoms and a history of exposure to a potential source. History of inadequately cooked meat consumption or contact with contaminated soil, clinical findings, and direct microscopic examination of tissues are helpful in the diagnosis of toxocariasis. Laboratory examination may reveal leukocytosis and eosinophilia [99]. Seropositivity may present in previous and asymptomatic infections. Therefore, positive serologic test results should be evaluated in light of the patient's clinical condition. Paired serum samples showing a significant increase in antibody levels over time may help confirm active infection.

Animal studies showed that the adult form of *T. canis* develops in the small intestine, and transmission occurs by larval migration through transplacental and transmammary routes [100–102]. Transmission of *T. canis* larvae via breast milk was demonstrated in mice [102, 103]. However, in humans, larvae invade tissues but do not develop into the adult form; hence, the transmission of toxocariasis through breast milk has not been demonstrated and is not a consideration [98, 104].

4.2 *Strongyloidiasis:* Strongyloides stercoralis *and* Strongyloides fuelleborni

The nematode *Strongyloides stercoralis* is the primary causative agent of strongyloidiasis in humans, whereas *Strongyloides fuelleborni* relatively rarely causes infections in humans [105, 106]. *Strongyloides stercoralis* is mainly distributed in tropical and subtropical areas. Infections with *S. fuelleborni* have been widely reported in sub-Saharan Africa [107, 108]. Transmission of strongyloidiasis has primarily been reported in rural areas in temperate climates. The main route of strongyloidiasis transmission is skin contact with contaminated soil; fecal-oral and human-to-human transmissions have also been reported [106, 107, 109, 110]. *Strongyloides stercoralis* and *S. fuelleborni* follow the same life cycles with the important difference that *S. stercoralis* larvae are excreted in feces, in contrast to the eggs seen with *S. fuelleborni* infestation [105].

Strongyloides stercoralis has a complex life cycle, alternating between free-living and parasitic cycles and causing autoinfection of hosts. When human skin comes into contact with filariform larvae of *S. stercoralis* from contaminated soil, the larvae penetrate the skin and travel through the bloodstream to the lungs, where they enter the alveoli. Then the larvae ascend the tracheobronchial tree and are swallowed by the host. Autoinfection in strongyloidiasis is important because untreated cases can lead to persistent infection, even many years later, and may contribute to developing a hyperinfection syndrome [111]. Autoinfection with *S. fuelleborni* does not occur because eggs do not hatch in the host intestine [108].

Symptoms of strongyloidiasis are usually subclinical and may persist for years [112]. Initially, a purpuric erythematous rash appears on the skin penetration area [105]. Dry cough may occur as the larvae migrate upward from the lungs through the trachea [105]. Gastrointestinal symptoms such as diarrhea, constipation, abdominal pain, and malnutrition may occur; respiratory failure and death have been reported in acute infection [112–115].

Chronic strongyloidiasis is mainly asymptomatic [112]. In rare cases, chronic strongyloidiasis may develop arthritis, cardiac arrhythmias, chronic malabsorption, intestinal obstruction, and asthma [114, 116]. If chronic strongyloidiasis is not treated, the mortality rate may be as high as 90% [105]. *Strongyloides fuelleborni* causes the so-called swollen belly syndrome in infants, associated with malnutrition, generalized edema, and a high mortality rate [115].

Strongyloidiasis should be suspected in patients with gastrointestinal, respiratory, and dermatologic manifestations, having relevant epidemiologic exposure, and living in places where *Strongyloides* spp. are endemic [117]. In chronic strongyloidiasis, eosinophilia or elevated immunoglobulin E levels may be detected. The definitive diagnosis of *S. stercoralis* infection is based on examining feces for larvae [117].

Animal studies have suggested that *S. stercoralis* might be transmitted by the transmammary route [118–120]; however, the such spread has not been documented in humans [120]. Human-to-human transmission of strongyloidiasis has been observed [121]. In particular, transmammarian transmission of *S. fuelleborni* has been reported in humans [122]. In an African study, *S. fuelleborni* eggs were found in the stools of 34% of 76 infants under 200 days of age. *Strongyloides* larvae were detected in the milk of one nursing mother. The authors postulated that these findings suggest that *S. fuelleborni* can be transmitted via breastfeeding [122]. Vince et al. [115] reported the clinical and laboratory findings of 13 infants whose median age was 8 weeks, with abdominal distension, respiratory distress, generalized edema, and gastrointestinal dysfunction. *Strongyloides fuelleborni* eggs were found in half of the stool examinations, and about half of the infants died. The authors suggested the possibility of two transmission routes, direct skin penetration and transmammary transmission of *S. fuelleborni,* although they could not detect the parasites in human milk.

4.3 Hookworm Infections: Necator americanus *and* Ancylostoma *Species*

Necator americanus and *Ancylostoma duodenale,* also called hookworms, are soil-transmitted helminths among the most common roundworms in humans [123]. *Ancylostoma ceylanicum* is another hookworm parasitizing in humans [124].

Necator americanus and *A. duodenale* live in the intestine of humans, and their eggs are excreted in feces [125, 126]. The hookworm eggs hatch and release immature larvae in the soil when the infected feces are mixed with the ground or used as fertilizer [127]. After maturation, the larvae can penetrate the skin of humans [128]. Hookworms are transmitted mainly by walking barefoot on contaminated soil [126, 128, 129]. The ingested hookworm larvae also can cause infection [128, 130]. After being ingested or penetrating the skin, the hookworm larvae spread through the human body via the bloodstream, reach the alveolar tissue, travel up the tracheo-bronchial tree, and are swallowed [131]. The larvae then enter the small intestine, develop into adult worms, live in the distal jejunum, and attach to the intestinal wall, causing blood loss [125, 131]. Most adult hookworms disappear after a few years [132].

Most people infected with hookworms have the asymptomatic form of the disease [133]. Some individuals experience gastrointestinal symptoms, particularly those experiencing their first infection [134]. In some cases, attachment of the hookworms to the jejunal wall causes blood loss, resulting in anemia, protein loss, growth retardation, and even decreased cognitive abilities [134]. The first intrauterine hookworm infection was reported in the first half of the twentieth century [135].

Studies showed that transmission of *Ancylostoma caninum* larvae to puppies is an important transmission route in naturally infected female animals [100, 136]. Some human studies concluded that transmammary transmission to infants is a possible route for human hookworm infections [137]. Nwosu [138] reported that examining fecal smears of 316 neonates in a human hookworm endemic area of southern

Nigeria showed that 33 (10%) were hookworm infected. Most neonatal infections (88%) were due to *A. duodenale*, although *N. americanus* was the more prevalent hookworm species in the area. The incidence of neonatal infections was 64% for the infants of mothers with *A. duodenale* infection. Nwosu concluded that these results indicate a possibility of a transmammary infection route for *A. duodenale*. Similarly, Setasuban et al. [139] reported that the prevalence of hookworm infection with *N. americanus* was 61% in 128 breastfeeding mothers. The examination of the breast milk of these mothers revealed the presence of *N. americanus* larvae in one case. The authors concluded that breast milk could potentially be a source of hookworm infection in humans.

The possible route of hookworm transmission to neonates and infants remains unclear and requires more studies [140, 141]. The parasites penetrate the skin and reach the intestinal wall, where they become sexually active and lay eggs after approximately 2 months [142]. In the literature, the youngest patients suffering from hookworm infection were 1 and 12 days old [141, 143]. From this point of view, hookworm larvae were likely transmitted transplacentally or via breastfeeding shortly after birth, as these two routes can provide a shorter time for transmission than the 2 months expected for the usual course of hookworm infections [140].

5 Conclusion

The global distribution of parasitoses and their transmission modes differ significantly. Parasitic infections may be acquired in different ways, including vertical, fecal-oral, and skin contact routes. Transmitting parasites to infants via breastfeeding is not expected with most parasitic infections. However, breastfeeding may provide a possible transmission route to infants in some parasitoses. Therefore, the possibility of transmitting parasites via breast milk should be kept in mind in infants of mothers with a suspected parasitic infection.

References

1. Andreas NJ, Kampmann B, Mehring L-DK. Human breast milk: a review on its composition and bioactivity. Early Hum Dev. 2015;91:629–35.
2. Garofalo R, Chheda S, Mei F, et al. Interleukin-10 in human milk. Pediatr Res. 1995;37:444–9.
3. Hurley WL, Theil PK. Perspectives on immunoglobulins in colostrum and milk. Nutrients. 2011;3:442–74.
4. Pabst HF. Immunomodulation by breast-feeding. Pediatr Infect Dis J. 1997;16:991–5.
5. Bertolli J, St Louis ME, Simonds RJ, et al. Estimating the timing of mother-to-child transmission of human immunodeficiency virus in a breast-feeding population in Kinshasa, Zaire. J Infect Dis. 1996;174:722–6.
6. Lawrence RM, Lawrence RA. Breast milk and infection. Clin Perinatol. 2004;31:501–28.
7. Myers BJ, Kuntz R, Wells W. Helminth parasites of reptiles, birds, and mammals in Egypt: VII. Check list of nematodes collected from 1948 to 1955. Can J Zool. 1962;40:531–8.

8. Bern C, Messenger LA, Whitman JD, Maguire JH. Chagas disease in the United States: a public health approach. Clin Microbiol Rev. 2019;33(1):e00023–19.

9. Pérez-Molina JA, Molina I. Chagas disease. Lancet. 2018;391:82–94.

10. Cura CI, Lattes R, Nagel C, et al. Early molecular diagnosis of acute Chagas disease after transplantation with organs from *Trypanosoma cruzi*-infected donors. Am J Transplant. 2013;13:3253–61.

11. Kessler DA, Shi PA, Avecilla ST, Shaz BH. Results of lookback for Chagas disease since the inception of donor screening at New York Blood Center. Transfusion. 2013;53:1083–7.

12. Herwaldt BL. Laboratory-acquired parasitic infections from accidental exposures. Clin Microbiol Rev. 2001;14:659–88.

13. Roca C, Málaga-Machaca ES, Verastegui MR, et al. IgG subclasses and congenital transmission of Chagas disease. Am J Trop Med Hyg. 2021;105:1187–92.

14. Beltrão Hde B, Cerroni Mde P, Freitas DR, et al. Investigation of two outbreaks of suspected oral transmission of acute Chagas disease in the Amazon region, Para State, Brazil, in 2007. Trop Dr. 2009;39:231–2.

15. Bern C. Chagas' disease. N Engl J Med. 2015;373:456–66.

16. Dias E, Laranja FS, Miranda A, Nobrega G. Chagas' disease; a clinical, epidemiologic, and pathologic study. Circulation. 1956;14:1035–60.

17. Rassi A Jr, Rassi A, Marin-Neto JA. Chagas disease. Lancet. 2010;375:1388–402.

18. Parise ME, Hotez PJ, Slutsker L. Neglected parasitic infections in the United States: needs and opportunities. Am J Trop Med Hyg. 2014;90:783–5.

19. Montgomery SP, Starr MC, Cantey PT, Edwards MS, Meymandi SK. Neglected parasitic infections in the United States: Chagas disease. Am J Trop Med Hyg. 2014;90:814–8.

20. Rassi A Jr, Rassi A, Little WC. Chagas' heart disease. Clin Cardiol. 2000;23:883–9.

21. Andrade ZA, Andrade SG, Oliveira GB, Alonso DR. Histopathology of the conducting tissue of the heart in Chagas' myocarditis. Am Heart J. 1978;95:316–24.

22. Moncayo A, Silveira AC. Current epidemiological trends for Chagas disease in Latin America and future challenges in epidemiology, surveillance and health policy. Mem Inst Oswaldo Cruz. 2009;104:17–30.

23. World Health Organization. Control of Chagas disease- Second report of the WHO Expert Committee. Geneva: World Health Organization. 2002:1–112. https://apps.who.int/iris/bitstream/handle/10665/42443/WHO_TRS_905.pdf?sequence=1&isAllowed=y. Accessed 28 Feb 2023.

24. Kun H, Moore A, Mascola L, et al. Transmission of *Trypanosoma cruzi* by heart transplantation. Clin Infect Dis. 2009;48:1534–40.

25. World Health Organization. WHA 63.20 Chagas disease: control and elimination. The 63rd World Health Assembly - governing bodies documentation (May 20, 2010). https://www.who.int/publications/i/item/wha63.20. Accessed 28 Feb 2023.

26. Bern C, Montgomery SP, Herwaldt BL, et al. Evaluation and treatment of Chagas disease in the United States: a systematic review. JAMA. 2007;298:2171–81.

27. Norman FF, López-Vélez R. Chagas disease and breast-feeding. Emerg Infect Dis. 2013;19:1561–6.

28. Bittencourt AL, Sadigursky M, Da Silva AA, et al. Evaluation of Chagas' disease transmission through breast-feeding. Mem Inst Oswaldo Cruz. 1988;83:37–9.

29. Ferreira CS, Martinho PC, Amato Neto V, Cruz RR. Pasteurization of human milk to prevent transmission of Chagas disease. Rev Inst Med Trop Sao Paulo. 2001;43:161–2.

30. Santos Ferreira C, Amato Neto V, Gakiya E, Bezerra RC, Alarcón RS. Microwave treatment of human milk to prevent transmission of Chagas disease. Rev Inst Med Trop Sao Paulo. 2003;45:41–2.

31. Schijman AG, Altcheh J, Burgos JM, et al. Aetiological treatment of congenital Chagas' disease diagnosed and monitored by the polymerase chain reaction. J Antimicrob Chemother. 2003;52:441–9.

32. Altcheh J, Moscatelli G, Moroni S, Garcia-Bournissen F, Freilij H. Adverse events after the use of benznidazole in infants and children with Chagas disease. Pediatrics. 2011;127:e212–8.
33. Miles MA. *Trypanosoma cruzi* milk transmission of infection and immunity from mother to young. Parasitology. 1972;65:1–9.
34. Campos R, Pinto PL, Moreira AA, et al. Experimental study on the transmission of Chagas' disease by milk. Rev Hos Clin Fac Med Sao Paulo. 1988;43:146–7.
35. Martins LP, Castanho RE, Nogueira AB, Silva OT, Gusmão AS. Incidence of *Trypanosoma cruzi* transmission through breastfeeding during acute experimental Chagas disease. Braz J Infect Dis. 2011;15:116–8.
36. Amato Neto V, Matsubara L, Campos R, et al. *Trypanosoma cruzi* in the milk of women with chronic Chagas disease. Rev Hosp Clin Fac Med Sao Paulo. 1992;47:10–1.
37. Centers for Disease Control and Prevention. Toxoplasmosis (*Toxoplasma* infection): epidemiology and risk factors (last reviewed: Sep 4, 2018). https://www.cdc.gov/parasites/toxoplasmosis/epi.html. Accessed 28 Feb 2023.
38. Spalding SM, Amendoeira MR, Klein CH, Ribeiro LC. Serological screening and toxoplasmosis exposure factors among pregnant women in South of Brazil. Rev Soc Bras Med Trop. 2005;38:173–7.
39. Bahia-Oliveira LM, Jones JL, Azevedo-Silva J, Alves CC, Oréfice F, Addiss DG. Highly endemic, waterborne toxoplasmosis in north Rio de Janeiro state, Brazil. Emerg Infect Dis. 2003;9:55–62.
40. Centers for Disease Control and Prevention. Toxoplasmosis (*Toxoplasma* infection): biology (last reviewed: Nov 10, 2020). https://www.cdc.gov/parasites/toxoplasmosis/biology.html. Accessed 28 Feb 2023.
41. Kochanowsky JA, Koshy AA. Toxoplasma gondii. Curr Biol. 2018;28:770–1.
42. Tenter AM, Heckeroth AR, Weiss LM. *Toxoplasma gondii*: from animals to humans. Int J Parasitol. 2000;30:1217–58.
43. Hide G. Role of vertical transmission of *Toxoplasma gondii* in prevalence of infection. Expert Rev Anti-Infect Ther. 2016;14:335–44.
44. Schlüter D, Barragan A. Advances and challenges in understanding cerebral toxoplasmosis. Front Immunol. 2019;10:242.
45. Tedford E, McConkey G. Neurophysiological changes induced by chronic *Toxoplasma gondii* infection. Pathogens. 2017;6:19.
46. Holland GN. Ocular toxoplasmosis: a global reassessment. Part I: epidemiology and course of disease. Am J Ophthalmol. 2003;136:973–88.
47. Neves ES, Bicudo LN, Curi AL, et al. Acute acquired toxoplasmosis: clinical-laboratorial aspects and ophthalmologic evaluation in a cohort of immunocompetent patients. Mem Inst Oswaldo Cruz. 2009;104:393–6.
48. O'Connell S, Guy EC, Dawson SJ, Francis JM, Joynson DH. Chronic active toxoplasmosis in an immunocompetent patient. J Infect. 1993;27:305–10.
49. Montoya JG, Liesenfeld O. Toxoplasmosis. Lancet. 2004;363:1965–76.
50. Hampton MM. Congenital toxoplasmosis: a review. Neonatal Netw. 2015;34:274–8.
51. Lawrence RM. Transmission of infectious diseases through breast milk and breastfeeding. In: Lawrence RA, Lawrence RM, Noble L, Rosen-Carole C, Stuebe AM, editors. Breastfeeding: a guide for the medical profession. 9th ed. Philadelphia, PA: Elsevier; 2021. p. 393–456.
52. McCabe RE, Brooks RG, Dorfman RF, Remington JS. Clinical spectrum in 107 cases of toxoplasmic lymphadenopathy. Rev Infect Dis. 1987;9:754–74.
53. Carter AO, Frank JW. Congenital toxoplasmosis: epidemiologic features and control. CMAJ. 1986;135:618–23.
54. de Chiari AC, Neves DP. [Human toxoplasmosis acquired by ingestion of goat's milk.] Mem Inst Oswaldo Cruz 1984;79:337–40. [article in Portuguese, abstract in English].
55. Valian HK, Mirhendi H, Mohebali M, et al. Comparison of the RE-529 sequence and B1 gene for *Toxoplasma gondii* detection in blood samples of the at-risk seropositive cases using ura-

cil DNA glycosylase supplemented loop-mediated isothermal amplification (UDG-LAMP) assay. Microb Pathog. 2020;140:103938.

56. Bonametti AM, Passos JN, Koga da Silva EM, Macedo ZS. Probable transmission of acute toxoplasmosis through breast feeding. J Trop Pediatr. 1997;43:116.

57. Sacks JJ, Roberto RR, Brooks NF. Toxoplasmosis infection associated with raw goat's milk. JAMA. 1982;248:1728–32.

58. Walsh CP, Hammond SE, Zajac AM, Lindsay DS. Survival of *Toxoplasma gondii* tachyzoites in goat milk: potential source of human toxoplasmosis. J Eukaryot Microbiol. 1999;46:73–4.

59. Riemann HP, Meyer ME, Theis JH, Kelso G, Behymer DE. Toxoplasmosis in an infant fed unpasteurized goat milk. J Pediatr. 1975;87:573–6.

60. Goldfarb J. Breastfeeding. AIDS and other infectious diseases. Clin Perinatol. 1993;20:225–43.

61. Langer H, Geissler H. Demonstration of *Toxoplasma* in aborted fetus and premature infants. Arch Gynakol. 1960;192:304–7.

62. Feldman HA. Toxoplasmosis. N Engl J Med. 1968;279:1431–7.

63. Sroka J, Wójcik-Fatla A, Dutkiewicz J. Occurrence of *Toxoplasma gondii* in water from wells located on farms. Ann Agric Environ Med. 2006;13:169–75.

64. Pettersen EK. Transmission of toxoplasmosis via milk from lactating mice. Acta Pathol Microbiol Immunol Scand B. 1984;92:175–6.

65. Secretaria de Vigilância em Saúde, Brasil. Surto intra familiar de toxoplasmose, Santa Vitoria do Palmar-RS, julho de 2005. Bol Eletrôn Epidemiol. 2006;6:1–7.

66. Khamsian EM, Hajimohammadi B, Eslami G, Fallahzadeh MH, Hosseini SS. *Toxoplasma gondii* in milk of human and goat from the desert area in central Iran. Iran J Parasitol. 2021;16:601–9.

67. Capobiango JD, Mitsuka-Breganó R, Monica TC, Ferreira FP, Reiche EM. Acute toxoplasmosis in a breastfed infant with possible transmission by water. Rev Inst Med Trop Sao Paulo. 2015;57:523–6.

68. Karanis P, Aldeyarbi HM, Mirhashemi ME, Khalil KM. The impact of the waterborne transmission of *Toxoplasma gondii* and analysis efforts for water detection: an overview and update. Environ Sci Pollut Res Int. 2013;20:86–99.

69. Saari M, Räisänen S. Transmission of acute toxoplasma infection. The survival of trophozoites in human tears, saliva, and urine and in cow's milk. Acta Ophthalmol. 1974;52:847–52.

70. World Health Organization. Schistosomiasis (updated: Feb 1, 2023). https://www.who.int/news-room/fact-sheets/detail/schistosomiasis. Accessed 28 Feb 2023.

71. Centers for Disease Control and Prevention. Schistosomiasis (Apr 11, 2018). https://www.cdc.gov/parasites/schistosomiasis/index.html. Accessed 28 Feb 2023.

72. Webster BL, Southgate VR, Littlewood DT. A revision of the interrelationships of *Schistosoma* including the recently described *Schistosoma guineensis*. Int J Parasitol. 2006;36:947–55.

73. Yi-Xin H. [Ecological characteristics of *Oncomelaniahupensis* and water conservancy combined with schistosomiasis prevention and control.] Zhongguo Xue Xi Chong Bing Fang Zhi Za Zhi. 2019;31:47–52. [article in Chinese, abstract in English].

74. Verjee MA. Schistosomiasis: still a cause of significant morbidity and mortality. Res Rep Trop Med. 2019;10:153–63.

75. Carbonell C, Rodríguez-Alonso B, López-Bernús A, et al. Clinical spectrum of schistosomiasis: an update. J Clin Med. 2021;10:5521.

76. Williams DS. Schistosomiasis. J Insur Med. 2008;40:248–9.

77. Dai SM, Guan Z, Zhang LJ, et al. Imported schistosomiasis, China, 2010-2018. Emerg Infect Dis. 2020;26:179–80.

78. Osakunor DNM, Woolhouse MEJ, Mutapi F. Paediatric schistosomiasis: What we know and what we need to know. PLoS Negl Trop Dis. 2018;12:e0006144.

79. Tukahebwa EM, Magnussen P, Madsen H, et al. A very high infection intensity of *Schistosoma mansoni* in a Ugandan Lake Victoria fishing community is required for association with highly prevalent organ related morbidity. PLoS Negl Trop Dis. 2013;7:e2268.

80. Wall KM, Kilembe W, Vwalika B, et al. Schistosomiasis is associated with incident HIV transmission and death in Zambia. PLoS Negl Trop Dis. 2018;12:e0006902.
81. Lingscheid T, Kurth F, Clerinx J, et al. Schistosomiasis in European travelers and migrants: analysis of 14 years Ttropnet surveillance data. Am J Trop Med Hyg. 2017;97:567–74.
82. Tracz ES, Al-Jubury A, Buchmann K, Bygum A. Outbreak of swimmer's itch in Denmark. Acta Derm Venereol. 2019;99:1116–20.
83. Colebunders R, Verstraeten T, Van Gompel A, et al. Acute schistosomiasis in travelers returning from Mali. J Travel Med. 1995;2:235–8.
84. Ross AG, Vickers D, Olds GR, Shah SM, McManus DP. Katayama syndrome. Lancet Infect Dis. 2007;7:218–24.
85. Bottieau E, Clerinx J, De Vega MR, et al. Imported Katayama fever: clinical and biological features at presentation and during treatment. J Infect. 2006;52:339–45.
86. Lambertucci JR. Acute schistosomiasis: clinical, diagnostic and therapeutic features. Rev Inst Med Trop Sao Paulo. 1993;35:399–404.
87. Yun X, Zhi-Hong G, Hui-Qun X. [Clinical features of 14 cases of cerebral schistosomiasis in Jiangxi Province.] Zhongguo Xue Xi Chong Bing Fang Zhi Za Zhi. 2017;29:740–2. [article in Chinese, abstract in English.]
88. Gryseels B, Polman K, Clerinx J, Kestens L. Human schistosomiasis. Lancet. 2006;368:1106–18.
89. Abel L, Demenais F, Prata A, Souza AE, Dessein A. Evidence for the segregation of a major gene in human susceptibility/resistance to infection by *Schistosoma mansoni*. Am J Hum Genet. 1991;48:959–70.
90. Kaatano GM, Min DY, Siza JE, et al. *Schistosoma mansoni*-related hepatosplenic morbidity in adult population on Kome Island, Sengerema District, Tanzania. Korean J Parasitol. 2015;53:545–51.
91. Haghighi L, Akbaribazm M, Arab-Mazar Z, Rahimi M. Vesical schistosomiasis and squamous cell carcinoma associated with *Schistosoma haematobium*: a re-emerging neglected tropical disease in Tehran, Iran. Urol Case Rep. 2020;30:101140.
92. Khalaf I, Shokeir A, Shalaby M. Urologic complications of genitourinary schistosomiasis. World J Urol. 2012;30:31–8.
93. Eissa AM, Saad MA, Abdel Ghaffar AK, el-Sharkaway IM, Kamal KA. Transmission of lymphocyte responsiveness to schistosomal antigens by breast feeding. Trop Geogr Med. 1989;41:208–12.
94. Noureldin MS, Shaltout AA. Anti-schistosomal IgE and its relation to gastrointestinal allergy in breast-fed infants of *Schistosoma mansoni* infected mothers. J Egypt Soc Parasitol. 1998;28:539–50.
95. Despommier D. Toxocariasis: clinical aspects, epidemiology, medical ecology, and molecular aspects. Clin Microbiol Rev. 2003;16:265–72.
96. Holland CV. Knowledge gaps in the epidemiology of *Toxocara*: the enigma remains. Parasitology. 2017;144:81–94.
97. Chen J, Liu Q, Liu GH, et al. Toxocariasis: a silent threat with a progressive public health impact. Infect Dis Poverty. 2018;7:59.
98. Centers for Disease Control and Prevention. Toxocariasis (also known as roundworm Infection): diagnosis (May 20, 2020). https://www.cdc.gov/parasites/toxocariasis/health_professionals/index.html. Accessed 28 Feb 2023.
99. Hotez PJ, Wilkins PP. Toxocariasis: America's most common neglected infection of poverty and a helminthiasis of global importance? PLoS Negl Trop Dis. 2009;3:400.
100. Burke TM, Roberson EL. Prenatal and lactational transmission of *Toxocara canis* and *Ancylostoma caninum*: experimental infection of the bitch before pregnancy. Int J Parasitol. 1985;15:71–5.
101. Dunsmore JD, Thompson RC, Bates IA. The accumulation of *Toxocara canis* larvae in the brains of mice. Int J Parasitol. 1983;13:517–21.

102. de Souza AP, Furtado RD, de Avila LF, et al. Transmammary infection in BALB/c mice with chronic toxocariasis. Parasitol Int. 2015;64:145–7.
103. Jin Z, Akao N, Ohta N. Prolactin evokes lactational transmission of larvae in mice infected with *Toxocara canis*. Parasitol Int. 2008;57:495–8.
104. Beaver PC. The nature of visceral larva migrans. J Parasitol. 1969;55:3–12.
105. Centers for Disease Control and Prevention. Strongyloides: biology (last reviewed: Jul 30, 2019). https://www.cdc.gov/parasites/strongyloides/biology.html. Accessed 28 Feb 2023.
106. Gonzales DJ, Chakraborty RK, Climaco A. Strongyloidiasis (updated: Sep 12, 2022). In: StatPearls [Internet]. Treasure Island (FL): StatPearls Publishing. https://www.ncbi.nlm.nih.gov/books/NBK430775/. Accessed 28 Feb 2023.
107. La Hoz RM, Morris MI. Intestinal parasites including *Cryptosporidium, Cyclospora, Giardia*, and *Microsporidia, Entamoeba histolytica, Strongyloides, Schistosomiasis,* and *Echinococcus*: guidelines from the American Society of Transplantation Infectious Diseases Community of Practice. Clin Transpl. 2019;33:e13618.
108. Thanchomnang T, Intapan PM, Sanpool O, et al. First molecular identification and genetic diversity of *Strongyloides stercoralis* and *Strongyloides fuelleborni* in human communities having contact with long-tailed macaques in Thailand. Parasitol Res. 2017;116:1917–23.
109. Sugiyama K, Hasegawa Y, Nagasawa T, Hitomi S. Exposure of medical staff to *Strongyloides stercolaris* from a patient with disseminated strongyloidiasis. J Infect Chemother. 2006;12:217–9.
110. Jones JM, Hill C, Briggs G, et al. Notes from the field: strongyloidiasis at a long-term-care facility for the developmentally disabled - Arizona, 2015. MMWR Morb Mortal Wkly Rep. 2016;65:608–9.
111. Mohammed S, Bhatia P, Chhabra S, Gupta SK, Kumar R. Pulmonary hyperinfection with *Strongyloides stercoralis* in an immunocompetent patient. Indian J Crit Care Med. 2019;23:481–3.
112. Mejia R, Nutman TB. Screening, prevention, and treatment for hyperinfection syndrome and disseminated infections caused by *Strongyloides stercoralis*. Curr Opin Infect Dis. 2012;25:458–63.
113. Ashford RW, Barnish G, Viney ME. *Strongyloides fuelleborni kelly*i: infection and disease in Papua New Guinea. Parasitol Today. 1992;8:314–8.
114. da Silva OA, Amaral CF, da Silveira JC, López M, Pittella JE. Hypokalemic respiratory muscle paralysis following *Strongyloides stercoralis* hyperinfection: a case report. Am J Trop Med Hyg. 1981;30:69–73.
115. Vince JD, Ashford RW, Gratten MJ, Bana-Koiri J. *Strongyloides* species infestation in young infants of Papua New Guinea: association with generalized oedema. 1979. P N G Med J. 2005;48:50–7.
116. Nazik S, Yıldız F. A case of rheumatoid arthritis with *Strongyloides stercoralis* hyperinfection. Turkiye Parazitol Derg. 2020;44:112–4.
117. Krolewiecki A, Nutman TB. Strongyloidiasis: a neglected tropical disease. Infect Dis Clin N Am. 2019;33:135–51.
118. Stone W, Smith FW. Infection of mammalian hosts by milk-borne nematode larvae: a review. Exp Parasitol. 1973;34:306–12.
119. Batte EG. Trans-colostral migration of *Stronglyoides ransomi* larvae in the pig. Wiad Parazytol. 1973;19:155–8.
120. Shoop WL, Michael BF, Eary CH, Haines HW. Transmammary transmission of *Strongyloides stercoralis* in dogs. J Parasitol. 2002;88:536–9.
121. Czachor JS, Jonas AP. Transmission of *Strongyloides steracolis* person to person. J Travel Med. 2000;7:211–2.
122. Brown RC, Girardeau HF. Transmammary passage of *Strongyloides* sp. larvae in the human host. Am J Trop Med Hyg. 1977;26:215–9.
123. Centers for Disease Control and Prevention. Hookworm (last reviewed: apr 29,2022). https://www.cdc.gov/parasites/hookworm/index.html. Accessed 28 Feb 2023.

124. Inpankaew T, Schär F, Dalsgaard A, et al. High prevalence of *Ancylostoma ceylanicum* hookworm infections in humans, Cambodia, 2012. Emerg Infect Dis. 2014;20:976–82.

125. Beaver P. [Observations on Necator infections resulting from exposure to three larvae.] Revista Iberica de Parasitologia. 1950:17:713–21. [article in Spanish].

126. Bartsch SM, Hotez PJ, Asti L, et al. The global economic and health burden of human hookworm infection. PLoS Negl Trop Dis. 2016;10:e0004922.

127. Humphries DL, Stephenson LS, Pearce EJ, The PH, Dan HT, Khanh LT. The use of human faeces for fertilizer is associated with increased intensity of hookworm infection in Vietnamese women. Trans R Soc Trop Med Hyg. 1997;91:518–20.

128. Sarinas P, Chitkara RK. Ascariasis and hookworm. Semin Respir Infect. 1997;12:130–7.

129. Jiraanankul V, Aphijirawat W, Mungthin M, et al. Incidence and risk factors of hookworm infection in a rural community of central Thailand. Am J Trop Med Hyg. 2011;84:594–8.

130. Bowman DD. Zoonotic hookworm infections (ancylostomiasis). In: Palmer SR, Torgerson PR, Brown DWG, editors. Zoonoses. 1st ed. Oxford: Oxford Medical Publications; 2011. p. 767–73.

131. Nawalinski TA, Schad GA. Arrested development in *Ancylostoma duodenale*: course of a self-induced infection in man. Am J Trop Med Hyg. 1974;23:895–8.

132. Beaver PC. Light, long-lasting *Necator* infection in a volunteer. Am J Trop Med Hyg. 1988;39:369–72.

133. Loukas A, Hotez PJ, Diemert D, et al. Hookworm infection. Nat Rev Dis Primers. 2016;2:16088.

134. Weatherhead JE, Hotez PJ. Worm infections in children. Pediatr Rev. 2015;36:341–52.

135. Nawa H. On a case with intrauterine hookworm infection. Jikken Iho. 1937;23:540–3.

136. Burke TM, Roberson EL. Prenatal and lactational transmission of *Toxocara cams* and *Ancylostoma caninum*: Experimental infection of the bitch at midpregnancy and at parturition. Int J Parasitol. 1985;15:485–90.

137. Donges J, Madecki O. The possibility of hookworm infection through breast milk. Germ Med Mon. 1968;13:391–2.

138. Nwosu AB. Human neonatal infections with hookworms in an endemic area of Southern Nigeria. A possible transmammary route. Trop Geogr Med. 1981;33:105–11.

139. Setasuban P, Punsri W, Meunnoo C. Transmammary transmission of *Necator americanus* larva in the human host. Southeast Asian J Trop Med Public Health. 1980;11:535–8.

140. Savioli L, Albonico M, Daumerie D, et al. Review of the 2017 WHO Guideline: preventive chemotherapy to control soil-transmitted helminth infections in at-risk population groups. An opportunity lost in translation. PLoS Negl Trop Dis. 2018;12:e0006296.

141. Yu SH, Jiang ZX, Xu LQ. Infantile hookworm disease in China. a review. Acta Trop. 1995;59:265–70.

142. Hotez PJ. Hookworms (*Necator americanus* and *Ancylostoma* spp.). In: Kliegman RM, St Geme III JW, Blum NJ, Shah SS, Tasker RC, Wilson KM, editors. Nelson textbook of pediatrics. 21st ed. Philadelphia, PA: Elsevier; 2020. p. 1878–81.

143. Tiwari L, James J, Chowdhary S, Sharma A, Puliyel JM. Severe anaemia owing to hookworm in a 12-day-old Nepalese infant. Ann Trop Paediatr. 2004;24:361–3.

Maternal Infections: Who Can and Who Cannot Breastfeed?

Gonca Keskindemirci and Gülbin Gökçay

1 Introduction

Breast milk is the most fabulous nutritional source for babies. In addition to being a food source, it contains antimicrobial, anti-infective, and bactericidal complexes such as secretory IgA (SlgA), immunoglobulins, lysozyme, lactoferrin, lactoperoxidase, casein, human alpha-lactalbumin made lethal to tumor cell (HAMLET), and cytokines. These features of breast milk protect breastfeeding children from many infectious diseases [1–11]. For example, lactoferrin inactivates virulence factors of various microorganisms. In addition, lactoferrin prevents the binding of some viruses to host cells [12]. Therefore, it is not rational to say that every virus found in breast milk can cause disease. In this respect, case reports are important in developing recommendations. The fear and anxiety of transmission of the maternal infection to the baby through breast milk and the lack of knowledge on this subject can cause the baby to be deprived of breast milk and put the child in great risk for infection. In the presence of maternal infection, the benefits of breastfeeding should be weighed against the known or anticipated risks of breastfeeding during a maternal infection. Maternal illnesses during which breastfeeding is contraindicated are extremely rare. Breastfeeding recommendations during maternal infectious diseases are discussed in detail in this chapter.

G. Keskindemirci (✉) · G. Gökçay
Division of Social Pediatrics, Department of Pediatrics, İstanbul Faculty of Medicine, İstanbul University, İstanbul, Türkiye

Department of Social Pediatrics, Institute of Child Health, Istanbul University, İstanbul, Türkiye

Ö. N. Şahin et al. (eds.), *Breastfeeding and Metabolic Programming*, https://doi.org/10.1007/978-3-031-33278-4_32

2 Bacterial Infections of the Mother and Breastfeeding

2.1 Botulism

Botulism occurs when the botulinum toxin passes into the circulation. Although the toxin is produced by *Clostridium botulinum,* it is also produced by *Clostridium butyricum* and *Clostridium baratii* [13]. At least seven toxins are known, and botulinum toxins A, B, and E are the most common pathogens [14]. Infant botulism is caused by the opening of *C. botulinum* spores in the intestine and the release of toxins when perhaps accidentally eating foods containing botulinum spores such as honey, especially under 12 months of age. At low pH, toxin production of *C. botulinum* decreases, and even at more acidic pH, toxin production stops. The fecal pH of breastfed infants is between 5.1 and 5.4, that is acidic, while the fecal pH of formula-fed infants varies between 5.9 and 8.0 [12]. Even if the nursing mother eats the botulism spores in honey, the spores are too large to pass into breast milk, so they are not expected to be in breast milk. Therefore, breast milk is not the source of bacterial spores or toxins that cause infant botulism. Matsumura et al. found that SIgA in breast milk binds the 16S toxin of *C. Botulinum* and prevents its entry into intestinal epithelial cells [15]. Continuation of breastfeeding or expressed breast milk should be recommended and supported in the light of available information [16, 17].

2.2 Brucellosis

Brucellosis is a zoonotic infectious disease. Transmission to humans occurs through contact with infected animals, infected animal carcasses, or ingestion of infected raw milk and dairy products [18]. Transmission of bacteria may also be occurred by breathing or through skin wounds or mucose membranes [19]. Some case reports showed that transplacental and breast milk transmission may occur from mother to infant [20–22]. When brucellosis is detected in the mother, the mother should express her breast for the continuity of breast milk, and the expressed milk should be discarded. Breastfeeding can be resumed after 48–96 hours of treatment given to the mother. Since breastfeeding will continue, antimicrobial agents compatible with breastfeeding should be used in treatment [3]. In the presence of brucella mastitis, there is no need to wean the breast milk, as it is thought that the baby is already exposed to the infection. The mother needs to be treated for the abscess [12].

2.3 *Tuberculosis*

Tuberculosis disease is caused by the complex bacilli of *Mycobacterium tuberculosis*. The main cause of tuberculosis in infants is prolonged close contact with an adult with pulmonary tuberculosis, mostly in their own home during the postpartum period. Sources of transmission can be mother or babysitter, nursery staff, relatives, friends, or neighbors. All household contacts should be evaluated in detail. Except for tuberculosis infection in the breast, tuberculosis bacillus could not be demonstrated in breast milk [12, 23]. Transmission is usually by respiratory droplets containing bacillus shed from adults or adolescents. Mothers found to be contagious should be isolated and should interrupt breastfeeding. Breast milk is not contraindicated, only isolation is required to prevent transmission from the mother via droplets [24]. Expressed breast milk can be used as long as there is no evidence of tuberculosis mastitis. Mothers who have negative sputum may breastfeed [12, 25, 26]. Small concentrations of tuberculosis drugs are excreted in breast milk; this is not considered a contraindication for breastfeeding. It is also important to note that the concentrations of tuberculosis drugs in breast milk are too low to be relied upon for the treatment of the infant [26, 27]. Rifampicin, used for the treatment, may give an orange color to all body fluids, including breast milk. This does not cause any harm [27].

3 Maternal Viral Infections and Breastfeeding

3.1 *Chickenpox*

Chickenpox is a contagious disease caused by the varicella-zoster virus (VZV). Rashes are considered contagious until they crust over. It can be transmitted by inhalation of infected droplets and contact with the virus from skin lesions. There are case reports showing the VZV DNA in breast milk [28–30]. On the other hand, in one case, it was reported that although the mother who had chickenpox lesions and who breastfed her infant, no chickenpox lesion was observed in her infant [29]. Perinatal infection can cause severe illness in infants if a maternal rash develops 5 days before and 2 days after delivery [12]. The reason for this is that the antibodies to be formed in the mother cannot pass placentally in sufficient amounts. Under these circumstances, the baby should be separated from the mother with chickenpox, and breastfeeding should be interrupted when the mother is contagious. Expressed milk can be given if there is no skin lesion on the breast [31, 32]. There is a need for more evidence on this subject.

3.2 Cytomegalovirus

Cytomegalovirus (CMV) is one of the largest viruses with a double-stranded DNA genome from the herpesviridae family. Although CMV has been found in the breast milk of mothers who had preterm infants, case reports of preterm infants acquiring CMV postnatally have not demonstrated long-term clinical sequelae. Preterms born at gestational age lower than 30–32 weeks and/or having birth weight below than 1000 g have greater risks of CMV acquisition via breast milk [33]. The decision of CMV-positive mothers to breastfeed preterm infants must be made considering the potential benefits of breast milk and the CMV transmission risk [34]. *Cytomegalovirus* was detected at varying rates in the milk of CMV-positive mothers using viral cultures or CMV DNA polymerase chain reaction (PCR). It is less isolated in colostrum than in mature milk [33, 35–37]. Different techniques are recommended to prevent contamination from breast milk. However, there is no standard guideline for preventing contamination [38, 39]. *Cytomegalovirus*-positive mothers can safely breastfeed their term babies [40]. *Cytomegalovirus* infection via breast milk transmission does not usually occur in term infants due to the protective maternal antibodies' transmission [34].

3.3 Ebola Virus Disease

Ebola virus disease (EVD) is spread through direct contact with blood and other body fluids including breast milk. Ebola virus has been detected in breast milk samples, but there is no data on when the virus is excreted in breast milk during the course of the disease. Therefore, breastfeeding is contraindicated in women with suspected or confirmed Ebola virus disease. The milk of mothers diagnosed with EVD is considered infectious waste and should be disposed according to medical waste rules. If the mother uses a breast pump, the pump parts should be disposable. Mothers diagnosed with the disease should also pay attention to hand hygiene in terms of possible contamination [12, 41]. When safe alternatives to breastfeeding and infant care are available, a mother with Ebola virus infection should not breastfeed and be in close contact with her infant [42]. Testing of human milk for the presence of Ebola virus RNA may help to make decisions about when breastfeeding can be safely resumed. Any child exposed to Ebola through breast milk should be closely monitored for a period of 21 days. If a breastfeeding woman and her child are both diagnosed with the disease, breastfeeding should be discontinued and the mother-baby couple be separated and appropriate breast milk (such as donor milk) or substitutes should be provided. However, if the mother and baby are diagnosed with EVD and if the child is less than 6 months old and there is no safe and appropriate breast milk or substitute, or if the child is not adequately cared for, the option of continuing to breastfeed may be considered. This decision should be taken on a case-by-case basis [12, 41].

3.4 Epstein-Barr Virus

Epstein-Barr virus (EBV) can lead to clinical pictures such as infectious mononucleosis, chronic fatigue syndrome, nasopharyngeal carcinoma, and Burkitt lymphoma. There is a concern that EBV may cause lifelong latent infection and has potential transmission from the mother to her infant. PCR demonstrated EBV DNA in breast milk and cervix [12, 43, 44]. However, it is also unknown how early breast milk can be an EBV infection source when compared with other sources in an infant's environment. More studies on the pathogenesis of EBV-associated tumors are needed in areas where these tumors are not rare before recommending avoiding breastfeeding during maternal infections in these places. In areas where nasopharyngeal carcinoma and Burkitt lymphoma are rare, maternal EBV infection in the mother is by no means a contraindication for breastfeeding [12].

3.5 Hepatitis A Virus

Hepatitis A virus (HAV) is from the Picornaviridae family. In addition to fecal–oral transmission of HAV, food- or water-borne epidemics have also been reported [45]. Although there are some case reports showing that HAV RNA are detected in breast milk, there is no clear evidence that breastfeeding can cause hepatitis A virus transmission from an infected mother [46]. Therefore, mothers with hepatitis A infection should not refrain from breastfeeding and breastfeeding should be continued [12].

3.6 Hepatitis B Virus

Hepatitis B virus (HBV), which contains double-stranded DNA, is from the Hepadnaviridae family. HBV is transmitted through parenteral exposure to contagious blood or body fluids. Transmission during childhood mostly occurs through perinatal transmission from infected mother to child. The virus is most commonly transmitted from mother to child during birth [47]. Hepatitis B surface antigen (HBsAg) has been found in breast milk, but HBsAg positivity has not been demonstrated in breastfed infants who received the full dose vaccine series and hepatitis B immunoglobulin [48–50]. Breastfeeding of an infant by an HBsAg-positive mother does not create any additional risk of getting HBV infection [51]. Babies of mothers with hepatitis B infection should be administered hepatitis B immunoglobulin together with the hepatitis B vaccine in the first 12 h after delivery. The vaccine series should be completed with the second dose that is administered 1–2 months after and then the third dose in the sixth month. If the baby was born under 2000 g and the mother has HBsAg positivity, vaccine and immunoglobulin are administered to the baby at birth. A three-dose series of vaccines is planned 1 month after the dose given at birth, 2 months later, and at the baby's sixth month, without counting the first vaccine at birth [51]. After completion of vaccination, infants born to HbsAg-positive women should have a serological evaluation at 9–12 months of age. Postponing breastfeeding until the baby is fully vaccinated is not considered. There is insufficient information about breastfeeding the baby when there are cracks bleeding in the breast of an HBsAg-positive mother. Some authorities recommended that the mother may pause breastfeeding until the bleeding stops in the crack of the nipple, express her milk, and continue breastfeeding when the bleeding stops [52]. On the other hand, an in vitro study showed that breast milk inhibits the infectivity of hepatitis B virus. In this study, lactoferrin was identified as a component in breast milk to bind to HbsAg and the authors stated that although the virus was detected in the mother's milk it did not cause maternal transmission [53]. Lactoferrin with a cationic structure is a potent inhibitor of enveloped and naked viruses in breast milk [54, 55]. Results of various studies showed that even before the presence of immunoprophylaxis against HBV, breastfeeding did not pose an additional risk for maternal HBV transmission [54–56]. Breastfeeding counseling is important to avoid nipple cracking and bleeding.

3.7   Hepatitis C Virus

Hepatitis C virus (HCV) infection is the most common cause of non-A and non-B hepatitis. There is no evidence of mother-to-infant hepatitis C transmission with breastfeeding. According to current guidelines, there is no contraindication about breastfeeding for maternal HCV infection [57]. Some authorities recommended that the mother should consider stopping breastfeeding from a breast with bleeding in the nipple crack but express her milk to maintain the breast milk production so can resume breastfeeding when the bleeding stops [12, 52, 57].

3.8   Herpes Simplex Virus Infections

There are two types of Herpes simplex virus (HSV) as HSV-1 and HSV-2. HSV-1 is mainly transmitted through mouth-to-mouth contact and causes herpes in the mouth. HSV-2 causes sexually transmitted infection leading to genital herpes. Herpes simplex virus can be transmitted via direct contact of the mothers' lesions to the infants. Transmission can be prevented with good hand hygiene and covering lesions with which the infant might come into contact. No transmission through breast milk has been reported. If there is no lesion in the mother's breasts, the mother can breastfeed her baby. When the mother has a herpetic lesion on the breast, she should temporarily avoid breastfeeding from the affected breast. Expressed milk from the affected breast may be used with high precautions to prevent contamination from the lesions

[31]. If there is no lesion in the other breast, she can breastfeed from that breast paying attention to covering the lesions on the affected breast completely [58–60].

3.9 Human Immunodeficiency Virus

World Health Organisation (WHO) reported that 37.7 million people had human immunodeficiency virus (HIV) infection in 2020 [61]. When protective measures are not applied to HIV-infected pregnant women at birth, HIV transmission to babies is observed at a rate of 14–45%. Human immunodeficiency virus can be transmitted through breast milk. However, taking antiretroviral treatment during pregnancy and being under the control of a physician, delivery by cesarean section at 38 weeks, postpartum antiretroviral prophylaxis to the baby, and not giving the mother's milk can prevent the transmission of infection to a large extent [62, 63]. However, although maternal antiretroviral therapy significantly reduces the risk of transmission through breast milk, it does not eliminate the risk [64]. World Health Organisation does not consider maternal HIV infection as an absolute contraindication for breastfeeding [65]. World Health Organisation recommends that breastfeeding should be evaluated according to some criteria such as socio-economic and cultural values, provision of health services, local epidemiological data, and the incidence of child and maternal deaths due to malnutrition. In resource-limited settings, infants of mothers with HIV infection should be breastfed exclusively for the first 6 months of life and breastfeeding should be continued at least 12 months with the addition of complementary foods. These mothers should be closely monitored to decrease the transmission risk. Comply with antiretroviral treatment of the mother and extended infant prophylaxis is very important in this respect. In settings where the risk of infant morbidity and mortality from infectious diseases and malnutrition is not high and alternative feeding regimens are sustainable, mothers with HIV infection should be recommended not to breastfeed. The decision of national health authorities should be taken into account under these circumstances [65, 66].

3.10 Human Papillomavirus

The human papillomavirus (HPV) is a DNA virus. There are many different species of HPV. which may cause cervical carcinoma, laryngeal papillomatosis, genital dysplasia and warts. It is mostly transmitted sexually. The origin of HPV-related laryngeal papilloma seen in infants is thought to originate from the birth canal. The breast of a mother is a rare site of involvement. There are studies detecting HPV DNA in breast milk [67, 68]. However, an increased association of HPV disease with breast milk has not been shown. Even in the rare occurrence of an HPV lesion on the breast, there are no data to support the suggestion of not breastfeeding or not using expressed breast milk. Mothers with HPV infection can breastfeed their infants.

3.11   Human T-Cell Leukemia Virus Type I infection

The first human retrovirus discovered is the human T-cell leukemia virus type 1 (HTLV-1), its infection is usually asymptomatic. At the onset, silent transmission happens, and the disease usually occurs later in life. The most important modes of transmission are breastfeeding, sexual relations, and blood transfusions [69, 70]. Among children, breastfed for less than 6 months, the prevalence was found to be lower than among those breastfed for 6 months or more [71]. Mother-to-infant transmission during the intrauterine or peripartum period is reported in less than 5% of cases [72]. Human T-Cell Leukemia Virus −1 infection causes serious diseases in humans, including uveitis, arthritis, infective dermatitis as well as adult myelopathy/tropical spastic paraparesis, T-cell leukemia, or lymphoma. Although HTLV-1 can be eliminated by freezing and thawing breast milk, this is not practical and there may be technological impossibilities in societies with low resources. In the light of current information, breastfeeding is contraindicated during HTLV-1 infection [73, 74].

3.12   Human T-Cell Leukemia Virus Type II infection

Human T-cell leukemia virus type II (HTLV-II) is endemic in certain geographic areas. Transmission primarily occurs via sexual intercourse, contaminated blood products, intravenous drug use, and breastfeeding. Human T-cell leukemia virus type-II has been associated with glomerulonephritis, arthritis, myelopathy, granulocytic leukemia, T-hairy cell leukemia, and some chronic neurological disorders similar to those caused by HTLV-I. Transmission of mother-to-infant has been shown in both formula-fed and breastfed infants. Based on current information, mothers who are HTLV-II seropositive should avoid breastfeeding [75, 76].

3.13   Influenza

Influenza is a contagious respiratory infection. Transmission occurs by droplet. Breastfeeding has been shown to protect infants against influenza viruses by activating natural antiviral mechanisms, particularly type 1 interferon. In addition, very high influenza-specific IgA was detected in the milk of mothers who received the influenza vaccine in the third trimester of pregnancy [6, 77]. A similar situation may occur during the influenza infection of the mother. Influenza infection of the mother is not an obstacle to breastfeeding and breastfeeding should be strongly recommended [12, 78].

3.14 Monkeypox

Monkeypox is a viral zoonotic disease belonging to the genus Orthopoxvirus of the family Poxviridae. Monkeypox spreads from person to person through close contact with someone who has a monkeypox rash, including face-to-face, skin-to-skin, mouth-to-mouth, or sexual contact. Environments can be contaminated with the monkeypox virus, for example, when an infectious person touches clothing, bedding, towels, objects, electronic devices, and surfaces. Anyone else touching these items could then become infected. It is also possible to breathe in spilled skin or become infected with the virus from clothing, bedding, or towels. The transmission can occur from a pregnant person to a fetus, through skin-to-skin contact after birth, or to an infant or child during close contact with a parent who has monkeypox. Although the asymptomatic infection has been reported, it is not clear whether people without any symptoms can transmit the disease. The incubation period is usually 6 to 13 days after exposure. Although most people recover within weeks, severe complications may occur especially in unvaccinated people. Most reported deaths are in young children and immunocompromised persons, such as people with poorly controlled HIV. The risk of infection will need to be carefully balanced with the potential harm and distress caused by interruption of breastfeeding and close parent-child contact. It is not yet known whether the monkeypox virus can be transmitted from parent to child through breast milk; this is an area that needs further study [79, 80]. World Health Organisation suggests that breastfeeding during monkeypox infection should be individually evaluated. Breastfeeding can be sustained with some precautions in some cases. Information for clean water and the preparation of breast milk substitutes must be given for cases if breastfeeding is not possible. Growth and developmental monitoring should be carried out for children. Breastfeeding counseling can be given for re-lactation [79].

3.15 Severe Acute Respiratory Syndrome-Associated Coronavirus Type 2 Infection: Coronavirus Disease 2019 (COVID-19)

Severe acute respiratory syndrome-associated coronavirus type 2 (SARS-CoV-2) is a virus from the coroviridae family that causes the coronavirus disease 2019 pandemic. Transmission from person to person is via droplets. Severe acute respiratory syndrome-associated coronavirus type 2 infections in infants and young children are usually mild but, although rare, can be a life-threatening illness. Although there are studies detecting SARS-CoV2 RNA or antigen in breast milk, there are no data on transmission to infants [81, 82]. In addition, it has been reported that SIgA, immunoglobulin G (IgG), and IgM against SARS-CoV2 are detected in breast milk [82, 83]. World Health Organisation reports that there is no harm in breastfeeding children during maternal infection with COVID-19. Considering that transmission is via droplets, it is necessary to apply necessary preventive measures such as hand washing especially before breastfeeding, and wearing a medical mask during breast-feeding should be applied. If a mother with proven or suspected COVID-19 coughs towards her breast, she should gently wash the breast with soap and warm water for at least 20 s before breastfeeding. However, routine washing the breast before each breastfeeding is not required [84].

4 Maternal Fungal Infections and Breastfeeding

4.1 Candidiasis

Candida albicans is the most common *Candida* species that is found commensally in the mucosal tissue of the mother and child. It can cause an irritating fungal infection in the baby-mother dyad, as breast and nipple pain in mothers and feeding difficulties in babies. Breastfeeding is not a contraindication during the infection. The treatment should begin with a topical agent for mild-to-moderate breast candidiasis and should continue for at least 2 weeks, even if there is significant improvement within 1 or 2 days [12, 85]. While the mother and baby are being treated for thrush, they can continue to breastfeed.

5 Parasitic Infections in the Mother and Breastfeeding

5.1 Malaria

Malaria is a mosquito-borne parasitic disease. There is no evidence of malaria transmission through breast milk. However, a nursing mother planning to travel to a malaria-prone geographic area should take every precaution to reduce the risk of infection. Standard preventive approaches include mosquito avoidance measures such as insect repellent, mosquito nets, and prophylactic antimalarial drugs. Nursing mothers should avoid applying insect repellent under their clothes or on the nipple and should carefully wash their hands before breastfeeding their babies [12].

5.2 Toxoplasmosis

Toxoplasmosis is one of the commonest infections in humans. The disease agent, *Toxoplasma gondii*, is widespread in nature. The cat is the host, but infection can occur in warm-blooded animals. There is no data on transmission through breast milk. Considering the protective properties of breast milk, there is no obstacle to breastfeeding during maternal toxoplasmosis [12].

6 Conclusion

The anti-infective properties of breast milk are well known. Breast milk or breast-feeding is contraindicated during few maternal infections. These are Ebola virus disease, HIV infection (changing according to the cases and countries), and HTLV type I and II infections. Cases in which breastfeeding and/or giving expressed human milk should be temporarily stopped are tuberculosis, brucellosis, and the presence of herpes simplex in the breast. In the case of maternal infections, the continuity of breastfeeding should be prioritized in terms of infant and maternal health. Under the circumstances of insufficient evidence polarity map management [86] should be used for decision making on the safety of breastfeeding during some maternal infections, and drug selection for treatment. Polarity map management can be applied by reviewing current epidemiological data and case reports; evaluating the risks and benefits of breastfeeding, and of stopping breastfeeding together with the mother and the family.

References

1. Palmeira P, Carneiro-Sampaio M. Immunology of breast milk. Rev Assoc Med Bras (1992). 2016;62:584–93.
2. Demers-Mathieu V, Mathijssen G, Dapra C, Do DM, Medo E. Active free secretory component and secretory IgA in human milk: do maternal vaccination, allergy, infection, mode of delivery, nutrition and active lifestyle change their concentrations? Pediatr Res. 2021;89:795–802.
3. Lawrence RA, Lawrence RM. Breastfeeding: a guide for the medical profession. 8th ed. Philadelphia, PA: Elsevier; 2015. p. 146–93.
4. Ollès P, Jollès J. Lysozyme from human milk. Nature. 1961;192:1187–8.
5. Arnold D, Di Biase AM, Marchetti M, et al. Antiadenovirus activity of milk proteins: lactoferrin prevents viral infection. Antivir Res. 2002;53:153–8.
6. Campione E, Cosio T, Rosa L, et al. Lactoferrin as protective natural barrier of respiratory and intestinal mucosa against coronavirus infection and inflammation. Int J Mol Sci. 2020;21:4903.
7. Özer B, Yaman H. Milk and milk products: microbiology of liquid milk. In: Encyclopedia of Food Microbiology. 2nd ed. Amsterdam: Elsevier; 2014.
8. Strömqvist M, Falk P, Bergström S, et al. Human milk kappa-casein and inhibition of Helicobacter pylori adhesion to human gastric mucosa. J Pediatr Gastroenterol Nutr. 1995;21:288–96.
9. Alamiri F, Riesbeck K, Hakansson AP. HAMLET, a protein complex from human milk has bactericidal activity and enhances the activity of antibiotics against pathogenic Streptococci. Antimicrob Agents Chemother. 2019;63:e01193–19.
10. Dawod B, Marshall JS. Cytokines and soluble receptors in breast milk as enhancers of oral tolerance development. Front Immunol. 2019;22:10–6.
11. Ogawa J, Sasahara A, Yoshida T, et al. Role of transforming growth factor-beta in breast milk for initiation of IgA production in newborn infants. Early Hum Dev. 2004;77:67–75.
12. Lawrence RM. Transmission of infectious diseases through breast milk and breastfeeding. In: Lawrence RA, Lawrence RM, editors. Breastfeeding: a guide for the medical profession. 9th ed. Philadelphia, PA: Elsevier; 2022. p. 393–456.
13. Centers for Disease Control and Prevention. Botulism. https://www.cdc.gov/botulism/general.html. Accessed 1 July 2022.

14. American Academy of Pediatrics. Clostridial infections. In: Kimberlin DW, Brady MT, Jackson MA, Long SS, editors. Red Book: 2018 Report of the Committee on Infectious Diseases. 31st ed. Itasca, IL: American Academy of Pediatrics; 2018. p. 266–9.

15. Matsumura T, Fujinaga Y, Jin Y, Kabumoto Y, Oguma K. Human milk SIgA binds to botulinum type B 16S toxin and limits toxin adherence on T84 cells. Biochem Biophys Res Commun. 2007;352:867–72.

16. Rosow LK, Strober JB. Infant botulism: review and clinical update. Pediatr Neurol. 2015;52:487–92.

17. California Department of Public Health. Infant Botulism Treatment and Prevention Program. Frequently Asked Questions (FAQs) About Infant Botulism, https://www.cdph.ca.gov › Programs › CID › DCDC. Accessed 2 July 2022.

18. American Academy of Pediatrics. Brucellosis. In: Kimberlin DW, Brady MT, Jackson MA, Long SS, editors. Red Book: 2018 Report of the Committee on Infectious Diseases. 31st ed. Itasca, IL: American Academy of Pediatrics; 2018. p. 238–40.

19. Centers for Disease Control and Prevention. Brucellosis, https://www.cdc.gov/brucellosis/transmission/index.html. Accessed 2 July 2022.

20. Palanduz A, Palanduz S, Güler K, Güler N. Brucellosis in a mother and her young infant: probable transmission by breast milk. Int J Infect Dis. 2000;4:55–6.

21. Arroyo Carrera I, López Rodríguez MJ, Sapiña AM, López Lafuente A, Sacristán AR. Probable transmission of brucellosis by breast milk. J Trop Pediatr. 2006;52:380–1.

22. Apa H, Keskin S, Gülfidan G, Yaman Y, Devrim I. An infant with acute brucellosis presenting with Coombs-positive autoimmune hemolytic anemia: is breastfeeding guilty for transmission? Vector Borne Zoonotic Dis. 2013;13:509–12.

23. Loveday M, Hlangu S, Furin J. Breastfeeding in women living with tuberculosis. Int J Tuberc Lung Dis. 2020;24(9):880–91.

24. World Health Organization. WHO operational handbook on tuberculosis: Module 1: Prevention: tuberculosis preventive treatment 22 March 2020 Guideline, https://www.who.int/health-topics/tuberculosis#tab=tab_1. Accessed 2 Aug 2022.

25. American Academy of Pediatrics. Tuberculosis. In: Kimberlin DW, Brady MT, Jackson MA, Long SS, editors. Red Book: 2018 Report of the Committee on Infectious Diseases. 31st ed. Itasca, IL: American Academy of Pediatrics; 2018. p. 786–815.

26. Queensland Government. Management of tuberculosis in pregnant women and newborn infants. The guideline, Version 3.2 November 2021, https://www.health.qld.gov.au/__data/assets/pdf_file/0030/444558/tb-guideline-pregnancy.pdf. Accessed 2 July 2022.

27. Centers for Disease Control and Prevention. Tuberculosis https://www.cdc.gov/tb/topic/treatment/pregnancy.htm. Accessed 2 July 2022.

28. Yoshida M, Tezuka T, Hiruma M. Detection of varicella-zoster virus DNA in maternal breast milk from a mother with herpes zoster. Clin Diagn Virol. 1995;4:61–5.

29. Karabayir N, Yaşa B, Gökçay G. Chickenpox infection during lactation. Breastfeed Med. 2015;10:71–2.

30. May JT. Antimicrobial factors and microbial contaminants in human milk: recent studies. J Paediatr Child Health. 1994;30:470.

31. American Academy of Pediatrics. Breastfeeding and the use of human milk. Pediatrics. 2012;129:827–41.

32. American Academy of Pediatrics. Cytomegalovirus Infection. In: Kimberlin DW, Brady MT, Jackson MA, Long SS, editors. Red Book: 2018 Report of the Committee on Infectious Diseases. 31st ed. Itasca, IL: American Academy of Pediatrics; 2018. p. 107–15.

33. Bardanzellu F, Fanos V, Reali A. Human breast milk-acquired cytomegalovirus infection: certainties, doubts and perspectives. Curr Pediatr Rev. 2019;15(1):30–41.

34. American Academy of Pediatrics. Cytomegalovirus infection. In: Kimberlin DW, Brady MT, Jackson MA, Long SS, editors. Red Book: 2018 Report of the Committee on Infectious Diseases. 31st ed. Itasca, IL: American Academy of Pediatrics; 2018. p. 310–7.

35. Bryant P, Morley C, Garland S, Curtis N. Cytomegalovirus transmission from breast milk in premature babies: Does it matter? Arch Dis Child Fetal Neonatal Ed. 2002;87:F75–7.
36. Hayes K, Danks DM, Gibas H, Jack I. Cytomegalovirus in human milk. N Engl J Med. 1972;287:177–8.
37. Reynolds DW, Stagno S, Hosty TS, Tiller M, Alford CA. Maternal cytomegalovirus excretion and perinatal infection. N Engl J Med. 1973;289:1–5.
38. Volder C, Work BJ, Hoegh SV, et al. Transmission of cytomegalovirus in fresh and freeze–thawed mother's own milk to very preterm infants: a cohort study. J Perinatol. 2021;41:1873–8.
39. Klotz D, Jansen S, Gebauer C, Fuchs H. Handling of breast milk by neonatal units: large differences in current practices and beliefs. Front Pediatr. 2018;6:235.
40. Hamprecht K, Goelz R. Postnatal cytomegalovirus infection through human milk in preterm infants transmission, clinical presentation, and prevention. Clin Perinatol. 2017;44:121–30.
41. World Health Organisation. Guidelines for the management of pregnant and breastfeeding women in the context of Ebola virus disease. 16 February 2020, https://www.who.int/publications/i/item/9789240001381. Accessed 8 July 2022.
42. American Academy of Pediatrics. Transmission of infectious agents via human milk. In: Kimberlin DW, Brady MT, Jackson MA, Long SS, editors. Red Book: 2018 Report of the Committee on Infectious Diseases. 31st ed. Itasca, IL: American Academy of Pediatrics; 2018. p. 109–15.
43. Junker AK, Thomas EE, Radcliffe A, Forsyth RB, Davidson AG, Rymo L. Epstein-Barr virus shedding in breast milk. Am J Med Sci. 1991;302(4):220–3.
44. Daud II, Coleman CB, Smith NA, et al. breast milk as a potential source of Epstein Barr virus transmission among infants living in a malaria-endemic region of Kenya. J Infect Dis. 2015;212:1735–42.
45. Sinha A, Dutta S. Waterborne & foodborne viral hepatitis: a public health perspective. Indian J Med Res. 2019;150:432–5.
46. Daudi N, Shouval D, Stein-Zamir C, Ackerman Z. Breast-milk hepatitis A virus RNA in nursing mothers with acute hepatitis A virus infection. Breastfeed Med. 2012;7:313–5.
47. World Health Organisation. Hepatitis B, https://www.who.int/news-room/fact-sheets/detail/hepatitis-b. Accessed 3 July 2022.
48. Zheng Y, Lu Y, Ye Q, Xia Y, Zhou Y, Yao Q, Wei S. Should chronic hepatitis B mothers breastfeed? a meta-analysis. BMC Public Health. 2011;11:502.
49. Chen X, Chen J, Wen J, et al. Breastfeeding is not a risk factor for mother-to-child transmission of hepatitis B virus. PLoS One. 2013;8(1):e55303.
50. Shi Z, Yang Y, Wang H, et al. Breastfeeding of newborns by mothers carrying hepatitis B virus: a meta-analysis and systematic review. Arch Pediatr Adolesc Med. 2011;16:837–46.
51. American Academy of Pediatrics. Immunization in preterm and low birth weight infant. In: Kimberlin DW, Brady MT, Jackson MA, Long SS, editors. Red Book: 2018 Report of the Committee on Infectious Diseases. 31st ed. Itasca, IL: American Academy of Pediatrics; 2018. p. 67–9.
52. Centers for Disease Control and Prevention. Hepatitis B or C infections. https://www.cdc.gov/breastfeeding/breastfeeding-special-circumstances/maternal-or-infant-illnesses/hepatitis.html. Accessed 3 July 2022.
53. Luo Y, Xiang K, Liu J, et al. Inhibition of in vitro infection of hepatitis B virus by human breastmilk. Nutrients. 2022;14:1561.
54. Dalmastri C, Valenti P, Visca P, Vittorioso P, Orsi N. Enhanced antimicrobial activity of lactoferrin by binding to the bacterial surface. Microbiologica. 1988;11:225–30.
55. He J, Furmanski P. Sequence specificity and transcriptional activation in the binding of lactoferrin to DNA. Nature. 1995;373:721–4.
56. Beasley R, Stevens CE, Shiao IS, Meng HC. Evidence against breastfeeding as a mechanism for vertical transmission of hepatitis B. Lancet. 1975;2:740–1.

57. American Academy of Pediatrics. Hepatitis C. In: Kimberlin DW, Brady MT, Jackson MA, Long SS, editors. Red Book: 2018 Report of the Committee on Infectious Diseases. 31st ed. Itasca, IL: American Academy of Pediatrics; 2018. p. 399–404.
58. World Health Organisation. Herpes simplex virus. https://www.who.int/news-room/fact-sheets/detail/herpes-simplex-virus#:~:text=Overview,transmitted%20and%20causes%20genital%20herpes. Accessed 4 July 2022.
59. Centers for Disease Control and Prevention. Herpes Simplex Virus (HSV). https://www.cdc.gov/breastfeeding/breastfeeding-special-circumstances/maternal-or-infant-illnesses/herpes.html. Accessed 3 July 2022.
60. D'Andrea MA, Spatz DL. Maintaining breastfeeding during severe infant and maternal HSV-1 infection: a case report. J Hum Lact. 2019 Nov;35(4):737–41.
61. World Health Organization. HIV/AIDS, https://www.who.int/data/gho/data/themes/hiv-aids. Accessed July10, 2022.
62. World Health Organization, Unicef. Guidance on global scale-up of the prevention of mother to child transmission of HIV: towards universal access for women, infants and young children and eliminating HIV and AIDS among children / Inter-Agency Task Team on Prevention of HIV Infection in Pregnant Women, Mothers and their Children. WHO, 2007, Switzerland, http://www.unicef.org/aids/files/PMTCT_enWEBNov26.pdf. Accessed 10 July 2022.
63. Mofenson L, Taylor AW, Rogers M, et al. Achievements in public health. Reduction in perinatal transmission of HIV infection- United States, 1985- 2005. MMWR Morb Mortal Wkly Rep. 2006;55:592–7.
64. Centers for Disease Control and Prevention. Human Immunodeficiency Virus (HIV). https://www.cdc.gov/breastfeeding/breastfeeding-special-circumstances/maternal-or-infant-illnesses/hiv.html#:~:text=In%20the%20United%20States%2C%20to,body%20fluids%2C%20including%20breast%20milk. Accessed 12 July 2022.
65. World Health Organization. Guideline: updates on HIV and infant feeding: the duration of breastfeeding, and support from health services to improve feeding practices among mothers living with HIV; 2016. https://apps.who.int/iris/bitstream/handle/10665/246260/9789241549707-eng.pdf. Accessed 12 July 2022.
66. World Health Organization. Advocacy brief: breastfeeding and HIV: global breastfeeding collective; 2019. https://apps.who.int/iris/handle/10665/279781. Accessed 12 July 2022.
67. Sarkola M, Rintala M, Grenman S. Human papillomavirus DNA detected in breast milk. Pediatr Infect Dis J. 2008;27:557–8.
68. Cazzaniga M, Gheit T, Casadio C. Analysis of the presence of cutaneous and mucosal papillomavirus types in ductal lavage fluid, milk and colostrum to evaluate its role in breast carcinogenesis. Breast Cancer Res Treat. 2009;114:599–605.
69. Gonçalves DU, Proietti FA, Ribas JG, et al. Epidemiology, treatment, and prevention of human T-cell leukemia virus type 1-associated diseases. Clin Microbiol Rev. 2010;23:577–89.
70. Proietti FA, Carneiro-Proietti BC. Catalan-Soares, and E. L. Murphy. Global epidemiology of HTLV-1 infection and associated diseases. Oncogene. 2005;24:6058–68.
71. Biggar RJ, Kim M, Hisada HC, et al. Human leukocyte antigen concordance and the transmission risk via breastfeeding of human T cell lymphotropic virus type I. J Infect Dis. 2006;93:277–82.
72. Kusuhara K, Sonoda S, Takahashi K, Tokugawa K, Fukushige J, Ueda K. Mother-to-child transmission of human T-cell leukemia virus type I (HTLV-1): a fifteen year follow-up study in Okinawa, Japan. Int J Cancer. 1987;40:755–7.
73. Fujito T, Nagata Y. HTLV-I transmission from mother to child. J Reprod Immunol. 2000;47:197–206.
74. Ando Y, Kakimoto K, Tanigawa T, et al. Effect of freeze-thawing breast milk on vertical HTLV-I transmission from seropositive mothers to children. Jpn J Cancer Res. 1989;80:405–7.
75. World Health Organization. Human T-lymphotropic virus type 1: technical report; 2021. https://www.who.int/publications/i/item/9789240020221. Accessed 4 July 2022.

76. Bittencourt AL. Vertical transmission of HTLV-I/II: a review. Rev Inst Med Trop Sao Paulo. 1998;40:245–51.
77. Melendi GA, Coviello S, Bhat N, Zea-Hernandez J, Ferolla FM, Polack FP. Breastfeeding is associated with the production of type I interferon in infants infected with influenza virus. Acta Paediatr. 2010;99:1517–21.
78. Schlaudecker EP, Steinhoff MC, Omer SB, et al. IgA and neutralizing antibodies to influenza a virus in human milk: a randomized trial of antenatal influenza immunization. PLoS One. 2013;8:e70867.
79. World Health Organization. (2022). Clinical management and infection prevention and control for monkeypox: interim rapid response guidance, 10 June 2022. https://www.who.int/publications/i/item/WHO-MPX-Clinical-and-IPC-2022.1. Accessed 12 July 2022.
80. UK Security Agency. Monkeypox outbreak: epidemiological overview, https://www.gov.uk/government/publications/monkeypox-outbreak-epidemiological-overview. Accessed 14 July 2022.
81. Krogstad P, Contreras D, Ng H, et al. No evidence of infectious Sars-Cov-2 in human milk: analysis of a cohort of 110 lactating women. medrxiv [Preprint]. 20217:2021.04.05.21254897.
82. Keskindemirci G, Karabayır N, İstanbullu Tosun A, et al. Severe acute respiratory syndrome coronavirus-2 antigens and antibodies in breast milk. J Ist Faculty Med. 2021;84(3):287–92.
83. Juncker HG, Romijn M, Loth VN, et al. Antibodies against sars-cov-2 in human milk: milk conversion rates in the Netherlands. J Hum Lact. 2021;37:469–76.
84. World Health Organisation. Frequently Asked Questions: Breastfeeding and COVID-19 For health care workers. https://www.who.int/publications/m/item/frequently-asked-questions-breastfeeding-and-covid-19. Accessed 14 July 2022.
85. National Health Service. Breastfeeding and Trush. https://www.nhs.uk/conditions/baby/breastfeeding-and-bottle-feeding/breastfeeding-problems/thrush/#:~:text=Treating%20thrush%20when%20you're,carefully%20after%20treating%20your%20baby. Accessed 14 July 2022.
86. Jones W. Professional responsibility and counseling. In: Jones W, editor. Breastfeeding and medication. Oxon: Routledge; 2013. p. 85–102.

Part V
Breastfeeding: Special Conditions and Issues

Nuray Bayar Muluk and Cemal Cingi

Programming the Gustatory and Olfactory Systems

Fatih Yucedag, Cemal Cingi, and Sergei Karpischenko

1   Introduction

Over the course of life, people alter in the tastes and smells that they most enjoy. Preferences for specific tastes or smells appear to begin from the stage of conception and continue right up until old age. There are many interacting factors, biological, social, cultural and environmental, which affect which foods an individual chooses, enjoys or wishes to eat. There are many questions that remain to be answered regarding food preferences, such as whether the key effects are genetically determined, result from metabolic programming or are shaped by the mother during pregnancy and any period of breastfeeding which follows. Does the local cuisine play an important part in establishing an individual's gastronomic preferences? Do familiarity and nostalgia play a part? And is it possible to begin to enjoy a flavour first encountered in adulthood? Besides these questions, there are the many effects of culture to consider. Geographic availability, food culture, socioeconomic status, religious dietary rules and affordability all play a major role, it seems. However, deciding which of these many factors is central to food choices is not a simple matter. Does biology determine the situation, or is it less straightforward than we might suppose?

F. Yucedag (✉)
Faculty of Medicine, Department of Otorhinolaryngology, Karamanoglu Mehmetbey University, Karaman, Türkiye

C. Cingi
Medical Faculty, Department of Otorhinolaryngology, Eskisehir Osmangazi University, Eskisehir, Türkiye
e-mail: cemal@ogu.edu.tr

S. Karpischenko
Department of Otorhinolaryngology, The First Pavlov State Medical University of Saint Petersburg, Saint Petersburg, Russia

© The Author(s), under exclusive license to Springer Nature Switzerland AG 2023
Ö. N. Şahin et al. (eds.), *Breastfeeding and Metabolic Programming*,
https://doi.org/10.1007/978-3-031-33278-4_33

It is clear that there are key biological determinants of food-seeking behaviour, including likes and dislikes, but the individual's experience of different foods during life also modulates this behaviour. The evidence appears to support the hypothesis that in childhood the preferred food choices are those which are highly sweet-tasting, salty or savoury, in addition to foods with a high calorific value. These preferences may be directed by social and environmental factors, but the individual's favourite flavours continue to have a very major influence on which foods are consumed, both in childhood and adulthood [1–3].

How foods taste and are perceived plays a vital role in establishing an individual's food preferences. Taste and favour have been demonstrated to be the key determinants of the foods enjoyed in early childhood [4]. Furthermore, the child's preferences for specific foods are the most powerful determiners of what foods children will accept [5, 6]. Accordingly, to appreciate exactly how children come to prefer specific flavours and accept particular food items, a knowledge of the development of gustatory and olfactory perception in early life is essential.

The perception of taste occurs due to stimulation of gustatory receptors, which are usually stated to consist of only five types, namely sweet, bitter, sour, salty and umami. The results of recent studies does, however, seem to support the possibility that other gustatory receptors may exist, capable of recognising lipids and calcium [7, 8]. Whereas gustatory sensation is limited to perceiving a restricted range of basic tastes, smell is responsive to thousands of different odoriferous compounds. Perceiving the flavour of any food depends on both gustatory and olfactory signals. The gustatory receptors are within the mouth, but odoriferous compounds stimulate receptors both orthonasally and retronasally. The ability of the child to perceive differences between flavours has already begun during foetal life, with both the olfactory and gustatory system having achieved full functional maturity at the time of birth. It is believed that the fact that the olfactory and gustatory systems already operate before birth means that the foetus is primed to expect to encounter certain tastes postnatally [9, 10].

2 Morphological and Functional Development

The taste-sensitive cells have already begun to develop and become functional by the end of the initial trimester of pregnancy. At week 10, papillae of different types are already identifiable, namely fungiform, foliate and circumvallate. Between the 8th and 13th weeks of gestation, synapse formation increases. As the second trimester starts, the taste buds are already fully capable of responding to tastes. There are very few differences between the number and distribution of taste buds in children or indeed adults and those in a foetus towards the end of the pregnancy [9, 11, 12].

The initial trimester is the period when the olfactory system first starts to develop. At week 8, the olfactory bulb can be clearly seen as an outgrowth of the forebrain, and primary olfactory receptors are already present. The presence of olfactory marker proteins by weeks 28–29 shows that the olfactory receptors are functionally mature by that point. There are nasal plugs present at first within the nasal passages, but after these structures disappear, between weeks 16 and 36, amniotic fluid can already reach the olfactory epithelium of the nose [13, 14].

After birth, the gustatory and olfactory systems keep developing, but there is little evidence on exactly how this occurs in humans, since studies where the development in individuals is tracked over time have not yet been undertaken. The evidence base at present indicates that the anatomical development of the gustatory and olfactory systems is more or less finished by the time of birth [13, 14], but the central nervous system becomes progressively more responsive to stimulation of the two systems as the individual grows. This situation implies that the nervous pathways involved in processing olfactory and gustatory perception continue to develop after birth [13, 14].

3   Prenatal Factors Affecting Development

The gustatory and olfactory system in human beings develop early in pregnancy (within the initial trimester) and these systems have already reached functional maturity when the child is born [11]. This situation allows infants to learn before birth which foods are safe to eat and likely to be available. Amniotic fluid contains molecules that can stimulate both the olfactory and gustatory systems and the foetus can detect such stimuli. Being exposed to specific flavours before birth influences the child's food preferences later in life. When newborn children are presented a choice between the mother's amniotic fluid, that of another woman or distilled water, they exhibit a preference for their own mother's smell [15, 16]. It has been proven that newborns whose mothers' diets in pregnancy featured regular garlic or anise have a preference for those specific flavours, whilst neonates who encountered carrot flavour *in utero* demonstrated a preference for carrot-flavoured cereal rather than plain cereal when they began to be weaned [17–20]. Animal models permit a more systematic examination of the mother's dietary intake. These models show that exposing the foetus to some flavours which young offspring usually avoid meant the offspring more readily accepted the flavour later. Furthermore, mothers whose diet was lipid-enriched in pregnancy produced offspring with a heightened preference for highly sweet and lipid-dense food items [20, 21].

4   Influences on Dietary Preferences at the Early Stage of Lactation

The behaviour of infants towards food is also shaped by the flavours present in milk, whether in breast milk or in artificial baby milk. Infants who receive breast feeding encounter a wide range of different flavour-bearing molecules. These molecules originate in the mother's diet [22]. Infants receiving artificial baby milk are exposed to a more restricted range of flavour molecules, although there are some differences in the taste of different types of formula milk [23].

When infants are exposed at a very young age to flavours they have not previously encountered, they are briefly drawn towards those specific flavours [24]. Infants exhibit a preference for their usual type of milk (whether breast milk or artificial baby milk). If a flavour is repeatedly present in milk, the short-term increased attraction towards a particular flavour comes to an end. This probably represents satiety or the fact that the flavour no longer possesses novelty [25–27]. However, in the long term, the dietary preferences of weaned infants or young children reflect similarities with the flavours encountered during the period of breast feeding or consumption of artificial baby milk. In certain cases, it has been possible to link children's dietary preferences up to the age of at least 10 years to the flavours and tastes encountered in the period before weaning occurred [27].

5 Influences Whilst Complementary Food Items and Drinks Are Introduced into Infants' Diets

Anecdotal evidence about infants' reactions to newly introduced food items at the age of between 5 and 7 months confirms the results of studies, which noted a positive reaction (such as willingly taking a mouthful or smiling) in a large majority (between around 88% and 91%) of infants offered novel complementary food items [20]. There was some effect of taste on the infants' reactions, so, that, for example, vegetables with added salt were preferred to unsalted versions [20], or fruit or naturally sweet vegetables provoked a more positive reaction that those with a more bitter taste [21]. Despite it being commonly claimed that better infant acceptance comes from starting vegetables before fruit, since children have a natural inclination towards sweeter items, this does not seem to be shown by the few studies which have set out to examine acceptance rates according to the timing of the items offered. It has been demonstrated that repeatedly giving infants fruit does not reduce their willingness or actual consumption of new vegetables, either in the short [21] or long [22] term. Indeed, another study [23] ascertained that giving fruit every day actually resulted in infants being more willing to eat carrots [23].

The willingness to try new food items, however, does diminish as time passes, which implies that becoming familiar with different tastes in early childhood is a key step in developing wide food preferences [17]. There is growing evidence to show that several factors are involved in how infants respond to new food items, in particular their taste preferences [20], age, how much they like eating generally, the ease with which satiety occurs, and whether they exhibit fussy behaviour around eating. Temperament is also a key factor [24, 25]. The studies on best practice in promoting a willingness to eat healthily in infants have mainly concentrated on three specific techniques, namely repeatedly offering the same item, introducing variety and use of associative learning.

5.1 Repeatedly Offering the Same Item and Introducing Dietary Variety

At the stage when complementary feeding is occurring, simply offering the same item several times makes infants eat more of the item and exhibit a more positive attitude towards that items, as noted by smiling, for example, at least in the short term [26–28]. It also appears that repetition of the same offering also increases acceptance of similar dietary items [21]. An infant who has got used to green beans, for instance, is more likely to accept the similar artichoke, but this effect does not extend to markedly different items, such as plums or apples [21]. It has also been shown that combining repetition with a range of different food items may lead to even higher levels of infant acceptance for new items. This effect may be linked to the manner in which the earlier exposure to tastes occurs, i.e. the variety of tastes in breast milk originating in the mother's dietary consumption. It is an adaptive way for the infant to decide what is safe to eat. A study which examined infants receiving artificial baby milk and complementary feeding found that altering the type of starchy vegetable from day to day over 9 days (peas, potato and squash) led to greater consumption of carrots later than when potato only was offered [23]. This type of exposure to a variety of food items also increased the infants' acceptance of a completely unrelated item, namely puréed chicken [23], compared to exposure of a single item, i.e. carrot. If this variety exposure method is employed using different types of fruit [27] or vegetable [29], a similar benefit is seen. Varying the items offered each day is more effective at encouraging acceptance than doing so at longer intervals (such as every 3 days) [29]. The technique of varying the items offered seems to have a long-lasting effect [29], but this effect is hard to separate from the effects of the mother having a varied diet, with resulting infant exposure to tastes occurring through breastfeeding, and more results are needed, given the inconsistent results of the published evidence to date [20, 21, 26, 30–32].

6 Conditioning Behaviour Through Association

Another way to teach infants to accept specific food items is by constantly presenting the item to be learnt together with a taste they have already acquired, i.e. by classical conditioning. There are two ways in which this can be accomplished. In flavour-flavour type conditioning, a new taste is paired with a taste that is already enjoyable for the infant. The new taste then becomes perceived in the same positive way as the familiar taste. In flavour-nutrient conditioning, the new taste is paired with an item that produces a pleasant feeling of satiation in the infant. Such items are generally rich in nutrients. The new item is then perceived as nutritious. The power of associative conditioning techniques to shape feeding behaviour has been demonstrated using animal models. For example, animals can be trained in this way to eat an item they normally reject. In one study rats were offered an excessively bitter or sour solution at the same time as glucose was directly infused into the stomach. The rats subsequently behaved in the same way towards an intrinsically pleasant solution of glucose and the bitter/sour solution [33]. This study illustrates nutrient-flavour conditioning in action, but rats have also been trained by flavour-flavour stimulus pairing [34]. It is probable that a similar associative conditioning process is the mechanism by which human infants learn to appreciate certain flavours whilst still breastfeeding, as the milk is presented alongside flavour molecules originating from the mother's diet. There are data which also seem to show that the time when rats are most sensitive to associative conditioning is just after weaning. As the animals approach puberty, they become less sensitive [35]. It appears likely therefore that human infants also have a greater sensitivity to associative conditioning at precisely the point where they need to move from gaining all their nutrition from breast milk to where the diet is at least partly composed of complementary food and drink items.

References

1. Ventura AK, Worobey J. Early influences on the development of food preferences. Curr Biol. 2013;23(9):R401–8. https://doi.org/10.1016/j.cub.2013.02.037.
2. Drewnowski A, Henderson SA, Hann CS, Barratt-Fornell A, Ruf- fin, M. Age and food preferences influence dietary intakes of breast care patients. Health Psychol. 1999;18:570–8.
3. Birch LL. Dimensions of preschool children's food preferences. J Nutr Educ. 1979;11:77–80.
4. Ganchrow JR, Mennella JA. The ontogeny of human flavor perception. In: Doty RL, editor. Handbook of Olfaction and Gustation. Marcel Dekker, Inc.: New York; 2003. p. 823–46.
5. Domel SB, Thompson WO, Davis HC, Baranowski T, Leonard SB, Baranowski J. Psychosocial predictors of fruit and vegetable consumption among elementary school children. Health Educ Res. 1996;11:299–308.
6. Resnicow K, Davis-Hearn M, Smith M, Baranowski T, Lin LS, Bara- nowski, J., Doyle, C., and Wang, D.T. Social-cognitive predictors of fruit and vegetable intake in children. Health Psychol. 1997;16:272–6.
7. Tordoff MG, Alarcón LK, Valmeki S, Jiang P. T1R3: a human calcium taste receptor. Sci Rep. 2012;2:496.
8. Mattes RD. Is there a fatty acid taste? Annu Rev Nutr. 2009;29:305–27.
9. Witt M. Anatomy and development of the human taste system. Handb Clin Neurol. 2019;164:147–71. https://doi.org/10.1016/B978-0-444-63855-7.00010-1.
10. Barlow LA. The sense of taste: development, regeneration, and dysfunction. WIREs Mech Dis. 2022;14(3):e1547. https://doi.org/10.1002/wsbm.1547. Epub 2021 Nov 30
11. Witt M, Reutter K. Embryonic and early fetal development of human taste buds: a transmission electron microscopical study. Anat Rec. 1996;246(4):507–23. https://doi.org/10.1002/(SICI)1097-0185(199612)246:4<507::AID-AR10>3.0.CO;2-S.
12. Hersch M, Ganchrow D. Scanning electron microscopy of developing papillae on the tongue of human embryos and fetuses. Chem Senses. 1980;5:331–41.
13. Roper SD, Chaudhari N. Taste buds: cells, signals and synapses. Nat Rev Neurosci. 2017;18(8):485–97. https://doi.org/10.1038/nrn.2017.68. Epub 2017 Jun 29. PMID: 28655883; PMCID: PMC5958546
14. Anzman-Frasca S, Ventura AK, Ehrenberg S, Myers KP. Promoting healthy food preferences from the start: a narrative review of food preference learning from the prenatal period through

early childhood. Obes Rev. 2018;19(4):576–604. https://doi.org/10.1111/obr.12658. Epub 2017 Dec 20

15. Schaal B, Marlier L, Soussignan R. Responsiveness to the odour of amniotic fluid in the human neonate. Biol Neonate. 1995;67:397–406.

16. Schaal B, Marlier L, Soussignan R. Olfactory function in the human fetus: evidence from selective neonatal responsiveness to the odor of amniotic fluid. Behav Neurosci. 1998;112:1438–49.

17. Hepper PG. Human fetal "olfactory" learning. Int J Prenatal Perinatal Psychol Med. 1995;7:147–51.

18. Schaal B, Marlier L, Soussignan R. Human foetuses learn odours from their pregnant mother's diet. Chem Senses. 2000;25:729–37.

19. Mennella JA, Jagnow CP, Beauchamp GK. Prenatal and post- natal flavor learning by human infants. Pediatrics. 2001;107:E88.

20. Schaal B, Orgeur P. Olfaction in utero: can the rodent model be generalized? Q J Exp Psychol. 1992;44:245–78.

21. Vucetic Z, Kimmel J, Totoki K, Hollenbeck E, Reyes TM. Maternal high-fat diet alters methylation and gene expression of dopamine and opioid-related genes. Endocrinology. 2010;151:4756–64.

22. Hausner H, Bredie WL, Molgaard C, Petersen MA, Moller P. Differential transfer of dietary flavour compounds into human breast milk. Physiol Behav. 2008;95:118–24.

23. Cook DA, Sarett HP. Design of infant formulas for meeting normal and special need. Pediatric nutrition: Infant feeding, deficiencies, disease. New York: Marcel Dekker, Inc; 1982.

24. Mennella JA, Beauchamp GK. The effects of repeated exposure to garlic-flavored milk on the nursling's behavior. Pediatr Res. 1993;34:805–8.

25. Mennella JA, Beauchamp GK. Mothers' milk enhances the acceptance of cereal during weaning. Pediatr Res. 1997;41:188–92.

26. Mennella JA, Beauchamp GK. Understanding the origin of flavor preferences. Chem Senses. 2005;30(Suppl 1):i242–i3.

27. Mennella JA, Kennedy JM, Beauchamp GK. Vegetable acceptance by infants: effects of formula flavors. Early Hum Dev. 2006;82:463–8.

28. Mennella JA, Castor SM. Sensitive period in flavor learning: effects of duration of exposure to formula flavors on food likes during infancy. Clin Nutr. 2012;31:1022–5.

29. Sausenthaler S, Koletzko S, Koletzko B, et al. Effect of hydro- lysed formula feeding on taste preferences at 10 years. Data from the German Infant Nutritional Intervention Program Plus Study. Clin Nutr. 2010;29:304–6.

30. Mennella JA, Beauchamp GK. Experience with a flavor in mother's milk modifies the infant's acceptance of flavored cereal. Dev Psychobiol. 1999;35:197–203.

31. Schwartz C, Chabanet C, Lange C, Issanchou S, Nicklaus S. The role of taste in food acceptance at the beginning of complementary feeding. Physiol Behav. 2011;104:646–52.

32. Barends C, de Vries JH, Mojet J, De Graaf C. Effects of repeated exposure to either vegetables or fruits on infant's vegetable and fruit acceptance at the beginning of weaning. Food Qual Prefer. 2013;29:157–65.

33. Barends C, de Vries JH, Mojet J, de Graaf C. Effects of starting weaning exclusively with vegetables on vegetable intake at the age of 12 and 23 months. Appetite. 2014;81:193–9.

34. Gerrish CJ, Mennella JA. Flavor variety enhances food acceptance in formula-fed infants. Am J Clin Nutr. 2001;73:1080–5.

35. Caton SJ, Blundell P, Ahern SM, et al. Learning to eat vegetables in early life: the role of timing, age and individual eating traits. PLoS One. 2014;9:e97609.

Abnormalities of Smell and Taste in Eating Behaviour Through Life

Muhammet Pamukcu, Cemal Cingi, and Glenis Scadding

1 Introduction

In the past, diagnosing and treating abnormalities of gustatory and olfactory perception presented several challenges, mainly because both normal and abnormal olfaction and gustation were little understood. Abnormalities can occur in primary disorders of smell or taste, or arise as a secondary effect of some other disease process. [1]

There are several adverse consequences that may occur secondary to olfactory or gustatory disorders, namely insufficient consumption of nutrients, less enjoyment of social eating and lower psychological welfare. Furthermore, there is an increased risk of accidental death from failure to smell smoke from a fire or ingesting food that is not fit to eat. Since around 80% of gustatory dysfunction is a manifestation of an underlying olfactory disorder, this chapter mainly addresses loss of smell, but adds extra information specific to loss of taste [1].Chemosensory perception begins to decline in humans when they reach their 40s [2]. Since the mean age in Western societies, such as the United States, is rising, it is inevitable that large and growing numbers of people will undergo olfactory and gustatory perceptual impairment linked to age [3]. Research from 2002 indicates a frequency of objectively verifiable

M. Pamukcu (✉)
Medical Faculty, Department of Otorhinolaryngology, Istanbul Altinbas University, İstanbul, Türkiye

C. Cingi
Medical Faculty, Department of Otorhinolaryngology, Eskisehir Osmangazi University, Eskisehir, Türkiye
e-mail: cemal@ogu.edu.tr

G. Scadding
Consultant Allergist & Rhinologist, RNENT Hospital, University College Hospital, London, UK

Ö. N. Şahin et al. (eds.), *Breastfeeding and Metabolic Programming*,
https://doi.org/10.1007/978-3-031-33278-4_34

441

loss of smell of 24.5% in those above the age of 53 years, and this frequency rises with increasing age, such that 62.5% of adults between the ages of 80 and 97 years have a degree of olfactory impairment. If these figures are reliable, there must be around 14 million US adults who have experienced loss of smell. Studies which asked adults to report spontaneously any loss of smell found no more than 9.5% of respondents actually did so. This discrepancy underlines the necessity for objective testing to be used to identify where loss of smell occurs [4].

2 Aetiology of Olfactory and Gustatory Dysfunction

2.1 Impairment of Sense of Smell

The sense of smell may be impaired at any point within the olfactory circuitry. Just as deafness may be classified into two principal types, i.e. conductive or sensorineural, so loss of smell falls into two main categories, namely conductive (transportive) and sensorineural. In transport-related (conductive) dysfunction, there is some impairment of contact between odoriferous molecules and receptors on the neuro-epithelial mucosa. Sensorineural-type olfactory impairment occurs due to dysfunction of the associated neural circuitry. The most frequently occurring reasons for a primary loss of smell are increasing age, sinonasal disorders, previous upper respiratory tract infections (URTI) and traumatic injury to the head [5].

2.1.1 Conductive Olfactory Impairment

Inflammation is the common factor in many cases of loss of smell of this type. Inflammation may be in the form of rhinitis, which may be allergic, acute or toxic in nature. Snorting cocaine may cause toxic rhinitis. Chronic rhinosinusitis leads to increasingly extensive involvement of the mucosae and this may render patients less able to smell, even when the disorder is actively treated by pharmacotherapeutic, surgical or allergological interventions [1].

A nasal mass may also obstruct the transport of odoriferous molecules to the olfactory epithelium. This is a situation observed in some cases of nasal polyposis, inverting papilloma or neoplasia of the nasal cavity. The most likely mass to act in this way is a polyp [1].

Obstruction of odour-bearing compounds from the olfactory epithelium may also be due to a developmental anomaly, such as an encephalocoele or dermoid cyst.

Individuals who have undergone larynx removal or tracheotomy also have an impaired sense of smell due to the associated reduction in air passing through the nasal cavity. Some paediatric patients who undergo tracheotomy and long-term cannulation may remain hyposmic despite the removal of the cannula. This appears to be due to under-stimulation of the sense of smell at a key developmental stage [1].

2.1.2 Central/sensorineural Loss of Smell

Both infection and inflammation can produce sensorineural olfactory impairments. Following an URTI due to a virus, olfactory neuroepithelial cells may be lost and their place taken by non-specialised respiratory epithelial cells. However, provided that stem cells remain intact, the olfactory neuroepithelial cells may eventually regrow, albeit this process has a variable timescale, from months to years. In some cases, regrowth does not occur even with intact stem cells. Sarcoidosis of the nervous system, granulomatosis with polyangiitis and multiple sclerosis are disorders capable of causing olfactory loss. Olfactory impairment seen in cases of chronic rhinosinusitis was originally categorised as conductive in nature, since it causes swelling of the mucosae and polyposis. The olfactory loss is now known to be of mixed type, however, since it promotes apoptosis by neuroepithelial cells, and these are not subsequently replaced [1].

The very fine olfactory filaments or the parenchymal tissues of the brain may be damaged by traumatic head injury, neurosurgery or subarachnoid haemorrhage, causing loss of smell [6]. Research undertaken by Bratt et al. on cases of cerebral trauma of at least moderate severity noted that, in a sample of 182 patients, 13.7% suffered some degree of loss of smell, whilst 8.2% lost the ability to smell altogether. The researchers established that loss of smell was associated with traumatic injury to the head resulting from falling, fracturing the basal skull or contusion formation within the cortex [7].

Park et al. carried out research using resting-state functional magnetic resonance imaging (rs-fMRI) to compare the brains of patients who sustained anosmia secondary to head trauma with normal healthy volunteers. In the cases group, the connectivity within the olfactory pathways was reduced. There was, however, greater connectivity between the olfactory regions and the brain as a whole. The cases exhibited a lesser degree of modularity and the entire brain functioned to a more efficient degree, the extent of this compensatory mechanism corresponding to how severe the traumatic injury was [8].

Olfactory abilities exhibit an age-related decline, which has been correlated with progressive loss of fibres within the olfactory bulb. According to one study, the mean number of mitral cells lost on an annual basis was 520, corresponding to a volume decrease of 0.19 mm^3 [9]. The reduction in olfactory bulb volume may be secondary to loss of neuroepithelial cells from the olfactory mucosa, or may arise from a generalised reduction in regeneration due to decreasing stem cell replication within the subventricular region.

There are several congenital syndromes which involve sensorineural olfactory loss, e.g. Kallmann syndrome, in which the olfactory system fails to develop and there is hypogonadotropic hypogonadism. The vomeronasal organ is absent in cases of Kallmann syndrome, according to the results of one study [1].

Endocrinological disorders, such as hypothyroidism, hypoadrenalism and diabetes mellitus, potentially also disturb the ability to smell normally [1].

Certain medications, administered systemically or via inhalation (such as aminoglycosides), and certain chemicals (such as formaldehyde) may also impair the ability to smell. There are multiple substances that change an individual's olfactory acuity, notably alcohol, tobacco, organic solvents and zinc compounds when used topically [10].

2.2 *Gustatory Dysfunction*

A major part of apparent gustatory perception is, in fact, a change in olfactory perception. The taste of food arises from several elements, in particular its appearance, smell, gustatory qualities, texture and how hot or cold it is. These different elements each separately contribute to what food tastes like to individuals as they begin to eat [1].

The gustatory perceptions associated with food are potentially strengthened by the way the tongue moves, which causes more taste buds to be exposed to the food. The phenomenon of sensory adaptation is much more prominent in gustatory than other types of perception. This explains how we can 'acquire' a taste for a specific food or drink.

Olfactory dysfunction is the underlying reason behind most gustatory disorders. Traumatic head injury, URTI and idiopathic causes are common aetiologies, but there are numerous diagnoses associated with taste disturbance. Indeed, lesions throughout the head and neck region, beginning in the oral cavity (mucosal disorders, injury to taste buds), cranial neuropathies and brainstem lesions all have the potential to create taste disorders.

Lesions in the mouth that affect gustatory perception include infections, inflammatory processes and radiation-induced mucosal inflammation. In the latter case, the loss of taste is likely to occur due to injury to the microvilli rather than the taste bud cells themselves, which are believed to resist radiotherapy-related injury.

Unsatisfactory mouth hygiene also accounts for many cases of reduced ability to taste or an unpleasant taste in the mouth. Infections by viruses, bacteria, fungus or parasites can all cause gustatory disorders through effects on the taste buds.

The process by which progressive hypogeusia occurs with advancing age is attributable to altered function of the plasma membrane of the taste cells, not loss of the taste buds as a whole. Ion exchange and specific receptors have been implicated in the process [3, 11].

It is known that more than 200 drugs can create gustatory disorders [12]. This fact is especially crucial for physicians to bear in mind when assessing cases, especially where polypharmacy is involved [1] (Table 1).

Gustatory abnormalities have also been linked to nutritional deficiency states. Low body stores of zinc, copper or nickel are potentially linked to changes in the sense of taste. These low levels may occur due to poor appetite, malabsorption or over-excretion by the kidneys [1].

Endocrinological diseases may also produce abnormalities in gustation or olfaction. Hypogeusia is linked to diabetes mellitus, Sjögren syndrome and pseudohypoparathyroidism. Gustatory perception is heightened by hypothyroidism

Table 1 Selected medications that are reported that as they alter smell or taste [13]. (Adopted from Ref. [13]

Antianxiety agents
Alprazolam (Xanax)
Buspirone (BuSpar)
Antibiotics
Ampicillin
Azithromycin (Zithromax)
Ciprofloxacin (Cipro)
Clarithromycin (Biaxin)
Enalapril (Vaseretic)
Griseofulvin (Grisactin)
Metronidazole (Flagyl)
Ofloxacin (Floxin)
Terbinafine (Lamisil)
Ticarcillan (Timentin)
Tetracycline
Anticonvulsants
Carbamazepine (Tegretol)
Phenytoin (Dilantin)
Antidepressants
Amitriptyline (Elavil)
Clomipramine (Anafranil)
Desipramine (Norpramin)
Antihistamines and decongestants
Chlorpheniramine
Loratadine (Claritin)
Pseudoephedrine
Antihypertensives and cardiac medications
Acetazolamide (Diamox)
Amiodarone (Pacerone)
Amiloride (Midamor)
Amiodarone (Cordarone)
Betaxolol (Betoptic)
Captopril (Capoten)
Diltiazem (Cardizem)
Enalapril (Lexxel, Vasotec, Vaseretic)
Hydrochlorothiazide (Esidix)
Nifedipine (Procardia)
Nitroglycerin
Propafenone (Rythmol)
Propranolol (Inderal)
Spironolactone (Aldactone)

(continued)

Table 1 (continued)

Tocainide (Tonocard)
Anti-inflammatory agents
Auranofin (Ridaura)
Beclomethasone (Beclovent, Beconase) Budesonide (Rhinocort)
Colchicine
Dexamethasone (Decadron)
Flunisolide (Nasalide, Aerobid)
Nortriptyline (Pamelor)
Fluticasone (Flonase)
Gold (Myochrysine)
Hydrocortisone
Penicillamine (Cuprimine)
Antimanic drugs
Lithium
Antimigrane agents
Dihydroergotamine (Migranal)
Naratriptan (Amerge)
Rizatriptan (Maxalt)
Sumatriptan (Imitrex)
Antineoplastics
Cisplatin (Platinol) Doxorubicin (Adriamycin)
Levamisole (Ergamisol)
Methotrexate (Rheumatrex)
Vincristine (Oncovin)
Antiparkinsonian agents
Levodopa (Larodopa; with carbidopa: Sinemet)
Antithyroid agents
Methimazole (Tapazole)
Propylthiouracil
Antiviral agents
Ganciclovir (Cytovene)
Interferon (Ruferon-A)
Zalcitabine (HIVID)
Bronchodilators
Biotolterol (Tornalate)
Pirbuterol (Maxair)
Lipid-lowering agents
Atorvastatin (Lipitor)
Fluvastatin (Lescol)
Lovastatin (Mevacor)
Pravastatin (Pravachol)

Table 1 (continued)

Muscle relaxants	
Baclofen (Lioresal)	
Dantrolene (Dantrium)	
Pancreatic enzyme preparations	
Pancrelipase (Cotazym)	
Smoking cessation aids	
Nicotine (Nicotrol)	
Doxepin (Sinequan)	
Imipramine (Tofranil)	

andadrenocortical insufficiency. Moreover, gustatory perception varies in women during the menstrual cycle and whilst pregnant [1].

3   Eating Behaviour

Animals must eat to survive, but eating may also be highly pleasurable. On the other hand, abnormal patterns of eating behaviour may lead to being undernourished, overfed or developing an eating disorder. How individuals behave when eating is influenced by several factors, such as seeking to achieve homeostasis, the brain's reward pathways, and, for children, their degree of motor, sensory, social and emotional development. The way a person was brought up, the social environment and the way food is presented all affect the subsequent eating behaviour [13].

Eating behaviour comes about through the complex interplay of different factors, such as social pressures, cultural influences, physiological demands, the environment as a whole and individual personality [14–16]. The development of eating habits owes a great deal to those surrounding a growing child, both the parents and wider society. In the developed world, eating behaviour has altered markedly in response to social change occurring worldwide [17]. The existence of plentiful food in developed economies means food is seen as just another object for consumers to buy, with its origins often little attended to. Over the last decades, eating habits have altered significantly. Many children have become used to eating alone, including in front of the television. By contrast, in poorer countries, food is often less nutritious [18] and offers less dietary variety [19]. The way families are composed and the lack of disposable income mean that younger children are frequently undernourished [20].

Infant feeding behaviour is predominantly biologically-driven. Infants innately prefer sweet-tasting food, rather than flavours that are bitter or sharp-tasting. This ensures the infant happily feeds on breast milk or substitute milk [17]. When children are weaned, the behaviour of their parents and societal norms become more significant. A recently published study of American infants noted that the period between 9 and 18 months was the most significant in terms of later eating behaviour [21]. Economically-deprived infants living in cities were nutritionally deficient in terms of vitamin D, zinc and iron. The study chose these markers because low levels are associated with a higher risk of lead toxicity. The researchers noted that children aged up to 2 years had adequate calorific intake, but protein was present in excess. With increasing age, these children ate a progressively poorer diet and larger and larger volumes of protein. These findings accord with the findings of national surveys investigating what American infants consume. The attitudes of parents to food were vital in explaining the infants' diets and the type of food they preferred to consume. Children who are repeatedly provided with specific items in the diet develop a fixed attitude towards those items and this then influences their eating behaviour at a later stage [17].

Nutritionally inadequate diets that are monotonous and unpalatable have an effect on young children's urge to eat and can cause reduced growth through inadequate intake [18, 19]. Overall in both North and South America, children whose growth is abnormally reduced leave a quarter of the food presented to them [18]. Children whose diet was grossly deficient at an early age are at a raised risk of infection, death and lower intellectual development [22]. For children to eat well and remain well-nourished in the future, a nutritionally satisfactory diet needs to be available and the parents need to be able to offer it to the growing child.

For children up to the age of 5 years, the family's socioeconomic status determines how adequate and how varied the diet is [19]. In Caribbean countries, biological parents who were married were most likely to allocate more resources to feeding children than non-related carers, single parents or unmarried couples [20]. In both North and South America, a higher level of resources was devoted to the needs of children by biological mothers than by parents who fostered or adopted children, or whose relationship was based on marriage to the child's relative. In developing countries, the way children eat reflects the influence of socioeconomic condition, how the child and carer are related and whether the food available is of adequate quality. As children grow up, inadequate diet takes an increasing toll on their health [20]. The same phenomenon is observable in developed nations, albeit the reasons for its occurrence are markedly different.

4 Developmental and Biological Aspects of Eating Behaviour

In the period between a child being an infant and starting school, eating behaviour undergoes rapid development. If eating occurs normally, the child gains an appropriate amount of weight and develops a healthy attitude towards eating in the future. There are a number of factors which interact to generate eating behaviour. This behaviour is affected by maturation of the nervous system, overall psychological and physical maturation, how parents and children interact and the surrounding social environment. A variety of different topics have been the subject of interest for researchers seeking to understand eating behaviour, such as the physiological mechanisms involved in energy balance, the role of perceptions in appetite, social determinants and how behaviour itself affects what food is preferred and when appetite is stimulated. Neuroscientific advances are illuminating when eating is driven by energetic considerations and when by pleasure-seeking. How eating behaviours arise differs between different age groups, such as early childhood, adolescence and adulthood, and this research is of value in treating eating problems in these groups [13].

4.1 Biological Aspects

The initiation of eating or prevention of eating may occur under physiological control. The following organs are all linked through a complex neuroendocrine network: hypothalamus, brain stem, gut, pancreas and fat tissue. When the body is in negative energy balance, gastric secretion of the peptide hormone, ghrelin, results in stimulation of the arcuate nucleus of the hypothalamus. This results in release of the orexigenic hormones agouti-related peptide, neuropeptide Y and orexin [23]. Following ingestion of food, pro-orexigenic peptide release is inhibited by the presence of insulin released by the pancreas, peptide YY from the gut and leptin from fat tissue. The release of orexin from the hypothalamus also ceases. The individual stops wishing to eat [24, 25]. Once energy balance becomes positive, cholecystokinin and leptin act on the arcuate nucleus to express pro-opiomelanocortin and CART (cocaine and amphetamine-regulated transcript), which also suppress the desire to eat more [26–28]. A low concentration of leptin stimulates appetite, whereas elevated levels suppress appetite [24]. Adiponectin is released by fat cells. The fasting state induces a high level of secretion, whereas obesity causes low levels to be released [29].

5 Reward System Influences on Eating Behaviour

Recent neuroscientific discoveries have begun to link both under- and over-eating to the brain's reward systems [30]. These systems appear to function alongside the endocrine regulation of energy intake [31, 32]. How reward systems initially develop in the brain is still a matter of conjecture, but it appears probable that from a very early age, children are driven towards activities that give pleasure or stimulate the reward system. If food elicits little pleasure, by being bland tasting, it is unlikely to be eaten to excess. Individuals do, however, often over-consume highly palatable items [33–37]. When highly palatable food is eaten, the mood tends to improve, an effect mediated through reward circuitry [38]. Areas of the brain involved in reward associated with food include the striatum, insula, anterior cingulate cortex and midbrain, namely the ventral tegmental area and substantia nigra [30]. Food-linked reward occurs via dopaminergic neurones [39]. Furthermore, clues as to a food's being palatable are processed in the orbito-frontal cortex, where smell, visual appearance, temperature, consistency, tanginess and fat content are assessed along-side gustatory perceptions [40–43]. There is a powerful neural response when eating starts, but this response weakens up to the point when the individual feels satiated by the food. Observation of how children as young as 2.5–5 years of age behave towards food indicates that the same mechanism is probably already functioning at that stage [44]. Although the neural responsivity towards an individual item may decline, other food items may still elicit a powerful reaction. Thus, the presence of multiple palatable items can promote over-eating [45]. In evolutionary terms, this response to the presence of multiple food items may have conferred an advantage at a period when nutrients were likely to be in poor supply

6 How Preferences for Particular Tastes and Smells Arise

Even in utero the foetus is already beginning to identify specific tastes or smells, since the foetus ingests amniotic fluid, in which there are dissolved taste-bearing molecules (such as alliaceous plants) ingested by the mother [46–49]. When cereal mixed with carrot juice was offered to infants in one study, the infants whose mothers had regularly consumed carrot juice in the final trimester demonstrated a clear preference for this food [50]. Researchers are currently interested in seeing whether children can be primed in utero to accept a healthier diet later in life [50, 51]. One good way to test the feasibility of this intervention would be to set up longitudinally-designed studies of mothers and infants where different types of maternal diet, including healthier options, are consumed [52–54]

Breastfed infants experience exposure to a range of tastes through molecules absorbed from the mother's diet [50]. Long before weaning occurs, this experience of different tastes begins to shape what infants subsequently enjoy eating, whether or not this remains a lasting effect. However, the majority of children choose sweet or salty items whenever available [55–61], a tendency that strengthens when these types of food are regularly available, but weakens a little as the child grows up [58–61]. Bitter-tasting food, such as many vegetables, is rarely immediately enjoyed by children, but if repeatedly offered, they may develop a taste for them. It has been shown that infants exposed at an early stage to soy and hydrolysed protein later accept these foods [62]. Children repeatedly offered a wide range of foods when very young do subsequently acquire a taste for certain items [63]. Indeed, in certain cultures, children are systematically exposed to powerful flavours early on to accustom them to consuming such items. Mexican children are generally given hotter and hotter chilli peppers to get used to them [64, 65]. Acquiring a taste for a flavour that initially appears unappealing can be significant for socialisation [66]. The tastes an individual prefers are influenced by previous exposure, stage of development and genetic factors [67]. There has been extensive research into perception of 6-n-propylthiouracil (PROP), a molecule with a bitter flavour. Perceiving this taste appears partly dependent on the TAS2R38 gene [68]. Inability to perceive PROP may make a child more willing to eat vegetables. This insensitivity to PROP is present in around 30% of individuals of European ancestry and varies in frequency globally [69]. Being able to taste PROP makes an individual less receptive to eating bitter foods and thus causes a lower consumption of vegetables, more avoidance of certain foods and a greater propensity to become obese in childhood [70–77].

References

1. Holbrook EH. Disorders of Taste and Smell. In: Meyers AD (Ed). Medscape. Updated: Jan 19, 2022. https://emedicine.medscape.com/article/861242-overview#a6. Accessed online at February 11, 2022.
2. Zhang C, Wang X. Initiation of the age-related decline of odor identification in humans: a meta-analysis. Ageing Res Rev. 2017;40:45–50.
3. Boesveldt S, Lindau ST, McClintock MK, Hummel T, Lundstrom JN. Gustatory and olfactory dysfunction in older adults: a national probability study. Rhinology. 2011;49(3):324–30.
4. Murphy C, Schubert CR, Cruickshanks KJ, Klein BE, Klein R, Nondahl DM. Prevalence of olfactory impairment in older adults. JAMA. 2002;288(18):2307–12.
5. Allis TJ, Leopold DA. Smell and taste disorders. Facial Plast Surg Clin North Am. 2012;20(1):93–111.
6. Martin GE, Junque C, Juncadella M, Gabarros A, de Miquel MA, Rubio F. Olfactory dysfunction after subarachnoid hemorrhage caused by ruptured aneurysms of the anterior communicating artery. J Neurosurg. 2009; https://doi.org/10.3171/2008.11.JNS08827.
7. Bratt M, Skandsen T, Hummel T, et al. Frequency and prognostic factors of olfactory dysfunction after traumatic brain injury. Brain Inj. 2018:1–7.
8. Park M, Chung J, Kim JK, Jeong Y, Moon WJ. Altered functional brain networks in patients with traumatic anosmia: resting-state functional MRI based on graph theoretical analysis. Korean J Radiol. 2019;20(11):1536–45.
9. Bhatnagar KP, Kennedy RC, Baron G, Greenberg RA. Number of mitral cells and the bulb volume in the aging human olfactory bulb: a quantitative morphological study. Anat Rec. 1987;218(1):73–87.
10. Tuccori M, Lapi F, Testi A, Ruggiero E, Moretti U, Vannacci A, et al. Drug-induced taste and smell alterations: a case/non-case evaluation of an italian database of spontaneous adverse drug reaction reporting. Drug Saf. 2011;34(10):849–59.
11. Wylie K, Nebauer M. "The food here is tasteless!" Food taste or tasteless food? Chemosensory loss and the politics of under-nutrition. Collegian. 2011;18(1):27–35.
12. Wang T, Glendinning J, Grushka M, Hummel T, Mansfield K. From the cover: drug-induced taste disorders in clinical practice and preclinical safety evaluation. Toxicol Sci. 2017;156(2):315–24.
13. Doty RL, Bromley SM. Effects of drugs on olfaction and taste. Otolaryngol Clin N Am. 2004;37(6):1229–54. https://doi.org/10.1016/j.otc.2004.05.002.
14. Lockyear PLB. Childhood Eating Behaviors: Developmental and Sociocultural Considerations. Medscape General Surgery. February 02, 2004. https://www.medscape.com/viewarticle/467523#vp_1. Accessed online at February 11, 2022.
15. Kittler PG, Sucher KP. Food and culture in America: a Nutritional Handbook. 2nd ed. West/Wadsworth; 1998.
16. Parraga IM. Determinants of food consumption. J Am Diet Assoc. 1990;90:661–4.
17. Westenhoefer J. Establishing good dietary habits ý capturing the minds of children. Public Health Nutr. 2001;4:125–9.
18. Lutter CK, Rivera JA. Nutritional status of infants and young children and characteristics of their diets. J Nutr. 2003;133:2941S–9S.

19. Onyango AW. Dietary diversity, child nutrition and health in contemporary African communities. Comp Biochem Physiol. 2003;136:61–9.
20. Bronte-Tinkew J, Dejong G. Children's nutrition in Jamaica: do household structure and household economic resource matter? Soc Sci Med. 2004;58:499–514.
21. Nolan K, Schell LM, Stark AD, Gomez MI. Longitudinal study of energy and nutrient intakes for infants from low-income, urban families. Public Health Nutr. 2002;5:405–12. Abstract
22. Wachs TD, Moussa W, Bishry Z, et al. Relations between nutrition and cognitive performance in Egyptian toddlers. Intelligence. 1993;17:151–72.
23. Inui A, Asakawa A, Bowers CY, Mantovani G, Laviano A, Meguid MM, et al. Ghrelin, appetite, and gastric motility: the emerging role of the stomach as an endocrine organ. FASEB J. 2004;18:439–56.
24. Margetic S, Gazzola C, Pegg GG, Hill RA. Leptin: a review of its peripheral actions and interactions. Int J Obes Relat Metab Disord. 2002;26:1407–33.
25. Konner AC, Klockener T, Bruning JC. Control of energy homeostasis by insulin and leptin: targeting the arcuate nucleus and beyond. Physiol Behav. 2009;97:632–8.
26. Mutt V. Historical perspectives on cholecystokinin research. Ann N Y Acad Sci. 1994;713:1–10.
27. Dockray GJ. Cholecystokinin and gut-brain signalling. Regul Pept. 2009;155:6–10.
28. Elmer PJ, Obarzanek E, Vollmer WM, Simons-Morton D, Stevens VJ, Young DR, et al. Effects of comprehensive lifestyle modification on diet, weight, physical fitness, and blood pressure control: 18-month results of a randomized trial. Ann Intern Med. 2006;144:485–95.
29. Gustafson B. Adipose tissue, inflammation and atherosclerosis. J Atheroscler Thromb. 2010;17:332–41.
30. Kenny PJ. Reward mechanisms in obesity: new insights and future directions. Neuron. 2011;69:664–79.
31. Lutter M, Nestler EJ. Homeostatic and hedonic signals interact in the regulation of food intake. J Nutr. 2009;139:629–32.
32. Saper CB, Chou TC, Elmquist JK. The need to feed: homeostatic and hedonic control of eating. Neuron. 2002;36:199–211.
33. Shomaker LB, Tanofsky-Kraff M, Zocca JM, Courville A, Kozlosky M, Columbo KM, et al. Eating in the absence of hunger in adolescents: intake after a large-array meal compared with that after a standardized meal. Am J Clin Nutr. 2010;92:697–703.
34. Wang GJ, Volkow ND, Telang F, Jayne M, Ma J, Rao M, et al. Exposure to appetitive food stimuli markedly activates the human brain. NeuroImage. 2004;21:1790–7.
35. Sunday SR, Sanders SA, Collier G. Palatability and meal patterns. Physiol Behav. 1983;30:915–8.
36. Zheng H, Lenard NR, Shin AC, Berthoud HR. Appetite control and energy balance regulation in the modern world: reward-driven brain overrides repletion signals. Int J Obes. 2009;33:S8–13.
37. Wang GJ, Volkow ND, Thanos PK, Fowler JS. Similarity between obesity and drug addiction as assessed by neurofunctional imaging: a concept review. J Addict Dis. 2004;23:39–53.
38. Macht M, Mueller J. Immediate effects of chocolate on experimentally induced mood states. Appetite. 2007;49:667–74.
39. Cornelius JR, Tippmann-Peikert M, Slocumb NL, Frerichs CF, Silber MH. Impulse control disorders with the use of dopaminergic agents in restless legs syndrome: a case-control study. Sleep. 2010;33:81–7.
40. Rolls ET. Taste, olfactory and food texture reward processing in the brain and obesity. Int J Obes. 2011;35:550–61.
41. Small DM. Taste representation in the human insula. Brain Struct Funct. 2010;214:551–61.
42. Berridge KC. 'Liking' and 'wanting' food rewards: brain substrates and roles in eating disorders. Physiol Behav. 2009;97:537–50.
43. Dagher A. The neurobiology of appetite: hunger as addiction. Int J Obes. 2009;33:S30–3.
44. Birch LL, Deysher M. Caloric compensation and sensory specific satiety: evidence for self regulation of food intake by young children. Appetite. 1986;7:323–31.

45. Rolls BJ, Rowe EA, Rolls ET, Kingston B, Megson A, Gunary R. Variety in a meal enhances food intake in man. Physiol Behav. 1981;26:215–21.
46. Mennella JA, Johnson A, Beauchamp GK. Garlic ingestion by pregnant women alters the odor of amniotic fluid. Chem Senses. 1995;20:207–9.
47. Mennella JA, Beauchamp GK. Maternal diet alters the sensory qualities of human milk and the nursling's behavior. Pediatrics. 1991;88:737–44.
48. Schaal B, Marlier L, Soussignan R. Human foetuses learn odours from their pregnant mother's diet. Chem Senses. 2000;25:729–37.
49. Mennella J, Beauchamp GK. The ontogeny of human flavor perception. In: Beauchamp G, Bartoshuk L, editors. Tasting and smelling. 2nd ed. San Diego, CA: Academic Press; 1997. p. 199–216.
50. Mennella JA, Jagnow CP, Beauchamp GK. Prenatal and postnatal flavor learning by human infants. Pediatrics. 2001;107:e88.
51. Cooke L, Fildes A. The impact of flavour exposure in utero and during milk feeding on food acceptance at weaning and beyond. *Appetite.* 2011 epub ahead of print.
52. Jackson RA, Stotland NE, Caughey AB, Gerbert B. Improving diet and exercise in pregnancy with Video Doctor counseling: a randomized trial. Patient Educ Couns. 2011;83:203–9.
53. Skouteris H, Hartley-Clark L, McCabe M, Milgrom J, Kent B, Herring SJ, et al. Preventing excessive gestational weight gain: a systematic review of interventions. Obes Rev. 2010;11:757–68.
54. Kinnunen TI, Pasanen M, Aittasalo M, Fogelholm M, Hilakivi-Clarke L, Weiderpass E, et al. Preventing excessive weight gain during pregnancy - a controlled trial in primary health care. Eur J Clin Nutr. 2007;61:884–91.
55. Ventura AK, Mennella JA. Innate and learned preferences for sweet taste during childhood. Curr Opin Clin Nutr Metab Care. 2011;14:379–84.
56. Birch LL. Development of food preferences. Annu Rev Nutr. 1999;19:41–62.
57. Schwartz C, Issanchou S, Nicklaus S. Developmental changes in the acceptance of the five basic tastes in the first year of life. Br J Nutr. 2009;102:1375–85.
58. Desor J, Greene L, Maller O. Preferences for sweet and salty in 9- to 15-year-old and adult humans. Science. 1975;190:686–7.
59. Desor JA, Beauchamp GK. Longitudinal changes in sweet preferences in humans. Physiol Behav. 1987;39:639–41.
60. De Graaf C, Zandstra EH. Sweetness intensity and pleasantness in children, adolescents, and adults - The genesis of sweet preference. Physiol Behav. 1999;67:513–20.
61. Beauchamp GK, Cowart BJ, Moran M. Developmental changes in salt acceptability in human infants. Dev Psychobiol. 1986;19:17–25.
62. Julie AM, Gary KB. Flavor experiences during formula feeding are related to preferences during childhood. Early Hum Dev. 2002;68:71–82.
63. Birch LL. The role of experience in children's food acceptance patterns. J Am Diet Assoc. 1987;87:S36–40.
64. Rozin P, Schiller D. The nature and acquisition of a preference for chili pepper by humans. Motiv Emot. 1980;4:77–101.
65. Mennella JA, Turnbull B, Ziegler PJ, Martinez H. Infant feeding practices and early flavor experiences in Mexican infants: an intra-cultural study. J Am Diet Assoc. 2005;105:908–15.
66. Wardle J. Parental influences on children's diets. Proc Nutr Soc. 1995;54:747–58.
67. Mennella JA, Pepino MY, Reed DR. Genetic and environmental determinants of bitter perception and sweet preferences. Pediatrics. 2005;115:e216–22.
68. Duffy VB, Davidson AC, Kidd JR, Kidd KK, Speed WC, Pakstis AJ, et al. Bitter receptor gene (TAS2R38), 6-n-propylthiouracil (PROP) bitterness and alcohol intake. Alcohol Clin Exp Res. 2004;28:1629–37.
69. Guo SW, Reed DR. The genetics of phenylthiocarbamide perception. Ann Hum Biol. 2001;28:111–42.

70. Fischer R, Griffin F, England S, Garn SM. Taste thresholds and food dislikes. Nature. 1961;23:1328.
71. Keller KL, Steinmann L, Nurse RJ, Tepper BJ. Genetic taste sensitivity to 6-n-propylthiouracil influences food preference and reported intake in preschool children. Appetite. 2002;38:3–12.
72. Drewnowski A, Henderson SA, Hann CS, Berg WA, Ruffin MT. Genetic taste markers and preferences for vegetables and fruit of female breast care patients. J Am Diet Assoc. 2000;100:191–7.
73. Dinehart ME, Hayes JE, Bartoshuk LM, Lanier SL, Duffy VB. Bitter taste markers explain variability in vegetable sweetness, bitterness, and intake. Physiol Behav. 2006;87:304–13.
74. Turnbull B, Matisoo-Smith E. Taste sensitivity to 6-n-propylthiouracil predicts acceptance of bitter-tasting spinach in 3–6-y-old children. Am J Clin Nutr. 2002;76:1101–5.
75. Lumeng JC, Cardinal TM, Sitto JR, Kannan S. Ability to taste 6-n-propylthiouracil and BMI in low-income preschool-aged children. Obesity (Silver Spring). 2008;16:1522–8.
76. Glanvill EV, Kaplan AR. Food Preference and Sensitivity of Taste for Bitter Compounds. Nature. 1965;205:851.
77. Tepper BJ, Keller KL, Ullrich NV. Genetic variation in taste and preferences for bitter and pungent foods: Implications for chronic disease risk. Challenges Taste Chem Biol. 2004;867:60–74.

Olfactory Influences on Human Feeding Behaviour, from Sense to Satiety

Soner Taşar, Cemal Cingi, and Dilyana Vicheva

1 Introduction

Smell is highly significant in how humans perceive food. Accordingly, olfactory disorders typically cause changes in patients' feeding behaviour. Olfactory and gustatory dysfunction may significantly impair patients' quality of life and alter the diet they choose to eat [1, 2]. The process of eating food consists of two principal stages, namely an anticipatory stage, wherein the food is seen and its aroma arouses orthonasal perception, and a consumption stage, where the food enters the mouth and any aroma is perceived in a retronasal fashion [3]. Everybody is familiar with the way a coryzal illness alters gustatory perception, and this experience illustrates how significant olfaction is for perceiving food or drink to be tasty [4]. Research has so far focused mainly on how individuals change their diet in response to olfactory dysfunction [5–7], rather than how food actually tastes to people in this situation [8]. Response inhibition is sensitive to unexpected changes in the environment triggered by emotional stimuli [9].

S. Taşar (✉)
Department of Otorhinolaryngology, Afyonkarahisar State Hospital, Afyonkarahisar, Türkiye

C. Cingi
Medical Faculty, Department of Otorhinolaryngology, Eskisehir Osmangazi University, Eskisehir, Türkiye
e-mail: cemal@ogu.edu.tr

D. Vicheva
Department of Otorhinolaryngology, Medical University of Plovdiv, Plovdiv, Bulgaria

Ö. N. Şahin et al. (eds.), *Breastfeeding and Metabolic Programming*,
https://doi.org/10.1007/978-3-031-33278-4_35

2   Sensory Qualities of Food and Drinks

When individuals eat or drink, they perceive certain sensory qualities of the food or drink prior to, during and after eating. These sensory perceptions are key to locating food, choosing what and how much to consume, and guide how satiated a person feels after eating. Learning about food also depends on these perceptions. Increasingly, the role of sensory qualities in food in guiding the intake of energy has been appreciated. The palatability of food is especially important [10]. The role of visual, olfactory and gustatory qualities of food in increasing an individual's consumption of that food is well-recognised. In laboratory-based trials, foods that are considered most palatable are consumed in the highest quantities [10, 11].

The experimental data therefore confirm that overeating a certain food is linked to the sensory qualities it possesses, especially those associated with greater palatability [10]. The palatability of a food relates to a situation where the sensory perceptions about that food are pleasurable in nature [12]. This pleasurable nature depends on previous experience of a food as nutritional and not dangerous to consume [13]. How palatable a food appears is not fixed [12], since it is affected by factors such as sensory-specific satiety [14] and alliaesthesia [15]. A food may appear more or less appealing, and therefore more or less likely to be consumed, depending on how much of the same stimulus has been received, and the current metabolic requirements of an individual [11].

3   Sensory Perceptions, Regulation of Dietary Consumption and Satiety

Chambers et al. [16] have extensively developed understanding of the Satiety Cascade framework, an idea originally proposed 25 years earlier [17]. First some type of food is selected, then this food is eaten to a level where satiation occurs, following which, as hunger evaporates, satiety occurs. Despite the fact that research frequently treats satiation and satiety as distinct topics, these phenomena are in fact connected by responses that overlap and mutually interact, as indeed are the thought processes and evaluation of the sensory qualities triggering appetite and the physiological responses following the food being swallowed and digestion beginning [17]. The peripheral nervous system transports information about the process of feeding and carries it to various centres within the central nervous system. The brain centres involved are related to homeostatic equilibrium, learning, reward and attention [18, 19]. It is through this processing of signals from feeding, interpreted in the light of more enduring metabolic settings, that individuals feel satiation and satiety [11].

The components involved in satiation were examined by Cecil, French and Read [20], who ascertained that a portion of soup of mass 425 g and containing 400kCal produced less and less satiation as elements normally involved in eating were taken away from the feeding process. If the soup was eaten by mouth in the knowledge that it was food, the degree of satiation was highest, whereas when fed the same soup directly into the stomach after being told the soup was actually just water, the experimental subjects reported least satiation. The early stages of the eating process play an important role, since animals (including humans) learn that certain sensory perceptions are associated with feeding, and these perceptions have an association with the signals subsequently coming from the gut showing the food was indeed nutritious. Perceptions linked to particular foods come to be associated with the presence of nutrients when a specific perception coincides regularly with nutrient absorption, and individuals subsequently learn to predict how satiating a particular food may be [21]. The associations between pre-ingestive and post-ingestive perceptions lead to preference for foods that deliver plentiful nutrients and allow an individual to decide whether a certain amount and type of food will satisfy his or her appetite [22]. These judgements affect which foods are chosen to be consumed. When food is present, it triggers a rapidly acting set of physiological responses (the cephalic phase), involving, for example, saliva production [23], stomach acid secretion [24] and release of particular gut signalling molecules [25]. The visual, olfactory and gustatory qualities of the food help the gut respond in such a way as to maximise the extraction of nutrients from it [24]. Thus, sensory perceptions occurring both prior to and whilst consuming food act to allow the maximum extraction of calorific value from the food. Food that appears palatable is also the food from which maximum value can be extracted, since the perception of its being tasty triggers an appropriate physiological state for optimal nutrient extraction [11].

If food continues to present the same sensory qualities, subjects begin to perceive further consumption of the food as less pleasant, whereas changing some sensory quality without altering the basic nature of the food can render it more appealing. For example, chocolates may be offered to a subject that differ only in their colour. Always offering the same colour leads to a decline in the perceived pleasure of eating, whereas new colours are perceived as more pleasurable to eat. The same level of appeal can be achieved by offering chocolates of various colours or by making them all the same colour, if that colour is already the individual's favourite colour. The effects of altering appearance and mouth-feel have also been investigated using pasta moulded in different shapes. Subjects offered a variety of shapes rated the experience even more pleasant than when the same favourite shape was on offer. This situation led to 14% more consumption. When food was altered only in terms of taste, not nutritional value, such as by adding salt, artificial sweetener or curry, 15% more food was consumed, compared with constantly presenting the same food, even when this was the subject's preferred choice. These kinds of trials reveal which sensory qualities most affect satiety and influence the level of consumption [26].

4 Odours

The smell of food is a key part of gustatory perception in humans. Smell forms part of taste and affects how particular flavours and textures are perceived [27]. Odours emanating from food reveal its presence and provide information about whether it can be eaten or not. Perceiving such odours may precede seeing the food [28]. This phenomenon is widely utilised by restaurants and other food outlets to encourage hungry people to enter their establishment [29]. Laboratory experiments have shown that merely presenting highly agreeable food odours, such as from bakeries, to individual subjects is sufficient to stimulate salivation [30–32]. Some authors reported that the pleasant (vs. control) odour impaired inhibition, as reflected in slower stop-signal reaction times and higher release errors, indicating greater mobilisation of inhibitory resources by pleasant stimuli [9]. Furthermore, it increases appetite, the amount individuals plan to eat, and may raise the level of consumption in specific people. This increased consumption is related to the body mass index [31, 33, 34], degree of self-restraint about diet [33, 35–37] and self-reported tendency to acting impulsively [38].

Although smelling food does increase appetite, when different odours that are rated as the same level of appeal and the same strength are presented, varying effects are observed in how much they increase appetite and influence food selection [39]. A study undertaken by Ramaekers et al. [40] noted that certain popular food odours present in particular environments (such as bread, tomato soup, roasted meat, chocolate or banana) did increase the wish to eat, but only of the food from which the odour usually emanates. In a different study, subjects were exposed to odours from fruit at a level where they were not consciously aware of the stimulus. When then offered food, the exposed individuals had a greater tendency to select items based on fruit and vegetables [41, 42]. These findings support the notion that food odours specifically increase appetite for the corresponding food. The mechanism may involve the odour being pleasurably associated mentally with the food or more specifically with the nutrients typically provided by such items. It has recently been shown that a diet low in protein alters the way the nervous system responds to the smell of particular savoury foods [43]. Nonetheless, there is a lack of direct proof for the hypothesis that a specific odour activates the body to choose the corresponding food based on its nutritional profile [11].

The majority of individuals presenting with disorders of olfaction volunteer the information that they take less pleasure in eating and find foods more bland, which then means they eat and prepare food differently from the way they did before the problem began [44].

There is conflicting evidence about how much salivation can be triggered by exposure to particularly pleasant food odours [45, 46]. Studies which report that salivation is not altered by the level of pleasure aroused by an odour may have employed odours of insufficient potency to trigger the extra salivation [8, 40].

5 Visual Qualities of Food

The initial sensory perceptions associated with a food are often visual in nature. Simply seeing food nearby can be sufficient to encourage individuals to begin eating [47]. Food manufacturers pay especial attention to how altering a product's appearance may increase its desirability. When foods, such as biscuits or chocolate bars, are presented as smaller pieces, subjects eat less [48, 49], but with no change in the item's perceived attractiveness [50]. The reason for the decreased consumption may relate to changes in how the volume is perceived [51] or may be due to decreasing the speed with which it is eaten. However, if food is divided in such a way as to increase the perceived variety, this does result in higher consumption [52]. The amount consumed also depends to a degree on the size of plate, dish etc. on which food is served. Larger plates and cups promote greater consumption in some but not all individuals, regardless of age. However, this tendency to eat more from a larger plate may vary from occasion to occasion [11, 53].

6 Conclusion

Not only does the texture of food provide sensory experiences in the mouth, it also influences judgements by individuals about how filling a food, or thirst-quenching a drink, is likely to be, which then affects how much the individual consumes. It has newly been discovered that food which takes more chewing, or is denser, is perceived as more satiating [54, 55]. Thus, the addition of agents that thicken a drink or make it appear creamier results in its being judged more potentially satisfying [56]. Notably, if foods have a creamy taste but not an altered texture, they are not judged more filling [55, 56], and thus individuals do not consume less of the product, unlike the situation where creamy flavour is matched with a thicker texture [57]. Thus texture has a key impact on oro-sensory perception, resulting in judgements that the food is more likely to satiate the individual's hunger by providing the anticipated nutrients [58].

In addition to influencing what food an individual may choose to eat, texture also appears to be key to experiencing satiety. More specifically, texture helps explain why solid food is perceived as providing greater satiation than calories supplied in liquid form. Numerous studies have reached the conclusion that, when the same nutrients are supplied as either a liquid, semi-solid or solid preparation, the liquid form does not sate the appetite and stop further eating to the extent the other two forms do [59–65]. These experiments were careful to keep the macronutrient composition and taste of the food the same and merely alter its fluidity. Since liquids pass through the stomach and undergo processing in the gut more swiftly than solids, post-ingestive factors may be significant in why the liquid seems less satiating [66]. Importantly, however, if the manner of consumption of a liquid is altered (eating with a spoon vs drinking), the same food produces greater satiation when consumed more slowly with the spoon. This suggests that more prolonged oral sensation of texture makes the same nutrient offering appear more satisfying [67].

Liquids consumed as a straightforward beverage do not elicit a long oro-sensory perception and this means the cephalic phase preparation for digestion is less extensive than with food that remains in the oral cavity whilst being masticated [68, 69]. Lengthening the time food is held in the oral cavity makes it more satiating and increases the release of gut peptides [70–73]. Cognitive factors also play a probable role, since individuals may see a soup or solid food as a 'proper meal', whereas a beverage may be considered a drink to quench thirst. This would then affect how satiating the food or beverage is perceived to be [74]. The most probable explanation is that solid food is more satiating than liquid due to cognitive, oral perceptive and post-ingestive factors all acting together [11, 59].

References

1. Hummel T, Nordin S. Olfactory disorders and their consequences for quality of life. Acta Otolaryngol. 2005;125(2):116–21.
2. Aschenbrenner K, Hummel C, Teszmer K, et al. The influence of olfactory loss on dietary behaviors. Laryngoscope. 2008;118(1):135–44.
3. Brillat-Savarin JA. La Physiologie du Goût ("Die Physiologie des Geschmacks oder Transcendentalgastronomische Betrachtungen, German 1865; translater Habs R, corrected Muehlgassner J) Edited by Leipzig, Philipp Reclam jun., 1826, p. chapter 8.
4. Spence C. Multisensory flavor perception. Cell. 2015;161(1):24–35.
5. Aschenbrenner K, Hummel C, Teszmer K, Krone F, Ishimaru T, Seo HS, Hummel T. The influence of olfactory loss on dietary behaviors. Laryngoscope. 2008;118(1):135–44.
6. Ilona C, Steven N. Hummel T, Olfactory disorders and quality of life—an updated review. Chem Senses. 2014;39:185–94.
7. Stefanie K, Nancy H, Sanne B. The influence of olfactory impairment in vital, independently living older persons on their eating behaviour and food liking. Food Qual Prefer. 2014;38:30–9.
8. Zang Y, Han P, Burghardt S, Knaapila A, Schriever V, Hummel T. Influence of olfactory dysfunction on the perception of food. Eur Arch Otorhinolaryngol. 2019;276(10):2811–7.
9. Javier A, Umberto C, Valentina P. Olfactory influences on reach-to-press movements in a stop-signal task. Cogn Emot. 2021;35(6):1214–122.
10. Sorensen LB, Moller P, Flint A, Martens M, Raben A. Effect of sensory perception of foods on appetite and food intake: a review of studies on humans. Int J Obes (London). 2003;27:1152–66.
11. McCrickerd K, Forde CG. Sensory influences on food intake control: moving beyond palatability. Obes Rev. 2016 Jan;17(1):18–29.
12. Yeomans MR. Taste, palatability and the control of appetite. Proc Nutr Soc. 1998;57:609–15.
13. Mela DJ. Eating for pleasure or just wanting to eat? Reconsidering sensory hedonic responses as a driver of obesity. Appetite. 2006;47:10–7.
14. Rolls BJ. Sensory-specific satiety. Nutr Rev. 1986;44:93–101.
15. Cabanac M. Sensory pleasure. Q Rev Biol. 1979;54:1–29.
16. Chambers L, McCrickerd K, Yeomans MR. Optimising foods for satiety. Trends Food Sci Technol. 2015;41:149–60.
17. Blundell JE, Rogers PJ, Hill AJ. Evaluating the satiating power of foods. Implications for acceptance and consumption. In: Colms J, Booth DA, Pangborn RM, Raunhardt O, editors. Food acceptance and nutrition. London: Academic Press; 1987. p. 205–19.
18. Berthoud HR. Interactions between the "cognitive" and "metabolic" brain in the control of food intake. Physiol Behav. 2007;91:486–98.
19. Toepel U, Bielser M-L, Forde C, et al. Brain dynamics of meal size selection in humans. NeuroImage. 2015;113:133–42.
20. Cecil JE, Francis J, Read NW. Relative contributions of intestinal, gastric, oro-sensory influences and information to changes in appetite induced by the same liquid meal. Appetite. 1998;31:377–90.
21. Sclafani A. Learned controls of ingestive behaviour. Appetite. 1997;29:153–8.

22. Brunstrom JM. Associative learning and the control of human dietary behavior. Appetite. 2007;49:268–71.
23. Wooley SC, Wooley OW. Salivation to sight and thought of food – new measure of appetite. Psychosom Med. 1973;35:136–42.
24. Feldman M, Richardson CT. Role of thought, sight, smell, and taste of food in the cephalic phase of gastric-acid secretion in humans. Gastroenterology. 1986;90:428–33.
25. Smeets PAM, Erkner A, De Graaf C. Cephalic phase responses and appetite. Nutr Rev. 2010;68:643–55.
26. Rolls BJ, Rowe EA, Rolls ET. How sensory properties of foods affect human feeding behavior. Physiol Behav. 1982;29(3):409–17.
27. Small DM, Prescott J. Odor/taste integration and the perception of flavor. Exp Brain Res. 2005;166:345–57.
28. Stevenson RJ. an initial evaluation of the functions of human olfaction. Chem Senses. 2010;35:3–20.
29. Chebat J-C, Michon R. Impact of ambient odors on mall shoppers' emotions, cognition, and spending: a test of competitive causal theories. J Bus Res. 2003;56:529–39.
30. Engelen L, deWijk RA, Prinz JF, van der Bilt A, Bosman F. The relation between saliva flow after different stimulations and the perception of flavor and texture attributes in custard desserts. Physiol Behav. 2003;78:165–9.
31. Ferriday D, Brunstrom JM. 'I just can't help myself': effects of food-cue exposure in overweight and lean individuals. Int J Obes. 2011;35:142–9.
32. Pangborn RM, Berggren B. Human parotid secretion in response to pleasant and unpleasant odorants. Psychophysiology. 1973;10:231–7.
33. Ferriday D, Brunstrom JM. How does food-cue exposure lead to larger meal sizes? Br J Nutr. 2008;100:1325–32.
34. Tetley A, Brunstrom J, Griffiths P. Individual differences in food-cue reactivity. The role of BMI and everyday portion-size selections. Appetite. 2009;52:614–20.
35. Coelho JS, Polivy J, Peter Herman C, Pliner P. Wake up and smell the cookies. Effects of olfactory food-cue exposure in restrained and unrestrained eaters. Appetite. 2009;52:517–20.
36. Fedoroff IDC, Polivy J, Herman CP. The specificity of restrained versus unrestrained eaters' responses to food cues: general desire to eat, or craving for the cued food? Appetite. 2003;41:7–13.
37. Fedoroff IDC, Polivy J, Herman CP. The effect of pre-exposure to food cues on the eating behavior of restrained and unrestrained eaters. Appetite. 1997;28:33–47.
38. Larsen JK, Hermans RCJ, Engels RCME. Food intake in response to food-cue exposure. Examining the influence of duration of the cue exposure and trait impulsivity. Appetite. 2012;58:907–13.
39. de Wijk RA, Zijlstra S. Differential effects of exposure to ambient vanilla and citrus aromas on mood, arousal and food choice. Flavour. 2012;1:24.
40. Ramaekers MG, Boesveldt S, Lakemond CMM, Van Boekel MAJS, Luning PA. Odors: appetizing or satiating development of appetite during odor exposure over time. Int J Obes. 2014;38:650–6.
41. Gaillet M, Sulmont-Rossé C, Issanchou S, Chabanet C, Chambaron S. Priming effects of an olfactory food cue on subsequent food-related behaviour. Food Qual Prefer. 2013;30:274–81.
42. Gaillet-Torrent M, Sulmont-Rossé C, Issanchou S, Chabanet C, Chambaron S. Impact of a non-attentively perceived odour on subsequent food choices. Appetite. 2014;76:17–22.
43. Griffioen-Roose S, Smeets PA, van den Heuvel E, Boesveldt S, Finlayson G, de Graaf C. Human protein status modulates brain reward responses to food cues. Am J Clin Nutr. 2014;100:113–22.
44. Croy I, Nordin S, Hummel T. Olfactory disorders and quality of life—an updated review. Chem Senses. 2014;39(3):185–94.
45. Proserpio C, de Graaf C, Laureati M, Pagliarini E, Boesveldt S. Impact of ambient odors on food intake, saliva production and appetite ratings. Physiol Behav. 2017;174:35–41.

46. Pangborn RM, Witherly SA, Jones F. Parotid and wholemouth secretion in response to viewing, handling, and sniffing food. Perception. 1979;8(3):339–46.
47. Wansink B. Environmental factors that increase the food intake and consumption volume of unknowing consumers. Annu Rev Nutr. 2004;24:455–79.
48. Marchiori D, Waroquier L, Klein O. smaller food item sizes of snack foods influence reduced portions and caloric intake in young adults. J Am Diet Assoc. 2011;111:727–31.
49. Marchiori D, Waroquier L, Klein O. Split them smaller item sizes of cookies lead to a decrease in energy intake in children. J Nutr Educ Behav. 2012;44:251–5.
50. Weijzen PL, Liem DG, Zandstra EH, de Graaf C. Sensory specific satiety and intake: the difference between nibble- and bar-size snacks. Appetite. 2008;50:435–42.
51. Wadhera D, Capaldi-Phillips ED. A review of visual cues associated with food on food acceptance and consumption. Eat Behav. 2014;15:132–43.
52. Geier A, Wansink B, Rozin P. Red potato chips: segmentation cues can substantially decrease food intake. Health Psychol. 2012;31:398–401.
53. Robinson E, Nolan S, Tudur-Smith C, et al. Will smaller plates lead to smaller waists? A systematic review and meta-analysis of the effect that experimental manipulation of dishware size has on energy consumption. Obes Rev. 2014;15:812–21.
54. Forde CG, van Kuijk N, Thaler T, de Graaf C, Martin N. Oral processing characteristics of solid savoury meal components, and relationship with food composition, sensory attributes and expected satiation. Appetite. 2013;60:208–19.
55. Hogenkamp PS, Stafleu A, Mars M, Brunstrom JM, de Graaf C. Texture, not flavor, determines expected satiation of dairy products. Appetite. 2011;57:635–41.
56. McCrickerd K, Chambers L, Brunstrom JM, Yeomans MR. Subtle changes in the flavour and texture of a drink enhance expectations of satiety. Flavour. 2012;1(20):1–11.
57. McCrickerd K, Chambers L, Yeomans MR. Does modifying the thick texture and creamy flavour of a drink change portion size selection and intake? Appetite. 2014;73:114–20.
58. Mars M, Hogenkamp PS, Gosses AM, Stafleu A, De Graaf C. Effect of viscosity on learned satiation. Physiol Behav. 2009;98:60–6.
59. Cassady BA, Considine RV, Mattes RD. Beverage consumption, appetite, and energy intake: what did you expect? Am J Clin Nutr. 2012;95:587–93.
60. Almiron-Roig E, Palla L, Guest K, et al. Factors that determine energy compensation: a systematic review of preload studies. Nutr Rev. 2013;71:458–73.
61. Flood-Obbagy JE, Rolls BJ. The effect of fruit in different forms on energy intake and satiety at a meal. Appetite. 2009;52:416–22.
62. Hulshof T, de Graaf C, Weststrate JA. The effects of preloads varying in physical state and fat-content on satiety and energyintake. Appetite. 1993;21:273–86.
63. Mattes RD, CampbellWW. Effects of food form and timing of ingestion on appetite and energy intake in lean young adults and in young adults with obesity. J Am Diet Assoc. 2009;109:430–7.
64. Mourao DM, Bressan J, Campbell WW, Mattes RD. Effects of food form on appetite and energy intake in lean and obese young adults. Int J Obes. 2007;31:1688–95.
65. Tournier A, Louis-Sylvestre J. Effect of the physical state of a food on subsequent intake in human subjects. Appetite. 1991;16:17–24.
66. Marciani L, Gowland PA, Spiller RC, et al. Gastric response to increased meal viscosity assessed by echo-planar magnetic resonance imaging in humans. J Nutr. 2000;130:122–7.
67. Martens MJI, Westerterp-Plantenga MS. Mode of consumption plays a role in alleviating hunger and thirst. Obesity. 2012;20:517–24.
68. Teff KL. Cephalic phase pancreatic polypeptide responses to liquid and solid stimuli in humans. Physiol Behav. 2010;99:317–23.
69. Teff KL, Devine J, Engelman K. Sweet taste – effect on cephalic phase insulin release in men. Physiol Behav. 1995;57:1089–95.
70. Andrade AM, Kresge DL, Teixeira PJ, Baptista F, Melanson KJ. Does eating slowly influence appetite and energy intake when water intake is controlled? Int J Behav Nutr Phys Act. 2012;9:1479–5868.

71. Kokkinos A, le Roux CW, Alexiadou K, et al. eating slowly increases the postprandial response of the anorexigenic gut hormones, peptide YY and glucagon-like peptide-1. J Clin Endocrinol Metab. 2010;95:333–7.
72. Li J, Zhang N, Hu L, et al. Improvement in chewing activity reduces energy intake in one meal and modulates plasma gut hormone concentrations in obese and lean young Chinese men. Am J Clin Nutr. 2011;94:709–16.
73. Wijlens AGM, Erkner A, Alexander E, Mars M, Smeets PAM, de Graaf C. Effects of oral and gastric stimulation on appetite and energy intake. Obesity. 2012;20:2226–32.
74. McCrickerd K, Chambers L, Yeomans MR. Fluid or fuel? The context of consuming a beverage is important for satiety. PLoS One. 2014;9:e100406.

Choanal Atresia

Rezzan Budak, Cemal Cingi, and Dennis Chua

1 Introduction

Choanal atresia refers to a condition in which the posterior nasal aperture is either completely obliterated or partially obstructed. It is often found in association with anomalous anatomy of the pterygoid processes of the sphenoid and abnormal development of the midface [1].

Choanal atresia occurs congenitally. The posterior nasal apertures become occluded through the growth of osseous or soft tissues or a combination thereof [2, 3]. If the aperture is completely closed at birth, the infant may asphyxiate and perish. As the child attempts to draw breath, the tongue reaches up to the palate and air can then no longer pass through the oral cavity either. The infant's desperate efforts to breathe cause significant retraction of the chest. If there are no facilities to manage the condition, cyanosis and death may supervene. A crying response provides temporary relief, as the airway then becomes patent. Upon cessation of crying, the oral airway again becomes obstructed and asphyxiation restarts [4].

Management of choanal atresia consists of emergency treatment followed by definitive correction as an elective procedure. Bilateral choanal atresia requires emergency intervention, which usually consists of insertion of an artificial airway in

R. Budak (✉)
Department of Otorhinolaryngology, Şehit Sait Ertürk State Hospital, Ankara, Türkiye

C. Cingi
Medical Faculty, Department of Otorhinolaryngology, Eskisehir Osmangazi University, Eskisehir, Türkiye
e-mail: cemal@ogu.edu.tr

D. Chua
Department of Otorhinolaryngology, ENT Surgeons Medical Centre, Mount Elizabeth Hospital, Singapore, Singapore

Ö. N. Şahin et al. (eds.), *Breastfeeding and Metabolic Programming*, https://doi.org/10.1007/978-3-031-33278-4_36

the mouth. This airway prevents the tongue sticking to the palate and preventing airflow. Once the airway is inserted, this usually buys a few weeks' grace to decide on definitive management, since infants usually tolerate it well [4].

2 Epidemiology

2.1 Incidence

The mean incidence of choanal atresia is 0.82 per 10,000 infants. The right is more often affected than the left. Cases occur twice as often unilaterally as bilaterally. The risk in a twin birth is mildly raised. The risk does not depend on the mother's age or the number of previous children she has had. Amongst cases of choanal atresia, 6% also have some form of chromosomal anomaly. In 5% of infants with choanal atresia, a single gene syndrome or condition can be identified [4].

2.2 Ethnic Factors

There is no difference in the incidence of choanal atresia between different ethnic groups [4].

2.3 Sex Differences

There are more girls than boys with choanal atresia, and this difference is statistically significant. It was estimated by Michalski et al. [5] that the ratio of female-to-male cases was 2.2, this estimate being based on evidence from the National Birth Defects Prevention Study (1997–2009).

3 Aetiology

During embryogenesis, the nasal cavity extends in a posterior direction as a result of the processes of the palate fusing in that direction. There is a membrane present at that stage which keeps the oral and nasal cavities separate. The membrane consists of an oral and nasal epithelium fused to each other. This membrane normally recanalises before Day 38, resulting in the formation of the choanae (also termed interior nares). If the membrane remains partially or completely fused, choanal atresia occurs. In a normal infant, the choanae are in fact located more posteriorly than the primordial posterior nares. However, absence of the primordial nares results in choanal atresia and gives an insight into why the abnormal fusion is further forward in the mouth than might otherwise be predicted on the basis of normal infant anatomy [2].

4 Pathogenesis

Although failure of the membrane separating the embryonic nasal and oral cavities to recanalise can partially explain how the condition occurs, it does not explain why the osseous tissues and midface are also abnormal. One possible alternative hypothesis is that abnormal secretion of local growth factors during development means the choanae begin to form, but are undersized or remain imperforate [6]. Indeed, in the majority of cases there is both an osseous and soft tissue component to the obstruction.

The competing hypotheses to account for choanal atresia may be listed as follows [4]:

- Failure of the oropharyngeal membrane to break down.
- Non-rupture of the oronasal membrane.
- The vertical and horizontal palatine processes may overgrow medially.
- There may be adhesions formed in the region where the choanae usually develop. These are pathological and consist of mesoderm.
- Mesodermal cells may grow in the wrong location following abnormal secretion of local factors.

5 Management of Choanal Atresia

The most valuable investigation to assess the extent of choanal atresia is CT imaging. In order to get the clearest scan, the oral cavity should be suctioned to remove accumulated mucus and a decongestant agent administered topically. The aims of imaging are the following [4]:

- Diagnostic confirmation of choanal atresia and the ability to differentiate between uni- and bi-lateral cases.
- Assessment of the extent of the lesion (by measuring how wide the vomer is and how wide an opening is present).
- Exclusion of the possibility that the nose is blocked at a different position.
- Evaluation of the relative osseous, membranous or mixed nature of the lesion.
- Highlighting any anomalies present within the nose or nasopharynx.

6 Presentation

How choanal atresia presents varies according to whether the lesion is uni- or bilateral. Patients who have one-sided atresia often do not present until later, when they experience one-sided rhinorrhoea and nasal blockage. In cases where the lesion is two-sided, the presentation in infancy involves an obstructed upper airway, clearly audible respiration and cyanosis which become more severe whilst feeding, but lessens in severity when crying starts [1].

The work-up should encompass a thorough physical examination, which may reveal further congenital abnormalities. It is possible to get some idea of how patent each choana is by means of a small-diameter feeding tube, but a full assessment necessitates use of flexible fibre optic endoscopy. It has recently been reported how an automatic tympanometer may be used in screening neonates for choanal atresia. As well as being straightforward to apply, this test is stated by the authors to detect 100% of cases where the nasal airway is unobstructed. It is important to remain vigilant, however, so as not to miss a case of two-sided choanal atresia.

The classical presentation of bilateral choanal atresia in a newborn child is a severely blocked airway and cyanosis which recur in a cyclical fashion. If an infant ceases to experience respiratory difficulties when crying, this is a strong indication that the underlying diagnosis is choanal atresia occurring bilaterally. One-sided cases may not come to clinical attention until patients are considerably older and complain of a one-sided discharge from the nose, or one-sided nasal stuffiness [4].

It is common in cases of choanal atresia for there to be an association with narrowing of the nasopharyngeal cavity, a wider vomer than usual, the nasal wall being displaced in a medial direction and arching of the bony palate. In cases where there is no abnormality of the chromosomes, 47% have some other developmental structural anomaly. To confirm whether the associated abnormality is part of a syndrome or is coincidental, the CHARGE acronym may be utilised. Caution may be needed, however, since it may be excessively relied on by clinicians. CHARGE is made up of the following components [4]:

- *C*oloboma affecting the eye (including iris or choroid). Smaller than usual eye size.
- *C*ardiac (*h*eart) anomalies, e.g. atrial septal defect (ASD), with or without a conotruncal disorder.
- *A*tretic choanae.
- *R*etardation in how the child grows and develops.
- *G*enitourinary anomalies, e.g. cryptorchidism, microphallus +/− hydronephrosis.
- Ear abnormalities. The child has auditory impairment. Any part of the three divisions of the ear (outer, middle and inner) may be affected.

It is important to remember that few of the cases of choanal atresia are caused by the CHARGE association.

The frequency with which each component of CHARGE occurs differs [4]. The most frequently occurring features are choanal atresia and learning disability (in 100% and 94%, respectively). Ear abnormalities are also common – 88% of cases, as is retarded growth – 87%. Genital hypoplasia occurs in three quarters (75%) of affected boys. Cardiac abnormality is only found in some 58% of those with CHARGE.

7   Differential Diagnosis

Other diagnoses to consider in cases of suspected choanal atresia are:

- Nasal septal deviation.
- Nasal septal dislocation.
- Haematoma of the septum.
- Oedema affecting nasal mucosae.
- Hypertrophic turbinates.
- Encephalocoele.
- Nasal dermoid.
- Hamartoma.
- Chordoma.
- Teratoma [4].

8   Malformations and Syndromes Occurring in Association with Choanal Atresia

Further congenital anomalies are found in half of patients with one-sided choanal atresia, but 60% of patients where the condition is two-sided [7]. Choanal atresia is sometimes seen in isolation, but it may also be a component of a more wide-reaching syndrome or association of anomalies, such as Treacher Collins, CHARGE (see earlier in this chapter for a full description), Kallmann syndrome or the VACTERL/ VATER association. In the latter condition, there are abnormalities of the vertebrae, the anus is atretic, there are cardiac anomalies, there is a fistulous connection between the trachea and oesophagus (with or without atresia of the oesophagus), renal defects and abnormalities of the radius and other limb abnormalities [8].

Thus, the following are potentially associated features for the clinician to pay attention to [9]:

- Deformity affecting the face, nose or palate.
- Extra digit(s).
- Congenital cardiac conditions.
- Coloboma affecting the iris and retina.

- Learning disability.
- External ear anomalies.
- Atretic oesophagus.
- Premature fusion of the skull bones.
- Fistulous connection between the trachea and oesophagus.
- Meningocoele.

9   Assessment and Diagnosis

Choanal atresia is the likely diagnosis where it is impossible to introduce a 5 or 6 French catheter via the nasal cavity into the oropharynx, which involves a length of more than 32 mm [9]. The flow of air though the nose can also be confirmed by noting how a wisp of cotton wool placed by the nostrils is displaced by the air current or a mirror fogs when expired water vapour condenses on it [7]. Diagnostic confirmation is possible by use of the nasal endoscope (rigid or flexible). This investigation shows either reduced or absent communication between the interior of the nose and the nasopharynx [1].

Computed tomographic imaging can be used for diagnostic confirmation of choanal atresia. A contrast agent is introduced into the nose for this purpose. The appearances are then of a narrowed nasal interior at the level of the pterygoid plate, i.e. posteriorly [1]. Previous reports have mentioned that the atresia was made up of approximately 90% bony and 10% membranous tissue. Computed tomographic imaging and histologic specimens show about 30% pure bone atresia and 70% mixed membranous and bone atresia with no purely membranous anomalies present.

Any infant in whom choanal atresia is diagnosed should also be referred to a cardiac and ophthalmology specialist for an opinion on potential related abnormalities [1].

10   Treatment

The emergency treatment of two-sided choanal atresia in infancy calls for insertion of an airway through the mouth and commencing feeding by gavage. The use of an oral airway, McGovern nipple or intubation are possible options to secure the airway [9].

Definitive surgical intervention may be accomplished by puncture performed transnasally with subsequent stenting or by using an endoscopic technique to resect the posterior portion of the nasal septum. This latter approach is also achieved transnasally and may not require stenting [10, 11]. Since straightforward trans-nasal puncture often results in the choanae reclosing later, it has become a less preferred approach [7, 12]. The use of the nasal endoscope has several benefits, such as providing clear visualisation of the operative field, and this permits careful removal of the atretic plate and vomer, minimising any injury to adjoining tissues [13]. Only if this approach is not feasible or the lesion recurs is the classic transpalatal approach undertaken. However, in all cases, even where the initial operation succeeds, the choanae may subsequently re-stenose.

10.1 Operative Treatment

Management of choanal atresia consists of emergency treatment followed by definitive correction as an elective procedure. Bilateral choanal atresia requires emergency intervention, which usually consists of insertion of an artificial airway in the mouth. This airway prevents the tongue sticking to the palate and preventing airflow. Once the airway is inserted, this usually buys a few weeks' grace to decide on definitive management, since infants usually tolerate it well. There is no single approach to repair that all surgeons agree on. Any case of a neonate with bilateral choanal atresia needs to be rapidly identified and a stable airway provided. Three feasible approaches are intubation, siting an oral airway or a McGovern nipple. Features of an ideal remedial procedure for choanal atresia include restoration of normal intranasal anatomy, no injury to structures which feature in how the face grows, adequate safety, short length of operation and no need for lengthy hospital admission during convalescence.

10.1.1 Procedures

Trans-nasal puncture is now rarely employed, with or without the operating microscope, since it is frequently unsuccessful and calls for further remedial interventions. The explanation for failure was the restricted view of the choanal region, in particular the bridge between the vomer and septum and where the bony lateral boundary narrows. Approaching the lesion transnasally is complicated if the septum is deviated, there is overgrowth of the turbinates or there is rhinorrhoea. It is also more complex in children beyond infancy, since the distance between the nostrils and the posterior choanae enlarges [4].

A transseptal approach calls for creating a window in the nasal septum at a point further forward that the atretic plate [4].

Approaching trans-palatally offers the surgeon easy access to the field and the results are highly successful, but the operation lasts longer. Potential problems with transpalatal repair include increased blood loss, potential for a fistulous connection to form via the palate, incorrect functioning of the palate and disturbance of subsequent maxillofacial development [4].

Use of an endoscope, which may include powered instrumentation, has the advantages of clear views and straightforward removal of osseous choanae. The endoscope may be introduced into the nose or behind the palate [14]. There are reports in the literature about specific surgical instrumentation utilised in cases of choanal atresia, notably the retrograde 110° Sekunda endoscope and protectors made of silicone [15].

Karligkiotis et al. investigated outcomes of endoscopic endonasal surgical repair of choanal atresia by a retrospective review of 84 cases. They concluded this method was both safe and efficacious. Some 96.3% of unilateral cases were successfully managed in this way, while for bilateral cases the figure was 86.2% [16]. Another option is for a two-person surgical team to approach via both the nose and mouth. This is a more straightforward operation and is able to provide sufficiently patent choanae for the patient to start breathing through the nose [17].

Endoscopic approaches continue to benefit from use of microdebrider technology. These instruments allow for a clearer field, and, when handled correctly, produce a lower degree of tissue damage. Nonetheless, surgeons should be aware that microdebriders may cause severe complications, such as inadvertently entering the brain or orbit by breaching certain layers, hence caution may be required.

The use of surgical lasers (especially carbon dioxide and potassium titanyl phosphate) makes surgery more straightforward and briefer, as well as causing lower levels of pain to the patient. Hospital admission for such procedures can be brief and there is the option to repeat a procedure if the first attempt fails. The key advantage is the lack of stenting required. Mitomycin C may be applied to the area around the repair, which is associated with greater patency and a lower incidence of remedial procedures, such as stenting, dilatation or subsequent revisions [2]. The studied by Karligkiotis et al. mentioned earlier [16] used a transnasal approach, removed portions of vomer and created flaps of mucoperiosteum. These features were felt to lessen the likelihood of the lesion re-stenosing. Given the efficacy of this approach, the use of mitomycin C or stenting was not felt necessary [16].

References

1. Isaacson GC. Congenital anomalies of the nose. In: Messner AH, Wilkie L (Eds). UpTodate. Last updated: Jan 10, 2022.
2. Kwong KM. Current updates on choanal atresia. Front Pediatr. 2015;3:52.
3. Andaloro C, La Mantia I. Choanal Atresia. (Updated 2022 May 1). In: StatPearls (Internet). Treasure Island (FL): StatPearls Publishing; 2022 Jan. Available from: https://www.ncbi.nlm. nih.gov/books/NBK507724/
4. Tewfik TL. Choanal Atresia. In: Meyers Ad (Ed). Medscape. Updated: Apr 02, 2021. https:// emedicine.medscape.com/article/872409-overview#a1. Accessed online at 3 July 2022.
5. Michalski AM, Richardson SD, Browne ML, et al. Sex ratios among infants with birth defects, National Birth Defects Prevention Study, 1997-2009. Am J Med Genet A. 2015;167A(5):1071–81.
6. Keller JL, Kacker A. Choanal atresia, CHARGE association, and congenital nasal stenosis. Otolaryngol Clin N Am. 2000;33:1343.
7. Szeremeta W, Parikh TD, Widelitz JS. Congenital nasal malformations. Otolaryngol Clin N Am. 2007;40:97.
8. Burrow TA, Saal HM, de Alarcon A, et al. Characterization of congenital anomalies in individuals with choanal atresia. Arch Otolaryngol Head Neck Surg. 2009;135:543.
9. Myer CM 3rd, Cotton RT. Nasal obstruction in the pediatric patient. Pediatrics. 1983;72:766.

10. Friedman NR, Mitchell RB, Bailey CM, et al. Management and outcome of choanal atresia correction. Int J Pediatr Otorhinolaryngol. 2000;52:45.
11. Cedin AC, Atallah AN, Andriolo RB, et al. Surgery for congenital choanal atresia. Cochrane Database Syst Rev 2012:CD008993.
12. Hengerer AS, Brickman TM, Jeyakumar A. Choanal atresia: embryologic analysis and evolution of treatment, a 30-year experience. Laryngoscope. 2008;118:862.
13. Eladl HM, Khafagy YW. Endoscopic bilateral congenital choanal atresia repair of 112 cases, evolving concept and technical experience. Int J Pediatr Otorhinolaryngol. 2016;85:40.
14. Assanasen P, Metheetrairut C. Choanal atresia. J Med Assoc Thail. 2009;92(5):699–706.
15. Morokhoev VI. (Endonasal surgery of choanal atresia). Vestn Otorinolaringol. 2010:10–5.
16. Karligkiotis A, Farneti P, Gallo S, et al. An Italian multicentre experience in endoscopic endonasal treatment of congenital choanal atresia: proposal for a novel classification system of surgical outcomes. J Craniomaxillofac Surg. 2017;45(6):1018–25.
17. Hassan M, AboEl-Ezz T, Youssef T. Combined transoral-transnasal approach in the repair of congenital posterior choanal atresia: clinical experience. J Otolaryngol Head Neck Surg. 2011;40(3):271–6.

Nasal Toilet in Infants

Ayşe Karaoğullarindan, Nuray Bayar Muluk, and Luisa Maria Bellussi

1 Introduction

Newborns and newborns must depend only on nose breathing; therefore, a healthy nasal passage is essential. Infants with nasal blockage may have feeding difficulties and dyspnea. Nasal saline rinse is an effective treatment for mucus-related nasal blockage [1]. In order to thin mucous, increase mucociliary clearance (MCC), decrease edema, and lessen antigen load in the nasal and sinus canals, it is thought that nasal saline irrigation (NSI) is effective [2, 3].

2 Nasal Saline Usage

Low-volume, high-volume, powered high-pressure, and powered nebulized devices are just a few examples of the many nasal saline delivery options now on the market. Many studies have looked at possible influences on irrigation reaching the paranasal sinuses, such as the size of the incision, the patient's head posture, and the kind of delivery device used [4–9].

Recent research has increased our knowledge of how factors like head position and surgical scope affect NSI distribution. Craig et al. 2017 used a cadaver research

A. Karaoğullarindan (✉)
Department of Otorhinolaryngology, Adana City Hospital, Adana, Türkiye

N. B. Muluk
Faculty of Medicine, Department of Otorhinolaryngology, Kırıkkale University, Kırıkkale, Türkiye

L. M. Bellussi
University of Siena- ENT Clinic, Siena, Italy

© The Author(s), under exclusive license to Springer Nature Switzerland AG 2023
Ö. N. Şahin et al. (eds.), *Breastfeeding and Metabolic Programming*,
https://doi.org/10.1007/978-3-031-33278-4_37

to investigate how head posture affects the ability of irrigation to reach the sphenoid sinuses [5]. By comparing the effectiveness of two positions for administering irrigation to the sphenoid sinuses, it was found that the nose-to-ceiling posture was superior [5]. Consider this option for stubborn sphenoid sinusitis [5]. In a 2017 cadaver research, Halderman et al. looked examined how middle turbinate (MT) excision affected the efficacy of a nasal nebulizer's fluid delivery [6]. Penetrance into the frontal and sphenoid sinuses was shown to rise after partial MT resection, whereas penetrance into all sinuses was found to increase after total MT resection [2, 6].

High-volume, low-pressure tools include NSI squeeze bottles and gravity-fed plant waterers. Users of these goods will need to regularly clean and maintain their own solutions. Squeeze bottles from NSI are a convenient and inexpensive replacement since they are widely available and inexpensive. When comparing high- and low-volume devices, the prevalence of pain, burning, and eustachian tube dysfunction is higher with the former [4]. Nevertheless, low-pressure, high-volume devices are now considered the "gold standard" for nasal saline administration in Chronic Rhinosinusitis (CRS) due to its favorable combination of cheap cost, accessibility, tolerance, and dispersion [2, 7, 10].

3   Nasal Saline Composition

Nasal saline's make-up depends on the tonicity of the sodium chloride used, the minerals and oligo-elements added, and the temperature. Our discussion will not extend to the use of other supplementary additions such as steroids, antibiotics, saccharides, or surfactants. Yet, it's worth noting that NSI is a crucial vehicle for delivering supplementary ingredients, especially off-label, high-dose topical steroids. The optimal composition of nasal saline has been the subject of much laboratory and clinical research. Data from basic science studies reveal that intranasal application of hypertonic saline (HS; >0.9%) reduces intranasal mucosal edema and increases ciliary beat frequency more effectively than other treatments [11]. Unfortunately, there is a dearth of high-quality clinical research comparing the efficacy of HS with isotonic saline (IS; 0.9%) for patients with CRS or postoperative Functional Endoscopic Sinus Surgery (FESS) [12]. Furthermore, HS is connected to more pain and intolerance among patients [13].

Comparing non-diluted IS saltwater solution with diluted IS seawater and standard IS, a 2016 in-vitro research by Bonnomet et al. found that the former more efficiently increased ciliary beat frequency and accelerated wound healing [14]. Moreover, consistent IS impaired epithelial cell functionality [14]. Comparison of the antibacterial activity of nasal secretions exposed to low-salt solution, IS, and HS was conducted by Woods et al. in 2015 [15]. Researchers found that compared to low-salt solution and HS, IS significantly reduced the antibacterial activity of nasal secretions [15].

4   Hygiene

The issue of NSI cleanliness is a vital one that has garnered widespread attention on occasion. To prevent illness, the CDC advises using cooled boiled water (boiling for at least 1 min or 3 min at an elevation >6500 ft.), water that has been microfiltered (1 m pore), or bottled (distilled or sterile) water. The primary amebic meningoencephalitis (PAM) most usually linked with NSI is caused by the thermophilic ameba Naegleria fowleri, which is generally found in warm freshwater [16, 17]. The danger seems to be greatest for young guys who have recently been exposed to freshwater in regions with a warm climate. These amoebas may invade the brain by entering the nasal cavity and then following olfactory nerves to the brain. By 7 days of exposure, neurologic symptoms normally manifest, and death typically occurs within 5 days of clinical presentation [17].

5   Mechanisms

A mucociliary layer borders the sinonasal cavity, shielding the respiratory tracts from dust and other particles in the air. This layer is one of the body's initial lines of defense against foreign organisms and is made up of pseudostratified ciliated columnar epithelial cells and goblet cells drenched in mucus. Ciliary motion then forces the whole mucous layer out of the sinuses and into the nasopharynx, where it has caught invading particles [18, 19]. When the ciliary transport system fails, sinus disorders like rhinosinusitis develop. This may be the result of a virus, bacteria, an allergy, or an irritant [20].

The term "nasal irrigation" refers to the process of using a sterile fluid to cleanse the nasal passages [21]. The solution might also include other medicinal ingredients, such as steroids or antibiotics. Saline, hypertonic solutions (like seawater), and alkaline solutions may all be used for the solution (sodium bicarbonate). Although several research have been conducted on nasal irrigation, the specific mechanism by which it is effective is still up for debate. Potential mechanisms of action of nasal irrigation include the following: [18, 22].

5.1   *Improving the Rate of Ciliary Activity*

The nasal mucus has two layers, a deeper sol layer and a thinner gel layer. Mucus acts as a trap for foreign particles including bacteria, viruses, fungus, and allergies. The pseudostratified columnar epithelium of the nose is where the cilia emerge to move the mucus. The mucus is swept back toward the nasopharynx by the beating cilia, which are more prevalent on the gel layer, and ultimately ingested. Hence, nasal irrigation may have a direct physical influence on ciliary transport of mucus towards the nasopharynx [22]. In order to improve mucociliary clearance, it is necessary to increase the frequency of ciliary beating [18, 23].

5.1.1 Softening Effect on Thick Secretions

With regular use, nasal irrigation may soften and dislodge crusty and viscous secretions from the nasal passages [11]. This may make the thick, persistent discharge less viscous and improve mucus clearance. This theory is supported by a research that showed vigorous nasal irrigation to be more effective than mild nose cleansing [24].

5.1.2 Removal of Inflammatory Mediators

Histamines, prostaglandins, and leukotrienes are only some of the inflammatory mediators that may be found in nasal mucus. It indicates that the concentration of defensins, an inflammatory mediator isolated from nasal mucus, rises in tandem with the severity of the inflammation. When the mucosa of the nasal cavity was stimulated by allergens, this inflammatory response was triggered. So, it stands to reason that nasal irrigation, by eliminating these inflammatory mediators, alleviates the acute symptoms of allergic rhinitis [18, 25].

6 Topical Nasal Saline Applications

In addition to perhaps helping, topical saline is cheap, unlikely to be hazardous, and won't slow healing. Nasal saline irrigation has been shown to reduce nasal secretions, boost mucociliary clearance, and cause vasoconstriction (decongestion) in the short term [26]. Inflammation of the nasal membranes and bleeds are two possible adverse effects [27].

Baby saline nasal drops and a bulb syringe are used to apply the solution topically. Use of a saline nasal spray or saline nasal irrigation (e.g., a squeeze bottle, a neti pot, or a nasal douche) may be appropriate for older children. Nasal irrigation with tap water has been linked to instances of amebic encephalitis; thus, it's crucial that saline irrigants be made from sterile or bottled water [17].

Saline eye drops and nasal sprays low-volume nebulizers (micronized nasal douches) and nasal drops are frequently favored for usage with young children to provide saline to the nose in a tiny amount (less than 5 mL each nostril) [28, 29]. Although high-pressure and high-volume saline may enter the sinuses, evidence shows that nasal sprays successfully reach the nasal cavity [30], which is critical when treating the nasal mucosa [30]. In comparison to low-volume devices, high-volume ones are linked to a higher rate of pain, burning, and eustachian tube dysfunction [2]. It is anticipated that the use of nasal saline sprays will boost compliance because of their simplicity of use, widespread acceptance, and convenience [2, 31]. In the United States, nasal spray was the preferred form of saline nasal irrigation among actively practicing family doctors (78% endorsed it) [32]. Adults and children may respond differently to saline solutions of varying tonicities; research suggests that hypertonic saline (HS) solutions (>0.9% NaCl) are linked with higher symptom improvement and MCC than isotonic saline (IS) solutions (0.9% NaCl) [11, 33, 34]. In addition to its mechanical impact, hypertonicity may alleviate nasal congestion and enhance mucociliary clearance (MCC) by decreasing mucosal oedema owing to osmotic pressure-induced water transfer across the mucosal epithelial membrane [11, 28].

Acute respiratory infections of the nose and throat Use of saline nasal sprays and drops is likely to alleviate symptoms of acute upper respiratory tract infection (URTIs) such the common cold and rhinosinusitis [35]. Faster resolution of nasal secretion and obstruction, as well as decreased usage of nasal decongestants and mucolytic medications, was seen in a trial of 390 children aged 6–10 years with URTI who used IS administered 6 times a day for 3 weeks through fine spray or medium-strength jet. There were no major side effects observed, and any that did occur were related to the jet's increased flow rate rather than the nasal saline solution or spray [36]. Baby nasal drops might be more convenient than nasal sprays for parents to use. Daily use of HS or IS nasal drops, with and without nasal aspirator usage, has been found in studies in children under 2 years old with URTI symptoms to substantially improve nasal symptoms compared to baseline or no therapy [37, 38], resulting in improvements in eating and sleeping [38]. Around 20% of children under the age of 5 will get an ear infection as a result of a normal cold, making it imperative that parents take preventative measures, including as providing their children with IS nasal drops and encouraging them to regularly aspirate their mucus [39]. No significant difference in respiratory symptoms was observed between normal saline drops, phenylephrine drops, or no treatment after 2 days in a small randomized controlled trial of infants aged 3 weeks to 2 years with URTI; a similar number of infants did not tolerate saline or phenylephrine drops [28, 40].

References

1. Mensink MHA, Wieringa N, Videler W, Klok T. Neustoilet bij zuigelingen met rinitis (Nasal toilet in infants with rhinitis: nasal passage crucial, so treat with xylometazoline). Ned Tijdschr Geneeskd. 2022;166:D6606. Dutch
2. Succar EF, Turner JH, Chandra RK. Nasal saline irrigation: a clinical update. Int Forum Allergy Rhinol. 2019;9(S1):S4–8. https://doi.org/10.1002/alr.22330.
3. Orlandi RR, Kingdom TT, Hwang PH. International Consensus Statement on Allergy and Rhinology: rhinosinusitis executive summary. Int Forum Allergy Rhinol. 2016;6(suppl 1):S3–S21.
4. Thomas WW 3rd, Harvey RJ, Rudmik L, Hwang PH, Schlosser RJ. Distribution of topical agents to the paranasal sinuses: an evidence-based review with recommendations. Int Forum Allergy Rhinol. 2013;3:691–703.

5. Craig JR, Palmer JN, Zhao K. Computational fluid dynamic modeling of nose-to-ceiling head positioning for sphenoid sinus irrigation. Int Forum Allergy Rhinol. 2017;7:474–9.
6. Halderman AA, Stokken J, Sindwani R. The effect of middle turbinate resection on topical drug distribution into the paranasal sinuses. Int Forum Allergy Rhinol. 2016;6:1056–61.
7. Abadie WM, McMains KC, Weitzel EK. Irrigation penetration of nasal delivery systems: a cadaver study. Int Forum Allergy Rhinol. 2011;1:46–9.
8. Chen PG, Murphy J, Alloju LM, Boase S, Wormald PJ. Sinus penetration of a pulsating device versus the classic squeeze bottle in cadavers undergoing sinus surgery. Ann Otol Rhinol Laryngol. 2017;126:9–13.
9. Manes RP, Tong L, Batra PS. Prospective evaluation of aerosol delivery by a powered nasal nebulizer in the cadaver model. Int Forum Allergy Rhinol. 2011;1:366–71.
10. Wormald PJ, Cain T, Oates L, Hawke L, Wong I. A comparative study of three methods of nasal irriga-tion. Laryngoscope. 2004;114:2224–7.
11. Talbot AR, Herr TM, Parsons DS. Mucociliary clearance and buffered hypertonic saline solution. Laryngoscope. 1997;107:500–3.
12. Chong LY, Head K, Hopkins C, et al. Saline irriga-tion for chronic rhinosinusitis. Cochrane Database Syst Rev. 2016;4:CD011995.
13. Kanjanawasee D, Seresirikachorn K, Chitsuthipakorn W, Snidvongs K. Hypertonic saline versus isotonicsaline nasal irrigation: systematic review and meta-analysis. Am J Rhinol Allergy. 2018;32:269–79.
14. Bonnomet A, Luczka E, Coraux C, de Gabory L. Non-diluted seawater enhances nasal ciliary beat frequency and wound repair speed compared to diluted sea-water and normal saline. Int Forum Allergy Rhinol. 2016;6:1062–8.
15. Woods CM, Tan S, Ullah S, Frauenfelder C, Ooi EH, Carney AS. The effect of nasal irrigation formulation on the antimicrobial activity of nasal secretions. Int Forum Allergy Rhinol. 2015;5:1104–10.
16. Piper KJ, Foster H, Susanto D, Maree CL, Thornton SD, Cobbs CS. Fatal Balamuthia mandrillaris brain infection associated with improper nasal lavage. Int J Infect Dis. 2018;77:18–22.
17. Yoder JS, Straif-Bourgeois S, Roy SL, et al. Primary amebic meningoencephalitis deaths associated with sinus irrigation using contaminated tap water. Clin Infect Dis. 2012;55:e79–85.
18. Abdullah B, Periasamy C, Ismail R. Nasal irrigation as treatment in sinonasal symptoms relief: a review of its efficacy and clinical applications. Indian J Otolaryngol Head Neck Surg. 2019;71(Suppl 3):1718–26. https://doi.org/10.1007/s12070-017-1070-0. Epub 2017 Jan 13
19. Cole P. Physiology of the nose and paranasal sinuses. Clin Rev Allergy Immunol. 1998;16(1):25–54.
20. Osguthorpe JD, Hadley JA. Rhinosinusitis: current concepts in evaluation and management. Med Clin North Am. 1999;83(1):27–41.
21. Papsin B, McTavish A. Saline nasal irrigation: its role as an adjunct treatment. Can Fam Physician. 2003;49:168–73.
22. Brown CL, Graham SM. Nasal irrigations: good or bad? Curr Opin Otolaryngol Head Neck Surg. 2004;12(1):9–13.
23. Boek WM, Graamans K, Natzijl H, van Rijk PP, Huizing EH. Nasal mucociliary transport: new evidence for a key role of ciliary beat frequency. Laryngoscope. 2002;112(3):570–3.
24. Seppey M, Schweri T, Hausler R. Comparative randomised clinical study of tolerability and efficacy of Rhinomer Force 3 versus a reference product in post-operative care of the nasal fossae after endonasal surgery. ORL J Otorhinolaryngol Relat Spec. 1996;58(2):87–92.
25. Georgitis JW. Nasal hyperthermia and simple irrigation for perennial rhinitis. Chest. 1994;106(5):1487–92.
26. Achilles N, Mösges R. Nasal saline irrigations for the symptoms of acute and chronic rhinosinusitis. Curr Allergy Asthma Rep. 2013;13:229.
27. Pappas DE. The common cold in children: management and prevention. In: Edwards MS, Torchia MM (Eds). UpToDate. Last updated: Apr 25, 2022.

28. Santorol E, Kalita P, Novak P. The role of saline nasal sprays or drops in nasal hygiene: a review of the evidence and clinical perspectives. Rhinology Online. 2021;4:1–16.
29. Head K, Snidvongs K, Glew S, Scadding G, Schilder AG, Philpott C, et al. Saline irrigation for allergic rhinitis. Cochrane Database Syst Rev. 2018;6:CD012597.
30. Wormald PJ, Cain T, Oates L, Hawke L, Wong I. A comparative study of three methods of nasal irrigation. Laryngoscope. 2004;114(12):2224–7.
31. Gutierrez-Cardona N, Sands P, Roberts G, Lucas JS, Walker W, Salib R, et al. The acceptability and tolerability of nasal douching in children with allergic rhinitis: a systematic review. Int J Pediatr Otorhinolaryngol. 2017;98:126–35.
32. Rabago D, Zgierska A, Peppard P, Bamber A. The prescribing patterns of Wisconsin family physicians surrounding saline nasal irrigation for upper respiratory conditions. WMJ. 2009;108(3):145–50.
33. Li CL, Lin HC, Lin CY, Hsu TF. Effectiveness of hypertonic saline nasal irrigation for alleviating allergic rhinitis in children: a systematic review and meta-analysis. J Clin Med. 2019;8(1):64.
34. Cordray S, Harjo JB, Miner L. Comparison of intranasal hypertonic Dead Sea saline spray and intranasal aqueous triamcinolone spray in seasonal allergic rhinitis. Ear Nose Throat J. 2005;84(7):426–30.
35. King D, Mitchell B, Williams CP, Spurling GK. Saline nasal irrigation for acute upper respiratory tract infections. Cochrane Database Syst Rev. 2015;4:CD006821.
36. Slapak I, Skoupa J, Strnad P, Hornik P. Efficacy of isotonic nasal wash (seawater) in the treatment and prevention of rhinitis in children. Arch Otolaryngol Head Neck Surg. 2008;134(1):67–74.
37. Montanari G, Ceschin F, Masotti S, Bravi F, Chinea B, Quartarone G. Observational study on the performance of the Narhinel method (nasal aspirator and physiological saline solution) versus physiological saline solution in the prevention of recurrences of viral rhinitis and associated complications of the upper respiratory tract infections (URTI), with a special focus on acute rhinosinusitis and acute otitis of the middle ear. Minerva Pediatr. 2010;62(1):9–16. 17–21
38. Koksal T, Cizmeci MN, Bozkaya D, Kanburoglu MK, Sahin S, Tas T, et al. Comparison between the use of saline and seawater for nasal obstruction in children under 2 years of age with acute upper respiratory infection. Turk J Med Sci. 2016;46(4):1004–13.
39. National Institute for Health and Care Excellence. Clinical Knowledge Summary: Common Cold 2016 (cited 2020 June). Available from: https://cks.nice.org.uk/common-cold.
40. Bollag U, Albrecht E, Wingert W. Medicated versus saline nose drops in the management of upper respiratory infection. Helv Paediatr Acta. 1984;39(4):341–5.

Newborn Nasal Congestion

Tarik Yagci, Riza Dundar, and Nuray Bayar Muluk

1 Introduction

Infections, especially those of a viral nature, and allergies are the most prevalent causes of nasal blockage and runny nose in babies and children. Nasal obstruction is often associated with viral upper respiratory tract infections (URTI) in newborns and babies. Nasal saline irrigation is thought to aid with URTI symptoms by clearing out any extra mucus, decreasing congestion, and allowing for easier breathing. According to the available research, nasal saline irrigation is very effective in relieving the symptoms of allergic rhinitis and acute sinusitis in children. Little information is recorded on the use of medical equipment. As compared to a control group treated with physiological saline solution alone, patients who underwent nasal aspiration with a medical device while experiencing viral rhinitis had a significantly reduced chance of developing acute otitis media and rhinosinusitis [1].

2 Acute Bacterial Rhinosinusitis (ABRS)

Children often have acute bacterial rhinosinusitis (ABRS). Secondary ABRS is thought to occur in between 6 and 9% of children with viral upper respiratory infections [2–7].

While though ABRS most often affects kids between the ages of 4 and 7, it may happen to kids as young as 1 year old (complications of ethmoid sinusitis

T. Yagci (✉) · R. Dundar
Medical Faculty, Department of Otorhinolaryngology, Bilecik Seyb Edebali University, Bilecik, Türkiye

N. B. Muluk
Medical Faculty, Department of Otorhinolaryngology, Kirikkale University, Kirikkale, Türkiye

Ö. N. Şahin et al. (eds.), *Breastfeeding and Metabolic Programming*,
https://doi.org/10.1007/978-3-031-33278-4_38

occasionally are observed in infants). Children less than 2 years of age are at lower risk of developing ABRS than older children. There are two main reasons why ABRS is less common in younger children. If an antibiotic is used to treat acute otitis media (AOM) in a young kid, the virus cannot progress to acute bacterial respiratory syndrome (ABRS). The second benefit is that there is less of a chance of a blockage occurring since the sinus ostia are bigger (compared to the body of the sinus) in younger children [2].

2.1 Pathogenesis

Most of the time, the paranasal sinuses are free of infection [8–10]. The membranes lining the nose are continuous with the membranes lining the sinus canals; therefore, they may be contaminated with germs that inhabit the nasal mucosa and nasopharynx. In most cases, mucociliary clearance is sufficient to eliminate the offending germs [11]. Changes in mucociliary clearance may allow vast numbers of germs into the sinuses, leading to illness. Conditions that influence mucociliary clearance include injury to the ciliary epithelium, changes in the number or function of cilia, changes in mucus production, viscosity, or ostia patency (e.g., upper respiratory infections, allergic rhinitis) [2, 12–14].

2.1.1 Predisposing Factors

Acute bacterial rhinosinusitis (ABRS) is most often associated with a history of viral upper respiratory infection (URI) [5, 7, 15]. Children who spend time in day care have a higher chance of contracting a viral URI [16]. Children who acquired ABRS had three times as many URIs per year as children who did not (compared to the control group's one URI per year). This was found in a study of 237 children aged 48–96 months who were observed for a year [7]. Sinusitis is a common complication of URIs, and respiratory syncytial virus has been found more often than other respiratory viruses in these cases. Several sections are devoted to the epidemiology of viral URI and its clinical symptoms [2].

3 Allergic Rhinitis

An immunoglobulin E (IgE)-mediated response to numerous indoor and outdoor allergens causes allergic rhinitis, which often manifests in early infancy. When an allergen that the body has already identified and processed to produce IgE is reintroduced, it triggers an IgE-mediated response. When two IgEs on the same mast cell bind to the same antigen, degranulation of the mast cell and the subsequent response are triggered. By degranulating, mediators including histamines and leukotrienes are released. It is the nasal passages that respond in the case of allergic rhinitis. To put it simply, the response is the same for every allergic reaction. Allergy rhinitis may develop sensitivity to indoor allergens in children older than 2 years old, whereas outdoor allergen sensitization is more typical in children aged 4–6 years. Developing a clinically significant allergy to indoor allergens is uncommon in children less than 2 years of age. False-positive results are more prevalent in infants and toddlers because of atopic dermatitis. Dust mites, pet dander, cockroaches, molds, and pollens are some of the most prevalent allergens found indoors [17].

3.1 Symptoms and Signs

In most cases, a patient's history of allergic rhinitis will be simple; however, they may have a more complicated presentation of symptoms in other cases. Patients who have just gotten a pet or who have noticeable changes in their symptoms throughout the year make for an easy diagnosis. If the patient is younger, they may come with a different set of symptoms; for example, the family may not understand the child's discomfort with the persistent stuffiness of his or her nose. Since pet dander is shed in the spring and reaccumulates in the autumn, a young kid may seem to have seasonal allergies when, in reality, the allergy is to pets. Symptoms may have been present for years in older children, and the kid may have learned to live with them. Symptoms of an upper respiratory disease might match those of allergies, leading patients to incorrectly believe they have an allergy. As rhinovirus activity increases in the autumn, this is particularly the case [17].

Allergic rhinitis in children may manifest itself in a variety of ways [17].

Symptoms of a cold or flu:

- Rhinitis, stuffy nose, and runny nose with postnasal drip
- Turbinates in the nose that are pale, with or without watery discharge

    - Sneezing again and over again
    - Palate, nostril, ocular, or eye itching

- Snoring

    - Frequent throat pain
    - Coughing and throat clearing all the time

- Headaches

4 Congenital Anomalies

4.1 Nasal Encephaloceles

Nasal encephaloceles, like nasal dermoids, are the end outcome of fusion problems at the nasal base throughout development. Brain, meninges, and/or cerebrospinal fluid may herniate through a nasal encephalocele and into the nasal cavity [1]. They have open lines of communication with the subarachnoid space and the ventricular system inside the brain. A failure in the anterior neuropore's closing during the fourth week of embryogenesis is assumed to be the root cause of this disorder, which affects around 1 in 4000 infants [18, 19].

Frontoethmoidal (common) and basal (less common) encephaloceles of the nose each account for 60 and 10%, respectively [19, 20]. Those born with frontoethmoidal cephaloceles will likely notice a skinned bump at their nose's nasopharynx. As a baby screams or strains, lesions that are still communicating with the subarachnoid space grow. Externally, a basal cephalocele is not noticeable. Symptoms of a herniated base or nasal blockage are a possible result [20–22].

Correction of nasal cephaloceles with surgery enhances appearance and reduces the likelihood of contracting meningitis [23]. The frontal craniotomy is the standard procedure for treating cephaloceles. When the dural defect has been sealed and the soft tissues and nose have been transected of any dysplastic tissue, only then can the nose be worked on [24]. It is conceivable, and maybe less morbid, to access small lesions in the skull base via the nasal passages [25, 26].

4.2 Nasal Gliomas

Nasal gliomas are ectopic glial tumors that develop in utero and are benign [27, 28]. It is believed that an issue with the anterior neuropore closure leads to their emergence. Nasal blockage is often caused by these lesions, which originate in the side of the nose [22]. They tend to show up close to the base of the skull and have unique CT and MRI characteristics that help distinguish them from nasal dermoids, polyps, encephaloceles, and hemangiomas [19, 21, 29]. The nature of the lesion should be established by computed tomography and magnetic resonance imaging before any biopsy or surgical excision is undertaken [19]. The most effective therapy is surgical removal [22]. A delay in treatment may result in infection and/or a change in the nasal bone and/or septum [25].

4.3 Choanal Atresia

As its name implies, choanal atresia is a condition in which the nasal cavity's back passageway is completely closed up. Bone abnormalities of the pterygoid plates and midfacial development abnormalities are often seen in patients with choanal atresia [25].

4.3.1 Pathogenesis

Choanal atresia may have its roots in the failure of the nose and the oropharynx to fuse due to the persistence of the oronasal membrane. The anomalies in the bones and midface that are often seen with this disorder are not addressed by this explanation. Little or imperforate choanae may also be the consequence of changes in local growth factors [30]. Occlusion caused by bone and membranous blockage occurs most often and may be severe [25].

4.3.2 Incidence

Just around 1 in every 7000 newborns is born with choanal atresia [19]. Girls are more likely to be affected than males [31]. Almost two-thirds of all instances involve just one party [32, 33].

4.3.3 Presentation

Choanal atresia may manifest itself in a variety of ways, depending on whether or not both airways are affected. Unilateral nasal obstruction and/or discharge is a common symptom of unilateral choanal atresia in adults. Upper airway blockage, loud breathing, or cyanosis that increases while feeding and lessens when the newborn cries are common symptoms of bilateral choanal atresia in infants [25].

4.3.4 Concomitant Congenital Malformations and Syndromes

Fifty percent and sixty percent of people with unilateral and bilateral choanal atresia, respectively, also have other congenital abnormalities [32]. Multiple congenital anomaly syndromes, such as Treacher Collins, CHARGE (coloboma of the iris or choroid, heart defect, atresia of the choanae, retarded growth and development, genitourinary abnormalities, and ear defects with associated deafness), Kallmann, VACTERL/VATER association (vertebral anomalies, anal atresia, cardiac defects, tracheoe [25, 34].

4.4 Abnormalities of the Nasal Septum

Nasal septal deformities may be present at birth. They may occur alone or in tandem with other congenital midface defects as cleft lip and palate [35]. Some researchers believe that regular vaginal births, as opposed to cesarean sections, are more likely to cause anterior deviations in an otherwise well-formed nasal septum due to effects of intrauterine pressure or intrapartum trauma [36].

The decision to do surgery to correct a congenital nasal septal deformity and when to do so are surrounded by much disagreement [37]. When a person is young, the nasal septum is a primary site of development for the middle face [38]. Maxillary hypoplasia has been linked to disturbance of this growth center in both animal studies [39] and longitudinal clinical observations. Based on this knowledge, any necessary remedial surgery should seek to cause as little interference with normal development centers as possible [25].

Nasal tip deviations caused by intrapartum pressure effects may correct themselves after delivery. Infants are obligatory nasal breathers; therefore, serious malformations in the nasal septum might potentially restrict their upper airway. Surgery to fix the issue may be required as early as the newborn's first few weeks of life. The nasal septum may be repositioned on the maxillary crest by intranasal stenting or surgical manipulation of the septal cartilage. In extreme circumstances, some writers have advocated for a conservative septoplasty in which cracked or malformed cartilages are removed [25, 40].

5 Conclusion

Infections, especially those of a viral nature, and allergies are the most prevalent causes of nasal blockage and runny noses in babies and children. Choanal atresia, nasal encephaloceles, gliomas, and abnormalities of the nasal septum are also kept in mind in newborn nasal problems.

References

1. Chirico G, Quartarone G, Mallefet P. Nasal congestion in infants and children: a literature review on efficacy and safety of non-pharmacological treatments. Minerva Pediatr. 2014;66(6):549–57.
2. Wald ER. Acute bacterial rhinosinusitis in children: clinical features and diagnosis. In: Kaplan SL, Wood RA, Isaacson GC, Torchia MM, editors. UpToDate; 2022. Last updated 11 Nov 2022.
3. Wald ER, Nash D, Eickhoff J. Effectiveness of amoxicillin/clavulanate potassium in the treatment of acute bacterial sinusitis in children. Pediatrics. 2009;124:9.
4. Wald ER, Guerra N, Byers C. Upper respiratory tract infections in young children: duration of and frequency of complications. Pediatrics. 1991;87:129.
5. DeMuri GP, Gern JE, Moyer SC, et al. Clinical features, virus identification, and sinusitis as a complication of upper respiratory tract illness in children ages 4-7 years. J Pediatr. 2016;171:133.
6. Marom T, Alvarez-Fernandez PE, Jennings K, et al. Acute bacterial sinusitis complicating viral upper respiratory tract infection in young children. Pediatr Infect Dis J. 2014;33:803.
7. DeMuri GP, Eickhoff JC, Gern JC, Wald ER. Clinical and virological characteristics of acute sinusitis in children. Clin Infect Dis. 2019;69:1764.
8. Arruda LK, Mimica IM, Solé D, et al. Abnormal maxillary sinus radiographs in children: do they represent bacterial infection? Pediatrics. 1990;85:553.

9. Evans FO Jr, Sydnor JB, Moore WE, et al. Sinusitis of the maxillary antrum. N Engl J Med. 1975;293:735.
10. Shapiro ED, Wald ER, Doyle W, Rohn D. Bacteriology of the maxillary sinus of rhesus monkeys. Ann Otol Rhinol Laryngol. 1982;91:150.
11. Cherry JD, Kuan EC, Shapiro NL. Rhinosinusitis. In: Feigin and Cherry's textbook of pediatric infectious diseases, 8th ed, Cherry JD, Harrison G, Kaplan SL, et al (Eds), Elsevier, Philadelphia 2018. p.137.
12. Carson JL, Collier AM, Hu SS. Acquired ciliary defects in nasal epithelium of children with acute viral upper respiratory infections. N Engl J Med. 1985;312:463.
13. Manning SC. Pediatric sinusitis. Otolaryngol Clin North Am. 1993;26:623.
14. Shapiro GG. The role of nasal airway obstruction in sinus disease and facial development. J Allergy Clin Immunol. 1988;82:935.
15. Revai K, Dobbs LA, Nair S, et al. Incidence of acute otitis media and sinusitis complicating upper respiratory tract infection: the effect of age. Pediatrics. 2007;119:e1408.
16. Wald ER, Dashefsky B, Byers C, et al. Frequency and severity of infections in day care. J Pediatr. 1988;112:540.
17. Becker JM. Pediatric allergic rhinitis. In: Jyonouchi H, editor. Medscape; 2023. Updated 14 Feb 2023. https://emedicine.medscape.com/article/889259-overview. Accessed 23 Feb 2023.
18. Saettele M, Alexander A, Markovich B, et al. Congenital midline nasofrontal masses. Pediatr Radiol. 2012;42:1119.
19. Myer CM 3rd, Cotton RT. Nasal obstruction in the pediatric patient. Pediatrics. 1983;72:766.
20. Hoving EW. Nasal encephaloceles. Childs Nerv Syst. 2000;16:702.
21. Levine MR, Kellis A, Lash R. Nasal glioma masquerading as a capillary hemangioma. Ophthal Plast Reconstr Surg. 1993;9:132.
22. Rahbar R, Resto VA, Robson CD, et al. Nasal glioma and encephalocele: diagnosis and management. Laryngoscope. 2003;113:2069.
23. Izquierdo JM, Gil-Carcedo LM. Recurrent meningitis and transethmoidal intranasal meningoencephalocele. Dev Med Child Neurol. 1988;30:248.
24. Turgut M, Ozcan OE, Benli K, et al. Congenital nasal encephalocele: a review of 35 cases. J Craniomaxillofac Surg. 1995;23:1.
25. Isaacson GC. Congenital anomalies of the nose. In: Messner AH, Wilkie L, editors. UpToDate; 2022. Last updated 10 Jan 2022.
26. Mohindra S, Mohindra S, Mahendru S, Patil NR. Endoscopic management of congenital nasal meningoencephaloceles: a short series of 15 paediatric cases. Childs Nerv Syst. 2020;36:3059.
27. Chang KC, Leu YS. Nasal glioma: a case report. Ear Nose Throat J. 2001;80:410.
28. Puppala B, Mangurten HH, McFadden J, et al. Nasal glioma. Presenting as neonatal respiratory distress. Definition of the tumor mass by MRI. Clin Pediatr (Phila). 1990;29:49.
29. Hoeger PH, Schaefer H, Ussmueller J, Helmke K. Nasal glioma presenting as capillary haemangioma. Eur J Pediatr. 2001;160:84.
30. Keller JL, Kacker A. Choanal atresia, CHARGE association, and congenital nasal stenosis. Otolaryngol Clin North Am. 2000;33:1343.
31. Lee WT, Koltai PJ. Nasal deformity in neonates and young children. Pediatr Clin North Am. 2003;50:459.
32. Szeremeta W, Parikh TD, Widelitz JS. Congenital nasal malformations. Otolaryngol Clin North Am. 2007;40:97.
33. Hengerer AS, Brickman TM, Jeyakumar A. Choanal atresia: embryologic analysis and evolution of treatment, a 30-year experience. Laryngoscope. 2008;118:862.
34. Burrow TA, Saal HM, de Alarcon A, et al. Characterization of congenital anomalies in individuals with choanal atresia. Arch Otolaryngol Head Neck Surg. 2009;135:543.
35. Yoon YJ, Perkiomaki MR, Tallents RH, et al. Association of nasomaxillary asymmetry in children with unilateral cleft lip and palate and their parents. Cleft Palate Craniofac J. 2003;40:493.

36. Alpini D, Corti A, Brusa E, Bini A. Septal deviation in newborn infants. Int J Pediatr Otorhinolaryngol. 1986;11:103.
37. Béjar I, Farkas LG, Messner AH, Crysdale WS. Nasal growth after external septoplasty in children. Arch Otolaryngol Head Neck Surg. 1996;122:816.
38. Grymer LF, Bosch C. The nasal septum and the development of the midface. A longitudinal study of a pair of monozygotic twins. Rhinology. 1997;35:6.
39. Meeuwis J, Verwoerd-Verhoef HL, Verwoerd CD. Normal and abnormal nasal growth after partial submucous resection of the cartilaginous septum. Acta Otolaryngol. 1993;113:379.
40. Emami AJ, Brodsky L, Pizzuto M. Neonatal septoplasty: case report and review of the literature. Int J Pediatr Otorhinolaryngol. 1996;35:271.

Newborn Epistaxis

Aykut Ceyhan, Nuray Bayar Muluk, and Desiderio Passali

1 Introduction

Epistaxis in infants under 2 years of age requires particular treatment, even though emergency doctors see patients with this symptom on a regular basis. Epistaxis is uncommon in this age range and may indicate a serious underlying etiology, such as severe systemic illness or nonaccidental trauma [1]. Thus, it is vital to examine the assessment and treatment of epistaxis in this age range [2].

2 Epidemiology

Epistaxis was responsible for 450,000 emergency department (ED) visits in the United States during a 10-year period, with maxima in the pediatric and elderly age categories [3]. Pediatric epistaxis is most prevalent in children between 3 and 8 years, with up to 60% of children suffering an episode before the age of 10 years [4]. Epistaxis, on the other hand, is uncommon in newborns and young children under 2 years old [1]. Epistaxis was seen in 15.9 instances of children under 2 in general practice [5]. Nonetheless, the incidence of epistaxis in the ED ranges from

A. Ceyhan (✉)
Department of Otorhinolaryngology, Kutahya Evliya Çelebi Training and Research Hospital, Kutahya, Türkiye

N. B. Muluk
Faculty of Medicine, Department of Otorhinolaryngology, Kırıkkale University, Kırıkkale, Türkiye

D. Passali
Department of Medical, Surgical and Neuroscience Sciences, and Department of Otorhinolaryngology, Univerity of Siena, Siena, Italy

Ö. N. Şahin et al. (eds.), *Breastfeeding and Metabolic Programming*, https://doi.org/10.1007/978-3-031-33278-4_39

2.1 to 10.4 instances per 10,000 children, with younger children (1.19–1.9 cases per 10,000 children) experiencing it less often [1, 6–8].

Epistaxis is a frequent pediatric complaint that affects around 30% of children aged 0 to 5 years and more than 50% of children beyond the age of 5 years [9–11]. The incidence of epistaxis decreases with age, although nearly half of all people with epistaxis had nosebleeds as children [12]. Epistaxis accounts for over 250,000 visits in the United States each year [13, 14]. Typically, the median age of presentation is between 7 and 8 years old (10). Epistaxis is uncommon in infants and toddlers (about 1 per 10,000) and should prompt evaluation of trauma (deliberate or accidental) or severe disease (e.g., thrombocytopenia). Epistaxis in a newborn baby without a logical cause might indicate child abuse [9].

3 Etiology

The etiology of epistaxis in newborns and young children is poorly understood due to its rarity [8]. Other local causes of epistaxis in children and adolescents include allergies, upper respiratory tract infections (URI), and medications/ drugs such as decongestants or cocaine, though pediatric epistaxis is typically a benign condition caused by dry nasal mucosa and minor trauma to the anterior septum [15, 16]. Severe or repeated epistaxis in children and teenagers should raise the possibility of a more severe underlying etiology, such as a nasopharyngeal tumor, a bleeding problem, or a vascular anomaly [16]. In contrast, the first occurrence of epistaxis in babies may indicate a serious systemic condition [17]. Infants also have URI, clotting problems, and trauma in their differential diagnosis. For example, a 10-year retrospective record analysis of 77,173 ED visits and 58,059 hospitalizations for patients 2 years of age revealed 16 incidences of epistaxis. The majority ($n = 8$) were linked to trauma, whereas 4 had thrombocytopenia, 2 had an upper respiratory infection, and 2 had an apparent life-threatening incident [1]. In a population-based study of newborns brought to the hospital with epistaxis, 36 cases were found during a 6-year period. Twenty-three of these patients had a known cause, including trauma ($n = 5$), coagulation disease ($n = 4$), congenital abnormality ($n = 2$), acute rhinitis ($n = 11$), and suffocation ($n = 1$) [8].

Epistaxis in children under 10 years of age is often minor, starts in the anterior nostril, and does not normally need cautery or packing to prevent bleeding (10). For the rare situation when cautery or packing is necessary, hospitalization is rarely recommended unless the kid has a significant underlying reason (i.e., local tumor, bleeding condition, or cancer) [9, 18].

3.1 Local Causes

In children who have epistaxis, injuries to the septum as a result of picking their noses are common but usually go unnoticed. This is because picking one's nose may cause bleeding within the nose. It is important to frequently inquire about the frequency of nose picking with both patients and their parents or main caregivers [9].

"Facial and Head Trauma" blunt facial trauma that leads to nasal fractures is most commonly caused by automobile accidents, sports injuries, intentional injuries, and home injuries and may result in significant bleeding. These types of injuries can also occur as a result of other types of head trauma [19]. After mid-face trauma, bone fragments have the potential to lacerate the anterior ethmoidal artery. This is because the anterior ethmoidal artery enters the nasal cavity via the delicate lamina papyracea of the ethmoid bone.

The presence of massive epistaxis after a head injury is indicative of an internal carotid pseudoaneurysm [20], but this condition may also present initially with moderate epistaxis or with recurring epistaxis that does not respond to conservative therapy and may occur weeks after the injury [20–26]. After a severe illness in the deep spaces of the neck, a youngster was found to have a pseudoaneurysm of the internal carotid artery in the cervical region [27]. Blunt head trauma may also result in carotid-cavernous sinus fistulae, which can then lead to cerebral bleeding, cranial nerve palsy, and stroke. Carotid-cavernous sinus fistulae can also cause blindness [28].

When epistaxis occurs on one side alone and is accompanied by foul-smelling nasal discharge, the presence of a foreign body must be presumptively diagnosed as present until it can be shown otherwise. Mucosal irritation, laceration, and/or ulceration may be caused by the foreign body. If the foreign material has been stuck in the nose for a very short amount of time (minutes to hours), the nosebleed may have been caused by the patient or the parent's effort to remove the foreign body. When a foreign body has been lodged in the nose for many days, the mucus-filled outflow from the nose will often have a bloody appearance. The floor of the nose, just below the inferior turbinate, is the area in which foreign things in the nose are most often discovered. Beads, rubber erasers, paper wads, pebbles, marbles, beans, peas, almonds, sponges, and chalk are some examples of common foreign things that may be found in the nose. But, button batteries are a more hazardous kind of nasal foreign body that may cause epistaxis. This condition is far less prevalent. They need to be removed very once in order to avoid necrosis of the surrounding tissue, permanent rupture of the septum, or a saddle nose deformity [9].

Patients who have an upper respiratory infection or an allergy may get epistaxis as a result of barotrauma, which may occur while scuba diving [9].

Changes in humidity, viral or bacterial upper respiratory infections, chronic rhinitis with frequent nose blowing and increased vascularity and friability of the nasal mucosa, chronic use of nasal sprays or drying agents, intentional or unintentional exposure to irritant inhalants or substances of abuse (for example, tobacco smoke, cocaine, heroin, volatile vapors), and chronic uveitis are all potential triggers for nasal mucosal irritation [9].

Upper respiratory infections caused by viruses and bacteria, such as sinusitis and systemic diseases that are accompanied by nasal congestion, cause inflammation of the nasal mucosa, which increases the risk of bleeding. It would suggest that nasal colonization with *Staphylococcus aureus* has a significant role in the development of the mucosal irritation that is associated with epistaxis in children [29]. In one research, *S. aureus* was cultured from the anterior nasal cavities of 24 of 42 (57%) children who had epistaxis, but only 6 of 19 (24%) children who had no history of nasal bleeding had *S. aureus* cultured from their nasal cavities [30].

Epistaxis may also be caused by skin infections that are localized, such as staphylococcal furuncles. Rare, persistent granulomatous infections such as nasal tuberculosis are granulomatous infections that may lead to nasal blockage and epistaxis [31]. Epistaxis is one of the most prevalent spontaneous bleeding symptoms of dengue hemorrhagic fever in children, occurring in 25% of kids who have been afflicted by the disease [32–34].

Neoplasms of the nasal cavity, also known as tumors, are often the source of unilateral symptoms in patients. These symptoms may include intermittent epistaxis, foul discharge, nasal obstruction, or a change in the sense of smell. Those who have vascular tumors like juvenile nasopharyngeal angiofibroma are more likely to have severe bleeding than other individuals [9].

Juvenile nasopharyngeal angiofibromas, hemangiomas, and pyogenic granulomas, as well as inverted papillomas, are examples of benign localized neoplasms that have the potential to produce epistaxis in children. Rare but significant causes of epistaxis in children include the presence of malignant neoplasms in the nasal cavity, sinuses, or nasopharynx. Rhabdomyosarcoma, mesenchymal chondrosarcoma, non-Hodgkin lymphoma, and nasopharyngeal carcinoma are some of the diseases that fall under this category [35–38].

Angiofibroma of the juvenile nasopharynx—Angiofibroma of the juvenile nasopharynx is a histologically benign but locally aggressive tumor that is notably vascular and has the potential to produce severe epistaxis [39]. Lesions that originate in the lateral nasopharynx and are hormonally sensitive are often seen in adolescents who are affected by this condition [40]. The maxillary artery is the primary contributor to the blood flow that the tumor receives. Although juvenile nasopharyngeal angiofibroma is a benign tumor, it has the potential to create significant issues due to its ability to invade the structures that are in close proximity to it [9].

3.2 *Systemic Causes*

Systemic causes of nosebleeds in children include bleeding diatheses, blood vessel problems, medicines, neoplasms, inflammatory illnesses, and hypertension. Epistaxis is seldom the lone symptom of a systemic illness. Children with constitutional symptoms, severe or recurring nosebleeds, and a family history of bleeding disorder or another inherited systemic illness should be evaluated for systemic disease [9].

3.2.1 Bleeding Disorders

Although an uncommon cause of epistaxis in children, bleeding disorders must be considered in children with recurrent, frequent, spontaneous epistaxis, and those with a prolonged, difficult-to-control nosebleed, especially in children with a family history of a bleeding disorder [41–43]. Platelet abnormalities and von Willebrand disease are the most common hematologic causes. Bleeding diseases include genetic and acquired coagulation disorders, platelet disorders, and blood vessel problems. Early laboratory assessment for a bleeding condition in a kid with protracted or recurrent spontaneous epistaxis and interpretation of data is covered in detail separately [9].

3.2.2 Medicines

Children on certain drugs, especially anti-inflammatory agents (aspirin) and anticoagulants, may have more frequent or difficult-to-control nosebleeds (e.g., those with complex congenital heart disease or thromboembolic disease). In addition, a variety of rodenticides include anticoagulants (warfarins and "superwarfarins") that may be accidentally swallowed by youngsters [44].

4 Evaluation and Therapy

Quick examination of general appearance, vital signs, airway stability, and mental state is required to identify children with respiratory or hemodynamic instability who need airway intervention and/or fluid resuscitation [45, 46]. Patients who are spitting or regurgitating blood to the extent that they cannot sustain oxygenation or their airway need airway assistance [45].

Immediately after rapid examination and stabilization, efforts are made to identify the cause of bleeding and stop it, often in cooperation with otolaryngology [47]. Patients with hemorrhagic diseases that may be treated with blood factors or platelets should be offered these medications. The rest of the assessment is conducted after the patient has been stabilized [45].

If bleeding is caused by excessive dryness in the house (e.g., from radiator heating), patients may benefit from humidifying the air using a cool mist vaporizer in the bedroom or, as an alternative, putting a metal basin filled with water on top of a radiator to humidify the ambient air. If required, cauterization or packing is done [48].

5 Conclusion

The etiology of epistaxis in newborns and young children is poorly understood due to its rarity. General local causes of epistaxis in children and adolescents include allergies, upper respiratory tract infections, and medications/drugs such as decongestants or cocaine, though pediatric epistaxis is typically a benign condition caused by dry nasal mucosa and minor trauma to the anterior septum.

References

1. McIntosh N, Mok JYQ, Margerison A. Epidemiology of oronasal hemorrhage in the first 2 years of life: implications for child protection. Pediatrics. 2007;120:1074–8.
2. DeLaroche AM, Tigchelaar H, Kannikeswaran N. A rare but important entity: epistaxis in infants. J Emerg Med. 2017;52(1):89–92. https://doi.org/10.1016/j.jemermed.2016.07.079. Epub 2016 Oct 4
3. Pallin DJ, Chng YM, McKay MP, Emond JA, Pelletier AJ, Camargo CA Jr. Epidemiology of epistaxis in US emergency departments, 1992 to 2001. Ann Emerg Med. 2005;46:77–81.
4. Davies K, Batra K, Mehanna R, Keogh I. Pediatric epistaxis: epidemiology, management & impact on quality of life. Int J Pediatr Otorhinolaryngol. 2014;78:1294–7.
5. McIntosh N, Chalmers J. Incidence of oronasal haemorrhage in infancy presenting to general practice in the UK. Br J Gen Pract. 2008;58:877–9.
6. Boscardini L, Zanetta S, Ballardini G, et al. Epistaxis in children under the age of two: possible marker of abuse/neglect? A retrospective study in North-Eastern Piedmont hospitals. Minerva Pediatr. 2013;65:71–5.
7. McIntosh N, Mok JYQ, Margerison A, et al. The epidemiology of oro-nasal haemorrhage and suffocation in infants admitted to hospital in Scotland over 10 years. Arch Dis Child. 2010;95:810–6.
8. Paranjothy S, Fone D, Mann M, et al. The incidence and aetiology of epistaxis in infants: a population-based study. Arch Dis Child. 2009;94:421–4.
9. Messner AH. Causes of epistaxis in children. In: Isaacson GC, Nagler J, Wiley JF (Eds). UpToDate. Last updated: Jan 11, 2023.
10. Shay S, Shapiro NL, Bhattacharyya N. Epidemiological characteristics of pediatric epistaxis presenting to the emergency department. Int J Pediatr Otorhinolaryngol. 2017;103:121.
11. Qureishi A, Burton MJ. Interventions for recurrent idiopathic epistaxis (nosebleeds) in children. Cochrane Database Syst Rev. 2012;CD004461.
12. Beran M, Petruson B. Occurrence of epistaxis in habitual nose-bleeders and analysis of some etiological factors. ORL J Otorhinolaryngol Relat Spec. 1986;48:297.
13. Béquignon E, Teissier N, Gauthier A, et al. Emergency Department care of childhood epistaxis. Emerg Med J. 2017;34:543.
14. Sethi RKV, Kozin ED, Abt NB, et al. Treatment disparities in the management of epistaxis in United States emergency departments. Laryngoscope. 2018;128:356.
15. Patel N, Maddalozzo J, Billings KR. An update on management of pediatric epistaxis. Int J Pediatr Otorhinolaryngol. 2014;78:1400–4.
16. Volk MS. Epistaxis. In: Schoem SR, Darrow DH, editors. Pediatric otolaryngology. Elk Grove Village, IL: American Academy of Pediatrics; 2012. p. 145–56.
17. Okada T, Sasaki F, Itoh T, et al. Bleeding disorder as the first symptom of biliary atresia. Eur J Pediatr Surg. 2005;15:295–9.
18. Tunkel DE, Anne S, Payne SC, et al. Clinical practice guideline: nosebleed (epistaxis). Otolaryngol Head Neck Surg. 2020;162:S1.

19. Desrosiers AE 3rd, Thaller SR. Pediatric nasal fractures: evaluation and management. J Craniofac Surg. 2011;22:1327.
20. Köroglu M, Arat A, Cekirge S, et al. Giant cervical internal carotid artery pseudoaneurysm in a child: endovascular treatment. Neuroradiology. 2002;44:864.
21. Dai A, Jurges E. The problem with nose bleeds. Emerg Med J. 2005;22:596.
22. Williams PM, Traquina DN, Wallace RC, Niezgoda JJ. Coil embolization of a ruptured carotid pseudoaneurysm presenting as epistaxis--pediatric otolaryngology: principles and practice. Am J Otolaryngol. 2000;21:38.
23. Reiber ME, Burkey BB. Intracavernous carotid pseudoaneurysm after blunt trauma: case report and discussion. Head Neck. 1994;16:253.
24. Roebuck JC, Pereira KD. Idiopathic internal carotid artery aneurysm rupture in an infant: a case report. Ear Nose Throat J. 2009;88:835.
25. Fontela PS, Tampieri D, Atkinson JD, et al. Posttraumatic pseudoaneurysm of the intracavernous internal carotid artery presenting with massive epistaxis. Pediatr Crit Care Med. 2006;7:260.
26. Deng D, Du J, Liu F, et al. Clinical characteristics of internal carotid artery pseudoaneurysms in the sphenoid sinus. Am J Otolaryngol. 2019;40:106.
27. da Silva PS, Waisberg DR. Internal carotid artery pseudoaneurysm with life-threatening epistaxis as a complication of deep neck space infection. Pediatr Emerg Care. 2011;27:422.
28. Wyrick D, Smith SD, Dassinger MS. Traumatic carotid-cavernous fistula presenting as massive epistaxis. J Pediatr Surg. 2013;48:883.
29. Kamble P, Saxena S, Kumar S. Nasal bacterial colonization in cases of idiopathic epistaxis in children. Int J Pediatr Otorhinolaryngol. 2015;79:1901.
30. Whymark AD, Crampsey DP, Fraser L, et al. Childhood epistaxis and nasal colonization with Staphylococcus aureus. Otolaryngol Head Neck Surg. 2008;138:307.
31. Batra K, Chaudhary N, Motwani G, Rai AK. An unusual case of primary nasal tuberculosis with epistaxis and epilepsy. Ear Nose Throat J. 2002;81:842.
32. Faridi MM, Aggarwal A, Kumar M, Sarafrazul A. Clinical and biochemical profile of dengue haemorrhagic fever in children in Delhi. Trop Dr. 2008;38:28.
33. Ahmed S, Arif F, Yahya Y, et al. Dengue fever outbreak in Karachi 2006 - a study of profile and outcome of children under 15 years of age. J Pak Med Assoc. 2008;58:4.
34. Kulkarni MJ, Sarathi V, Bhalla V, et al. Clinico-epidemiological profile of children hospitalized with dengue. Indian J Pediatr. 2010;77:1103.
35. Uppaluri SA, Yin LH, Goh GH. Maxillary mesenchymal chondrosarcoma presenting with epistaxis in a child. J Radiol Case Rep. 2015;9:33.
36. Zagolski O, Dwivedi RC, Subramanian S, Kazi R. Non-Hodgkin's lymphoma of the sino-nasal tract in children. J Cancer Res Ther. 2010;6:5.
37. Roganović J, Matijašić N, Mascarin M. Pediatric advanced stage nasopharyngeal carcinoma - case report. Acta Med Acad. 2015;44:186.
38. Fyrmpas G, Wurm J, Athanassiadou F, et al. Management of paediatric sinonasal rhabdomyosarcoma. J Laryngol Otol. 2009;123:990.
39. Gullane PJ, Davidson J, O'Dwyer T, Forte V. Juvenile angiofibroma: a review of the literature and a case series report. Laryngoscope. 1992;102:928.
40. Mulbury PE. Recurrent epistaxis. Pediatr Rev. 1991;12:213.
41. Sandoval C, Dong S, Visintainer P, et al. Clinical and laboratory features of 178 children with recurrent epistaxis. J Pediatr Hematol Oncol. 2002;24:47.
42. Medeiros D, Buchanan GR. Major hemorrhage in children with idiopathic thrombocytopenic purpura: immediate response to therapy and long-term outcome. J Pediatr. 1998;133:334.
43. Katsanis E, Luke KH, Hsu E, et al. Prevalence and significance of mild bleeding disorders in children with recurrent epistaxis. J Pediatr. 1988;113:73.
44. Watt BE, Proudfoot AT, Bradberry SM, Vale JA. Anticoagulant rodenticides. Toxicol Rev. 2005;24:259.

45. Messner AH. Evaluation of epistaxis in children. In: Isaacson GC, Nagler J, Wiley JF (Eds). UpToDate. Last updated: Jan 11, 2023.
46. Delgado EM, Nadel FM. Epistaxis. In: Shaw KN, Bachur RG, editors. Fleisher and Ludwig's textbook of pediatric emergency medicine. 8th ed. Philadelphia, PA: Wolters Kluwer; 2021. p. 166.
47. Svider P, Arianpour K, Mutchnick S. Management of Epistaxis in Children and Adolescents: Avoiding a Chaotic Approach. Pediatr Clin N Am. 2018;65:607.
48. Nguyen QA. Epistaxis Treatment & Management. In: Meyers AD (Ed). Medscape. Updated: Apr 13, 2022. https://emedicine.medscape.com/article/863220-treatment#d11. Accessed online at February 23, 2023.

Could Breastfeeding be a Protective Factor for Sinusitis?

Nagehan Dilsad Erdogdu Küçükcan, Cemal Cingi, and Codrut Sarafoleanu

1 Introduction

In most cases, human milk is the healthiest option for babies and young children [1]. Human milk also offers immunologic protection against numerous childhood illnesses [2]. The American Academy of Pediatrics stresses the benefits of breastfeeding and suggests that it be practiced for at least 12 months, and for as long beyond that as the mother and child choose [3]. Human milk is known to defend against infections thanks to the presence of a number of molecules and chemicals that have antibacterial, anti-inflammatory, immunomodulatory, and bioactive properties [1]. Mucosal maturation, gut microbiota balance, antigen attachment disruption, newborn immune system stimulation, and reduced exposure to pathogens via food antigens are some potential ways nursing protects against infectious illness [4, 5].

Whether or not human milk ingestion in infancy protects against illnesses even after breastfeeding has ended is not well known. Breastfeeding has been linked to a lower risk of several health problems, including a lifetime reduction in the likelihood of needing a tonsillectomy, acute appendicitis, and recurrent tonsillitis [6–10]. When comparing breastfed and non-breastfed children, researchers found that the former had much lower rates of wheezing sickness 6–7 years after nursing ended [11–13]. Moreover, Wilson et al. [13] showed that infants nursed exclusively for

N. D. E. Küçükcan (✉)
Department of Otorhinolaryngology, Çukurova State Hospital, Adana, Türkiye

C. Cingi
Medical Faculty, Department of Otorhinolaryngology, Eskisehir Osmangazi University, Eskisehir, Türkiye
e-mail: cemal@ogu.edu.tr

C. Sarafoleanu
Sfanta Maria Clinical Hospital ENT&HNS Department, University of Medicine and Pharmacy "Carol Davila", Bucharest, Romania

© The Author(s), under exclusive license to Springer Nature Switzerland AG 2023
Ö. N. Şahin et al. (eds.), *Breastfeeding and Metabolic Programming*, https://doi.org/10.1007/978-3-031-33278-4_40

15 weeks had more excellent protection against respiratory tract infections for 7 years than children not breastfed. While Saarinen [14] found that breastfeeding for 3–4 months reduced the risk of otitis media up to age 3 years, Howie et al. [15] found that breastfeeding for at least 13 weeks was not associated with an ear infection but was associated with a significantly lower prevalence of gastrointestinal (GI) disease in the first 2 years of life compared with those who were never breastfed or breastfed for 13 weeks [16].

2 Human Milk Immune Factors

The immune components included in human milk help protect infants from the illness. However, how human milk achieves its protective properties beyond infancy and nursing is unknown. Several researchers have hypothesized that breast milk's immunologic elements shape infants' immune system development in ways that affect the etiology of disease later in life. The thymus is an essential immune system organ because it ensures that T cells usually mature. At 4 months, babies breastfed entirely had considerably bigger thymus glands than those partly breastfed or given formula solely, as measured by ultrasonography.

Further research by Jeppesen et al. [17] confirmed their association between nursing and a larger thymus and discovered a link between breastfeeding and CD8+ T cells. Previous episodes of otitis media were identified by Alho et al [18] as a significant risk factor for recurrent otitis media, with increased chances (odds ratio [OR]: 3.74 (95% CI: 3.40–4.10)) if the most recent episode had occurred during the preceding 3 months. This discovery provides further evidence that the preventive benefits of breastfeeding against future ear infections may be partly mediated by a reduced risk of developing otitis media in early childhood [16].

Secretory IgA against microbes to which the mother has been exposed; antibacterial and antiviral agents like lactoferrin, lysozyme, and certain fatty acids; a large number of leukocytes; and oligosaccharides, which act as analogs of microbial epithelial receptors and, thus, decoys for potential pathogens are just some of the properties that may make breast milk protective against acute illness [19–23]. Increased expression of T cells has been linked to a more prominent thymus in breastfed babies compared to those not [23–25]. Furthermore, the gut microbiome of breastfed infants has been shown to contain a greater diversity of beneficial bacteria (particularly Bifidobacteria and Lactobacilli), which may have implications for the production of additional antimicrobial compounds, the reduction of intestinal permeability, the competition with harmful bacteria for nutrients and binding sites, the maturation and stimulation of local and systemic immune responses, and so on [19, 22, 26, 27].

In addition to its nutritional value, human milk is a complex, living biological material. Macro- and micronutrients are not the only things found in human milk; there are also growth factors, immunoprotective compounds, and live cells [28–30].

Biological activity occurs at mucosal surfaces, where many of these components remain intact despite exposure to digesting enzymes in the newborn GI tract [28].

Biologically active components include [28]:

- *Antimicrobial activity*—Immunoglobulins (particularly secretory IgA), lysozyme, lactoferrin, free fatty acids and monoglycerides, human milk bile salt-stimulated lipase, mucins, white blood cells, stem cells, and human milk oligosaccharides all have antibacterial action (prebiotic and antimicrobial activities). These antimicrobial effects defend against necrotizing enterocolitis and other illnesses that might affect the digestive system (NEC).
- Immunomodulatory activity—Platelet-activating factor (PAF) acetylhydrolase, interleukin-10 polyunsaturated fatty acids glycoconjugates all have immuno-modulatory action. These elements aid in warding off NEC [31–34].
- Factors that promote gastrointestinal development and function factors - Protein-digesting enzymes (proteases), growth-promoting hormones (such as cortisol, somatomedin C, insulin-like growth factors, insulin, and thyroid hormone), growth-promoting growth factors (such as epidermal growth factor and nerve growth factor), gastrointestinal mediators (such as neurotensin and motilin), and amino acids that stimulate enterocyte growth (such as taurine and glutamine) all play essential roles in the digestive tract [35–40]. The microbiota and virome in the stomach benefit from exposure to human breast milk [28, 41, 42].

3 Breastfeeding, Respiratory Infections, and Sinusitis

According to the extensive body of research that investigates this connection, breastfeeding has been shown to reduce the risk of infants developing respiratory problems. The incidence of wheezing in infants has been demonstrated to decrease in correlation with increased breastfeeding time [43, 44]. A dose-response relationship between breastfeeding and a reduced incidence of dry cough, wheezing, shortness of breath, and persistent phlegm was found in Dutch research [45].

Consequently, it is plausible that nursing mothers' heightened awareness of and reporting upper respiratory symptoms accounts for the apparent impact of breastfeeding on the risk of respiratory infection. However, there may be some causal connection. Regular close physical contact between newborns and mothers while nursing may promote the spread of respiratory infections. On the other hand, moms whose kids have respiratory issues more often may choose to breastfeed longer to provide their kids with the purported health advantages of breast milk. Possible explanations for this discrepancy include that breastfed children are more likely to experience a mild respiratory illness, such as a cold, than their non-breastfed counterparts and that this illness is less likely to progress to a more severe one serious stage, such as fever or otitis media [19].

Frank et al. [19] showed that breastfeeding protected against respiratory illnesses accompanied by a high temperature in the breastfed infant between the ages of 3 and 6 months. While this research does not find a reduction in total respiratory infectious episodes among breastfed babies aged 3–6 months, it does suggest that respiratory infections in breastfed infants may be less severe than those in non-breastfed infants. Although this study found that continuing to breastfeed past the age of 6 months reduced the risk of conjunctivitis and tracheitis/laryngitis, it found that children who were breastfed past the age of 6 months had higher rates of all respiratory infections than children who were not breastfed past the age of 6 months, including the most common respiratory infection, the common cold.

Whether nursing also prevents respiratory issues later in life is less well documented. Elliott et al. [45] found no significant connection between breastfeeding and wheezing in the large Avon Longitudinal Study of Parents and Children (ALSPAC) cohort after accounting for the first 3 years of life and adjusting for other factors. Sears [46] found no evidence that breastfeeding protects against asthma in a study that followed children for 9 to 26 years. However, Grabenhenrich et al. [47] found no link between breastfeeding and asthma after tracking a birth cohort of 1,314 neonates from birth to age 20 across five German cities. It is plausible. However, baby feeding habits are connected with respiratory symptoms in adulthood, even without an asthma diagnosis, given that wheezing and coughing in early life are associated with later respiratory symptoms [48].

With children, coughing is most prevalent around 50, and respiratory illnesses often cause it. Recurrent cough in infancy is a risk factor for later asthma, although this symptom has received less attention than wheezing [48]. Nevertheless, chronic cough in adults could be an indicator of airway blockage. Recurrent cough, defined as "usual cough on most days for three consecutive months or more over the last year," was associated with moderate-to-severe obstruction and self-reported fair or poor health in the older National Health and Nutrition Examination Survey group [49]. Compared to people without symptomatic mild obstruction, those with symptomatic mild obstruction had a quicker drop in FEV1 and higher healthcare service use for respiratory outcomes [50]. These findings highlight the need to study the early life predictors of adult-onset chronic respiratory symptoms, which may be risk factors for morbidity and poor quality of life even without a diagnosis. Cigarette smoking is linked to chronic cough [51], which may be a precursor to airflow blockage [52]. Adjusting for smoking status in Gerhart et al.'s [53] research did not change the association between breastfeeding and chronic cough.

For unknown biological reasons, infant feeding patterns are linked to chronic cough in adults. Some evidence suggests respiratory diseases in infancy may raise the risk for later respiratory problems, and breastfeeding may mitigate this risk. Nevertheless, in this cohort, wheezing lower respiratory tract infections (LRIs) and Respiratory Syncytial Virus (RSV) LRIs were not linked to chronic cough in adulthood, showing that these factors do not explain the association between baby feeding and chronic cough in adults. Second, some components of human milk are associated with epigenetic changes in infancy. However, the mechanisms involved are still unclear [54]. It is still unknown whether or not these epigenetic changes are linked to an increased risk for cough or other respiratory symptoms later in life.

According to other research, giving an infant a bottle, especially before bedtime and in the crib [55], maybe just as significant as the bottle's contents in terms of posing a risk for infant cough and wheezing. Soto-Ramirez et al. [56] found that bottle-fed infants, even when they were also given human milk, were more likely to develop respiratory problems like coughing and wheezing later on in infancy, which suggests that bottle feeding may cause regurgitation and aspiration, which turn may cause an increase in mucus production in the airways. There was no association between an infant's first cough and subsequent recurrent cough in the Tucson Children's Respiratory study, regardless of whether the children were exclusively breastfed or transitioned to bottle feeding at any point. Several studies have shown increased FEV1/Forced Vital Capacity (FVC) [57] and greater lung capacities in adolescence [58, 59] among breastfed children.

Colds/upper respiratory tract infections (66%), ear infections (25%), and throat infections (24%) were the most prevalent types of illnesses reported by Li et al. [60]. Breastfeeding was not linked to an increased risk of getting a cold, bronchitis, pneumonia, or urinary tract infections. Breastfeeding length, exclusivity, and timing of supplementation with formula were all significantly associated with lower rates of ear, throat, and sinus infections and more doctor visits (P 0.05). Breastfed children for 9 months had decreased chances of ear, throat, and sinus infections in the preceding year compared with those nursed for >0–3 months (adjusted odds ratio [aOR]: 0.69 [95% confidence interval [CI]: 0.48–0.98]; P 0.001). Sinus infections were less likely among infants whose mothers produced breast milk at a high intensity (>66.6%) compared to those whose mothers produced breast milk at a low intensity (33.3%) during the first 6 months (adjusted odds ratio [aOR]: 0.53 (95% confidence interval [CI]: 0.35–0.79). Their findings suggested that nursing may protect ear, throat, and sinus infections far beyond infancy.

Studies conducted on various populations have shown that breastfed infants have a decreased chance of developing respiratory illnesses. Research out of the United Kingdom found that babies who were exclusively breastfed for 6 months compared to those who were nursed for less than 4 months had a reduced chance of developing lower respiratory tract infections [61]. Other American and European researchers found that children between the ages of 3 and 6 months old had a 20% lower chance of acquiring a respiratory illness when they were breastfed [62]. It has been projected that if breastfeeding rates were increased in the United States to meet current guidelines, about 21,000 cases of hospitalization and 40 cases of mortality from lower respiratory tract infections would be avoided in the first year of life [28, 63].

4 Conclusion

Breastfeeding affects young children's acute diseases. They have fewer throat infections [60, 64–67], respiratory illnesses [64–66, 68–70], sinus infections [67], and even hospitalizations [71] in their childhood and later in life.

References

1. Lawrence RA, Lawrence LM. Breastfeeding: a guide for the medical profession. 7th ed. Elsevier Mosby: Maryland Heights, MO; 2011.
2. Ip S, Chung M, Raman G, Chew P, Magula N, DeVine D, Trikalinos T, Lau J. Breastfeeding and maternal and infant health outcomes in developed countries. Evid Rep Technol Assess (Full Rep). 2007;(153):1–186.
3. Section on Breastfeeding. Breastfeeding and the use of human milk. Pediatrics. 2012;129(3). Available at: www.pediatrics.org/cgi/content/full/129/3/e827
4. Oddy WH. Breastfeeding protects against illness and infection in infants and children: a review of the evidence. Breastfeed Rev. 2001;9(2):11–8.
5. Bachrach VR, Schwarz E, Bachrach LR. Breastfeeding and the risk of hospitalization for respiratory disease in infancy: a meta-analysis. Arch Pediatr Adolesc Med. 2003;157(3):237–43.
6. Pearce MS, Thomas JE, Campbell DI, Parker L. Does increased duration of exclusive breastfeeding protect against Helicobacter pylori infection? The Newcastle Thousand Families Cohort Study at age 49-51 years. J Pediatr Gastroenterol Nutr. 2005;41(5):617–20.
7. Malaty HM, Logan ND, Graham DY, Ramchatesingh JE. Helicobacter pylori infection in pre-school and school-aged minority children: effect of socioeconomic indicators and breastfeeding practices. Clin Infect Dis. 2001;32(10):1387–92.
8. Rothenbacher D, Bode G, Brenner H. History of breastfeeding and Helicobacter pylori infection in pre-school children: results of a population-based study from Germany. Int J Epidemiol. 2002;31(3):632–7.
9. Pisacane A, de Luca U, Impagliazzo N, Russo M, De Caprio C, Caracciolo G. Breast feeding and acute appendicitis. BMJ. 1995;310(6983):836–7.
10. Pisacane A, Impagliazzo N, De Caprio C, Criscuolo L, Inglese A, Pereira de Silva MC. Breast feeding and tonsillectomy. BMJ. 1996;312(7033):746–7.
11. Burr ML, Limb ES, Maguire MJ, et al. Infant feeding, wheezing, and allergy: a prospective study. Arch Dis Child. 1993;68(6):724–8.
12. Porro E, Indinnimeo L, Antognoni G, Midulla F, Criscione S. Early wheezing and breast feeding. J Asthma. 1993;30(1):23–8.
13. Wilson AC, Forsyth JS, Greene SA, Irvine L, Hau C, Howie PW. Relation of infant diet to childhood health: seven year follow up of cohort of children in Dundee infant feeding study. BMJ. 1998;316(7124):21–5.
14. Saarinen UM. Prolonged breast feeding as prophylaxis for recurrent otitis media. Acta Paediatr Scand. 1982;71(4):567–71.
15. Howie PW, Forsyth JS, Ogston SA, Clark A, Florey CD. Protective effect of breast feeding against infection. BMJ. 1990;300(6716):11–6.
16. Li R, Dee D, Li CM, Hoffman HJ, Grummer-Strawn LM. Breastfeeding and risk of infections at 6 years. Pediatrics. 2014;134 Suppl 1(Suppl 1):S13–20. https://doi.org/10.1542/peds.2014-0646D.
17. Jeppesen DL, Hasselbalch H, Lisse IM, Ersbøll AK, Engelmann MD. T-lymphocyte subsets, thymic size and breastfeeding in infancy. Pediatr Allergy Immunol. 2004;15(2):127–32.
18. Alho OP, Kilkku O, Oja H, Koivu M, Sorri M. Control of the temporal aspect when considering risk factors for acute otitis media. Arch Otolaryngol Head Neck Surg. 1993;119(4):444–9.
19. Frank NM, Lynch KF, Uusitalo U, Yang J, Lönnrot M, Virtanen SM, Hyöty H, Norris JM, TEDDY Study Group. The relationship between breastfeeding and reported respiratory and gastrointestinal infection rates in young children. BMC Pediatr. 2019;19(1):339. https://doi.org/10.1186/s12887-019-1693-2.
20. Newburg DS. Oligosaccharides in human milk and bacterial colonization. J Pediatr Gastroenterol Nutr. 2000;30(Sup 2):S8–S17. https://doi.org/10.1097/00005176-200003002-00003.

21. Turfkruyer M, Verhasselt V. Breast milk and its impact on maturation of the neonatal immune system. Curr Opin Infect Dis. 2015;28:199–206. https://doi.org/10.1097/QCO.0000000000000165.
22. Castanys-Munoz E, Martin MJ, Vazquez E. Building a beneficial microbiome from birth. Adv Nutr. 2016;7:323–30. https://doi.org/10.3945/an.115.010694.
23. Jackson KM, Nazar AM. Breastfeeding, the immune response, and long-term health. J Am Osteopath Assoc. 2006;106(4):203–7.
24. Hasselbalch H, Engelmann MDM, Ersboll AK, Jeppesen DL, Fleischer-Michaelsen K. Breastfeeding influences thymic size in late infancy. Eur J Pediatr. 1999;158:964–7. https://doi.org/10.1007/s004310051258.
25. Jeppesen DL, Hasselbalch H, Lisse IM, Ersboll AK, Engelmann MDM. T-lymphocyte subsets, thymic size and breastfeeding in infancy. Pediatr Allergy Immunol. 2004;15:127–32. https://doi.org/10.1111/j.1399-3038.2004.00032.x.
26. Beattie LM, Weaver LT. Mothers, babies and friendly bacteria. Arch Dis Child Fetal Neonatal Ed. 2011;96(3):F160–3.
27. Wall R, Ross RP, Ryan CA, Hussey S, Murphy B, Fitzgerald GF, Stanton C. Role of gut microbiota in early infant development. Clin Med Pediatr. 2009;3:45–54. https://doi.org/10.4137/CMPed.S2008.
28. Meek JY. Infant benefits of breastfeeding. In: Abrams SA, Hoppin AG (Eds). UpToDate. Last updated: Nov 21, 2022.
29. Andreas NJ, Kampmann B, Mehring L-DK. Human breast milk: a review on its composition and bioactivity. Early Hum Dev. 2015;91:629.
30. Ballard O, Morrow AL. Human milk composition: nutrients and bioactive factors. Pediatr Clin N Am. 2013;60:49.
31. Garofalo R, Chheda S, Mei F, et al. Interleukin-10 in human milk. Pediatr Res. 1995;37:444.
32. Fituch CC, Palkowetz KH, Goldman AS, Schanler RJ. Concentrations of IL-10 in preterm human milk and in milk from mothers of infants with necrotizing enterocolitis. Acta Paediatr. 2004;93:1496.
33. Caplan MS, Jilling T. The role of polyunsaturated fatty acid supplementation in intestinal inflammation and neonatal necrotizing enterocolitis. Lipids. 2001;36:1053.
34. Caplan MS, Lickerman M, Adler L, et al. The role of recombinant platelet-activating factor acetylhydrolase in a neonatal rat model of necrotizing enterocolitis. Pediatr Res. 1997;42:779.
35. Lucas A, Bloom SR, Aynsley-Green A. Gut hormones and 'minimal enteral feeding'. Acta Paediatr Scand. 1986;75:719.
36. Rodriguez-Palmero M, Koletzko B, Kunz C, Jensen R. Nutritional and biochemical properties of human milk: II. Lipids, micronutrients, and bioactive factors. Clin Perinatol. 1999;26:335.
37. Sheard NF, Walker WA. The role of breast milk in the development of the gastrointestinal tract. Nutr Rev. 1988;46:1.
38. Dvorak B, Halpern MD, Holubec H, et al. Epidermal growth factor reduces the development of necrotizing enterocolitis in a neonatal rat model. Am J Physiol Gastrointest Liver Physiol. 2002;282:G156.
39. Clark JA, Lane RH, Maclennan NK, et al. Epidermal growth factor reduces intestinal apoptosis in an experimental model of necrotizing enterocolitis. Am J Physiol Gastrointest Liver Physiol. 2005;288:G755.
40. Berseth CL, Michener SR, Nordyke CK, Go VL. Postpartum changes in pattern of gastrointestinal regulatory peptides in human milk. Am J Clin Nutr. 1990;51:985.
41. Stiemsma LT, Michels KB. The Role of the Microbiome in the Developmental Origins of Health and Disease. Pediatrics. 2018;141:e20172437.
42. Liang G, Zhao C, Zhang H, et al. The stepwise assembly of the neonatal virome is modulated by breastfeeding. Nature. 2020;581:470.
43. Wright AL, Holberg CJ, Martinez FD, et al. Breast feeding and lower respiratory tract illness in the first year of life. Group Health Medical Associates. BMJ. 1989;299:946–9.

44. Cushing AH, Samet JM, Lambert WE, et al. breastfeeding reduces risk of respiratory illness in infants. Am J Epidemiol. 1998;147:863–70.

45. Elliott L, Henderson J, Northstone K, et al. Prospective study of breastfeeding in relation to wheeze, atopy, and bronchial hyperresponsiveness in the Avon Longitudinal Study of Parents and Children (ALSPAC). J Allergy Clin Immunol. 2008;122:49–54.

46. Sears MR, Greene JM, Willan AR, et al. Long-term relation between breastfeeding and development of atopy and asthma in children and young adults: a longitudinal study. Lancet. 2002;360:901–7.

47. Grabenhenrich LB, Gough H, Reich A, et al. Early-life determinants of asthma from birth to age 20 years: a German birth cohort study. J Allergy Clin Immunol. 2014;133:979–88.

48. Oren E, Rothers J, Stern DA, et al. Cough during infancy and subsequent childhood asthma. Clin Exp Allergy. 2015;45:1439–46.

49. Wheaton AG, Ford ES, Thompson WW, et al. Pulmonary function, chronic respiratory symptoms, and health-related quality of life among adults in the United States-- National Health and Nutrition Examination Survey 2007-2010. BMC Public Health. 2013;13:854.

50. Bridevaux PO, Gerbase MW, Probst-Hensch NM, et al. Long-term decline in lung function, utilisation of care and quality of life in modified GOLD stage 1 COPD. Thorax. 2008;63:768–74.

51. Cerveri I, Brusasco V. Revisited role for mucus hypersecretion in the pathogenesis of COPD. Eur Respir Rev. 2010;19:109–12.

52. Blanc FX, Macedo P, Hew M, et al. Capsaicin cough sensitivity in smokers with and without airflow obstruction. Respir Med. 2009;103:786–90.

53. Gerhart KD, Stern DA, Guerra S, et al. Protective effect of breastfeeding on recurrent cough in adulthood. Thorax. 2018;73:833–9.

54. Verduci E, Banderali G, Barberi S, et al. Epigenetic effects of human breast milk. Nutrients. 2014;6:1711–24.

55. Celedón JC, Litonjua AA, Ryan L, et al. Bottle feeding in the bed or crib before sleep time and wheezing in early childhood. Pediatrics. 2002;110:e77.

56. Soto-Ramírez N, Karmaus W, Zhang H, et al. Modes of infant feeding and the occurrence of coughing/wheezing in the first year of life. J Hum Lact. 2013;29:71–80.

57. Owens L, Laing IA, Zhang G, et al. Can risk factors for COPD be traced back to infancy? The Perth infant asthma follow up study. Eur Respir J. 2016;48:OA3305.

58. Guilbert TW, Stern DA, Morgan WJ, et al. Effect of breastfeeding on lung function in childhood and modulation by maternal asthma and atopy. Am J Respir Crit Care Med. 2007;176:843–8.

59. Dogaru CM, Strippoli MP, Spycher BD, et al. breastfeeding and lung function at school age: does maternal asthma modify the effect? Am J Respir Crit Care Med. 2012;185:874–80.

60. Duncan B, Ey J, Holberg CJ, Wright AL, Martinez FD, Taussig LM. Exclusive breastfeeding for at least 4 months protects against otitis media. Pediatrics. 1993;91(5):867–72.

61. Quigley MA, Carson C, Sacker A, Kelly Y. Exclusive breastfeeding duration and infant infection. Eur J Clin Nutr. 2016;70:1420.

62. Frank NM, Lynch KF, Uusitalo U, et al. The relationship between breastfeeding and reported respiratory and gastrointestinal infection rates in young children. BMC Pediatr. 2019;19:339.

63. Bartick MC, Schwarz EB, Green BD, et al. Suboptimal breastfeeding in the United States: Maternal and pediatric health outcomes and costs. Matern Child Nutr. 2017;13:e12366.

64. Chantry CJ, Howard CR, Auinger P. Full breastfeeding duration and associated decrease in respiratory tract infection in US children. Pediatrics. 2006;117(2):425–32. https://doi.org/10.1542/peds.2004-2283.

65. Philipsen Hetzner NM, Razza RA, Malone LM, Brooks-Gunn J. Associations among feeding behaviors during infancy and child illness at two years. Matern Child Health J. 2009;13(6):795–805. https://doi.org/10.1007/s10995-008-0401-x.

66. Hatakka K, Piirainen L, Pohjavuori S, Poussa T, Savilahti E, Korpela R. Factors associated with acute respiratory illness in day care children. Scand J Infect Dis. 2010;42(9):704–11. https://doi.org/10.3109/00365548.2010.483476.

67. Ruowei L, Dee D, Li CM, Hoffman HJ, Grummer-Strawn LM. Breastfeeding and risk of infections at 6 years. Pediatrics. 2014;134(Suppl 1):S13–20.
68. Tiewsoh K, Lodha R, Pandey RM, Broor S, Kalaivani M, Kabra SK. Factors determining the outcome of children hospitalized with severe pneumonia. BMC Pediatr. 2009;9:15. https://doi.org/10.1186/1471-2431-9-15.
69. Quigley MA, Kelly YJ, Sacker A. Breastfeeding and hospitalization for diarrheal and respiratory infection in the United Kingdom millennium cohort study. Pediatrics. 2007;119(4):e837–42. https://doi.org/10.1542/peds.2006-2256.
70. Yamakawa M, Yorifuji T, Kato T, Inoue S, Tokinobu A, Tsuda T, Doi H. Long-term effects of breastfeeding on children's hospitalization for respiratory tract infections and diarrhea in early childhood in Japan. Matern Child Health J. 2015;19:1956–65. https://doi.org/10.1007/s10995-015-1703-4.
71. Paricio Talayero JM, Lizan-Garcia M, Otero Puime A, Benlloch Muncharaz MJ, Beseler Soto B, Sanchez-Palomares M, Santos Serrano L, Landa RL. Full breastfeeding and hospitalization as a result of infections in the first year of life. Pediatrics. 2006;118(1):e92–9. https://doi.org/10.1542/peds.2005-1629.

Could Breastfeeding Be a Protective Factor for Sleep Apnea?

Saltuk Bugra Kilinc, Nuray Bayar Muluk, and Suela Sallavaci

1 Introduction

Obstructive sleep apnea (OSA) is more than expected in children, such as 1–6% of children and adolescents have obstructive sleep apnea [1]. Most of the kids that get it are between the ages of 2 and 8. The likelihood of upper airway collapse, and therefore of pediatric OSA, may be decreased or raised by a number of variables. Obesity is a major contributor to the risk. The incidence of OSA rises to 19–61% when the population is broken down into obese children [2–5]. According to studies, the chance of developing OSA increases by 10–12% for every percentage point over the 50th percentile that a person's body mass index (BMI) resides in [6, 7]. There is a possibility of upper airway reduction with adenoids and tonsils that have grown too large; therefore, this condition has been described as a risk factor as well. Pediatric obstructive sleep apnea is often treated by adenotonsillectomy [8]. While inflammation of the nasal mucosa is thought to cause congestion, which in turn may raise airway resistance, allergic rhinitis (AR) is also considered a risk factor [9]. Moreover, maxillofacial anomalies and malocclusion have been linked to pediatric OSA [10]. Changes in the size, location, or shape of the jaws and/or tongue may limit the upper airway, increasing the risk of blockage [9].

S. B. Kilinc (✉)
Department of Otorhinolaryngology, Yozgat Sarıkaya State Hospital, Yozgat, Türkiye

N. B. Muluk
Faculty of Medicine, Department of Otorhinolaryngology, Kırıkkale University, Kırıkkale, Türkiye

S. Sallavaci
Department of Otorhinolaryngology, University Hospital Centre "Mother Teresa", Tirana, Albania

Ö. N. Şahin et al. (eds.), *Breastfeeding and Metabolic Programming*, https://doi.org/10.1007/978-3-031-33278-4_41

2 Mechanisms

2.1 Breastfeeding and Occlusion

The structural difference in feeding methods is another factor that lends biological validity to the link between breastfeeding and malocclusion. As compared to the mother's nipple, which properly conforms to the internal contour of the oral cavity, allowing the oral seal to occur without undue pressures, the nipple of the baby feeding bottle is often less flexible [11, 12]. As a consequence, bottle feeding may have an impact on factors such as the development of the palate (transverse, vertical, and sagittal growth) and the nasal airway (facilitating breathing). This breastfeeding-malocclusion connection was studied in two separate systematic reviews and meta-analyses [13, 14]. Breastfeeding for a longer period of time has been linked to a reduced risk of nonspecific malocclusion, according to a large body of research. Breastfed infants were shown to have a 46% lower risk of developing a malocclusion than formula-fed infants (odds ratio [OR]: 0.54; 95% confidence interval [CI]: 0.38–0.77) [13]. We found moderate evidence for every kind of malocclusion. This is due to the limited amount of studies that have been conducted on the topic and the fact that almost all of these research relied on retrospective questionnaires or interviews with parents to get their information on nursing, both of which are susceptible to memory bias. Although if there isn't unanimous agreement, it seems that breastfed infants are less likely to have a posterior crossbite, an anterior open bite, a greater overjet, dental Class II, a smaller and deeper palate, and a higher-angled face. The correlation weakens significantly with longer periods of nursing. The transverse dimension in primary and mixed dentition showed this to be true [14]. Children who were not breastfed had a posterior crossbite ratio 1.70 (95% CI: 1.22–2.39), 3.76 (95% CI: 2.01–7.03), and 8.78 (95% CI: 1.67–46.1) times higher than breastfed children of the same ages. It has been found that, compared to partially breastfed infants, exclusively breastfed infants have a significantly younger mean age of emergence of deciduous teeth [15], which may lend further support to the idea that breastfeeding plays a positive role in fostering oral development in infancy and early childhood.

Craniofacial characteristics have been shown to influence the retropalatal and retroglossal region of the upper airways. Children with sleep-disordered breathing (SDB) often have a face that is too long and narrow for their skull, jaws that are rotated too far back, a narrow and high palate, a posterior crossbite, a short lower arch, and significant crowding in the maxilla and mandible [16–19]. Moreover, it has been shown that dental agenesis or early extractions impair the development of the oral cavity, resulting to a long, narrow face and the collapsibility of the airways when sleeping [20]. Children between the ages of one and six who are bottle-fed have an alarmingly high chance of developing dental caries [21], which may lead to the premature loss of baby teeth. The existence of a short lingual frenulum has also been linked to altered jaw growth. Having a short lingual frenulum is also linked to issues with sucking and swallowing as a baby, as well as mouth breathing, tongue position changes, and a restricted airway in the upper respiratory tract [20].

2.2 *Breastfeeding, Breathing, and Muscles' Development*

Proper stimulation of orofacial development requires early maturation of the synchronization between nasal breathing and nursing. Because the mandible is so tiny at birth, newborns must breathe through their noses, and the tongue must expand in a protruded posture to provide enough room at the back of the throat for breathing. A similar arrangement exists between the posterior part of the tongue and the epiglottitis, which serves to shield the lower respiratory system from food particles and liquids during swallowing. As you swallow, the bolus goes down your throat and into your stomach, where it can't enter your trachea and cause an obstruction. In order to get the milk bolus from beneath the soft palate and into the throat, the tongue must travel upwards while sucking. After the baby has had enough milk, the reflex of swallowing kicks in and, for approximately half a second, the baby stops breathing [11]. Saturation with oxygen naturally drops when nursing, but rises in the first 3 months following delivery for physiological reasons. Oxygen saturation levels were found to be considerably lower during bottle feeding, indicating a diminished capacity of newborns to adjust throughout the suck-swallow-breathe cycle compared to breastfed children [22]. Hence, bottle feeding may encourage mouth breathing because it disrupts the delicate balance necessary for the development of an infant's upper airway.

2.3 *Hypothesis in Immunology*

Breast milk aids in the maturation of an infant's still-developing immune system by providing a variety of antibacterial and anti-inflammatory chemicals. As enlarged tonsils and adenoids play a major role in the development of OSA, there is strong evidence that infants who are completely breastfed are less likely to have respiratory tract infections than children who are only partly or never breastfed [23, 24]. Growing data suggests that respiratory virus exposures in infancy may increase persistent inflammation and hypertrophy of tissues in the upper airways, lending credence to this idea. The primary effect is changes to the airway that may trigger SDB in children. In pre- and early-school years, when the size of the adenoids and tonsils overflows into the diameter of the throat, breathing difficulties are common [25]. Tonsils in children with obstructive sleep apnea (OSA) and recurrent tonsillitis (RT) have two very divergent disease pathways [26]. Tonsillar parenchymal extrafollicular region expression of reactive molecules was much higher and more widespread in OSA than in non-OSA individuals [26]. Moreover, OSA was associated with elevated levels of the neurogenic inflammatory markers nerve growth factor, neurokinin 1, and Substance P, in comparison to RT [27]. The neurogenic inflammation is a pathogenic relationship between viral infections and chronic inflammatory disorders [27]. Therefore, early exposure to respiratory viruses may result in long-term changes in the immune modulation of adenotonsillar tissues and may predispose to accelerated tissue proliferation in response to further stimuli such as upper airway flutter and collapse, recurring hypoxia and re-oxygenation, allergens, and other microorganisms [28]. Tonsils removed for OSA and RT revealed striking differences [28].

3 Risk Factors

More than one study has linked obesity to an increased risk of pediatric obstructive sleep apnea syndrome (OSAS) [29–32]. For kids, Xu et al. [33] found a strong correlation between having a body mass index (BMI) over the 95th percentile and developing OSAS. Nevertheless, Katz et al. found that the neck to waist ratio, an indicator of how fat is distributed throughout the body, is a predictor of OSA in overweight and obese children and teenagers [34]. Neck circumference less than 30 centimeters, neck-to-height ratio less than 0.25, and waist-to-hip ratio less than 0.95 were also reported to be risk factors for obstructive sleep apnea by Xu et al. [33]. Nevertheless, when waist size, hip size, and the ratio of the two were included into the multiple regression analysis, neck circumference no longer had a significant role. This is due to the fact that the average ages of our research population's OAS and non-OAS participants were 5.7 and 6 years old, respectively. Adipose buildup around the neck and waist is thought to be less of a factor in younger children since they are less likely to be obese.

As an additional risk factor for OSA, preterm delivery has been studied. Preterm children, ages 8–11, had almost three times the rate of SDB as term-born children, according to research by Rosen et al. [35]. Preterm birth has been linked to an increased risk of OSAS in school-aged children, as documented by Tapia et al. [36]. Moreover, preterm children's exposures in the prenatal environment may raise their risk for SDB; these exposures may affect the maturation of respiratory control or the size of their upper airways [35]. Using univariate analysis, Xu et al. [33] found a positive correlation between preterm birth and OSAS; however, this correlation was not statistically significant after controlling for other factors. While our sample was clinically based, only a small percentage of our subjects were born prematurely (7% in OSAS and 5% in controls). Hence, further research into the role of preterm birth in the general population is required.

As allergic rhinitis is linked to at least partial nasal channel blockage, it has been described as a risk factor of OSAS. According to a recent meta-analysis, most studies have shown a statistically significant link between AR and SDB [37]. Having chronic sinusitis or rhinitis has been linked to an increased likelihood of obstructive sleep apnea and snoring in the general pediatric population [38–40]. Children who were evaluated for adenotonsillectomy as inpatients at a hospital did not have an increased risk of AR or obstructive sleep apnea based on the findings of Weinstock et [41]. OSAS may be more difficult to attribute to AR if enlarged tonsils and adenoids are a primary cause of the condition [33].

4 Breastfeeding and Sleep Apnea

It is becoming clear that breastfeeding may help prevent snoring in children. This theory has biological support from observations of the different mechanical effects of breastfeeding and bottle feeding on infants' still-developing oral tissues [22]. In two cohort studies, researchers discovered that children who were breastfed for at least portion of their first 6 years were less likely to develop a snoring habit later in life [42, 43]., Breastfeeding for the required 6 months or more, as opposed to less than 6 months, was not linked to an increased risk of regular snoring in children aged 1 to 14 in previous research, including our own [39, 44–46]., This shows that the frequency and length of breastfeeding during the first few months of life may be more essential than the duration of feeding in avoiding habitual snoring in young children (critical timing of exposure) Breastfeeding may prevent snoring and sleep apnea [47], a possible benefit mediated by the physical influence of the breast in the mouth on oropharyngeal development. Breastfeeding may help prevent jaw deformities [48, 49] and is associated with fewer malocclusions [50] compared to bottle feeding. In addition, some cross-sectional studies have employed cephalometry and orthodontic casts to determine links between face structure and childhood snoring and OSA [51–53]. Upper airway obstruction and sleep apnea are linked to factors including a long, narrow face (dolichocephaly), [17] a narrow palate, [17, 45, 54], overcrowding of teeth [17], a maxillary constriction with a cross-bite [17, 45], an overjet [54], and a deep palatal height [45]. Adults with snoring and OSA are found to have the same craniofacial anomalies, and it is believed that these conditions developed at some point during infancy. Hence, [55] if breastfeeding influences orofacial development in the first few months of life, this might alter whether the kid has an anatomical predisposition to SDB; this is a credible biological explanation. In addition, Montgomery-Downs has proposed an immunological hypothesis to explain the link between breastfeeding and snoring, arguing that the immunoglobulins provided by breastfeeding protect against infection with respiratory viruses, thereby reducing inflammation that could otherwise cause sleep-disordered breathing [56]. Another theory suggests that the peristaltic motion of the tongue below the breast during breastfeeding aids in the development and coordination of oropharyngeal muscles necessary for swallowing, as opposed to the sucking action associated with bottle-feeding. Breastfeeding for more than a month and exclusive breastfeeding for more than 3 months substantially reduced the incidence of observed sleep apnea in children aged 8 years, according to a study by Brew et al. [57]. The Avon Longitudinal Study of Parents and Children (ALSPAC) research did not discover a link between breastfeeding and sleep apnea at any age, thus our findings contradict that [42]. Nevertheless, our results are consistent with a research of children who snore who were recruited clinically and who had their sleep objectively evaluated using polysomnography and whose breastfeeding data was acquired retrospectively. The severity of SDB was shown to be lower in those who breastfed for at least 2 months. Breastfeeding was related with a lower risk of OSAS ($n = 58$) [33]. Similar findings were found in a single prior investigation that reported breastfeeding to be a risk factor of regular snoring [38]. In addition, our study's supplementary analysis showed that parents with lower levels of education were more likely to breastfeed their children than parents with higher levels of education. Snoring and SDB have both been linked to lower socioeconomic position, according to earlier research [43, 58, 59]. Less access to health care, changes in health-related behaviors, and exposure to environmental toxicants were all proposed as probable causes of this association. Even after taking into account the participants' levels of education, breastfeeding was shown to be a substantial risk factor in this research. We hypothesized that there was a strong correlation between parental education and socioeconomic position, but that one did not always guarantee the other. There was a reduction in the risk of SDB among children born to academic professionals and farmers, according to a prior research [48]. Hence, more research on the association between breastfeeding and OSAS should focus on potential confounders such socioeconomic level, parental employment, access to health services, inflammation, environmental exposure, and health-related behaviors [33].

5   Conclusion

Obstructive sleep apnea is more than expected in children, such as 1–6% of children and adolescents have obstructive sleep apnea. It is becoming clear that breastfeeding may help prevent snoring in children. This theory has biological support from observations of the different mechanical effects of breastfeeding and bottle feeding on infants' still-developing oral tissues. In addition, Montgomery-Downs has proposed an immunological hypothesis to explain the link between breastfeeding and snoring, arguing that the immunoglobulins provided by breastfeeding protect against infection with respiratory viruses, thereby reducing inflammation that could otherwise cause sleep-disordered breathing.

References

1. Storari M, Yanez-Regonesi F, Denotti G, Paglia L, Viscuso D. Breastfeeding and sleep-disordered breathing in children: systematic review and proposal of underlying interaction models. Eur J Paediatr Dent. 2021 Dec;22(4):309–13.
2. Verhulst SL, Schrauwen N, Haentjens D, Suys B, Rooman RP, Van Gaal L, et al. Sleep-disordered breathing in overweight and obese children and adolescents: prevalence, characteristics and the role of fat distribution. Arch Dis Child. 2007;92(3):205–8.

3. Wing YK, Hui SH, Pak WM, Ho CK, Cheung A, Li AM, et al. A controlled study of sleep related disordered breathing in obese children. Arch Dis Child. 2003;88(12):1043–7.

4. Kalra M, Inge T, Garcia V, Daniels S, Lawson L, Curti R, et al. Obstructive sleep apnea in extremely overweight adolescents undergoing bariatric surgery. Obes Res. 2005;13(7):1175–9.

5. Siegfried W, Siegfried A, Rabenbauer M, Hebebrand J. Snoring and sleep apnea in obese adolescents: effect of long-term weight loss-rehabilitation. Sleep Breath. 1999;3(3):83–8.

6. Hannon TS, Rofey DL, Ryan CM, Clapper DA, Chakravorty S, Arslanian SA. Relationships among obstructive sleep apnea, anthropometric measures, and neurocognitive functioning in adolescents with severe obesity. J Pediatr. 2012;160:732–5.

7. Tan HL, Gozal D, Kheirandish-Gozal L. Obstructive sleep apnea in children: a critical update. Nat Sci Sleep. 2013;5:109–23.

8. Venekamp RP, Hearne BJ, Chandrasekharan D, Blackshaw H, Lim J, Schilder AGM. Tonsillectomy or adenotonsillectomy versus non-surgical management for obstructive sleep-disordered breathing in children. Cochrane Database Syst Rev. 2015;10:CD011165.

9. Gulotta G, Iannella G, Vicini C, Polimeni A, Greco A, de Vincentiis M, et al. Risk factors for obstructive sleep apnea syndrome in children: state of the art. Int J Environ Res Public Health. 2019;16(18):3235.

10. Pirelli P, Saponara M, De Rosa C, Fanucci E. Orthodontics and obstructive sleep apnea in children. Med Clin North Am. 2010;94(3):517–29.

11. Sanches MT. Clinical management of oral disorders in breastfeeding. J Pediatr. 2004;80:155–62.

12. Agarwal M, Ghousia S, Konde S, Rai S. Breastfeeding: nature's safety net. Int J Clin Pediatr Dent. 2012;5(1):49–53.

13. Peres KG, Cascaes AM, Giacomelli Nascimento G, Gomes VC. Effect of breastfeeding on malocclusions: a systematic review and metaanalysis. Acta Paediatr. 2015;104:54–61.

14. Boronat-Catalá M, Montiel-Company JM, Bellot-Arcís C, Almerich-Silla JM, Catalá-Pizarro M. Association between duration of breastfeeding and malocclusions in primary and mixed dentition: a systematic review and meta-analysis. Sci Rep. 2017;7(1):5048.

15. Folayan MO, Sowole CA. Association between breastfeeding and eruption of the first tooth in preschool children in Nigeria. Eur J Paediatr Dent. 2013;14(1):51–4.

16. Löfstrand-Tideström B, Thilander B, Ahlqvist-Rastad J, Jakobsson O, Hultcrantz E. Breathing obstruction in relation to craniofacial and dental arch morphology in 4-year-old children. Eur J Orthod. 1999;21(4):323–32.

17. Huynh N, Morton PD, Rompre PH, Papadakis A, Remise C. Associations between sleep-disordered breathing symptoms and facial and dental morphometry, assessed with screening examinations. Am J Orthod Dentofac Orthop. 2011;140:762–70.

18. Marino A, Malagnino I, Ranieri R, Malagola C, Villa MP. Craniofacial morphology in preschool children with obstructive sleep apnoea syndrome. Eur J Paediatr Dent. 2009;10(4):181–4.

19. Galeotti A, Festa P, Viarani V, Pavone M, Sitzia E, Piga S, et al. Correlation between cephalometric variables and obstructive sleep apnoea severity in children. Eur J Paediatr Dent. 2019;20(1):43–7.

20. Guilleminault C, Abad VC, Chiu HY, Peters BR, Quo S. Missing teeth and pediatric obstructive sleep apnea. Sleep Breath. 2016;20(2):561–8.

21. Bahuguna R, Younis Khan S, Jain A. Influence of feeding practices on dental caries. A case–control study. Eur J Paediatr Dent. 2013;14(1):55–8.

22. Sakalidis VS, Geddes DT. Suck-swallow-breathe dynamics in breastfed infants. J Hum Lact. 2016;32(2):201–11.

23. Hornell A, Lagstrom H, Lande B, Thorsdottir I. Breastfeeding, introduction of other foods and effects on health: a systematic literature review for the 5th Nordic Nutrition Recommendations. Food Nutr Res. 2013;57:20823.

24. Kramer MS, Kakuma R. Optimal duration of exclusive breastfeeding. Cochrane Database Syst Rev. 2012;8:CD003517.

25. Handelman CS, Osborne G. Growth of the nasopharynx and adenoid development from one to eighteen years. Angle Orthod. 1976;46(3):243–59.

26. Goldbart AD, Goldman JL, Li RC, Brittian KR, Tauman R, Gozal D. Differential expression of cysteinyl leukotriene receptors 1 and 2 in tonsils of children with obstructive sleep apnea syndrome or recurrent infection. Chest. 2004;126:13–8.
27. Piedimonte G. Contribution of neuroimmune mechanisms to airway inflammation and remodeling during and after respiratory syncytial virus infection. Pediatr Infect Dis J. 2003;22(2):S66–75.
28. Yeshuroon-Koffler K, Shemer-Avni Y, Keren-Naus A, Goldbart AD. Detection of common respiratory viruses in tonsillar tissue of children with obstructive sleep apnea. Pediatr Pulmonol. 2015;50(2):187–95.
29. Sateia MJ. International classification of sleep disorders-third edition: highlights and modifications. Chest. 2014;146:1387–94.
30. Kaditis AG, Alexopoulos EI, Hatzi F, et al. Adiposity in relation to age as predictor of severity of sleep apnea in children with snoring. Sleep Breath. 2008;12:25–31.
31. Kohler MJ, Thormaehlen S, Kennedy JD, et al. Differences in the association between obesity and obstructive sleep apnea among children and adolescents. J Clin Sleep Med. 2009;5:506–11.
32. Bhatia R, Lesser DJ, Oliveira FG, et al. Body fat composition: apredictive factor for sleep related breathing disorder in obese children. J Clin Sleep Med. 2015;11:1039–45.
33. Xu Z, Wu Y, Tai J, et al. Risk factors of obstructive sleep apnea syndrome in children. J Otolaryngol Head Neck Surg. 2020;49:11. https://doi.org/10.1186/s40463-020-0404-1.
34. Katz SL, Vaccani JP, Barrowman N, Momoli F, Bradbury CL, Murto K. Does neck-to-waist ratio predict obstructive sleep apnea in children? J Clin Sleep Med. 2014;10:1303–8.
35. Tagaya M, Nakata S, Yasuma F, et al. Relationship between adenoid size and severity of obstructive sleep apnea in preschool children. Int J Pediatr Otorhinolaryngol. 2012;76:1827–30.
36. Rosen CL, Larkin EK, Kirchner HL, et al. Prevalence and riskfactors for sleep-disordered breathing in 8- to 11-year-old children:association with race and prematurity. J Pediatr. 2003;142:383–9.
37. Lin SY, Melvin TA, Boss EF, Ishman SL. The association between allergic rhinitis and sleep-disordered breathing in children: a systematic review. Int Forum Allergy Rhinol. 2013;3:504–9.
38. Chng SY, Goh DY, Wang XS, Tan TN, Ong NB. Snoring and atopic disease: a strong association. Pediatr Pulmonol. 2004;38:210–6.
39. Kuehni CE, Strippoli MP, Chauliac ES, Silverman M. Snoring in preschool children: prevalence, severity and risk factors. Eur Respir J. 2008;31:326–33.
40. Bixler EO, Vgontzas AN, Lin HM, et al. Sleep disordered breathing in children in a general population sample: prevalence and risk factors. Sleep. 2009;32:731–6.
41. Weinstock TG, Rosen CL, Marcus CL, et al. Predictors of obstructive sleep apnea severity in adenotonsillectomy candidates. Sleep. 2014;37:261–9.
42. Bonuck K, Chervin RD, Cole TJ, Emond A, Henderson J, et al. Prevalence and persistence of sleep disordered breathing symptoms in young children: a 6-year population-based cohort study. Sleep. 2011;34:875–84.
43. Beebe DW, Rausch J, Byars KC, Lanphear B, Yolton K. Persistent snoring in preschool children: predictors and behavioral and developmental correlates. Pediatrics. 2012;130:382–9.
44. Li AM, Au CT, So HK, Lau J, Ng PC, et al. Prevalence and risk factors of habitual snoring in primary school children. Chest. 2010;138:519–27.
45. Lofstrand-Tidestrom B, Thilander B, Ahlqvist-Rastad J, Jakobsson O, Hulcrantz E. Breathing obstruction in relation to craniofacial and dental arch morphology in 4-year-old children. Eur J Orthod. 1999;21:323–32.
46. Marshall N, Almqvist C, Grunstein R, Marks GB. Predictors for snoring in children with rhinitis at age 5. Pediatr Pulmonol. 2007;42:584–91.
47. Brew BK, Marks GB, Almqvist C, Cistulli PA, Webb K, Marshall NS. Breastfeeding and snoring: a birth cohort study. PLoS One. 2014;9(1):e84956. https://doi.org/10.1371/journal.pone.0084956.
48. Sanchez-Molins M, Carbo JG, Gaig CL, Torrent JM. Comparitive study of the craniofacial growth depending on the type of lactation received. Eur J Paediatr Dent. 2010;11:87–92.

49. Diouf J, Ngom P, Badiane A, Cisse B, Ndoye C, et al. Influence of the mode of nutritive and non-nutritive sucking on the dimensions of primary dental arches. Int Orthod. 2010;8:372–85.
50. Palmer B. Snoring and sleep apnoea: how it can be prevented in childhood. Breastfeed Rev. 2006;14:11–4.
51. Montaldo L, Montaldo P, Cuccaro P, Caramico N, Minervini G. Effects of feeding on non-nutritive sucking habits and implications on occlusion in mixed dentition. Int J Paediatr Dent. 2011;21:68–73.
52. Vazquez-Nava F, Quezada-Castillo JA, Oviedo-Trevino S, Saldivar-Gonzalez AH, Sanchez-Nuncio HR, et al. Association between allergic rhinitis, bottle feeding, non-nutritive sucking habits, and malocclusion in the primary dentition. Arch Dis Child. 2006;91:836–40.
53. Labbok M, Hendershot G. Does breastfeeding protect against malocclusion? An analysis of the 1981 Child Health Supplement to the National Health Interview Survey. Am J Prev Med. 1987;3:227–32.
54. Pirila-Parkkinen K, Pirttiniemi P, Nieminen P, Tolonen U, Pelttari U, et al. Dental arch morphology in children with sleep-disordered breathing. Eur J Orthod. 2009;31:160–7.
55. Darendeliler MA, Cheng L, Pirelli P, Cistulli PA. Dentofacial orthopedics. In: Lavigne G, Cistulli PA, editors. Sleep medicine for dentists: a practical overview. Sydney: Quintessence Publishing Co; 2009. p. 85–91.
56. Montgomery-Downs HE, Crabtree VM, Capdevila OS, Gozal D. Infant-feeding methods and childhood sleep-disordered breathing. Pediatrics. 2007;120:1030–5.
57. Woolridge M. The 'anatomy' of infant sucking. Midwifery. 1986;2:164–71.
58. Urschitz MS, Guenther A, Eggebrecht E, et al. Snoring, intermittent hypoxia and academic performance in primary school children. Am J Respir Crit Care Med. 2003;168:464–8.
59. Montgomery-Downs HE, Jones VF, Molfese VJ, Gozal D. Snoring in preschoolers: associations with sleepiness, ethnicity, and learning. Clin Pediatr (Phila). 2003;42:719–26.

The Role of Breastfeeding on the Development and Prevention of Allergic Diseases

Özlem Sancaklı, Demet Can, and Hesham Negm

1 Introduction

Globally, there are more than 300 million patients with asthma. The prevalence of atopic disorders in general, including allergic rhinitis, allergic eczema and food allergies, lies between 1 in 10 and 3 in 10 of the population of the entire world [1, 2]. Since allergic disorders have increased in frequency so rapidly within the last half-century, and atopic disorders reduce health-related quality of life to so marked a degree, it has become a priority to determine environmental or modifiable risk factors for atopy. It is not yet fully understood why there has been such a sudden rise in atopy, but the 'hygiene hypothesis' continues to be the most favoured working explanation [3]. According to this theory, atopy results from dysequilibrium between two kinds of immune response – one associated with response to infective pathogens, the other producing allergic reactions [4]. Competing explanations for atopy include the way diets have significantly altered in the recent past [5].

2 Constituents in Breast Milk

Breast milk is undoubtedly the ideal food for infants in the first stage of life, offering the best mixture of nutrients for the child to grow and develop normally. The composition of breast milk has been shaped over time by evolutionary pressures unique to humans and the result is a medium that offers the most guaranteed way to meet

Ö. Sancaklı (✉) · D. Can
Department of Pediatrics, Division of Allergy and Immunology, Izmir Dr. Behcet Uz
Children's Hospital, Izmir, Türkiye

H. Negm
Faculty of Medicine, Department of Otorhinolaryngology, Cairo University, Cairo, Egypt

Ö. N. Şahin et al. (eds.), *Breastfeeding and Metabolic Programming*,
https://doi.org/10.1007/978-3-031-33278-4_42

the child's physiological needs and a method of feeding that encourages healthy psychological development. Amongst many proven benefits, breast milk has been shown to increase cognitive maturation and promote the development of emotional and social responses [6]. The reason that breast milk is associated with improved cognitive abilities is likely to be due to the aliphatic acid component in milk, whereas social and emotional benefits associated with breastfeeding are mediated through the reinforcement effect of oxytocin, which also plays a part in promoting other adaptive behavioural responses [7]. When assigning causation, however, it is important to recognise the existence of confounding variables, namely the overall higher socioeconomic level and greater educational achievement on average of mothers who breastfeed. In addition, both smoking and obesity are less common in this group of mothers. These differences alone may be sufficient to explain the benefits on infant development. The constituents of breast milk alter over time, not only at different times of day and over the course of the lactation period, but even within a single feed. It also differs from woman to woman and between different populations [8]. The initial breast secretion is termed colostrum. This earliest milk is synthesised in a small volume in the first days following birth and contains abundant immune-related molecules and cells, in particular secretory immunoglobulin A, lactoferrin and leucocytes, in addition to hormones directing development, e.g. epidermal growth factor [8, 9]. Following the colostrum stage, there are continuous changes in the content of breast milk for the entire period of lactation. These alterations mirror the neonate or infant's requirements for nutrition as growth proceeds. Transitional stage milk shares some of the features of colostrum, although there is a greater volume available to match the increasing nutritional demands of the fast-developing baby. Transition milk is synthesised usually from around the fifth postpartum day to about the 14th day. In any case, the composition of breast milk is fully mature at between 4 and 6 weeks after delivery [5].

2.1 Macro- and Micronutritional Composition of Breast Milk

Breast milk provides vital support to the vulnerable neonate's immature immune system by transfer of both pathogen-killing humoral and cellular components and signals that prevent unwanted inflammatory reactions. Breast milk also steers the infant's immune system towards normal development. There are also certain constituents with prebiotic activity, the presence of which favours the development of a balanced gut bacterial flora, especially oligosaccharides, which are metabolised by particular microbes. The milk also has its own bacterial content, which helps to seed the intestine with a beneficial initial flora [10]. Infants who are born at term and delivered via the vagina then breastfed appear to carry the healthiest intestinal microbiome. In these infants, Bifidobacteria predominate, with fewer potential pathogens, such as *Clostridium difficile* or *Escherichia coli* [11, 12].

The principal constituents in human milk are carbohydrates and aliphatic acids. They are the principal macronutrients in milk. The macronutrient which differs to the greatest extent in different samples is lipid, often present as high concentrations of palmitic or oleic acid [13]. Lactose, a disaccharide, is the main sugar present, although a number of other carbohydrates are also significant, such as the human milk oligosaccharides (HMOs), which may be present at a concentration around 1 g/dL. The exact concentration depends on both the stage in breastfeeding and the mother's genetic make-up. The HMOs are unusual in that they are not digested by the infant but rather act as decoy soluble receptors that prevent pathogens from gaining attachment through binding to epithelial receptors within the neonatal gut [8]. Despite breast milk being the gold standard for infant nutrition, it may fail to supply the full recommended daily allowances (RDA) for specific vitamins, if the mother has inadequate dietary intake or her own stores are low [14]. The vitamin for which this most applies is vitamin D. It is possible for the infant to manufacture vitamin D endogenously, provided he or she is exposed to enough sunlight, but the American Academy of Paediatrics (AAP) does advocate supplying additional vitamin D to infants during lactation. Furthermore, the AAP advises that vitamin K be injected into the neonate shortly after delivery to prevent haemorrhagic disease of the newborn, which may occur because breast milk contains only a minimum concentration of vitamin K [5, 8].

2.2 Compounds in Breast Milk Which Are Bioactive

There are numerous factors in breast milk which possess bioactivity. In particular, there are a number of molecules which assist with the maturation and competence of the neonatal immune system, such as various enzymes, hormones, growth factors, lactoferrin, immunoglobulins and immune signalling molecules. The proteins present at the highest concentrations are casein, α-lactalbumin, lactoferrin, sIgA, lysozyme and serum albumin [15]. The iron-binding activity of lactoferrin prevents pathogens from attaching to the intestinal epithelium. It is a glycoprotein which reduces the bioavailability of iron to microbes in the gut. The cytokines, immunoglobulins and lysozyme are identical with the mature adult forms. Maternal immunoglobulins, especially in the form of sIgA, are transferred to the neonate via human milk. They function in concert with lactoferrin to inhibit pathogenic attachment to the gut lining. Lysozyme has a direct bactericidal action. Cytokines fine-tune the inflammatory responses in the gut. These molecules are of soluble, glycoprotein type. Their role is to bind to certain receptors on cell membranes and direct how the immune system matures and responds to perceived threats [16]. One particular cytokine found in breast milk is transforming growth factor-β (TGF-β). This molecule plays a potential role in how the infant's immunity develops and matures. Researchers have found that TGF-β exerts an important role in normal immune system development through stimulating synthesis of immunoglobulin A and inducing tolerance of specific compounds in the mouth [17, 18]. The adaptive immune responses do not develop immediately after birth and thus the ability of the infant to ward off infections depends on the innate immune defences of the gut bolstered by the support of immunologically active compounds in breast milk [5].

3 How Might Being Breastfed Prevent the Development of Atopy?

3.1 When Should Solid Foods be Introduced?

There is accumulating evidence to show that not introducing solid food into the infant diet up to the age of 6 months may be harmful in terms of increasing the risk of atopic disorders, including allergic dermatitis. Furthermore, the data support the notion that continuing to breastfeed whilst introducing solids into the infant diet can both confer a protective effect and let tolerance develop. There is a lack of consensus in the published recommendations on how to prevent allergy. Mostly they advise not giving an infant allergenic food before the age of 1 year, but some recommendations state the opposite, such as the advice to start between the ages of 4 and 6 months [19], or not prior to the age of 6 months [20]. According to an article by Prescott et al., introducing specific allergenic foods at an early stage into the infant diet potentially aids the development of tolerance and is not unduly risky [21]. There are also experts who view introducing allergenic foods at a later stage as counter-productive, as it raises the risk of hypersensitivity [22]. It was demonstrated by Koplin et al. [22] that introducing egg into the infant diet between the ages of 4 and 6 months was less risky than after the age of 1 year (odds ratio [OR]: 3.4, 95% confidence interval [CI]: 1.8–6.5). This result emerged after adjustment for confounding variables. The findings about cooked egg are of major significance for how clinicians should advise parents and for the direction of future research. It appears that introducing egg between the ages of 4 and 6 months may actually prevent development of an allergy, whereas introducing this item later risks provoking an allergy. If these results are confirmed by future studies, there will be a major change to the current dietary advice offered to parents, i.e. not to expose the child to allergenic foods before the age of 1 year [18].

Allergic responses to peanuts in paediatric patients living in the West are twice as common currently as they were a decade ago. This has stimulated research examining ways to stop the development of such allergic responses in children aged under 1 year [23]. It was found that offering peanuts to children at high risk of allergy at an early age was actually protective against the subsequent development of a peanut allergy, as well as changing how the immune system responded to peanut allergens. Accordingly, advice offered to parents in the USA about peanuts has now been altered [18, 24].

3.2   Constituents in Breast Milk

Breastfeeding reduces the incidence of wheezing in infants [25], with a number of constituents of breast milk having been considered potentially responsible for this benefit [26]. Very many constituents in breast milk may explain this effect, namely bioactive enzymes, hormones, growth factors, immunoglobulins or immune signalling molecules. There is evidence that all these constituents strengthen infant immunity [27, 28], thereby fulfilling a key role in the child's healthy development. There are multiple putative mechanisms by which breast milk constituents influence the pathogenesis of asthma. Breastfed infants are relatively better able to withstand respiratory pathogenic infections [29], and this may help to explain how breastfeeding modulates the development of asthma from an early age. Breast milk potentially directly attacks invading microbes, acting to support the not yet fully competent immune system of infants [30]. Although this overall effect is well-established, the exact means by which the protection is conferred by specific breast milk constituents still awaits clarification [18].

3.3   Human Milk Composition

There has frequently been uncertainty in the findings of studies focused on the relationship between atopy and breast milk. This is likely a reflection of the highly complex nature of the phenomenon under study – breast milk composition, the environment of the infant gut and the maturing immune system. Indeed, it is possible that whilst some constituents of human milk are protective against atopy, other elements may actually trigger allergic development [18].

There are a number of constituents in human milk that may affect the infant immune system, such as several antigenic compounds, immune signalling molecules (both cytokines and chemokines), antibodies and polyunsaturated fatty acids [31]. There is transfer of maternal sIgA to the infant via breast milk, including colostrum. One potential benefit of this transfer is that the infant then develops a degree of passive immunity. Infants fed breast milk containing a low concentration of sIgA are more likely to develop allergic hypersensitivity to bovine milk. When the breast milk (colostrum and mature milk) of mothers with allergy is compared with milk from non-allergic mothers, the former is lower in sIgA targeting ovalbumin. However, there was no link between the ovalbumin sIgA levels in milk and the subsequent allergic status of infants [18, 32].

3.4   Probiotics

Certain strains of probiotics alter the level of TGF-β in breast milk. However, *Lactobacillus reuteri* lowers the level [33]. Since the level of TGF-β in breast milk has a powerful role in immunomodulation, the area of probiotics is worthy of more detailed research [18].

3.5   Microbial Flora of the Intestines

Modern lifestyles are more hygienic than those in the past and this has resulted in alterations to the infant intestinal microbiota. This in turn may affect the development of immunological disorders, including allergies and asthma [34]. Human adults have a gut flora with hundreds of different species of bacteria present, the majority being anaerobes. The microbial flora is a complex system. Its composition changes as the infant and child grows. The initial colonisers are facultative or aerobic species, but these are succeeded by an ever more anaerobic flora. The establishment of commensal flora drives much of the development of the immune system [18].

When infants are breastfed for the first 4–6 months of life, this leads to benefit in terms of establishing a healthy intestinal flora. Breast milk contains bifidobacteria and lactate-metabolising bacterial species which contribute to a healthy microbiota [35]. Furthermore, milk supplies oligosaccharides containing galactose, that can be metabolised by beneficial species, especially bifidobacteria. There are several different types of these oligosaccharides in human milk. There are also several other components of breast milk which regulate the intestinal flora, namely specific nucleotides, immunoglobulin A and compounds, notably lactoferrin, which are inhibitory to bacterial growth [18].

The transfer of beneficial microbes occurs through breastfeeding. It is important for the infant gut to contain a varied flora for normal immune development to occur. The microbiota differ between infants who are breastfed and those receiving formula milk; however, these differences have reduced as a result of improvements in the composition of formula milk [34]. In both cases, bifidobacteria and lactobacilli can be isolated from the intestines. One difference is the higher level of *Clostridium difficile*, Bacteroides, enterococci and Enterobacteriaceae in children fed formula, whereas Staphylococci are present in greater numbers in children who are breastfed. Overall, formula feeding results in a smaller range of bacterial species. At present, there is a need for more detailed research investigating how microbial diversity interacts with normal development, including any protective effect on atopy arising from greater microbial diversity [18].

4   How Are Breastfeeding and Allergic Disorders Related?

Asthma, in common with other allergic disorders, arises due to multiple interactions between the genes of a patient and the surrounding environment. There are known environmental factors of importance, such as passive smoking, the diet in early life and allergenic triggers at home, such as house dust mites and pet dander. The vital period for normal development is the initial 1000 days. If the immune system does not encounter specific microbes at this stage, the infant or child may end up primed to develop allergic disorders in the longer term. Currently, the data available support the notion that breastfeeding may protect against developing allergic disorders in childhood, albeit there has been considerable debate over many years as to how extensive such a protective effect may be.

Although there have been a number of high-quality studies on breastfeeding, the evidence for benefit in non-communicable disorders (a category that also includes disorders affecting the immune system) still does not support definite conclusions. One explanation put forward for this apparent paradox is that breast milk varies in composition to a wide degree, and therefore those constituents which can stimulate an immune response also vary considerably [36]. Some researchers conclude that breast feeding reduces the risk of allergic disorders [37], whilst some other evidence has been interpreted to imply either breastfeeding confers no benefit against subsequent atopy, or even raises the likelihood of allergy [38]. These inconsistent conclusions arise through studies of different design, implicit biases in certain studies and the variation in the constituents of human milk [39]. Genetic factors may also play a role. Indeed, the complexity of interactions involved makes it possible for a breast-fed infant to be at lower or higher risk of sensitisation and subsequent atopy. There is also the effect of the mother's diet on breast milk composition, which may also alter its potential to trigger an allergic response [40]. Ethical considerations mean that a study where breastfeeding was the manipulable variable remains unacceptable. Thus, the only data available come from studies based on observation, which are less robust methodologically. Nonetheless, there are many other reasons to prefer breastfeeding and thus the World Health Organization (WHO) and European Society for Paediatric Gastroenterology, Hepatology and Nutrition (ESPGHAN) both advise mother to breastfeed infants exclusively for the initial 4 to 6 months. They note that for infants with a very high risk of subsequent allergy, the action most likely to reduce this risk is a decision to breastfeed. A study undertaken by Guilbert et al. [41] indicated that, when adolescents who had been exclusively breastfed for at least 4 months were compared with those who had received formula milk up to the age of 2 months, respiratory function was inferior in the latter group. Lodge et al. undertook a systematic review and meta-analysis recently [41]. These authors noted that breastfed children had a reduced risk of childhood asthma, but there was little evidence to support a protective effect on allergic eczema up to the age of 2 years or allergic rhinitis up to the age of 5 years. There was no association between breastfeeding and subsequent food allergy [5].

4.1   Breastfeeding and Asthma

Research examining how being breastfed is related to the risk of becoming asthmatic has likewise resulted in seemingly inconsistent results. Being exclusively breastfed up to the age of 3 or 4 months has an association with a lower likelihood of developing wheeze up to the age of around 6 years. This advantage seems to be most noticeable up to the age of 2 years. If the mother herself has asthma and the child is at raised risk, breastfeeding may even raise the risk of asthma in the offspring [42].

When used as a marker to indicate a developing asthmatic tendency, wheeze refers to several related respiratory problems, including coughing, dyspnoea, wheeze proper and shortness of breath. It is important to recall that wheeze has a differing pathological significance at different stages in a child's life, since asthma-like symptoms arise from different causes. Up to the age of 1 or 2 years, wheezing frequently results from infections of the upper respiratory tract. Infants who tend to wheeze frequently improve over time and the symptoms is not invariably associated with an asthmatic tendency. On the other hand, once children are attending school or enter adolescence, a tendency to wheeze is a more fixed characteristic and indicates a likely cause of allergic asthma [42].

Since it has been demonstrated that breastfed infants suffer a lower rate of respiratory tract infections, and since wheezing is strongly associated with such events, breastfeeding is expected to lower upper respiratory tract infection (URTI)-associated wheezing in infants [43–46]. A systematic review and meta-analysis that collated studies examining asthma in breastfed infants noted that the practice was most beneficial up to the age of 2 years, and this protection did not depend on how long breastfeeding occurred or whether formula was also given. The study used the terms 'asthma ever' and 'recent asthma' and accepted wheeze, bronchiolitis and bronchitis under its definition of asthmatic conditions [47]. Breastfeeding offered less protection as the child's age increased, and this accords with the observation from many studies that breastfeeding does not reduce the risk of asthma in those children at highest risk [48–50]. A different systematic review and meta-analysis [51] gathered the results of 29 studies to enquire whether the length of time breastfeeding occurred had any effect on the likelihood of becoming asthmatic. The authors concluded that more prolonged breastfeeding reduced the frequency of asthma in children aged between 5 and 18 years. The benefit from breastfeeding was highest if the child was raised in a medium or low-income country. Finally, a third article of this type [52] which compiled results from 31 studies noted that breastfeeding of any type and lasting any period was not associated with the development of wheeze. All the data related to children over the age of 5 years. This negative result also came out of a Norwegian study involving a cohort of the entire country, where the risk of asthma at age 7 years was not linked in any way to how long the child had been breastfed [42, 53].

4.2 The Relationship Between Breastfeeding and Allergic Rhinitis

How breastfeeding and allergic rhinitis may be related is a matter of ongoing debate. The studies undertaken between 1966 and 2000 looking at the relationship between being exclusively breastfed for 3 months or more and subsequent allergic rhinitis, and where a prospective design was employed, have been collated and a systematic review and meta-analysis performed. The follow-up lasted 2 years and 3 months [54]. This analysis was affected by diagnostic challenges in young children, in whom rhinitis is often infective rather than allergic in type. Furthermore, allergic rhinitis usually starts after the age of 3 years. When the results of 6 studies were pooled, breastfeeding seemed to lower the risk of allergic rhinitis although this result lacked statistical significance (OR: 0.74, 95% CI: 0.54–1.01) [54]. A different meta-analysis and systematic review did find that being breastfed for longer was associated with lower risk of allergic rhinitis, up to and including the age of 5 years, but the association was weak [24]. A cohort study involving the offspring of asthmatic mothers, which has since been reported [42, 48], noted that exclusive breastfeeding had no effect on the likelihood of the infant becoming sensitised to 12 frequently encountered airborne allergens up to the age of 6 years, nor on the likelihood of allergic rhinitis at age 7 years.

4.3 Breastfeeding and Food Allergy

The evidence base for how breastfeeding affects the development of hypersensitivity to food consists of a few studies, the findings from which may be subject to several potential confounding variables, namely how long breastfeeding occurred and whether or not it was supplemented by formula and the presence of other allergic disorders, such as allergic eczema or asthma [55–57].

A systematic review published in 2004 concluded that infants who were exclusively breastfed for a minimum period of 4 months were at a reduced risk of being allergic to bovine milk up to the age of 1.5 years [58]. A Taiwanese cohort study which enrolled small numbers found that hypersensitivity to bovine milk was lower below the age of 2 years in children who were exclusively breastfed for a minimum of 4 months than in those who were either breastfed for less time or had additional formula feeds [59].

A study of observational design that appeared after the Taiwanese study cited indicated that for children with allergic eczema, breastfeeding was associated with a higher incidence of egg allergy and sensitisation than formula feeding. The criteria for diagnosing allergy were a specific IgE level of at least 2 kU/L, and for sensitisation, at least 0.7 kU/L [57]. The family histories of the two groups of infants were not significantly different with regard to allergic disorders. How egg sensitisation occurred could not be definitely demonstrated, although the findings of this study suggest it was via breast milk. The two groups did not, however, differ at the level of statistical significance in terms of sensitisation or actual allergy to bovine or soy milk. A further study of observational design which examined children whose mothers were asthmatic [48] concluded that the length of time for which the children had been exclusively breastfed was not associated with any of 10 common allergens found in food, at least up to the age of 6 years. It is important to note, however, that sensitisation, defined in terms of expression of IgE to particular food antigens, does not invariably imply a food allergy. This doubt about true allergy status especially exists where there is no previous history of allergic response or allergy has not been confirmed by a specialist using a controlled food challenge [42].

References

1. Pawankar R, Canonica G, Holgate S, Lockey R, Blaiss M. WAO white book on allergy. Milwaukee Wi World Allergy Organ. 2011;3:156–7.
2. Prescott SL, Pawankar R, Allen KJ, Campbell DE, Sinn JK, Fiocchi A, Ebisawa M, Sampson HA, Beyer K, Lee B-W. A global survey of changing patterns of food allergy burden in children. World Allergy Organ J. 2013;6:1–12. https://doi.org/10.1186/1939-4551-6-21.
3. Strachan DP. Hay fever, hygiene, and household size. BMJ Br Med J. 1989;299:1259. https://doi.org/10.1136/bmj.299.6710.1259.
4. Munblit D, Peroni DG, Boix-Amorós A, Hsu PS, Land BVT, Gay MC, Kolotilina A, Skevaki C, Boyle RJ, Collado MC. Human milk and allergic diseases: an unsolved puzzle. Nutrients. 2017;9:894. https://doi.org/10.3390/nu9080894.
5. Nuzzi G, Di Cicco ME, Peroni DG. Breastfeeding and allergic diseases: what's new? Children (Basel). 2021;8(5):330. https://doi.org/10.3390/children8050330.
6. Julvez J, Guxens M, Carsin AE, Forns J, Mendez M, Turner MC, Sunyer J. A cohort study on full breastfeeding and child neuropsychological development: the role of maternal social, psychological, and nutritional factors. Dev Med Child Neurol. 2014;56:148–56. https://doi.org/10.1111/dmcn.12282.
7. Krol KM, Grossmann T. Psychological effects of breastfeeding on children and mothers. Bundesgesundheitsblatt Gesundheitsforschung Gesundheitsschutz. 2018;61:977–85. https://doi.org/10.1007/s00103-018-2769-0.
8. Ballard O, Morrow AL. Human milk composition: nutrients and bioactive factors. Pediatr Clin. 2013;60:49–74.
9. Kulski J, Hartmann P. Changes in human milk composition during the initiation of lactation. Aust J Exp Biol Med Sci. 1981;59:101–14. https://doi.org/10.1038/icb.1981.6.
10. Dzidic M, Boix-Amorós A, Selma-Royo M, Mira A, Collado MC. Gut microbiota and mucosal immunity in the neonate. Med Sci. 2018;6:56. https://doi.org/10.3390/medsci6030056.
11. Peroni DG, Nuzzi G, Trambusti I, Di Cicco ME, Comberiati P. Microbiome composition and its impact on the development of allergic diseases. Front Immunol. 2020;11:700. https://doi.org/10.3389/fimmu.2020.00700.
12. Penders JTC, Vink C, Stelma FF, Snijders B, Kummeling I, van den Brandt PA, Stobberingh EE. Factors influencing the composition of the intestinal microbiome in early infancy. Pediatrics. 2006;118:511–21. https://doi.org/10.1542/peds.2005-2824.
13. Saarela T, Kokkonen J, Koivisto M. Macronutrient and energy contents of human milk fractions during the first six months of lactation. Acta Paediatr. 2005;94:1176–81. https://doi.org/10.1111/j.1651-2227.2005.tb02070.x.
14. Greer FR. Do breastfed infants need supplemental vitamins? Pediatr Clin N Am. 2001;48:415–23. https://doi.org/10.1016/S0031-3955(08)70034-8.

15. Lönnerdal B. Human milk proteins. Prot Infants Hum Milk. 2004;554:11–25.
16. Srivastava MD, Srivastava A, Brouhard B, Saneto R, Groh-Wargo S, Kubit J. Cytokines in human milk. Res Commun Mol Pathol Pharm. 1996;93:263–87.
17. Ogawa J, Sasahara A, Yoshida T, Sira MM, Futatani T, Kanegane H, Miyawaki T. Role of transforming growth factor-β in breast milk for initiation of IgA production in newborn infants. Early Hum Dev. 2004;77:67–75. https://doi.org/10.1016/j.earlhumdev.2004.01.005.
18. Oddy WH. Breastfeeding, childhood asthma, and allergic disease. Ann Nutr Metab. 2017;70:26–36. https://doi.org/10.1159/000457920.
19. Prescott SL, Tang MLK. The Australasian Society of Clinical Immunology and Allergy position statement: summary of allergy prevention in children. Med J Aust. 2005;182:464–7.
20. World Health Organization: Global Strategy for Infant and Young Child Feeding. Geneva; 2003.
21. Prescott SL, Smith P, Tang M, Palmer DJ, Sinn J, Huntley SJ, et al. The importance of early complementary feeding in the development of oral tolerance: concerns and controversies. Pediatr Allergy Immunol. 2008;19:375–80.
22. Koplin JJ, Osborne NJ, Wake M, Martin PE, Gurrin LC, Robinson MN, et al. Can early introduction of egg prevent egg allergy in infants? A population-based study. J Allergy Clin Immunol. 2010;126:807–13.
23. Du Toit G, Roberts G, Sayre PH, Bahnson HT, Radulovic S, Santos AF, et al. Randomized trial of peanut consumption in infants at risk for peanut allergy. N Engl J Med. 2015;372:803–13.
24. Togias A, Cooper SF, Acebal ML, Assa'ad A, Baker JR Jr, Beck LA, et al. Addendum guidelines for the prevention of peanut allergy in the United States: report of the National Institute of Allergy and Infectious Diseases - sponsored expert panel. J Allergy Clin Immunol. 2017;139:29–44.
25. Oddy WH, Sly PD, de Klerk NH, Landau LI, Kendall GE, Holt PG, et al. Breast feeding and respiratory morbidity in infancy: a birth cohort study. Arch Dis Child. 2003;88:224–8.
26. Field CJ. The immunological components of human milk and their effect on immune development in infants. J Nutr. 2005;135:1–4.
27. Newburg DS, Walker WA. Protection of the neonate by the innate immune system of developing gut and of human milk. Pediatr Res. 2007;61:2–8.
28. Garofalo RP, Goldman AS. Expression of functional immunomodulatory and anti-inflammatory factors in human milk. Clin Perinatol. 1999;26:361–78.
29. Oddy WH, de Klerk NH, Sly PD, Holt PG. The effects of respiratory infections, atopy and breastfeeding on childhood asthma. Eur Respir J. 2002;19:899–905.
30. Hanson LÅ. Breastfeeding provides passive and likely longlasting active immunity. Ann Allergy Asthma Immunol. 1998;81:523–37.
31. Friedman NJ, Zeiger RS. The role of breast-feeding in the development of allergies and asthma. J Allergy Clin Immunol. 2005;115:1238–48.
32. Saarinen KM, Vaarala O, Klemetti P, Savilahti E. Transforming growth factor-β1 in mothers' colostrum and immune responses to cows' milk proteins in infants with cows' milk allergy. J Allergy Clin Immunol. 1999;104:1093–8.
33. Rautava S. Potential uses of probiotics in the neonate. Semin Fetal Neonatal Med. 2007;12:45–53.
34. Adlerberth I, Wold AE. Establishment of the gut microbiota in Western infants. Acta Paediatr. 2009;98:229–38.
35. Martín R, Olivares M, Marín ML, Fernández L, Xaus J, Rodríguez JM. Probiotic potential of 3 Lactobacilli strains isolated from breast milk. J Hum Lact. 2005;21:8–17.
36. D'Alessandro A, Scaloni A, Zolla L. Human milk proteins: an interactomics and updated functional overview. J Proteome Res. 2010;9:3339–73. https://doi.org/10.1021/pr100123f.
37. Davis MK. Breastfeeding and chronic disease in childhood and adolescence. Pediatr Clin. N. Am. 2001;48:125–41. https://doi.org/10.1016/S0031-3955(05)70289-3.
38. Giwercman C, Halkjaer LB, Jensen SM, Bønnelykke K, Lauritzen L, Bisgaard H. Increased risk of eczema but reduced risk of early wheezy disorder from exclusive breast-feeding in

high-risk infants. J Allergy Clin Immunol. 2010;125:866–71. https://doi.org/10.1016/j.jaci.2010.01.026.

39. Munblit D, Treneva M, Peroni DG, Colicino S, Chow LY, Dissanayeke S, Pampura A, Boner AL, Geddes DT, Boyle RJ. Immune components in human milk are associated with early infant immunological health outcomes: a prospective three-country analysis. Nutrients. 2017;9:532. https://doi.org/10.3390/nu9060532.

40. Munblit D, Boyle R, Warner J. Factors affecting breast milk composition and potential consequences for development of the allergic phenotype. Clin Exp Allergy. 2015;45:583–601. https://doi.org/10.1111/cea.12381.

41. Lodge CJ, Tan D, Lau M, Dai X, Tham R, Lowe AJ, Bowatte G, Allen K, Dharmage SC. Breastfeeding and asthma and allergies: a systematic review and meta-analysis. Acta Paediatr. 2015;104:38–53. https://doi.org/10.1111/apa.13132.

42. Fleischer DM. The impact of breastfeeding on the development of allergic disease. In: Sicherer SH, TePas E (Eds). UpToDate. Last updated: Aug 28, 2020.

43. Elliott L, Henderson J, Northstone K, et al. Prospective study of breast-feeding in relation to wheeze, atopy, and bronchial hyperresponsiveness in the Avon Longitudinal Study of Parents and Children (ALSPAC). J Allergy Clin Immunol. 2008;122:49.

44. Wright AL, Holberg CJ, Martinez FD, et al. Breast feeding and lower respiratory tract illness in the first year of life. Group Health Medical Associates. BMJ. 1989;299:946.

45. Holberg CJ, Wright AL, Martinez FD, et al. Risk factors for respiratory syncytial virus-associated lower respiratory illnesses in the first year of life. Am J Epidemiol. 1991;133:1135.

46. Howie PW, Forsyth JS, Ogston SA, et al. Protective effect of breast feeding against infection. BMJ. 1990;300:11.

47. Dogaru CM, Nyffenegger D, Pescatore AM, et al. Breastfeeding and childhood asthma: systematic review and meta-analysis. Am J Epidemiol. 2014;179:1153.

48. Jelding-Dannemand E, Malby Schoos AM, Bisgaard H. Breast-feeding does not protect against allergic sensitization in early childhood and allergy-associated disease at age 7 years. J Allergy Clin Immunol. 2015;136:1302.

49. Wright AL, Holberg CJ, Taussig LM, Martinez FD. Factors influencing the relation of infant feeding to asthma and recurrent wheeze in childhood. Thorax. 2001;56:192.

50. Sears MR, Greene JM, Willan AR, et al. Long-term relation between breastfeeding and development of atopy and asthma in children and young adults: a longitudinal study. Lancet. 2002;360:901.

51. Lodge CJ, Tan DJ, Lau MX, et al. Breastfeeding and asthma and allergies: a systematic review and meta-analysis. Acta Paediatr. 2015;104:38.

52. Brew BK, Allen CW, Toelle BG, Marks GB. Systematic review and meta-analysis investigating breast feeding and childhood wheezing illness. Paediatr Perinat Epidemiol. 2011;25:507.

53. Lossius AK, Magnus MC, Lunde J, Størdal K. Prospective cohort study of breastfeeding and the risk of childhood asthma. J Pediatr. 2018;195:182.

54. Mimouni Bloch A, Mimouni D, Mimouni M, Gdalevich M. Does breastfeeding protect against allergic rhinitis during childhood? A meta-analysis of prospective studies. Acta Paediatr. 2002;91:275.

55. Greer FR, Sicherer SH, Burks AW, et al. The effects of early nutritional interventions on the development of atopic disease in infants and children: the role of maternal dietary restriction, breastfeeding, hydrolyzed formulas, and timing of introduction of allergenic complementary foods. Pediatrics. 2019;143:e20190281.

56. Høst A, Halken S, Muraro A, et al. Dietary prevention of allergic diseases in infants and small children. Pediatr Allergy Immunol. 2008;19:1.

57. Han Y, Chung SJ, Kim J, et al. High sensitization rate to food allergens in breastfed infants with atopic dermatitis. Ann Allergy Asthma Immunol. 2009;103:332.

58. Muraro A, Dreborg S, Halken S, et al. Dietary prevention of allergic diseases in infants and small children. Part III: Critical review of published peer-reviewed observational and interventional studies and final recommendations. Pediatr Allergy Immunol. 2004;15:291.

59. Liao SL, Lai SH, Yeh KW, et al. Exclusive breastfeeding is associated with reduced cow's milk sensitization in early childhood. Pediatr Allergy Immunol. 2014;25:456.

Breastfeeding and Atopic Dermatitis

Sait Karaman and Demet Can

1 Introduction

Up to the age of 6 months, the best way for infants born at term to be fed is by breast milk only [1]. Universal breastfeeding is recommended by both national governments and doctors' professional associations worldwide, since breast milk offers multiple advantages: nutritional, functional, immune-protective and psychological. Breastfeeding helps the gut to develop healthily, confers immunity against many pathogens and improves the infant's emotional health [1–4]. Furthermore, epidemiological data support the conclusion that breastfed infants have a lower risk of several paediatric conditions linked to the immune system, namely inflammatory and autoimmune diseases and neoplasia, which may indicate breastfeeding has long-term effects on how the immune system works [5].

In every infant, the recommendation is to continue breastfeeding up to the age of 4–6 months, as a minimum [1, 6–8]. Due to the multiple advantages breastfeeding offers, both maternal and for infants, the WHO (World Health Organisation) advises that infants should receive only breast milk up to the age of 6 months, to ensure the best chance of normal healthy growth and development [8].

It is the recommendation of both the American Academy of Allergy, Asthma & Immunology and the European Academy of Allergy and Clinical Immunology that infants receive breast milk only up to the age of 4–6 months in order to reduce the risk of developing a primary atopic disorder [6, 9]. The assertion that breastfeeding can lower the incidence of allergy has been made for at least the last seven decades.

S. Karaman (✉)
Department of Pediatrics, Division of Allergy and Immunology, Manisa City Hospital, Manisa, Türkiye

D. Can
Department of Pediatrics, Division of Allergy and Immunology, Izmir Dr. Behcet Uz Children's Hospital, Izmir, Türkiye

Ö. N. Şahin et al. (eds.), *Breastfeeding and Metabolic Programming*, https://doi.org/10.1007/978-3-031-33278-4_43

531

However, whilst multiple studies have examined the relationship between breast-feeding and atopic disorders, such as allergic dermatitis, the conclusions researchers reach have remained somewhat inconsistent [10].

2 Immunological Properties of Human Milk

There are several components of breast milk which perform an active immune function, such as antibodies, antimicrobial enzymes and certain white cells. There are also some molecules which inhibit inflammation or increase tolerance, for example polyunsaturated long-chain fatty acids (PUFA), platelet-activating factor (PAF) acetylhydrolase and interleukin-10 (IL-10). Moreover, several molecules which exert a modulatory role on the innate immune defences through stimulation or inhibition of specific receptors, such as CD-14 and other factors interacting with toll-like receptors, have been characterised in breast milk [11–16]. Nonetheless, in the majority of studies so far published, it is unclear how the presence of these breast milk constituents affects the allergic state of either the mother or child [5, 17, 18].

3 Atopic Dermatitis (AD)

Atopic dermatitis is a dermatological disorder of chronic type involving inflammation and itching of the skin, usually distributed over the facial (especially malar) and cervical areas and limbs, but rarely found in the groin or axillae. See accompanying illustration. Although this condition generally has its onset in young infants, it is also common in adulthood. Atopic dermatitis is typically accompanied by raised serological titres of immunoglobulin E (IgE). Atopic dermatitis frequently precedes the development of other atopic conditions, which occur in the characteristic sequence: food allergy, asthma and allergic rhinitis. This has led some experts to propose that atopic dermatitis is the first step in the development of allergic reactions at various epithelial interfaces, namely the gastrointestinal tract and airways. This theory is termed the 'atopic march' [19–21].

The sole symptomatic presentation of atopic dermatitis is a continuous pruritic itch. There are generally periods where the atopic dermatitis flares up, interspersed with periods of remission. The triggers for exacerbations are usually obscure [19].

The main abnormalities on physical examination are as follows [19]:

- Xerosis (skin dryness).
- Lichenification (the skin becomes thickened and its markings more prominent).
- Areas of eczematous inflammation.

The appearances of the lesions and their distribution varies with the age of the patient, being different in infancy, childhood and adulthood.

In addition, the following clinical features often co-occur in cases of atopic dermatitis [19]:

- Itching.
- The patient is very young when the disorder first presents.
- The condition is chronic and relapsing in nature.
- IgE is central to the pathology.
- There is a raised blood eosinophil count.
- Lesions may be superinfected with *Staphylococcus aureus.*
- The patient either also suffers from asthma or allergic rhinitis, or there is a positive family history of atopy in a first-degree relative.

3.1 Diagnosing Atopic Dermatitis

According to the guidelines promulgated by the American Academy of Dermatology (AAD) since 2014, the following diagnostic criteria should be considered when diagnosing atopic dermatitis (AD) [22]:

Unless the following features are noted, the diagnosis of AD cannot be made:

- Itching.
- Eczematous rash. The condition may be acute, subacute or chronic.
- Furthermore:
  - The lesions must have the appropriate morphological appearances and follow the expected distribution according to the patient's age, i.e. affecting the face, neck and extensor surfaces in children or the flexures in all patients, but not affecting the groin or axilla.
  - The lesions must be chronic or follow a relapsing course.

Additionally, the following features are considered highly consistent with AD [19]:

- The condition begins early in life.
- There is a history of atopy in the patient or a relative and IgE levels are raised.
- Skin dryness is present.

There are also a number of features which do not specifically indicate AD, but are also found in the condition, namely [19]:

- Vascular reflexes are abnormal. This presents as pallor of the face, or delayed blanching.
- Keratosis pilaris, pityriasis alba, hyperlinear palms or ichthyosis.
- Changed appearances around the eyes and/or mouth.
- Other areas of changed skin appearance, such as around the pinna.
- Perifollicular accentuation, lichenification or prurigo.

4   Breastfeeding and Its Relationship to AD

The pathogenesis of asthma and other atopic disorders involves many complicated interactions, involving both genetic predisposition and environmental triggers. The environmental triggers include early weaning, breathing second-hand cigarette smoke and allergens found in homes (namely house dust mites or pet animal dander). The initial 1000 days following birth are a period of vital importance for healthy development of the immune system. If anything interferes with the normal interactions between microbes and the maturing immune system during this initial period, there is a possibility of long-term damage, rendering the infant at risk of allergic disorders. The current evidence points to a role for some constituents of breast milk in avoiding development of allergies, albeit the exact role of breast milk in prevention of atopic diseases remains controversial. Even though the evidence is gathering from studies of robust methodological design, the extent to which breast milk protects against several non-infectious diseases, including those involving the immune system, is still not clear from the results so far. One potential explanation that has been advanced is that the varying findings reflect the heterogeneity within breast milk, which may contain widely varying concentrations of particular bioactive constituents [23]. Whilst the results of some studies do indicate that breastfeeding significantly protects against atopic disorders [24], other studies have disputed this finding, with some experts asserting that breastfeeding may even increase the incidence [25]. Much of the inconsistency in the findings likely stems from different methodologies used in the studies involved, some inherent biases and the fact that breast milk plays complex immune roles [26]. Genetics may also be significant in this regard. Because of these different factors, it is possible that breastfeeding may protect some infants against atopic diseases, whilst triggering sensitisation in others. Furthermore, the dietary intake of the mother may also alter the immune function of milk, which then affects how children go on to develop allergies [27]. For ethical reasons, a study which randomised whether an infant was breastfed or not would not receive approval, and this then means that the evidence base consists of observational-type studies, which are of lower evidential value. Despite the incomplete picture gathered so far, it does appear clear that failure to endorse breastfeeding would risk significant potential harm in terms of missed opportunities to prevent atopic disorders. This is the reasoning behind the advice by the World Health Organisation (WHO) and European Society for Paediatric Gastroenterology Hepatology and Nutrition (ESPGHAN) that infants up to the age of 4 or 6 months should be exclusively breastfed. A study undertaken by Guilbert et al. [28] demonstrated superior respiratory function in infants receiving exclusively breast milk up to a minimum age of 4 months compared to those who received artificial baby milk before the age of 2 months. The recent article by Lodge et al., consisting of a systematic review and meta-analysis, showed that breastfed children had a lower risk of developing asthma. The risk of AD up to the age of 2 years, or allergic rhinitis up to the age of 5 years, may also be reduced, but the evidence for this conclusion is not very compelling. There appeared to be no relationship between breastfeeding and the risk of developing food allergies [29].

The majority of studies examining the relationship between breastfeeding and AD consist of follow-up of cohorts from birth or cross-sectional surveys. One study of observational type, which enrolled in excess of 200,000 infants across many different countries was ISAAC (the International Study of Asthma and Allergies in Childhood). This study concluded that breastfeeding did not reduce the incidence of AD in children aged between 6 and 7 years, albeit there was some protective effect against the most severe degree of AD [30]. Lodge et al. reviewed the literature and performed a meta-analysis of published data [31]. This revealed that exclusive breastfeeding for at least 3 or 4 months did result in a reduced incidence of AD, but this reduced incidence did not persist for longer than 2 years. According to the same article, many of the earlier studies which concluded that breastfeeding reduces the risk of AD involved small numbers of participants and failed to eliminate possible biases.

There are several studies, however, which have demonstrated a reduction in the incidence of AD occurring in childhood when infants were breastfed. A study of cohort design, which followed 4089 children from birth, found that a period of breastfeeding lasting a minimum of 4 months lowered the incidence of AD and resulted in allergic march only occurring at the age of 4 years [32]. One study, with a cross-sectional design and based in developing countries concluded that a lengthy period of being breastfed was protective against several atopic disorders, including AD, and this protective effect was irrespective of whether the mother herself suffered from atopy [33]. A study with a prospective methodology used randomisation to assign 17,046 healthy mothers, whose children were born at term, to one of two groups: one received usual follow-up, whilst patients in the other group received supportive advice about breastfeeding. The group where the extra support was provided had a 46% lower incidence of AD than the other, unsupported group. However, the result was very close to the limit for being deemed statistically significant [34]. A study from Taiwan using a cohort design and with 186 participants concluded that infants breastfed for a minimum of 6 months, whether exclusive or not, had a lower incidence of AD in early childhood than other children [35]. The results of some 18 studies were pooled for a meta-analysis and a systematic review was undertaken, the results of which showed that exclusively breastfed infants were at lower risk of AD, even with a family history of atopic disease [36]. The protective benefit is lower in children more generally and barely perceptible unless the child has a first degree relative with an atopic disposition [36]. Another study followed up a cohort of infants, all of whom were born at term and were healthy. Some 865 infants received breastfeeding only, whilst 256 were given at least some artificial baby milk. The infants were observed up to the age of 1 year. For those children with risk factors for atopic disorders, being exclusively breastfed for a minimum of 4 months stopped AD from occurring up to the age of 1 year [10, 37].

Other evidence in the literature, however, suggests no benefit from breastfeeding in terms of preventing AD. A recent article in *Allergy, Asthma and Immunology Research* examined once again how breastfeeding and AD are related in young children [38]. Lee et al. investigated 2015 young children between the ages of 1 and 3 years, who were enrolled in the Korea National Health and Nutrition Examination Survey. Breastfeeding and AD did not appear to be related at all. Furthermore, the duration of breastfeeding tends to be longer if the mother or father has an atopic disorder and the decision to breastfeed is also more popular in this group. Other studies have also made similar observations [39].

Lin et al. [40] concluded that it was still a matter of debate what relationship, if any, exists between breastfeeding and AD. This conclusion was based on 27 studies, the data from which were included in a meta-analysis. The odds ratios calculated from the pooled data for breastfeeding of any type were 1.01 (95% confidence interval [CI]: 0.93–1.10), and for exclusive breastfeeding, 0.99 (95% Confidence interval (CI): 0.88–1.11). There was a high degree of heterogeneity in the study types (total: $P < 0.01$ or $I^2 = 65.2\%$; exclusive: $P < 0.01$ or $I^2 = 72.3\%$). The data suggest that breastfed infants with a family history of atopy are mildly protected against developing AD (total: relative risk [RR] 0.85, 95% CI: 0.74–0.98; exclusive: RR 0.83, 95% CI: 0.70–0.97). For infants without a positive atopic family history, the protective effect for exclusively breastfed infants was less than that seen in those with a positive family history (RR: 1.19, 95% CI: 1.02–1.40). The protective effect started to disappear when looking at breastfed infants as a whole, regardless of exclusivity (RR: 1.11, 95% CI: 0.94–1.31). Thus, overall, Lin et al. assert, breastfeeding does not affect the risk of AD. In some subgroups there is a protective effect, namely those infants with a positive family history of atopy, whether exclusively breastfed or not. However, if the family history of atopy is not present, the protective effect disappears. In any case, the data are too heterogeneous to make firm conclusions about any relationship between AD and breastfeeding.

References

1. Section on Breastfeeding. Breastfeeding and the use of human milk. Pediatrics. 2012;129:e827.
2. Department of Health and Human Services, Office on Women's Health. Breastfeeding: HHS Blueprint for Action on Breastfeeding. US Department of Health and Human Services, Washington, DC; 2000.
3. American College of Obstetricians and Gynecologists. Breastfeeding: maternal and infant aspects. ACOG Educational Bulletin 258, American College of Obstetricians and Gynecologists, Washington, DC; 2000.
4. Greer FR, Sicherer SH, Burks AW, et al. The effects of early nutritional interventions on the development of atopic disease in infants and children: the role of maternal dietary restriction, breastfeeding, hydrolyzed formulas, and timing of introduction of allergenic complementary foods. Pediatrics. 2019;143
5. Fleischer DM. The impact of breastfeeding on the development of allergic disease. In: Sicherer SH, TePas E (Eds). UpToDate. Last updated: Oct 16, 2022.
6. Muraro A, Halken S, Arshad SH, Beyer K, Dubois AE, Du Toit G, et al. EAACI food allergy and anaphylaxis guidelines. Primary prevention of food allergy. Allergy. 2014;69:590–601.
7. Chan ES, Cummings C Canadian Paediatric Society, Community Paediatrics Committee and Allergy Section. Dietary exposures and allergy prevention in high-risk infants: a joint state-

ment with the Canadian Society of Allergy and Clinical Immunology. Paediatr Child Health. 2013;18:545–54.

8. Vandenplas Y, Abuabat A, Al-Hammadi S, Aly GS, Miqdady MS, Shaaban SY, et al. Middle east consensus statement on the prevention, diagnosis, and management of cow's milk protein allergy. Pediatr Gastroenterol Hepatol Nutr. 2014;17:61–73.

9. Fleischer DM, Spergel JM, Assa'ad AH, Pongracic JA. Primary prevention of allergic disease through nutritional interventions. J Allergy Clin Immunol Pract. 2013;1:29–36.

10. Kim JH. Role of breast-feeding in the development of atopic dermatitis in early childhood. Allergy Asthma Immunol Res. 2017;9(4):285–7. https://doi.org/10.4168/aair.2017.9.4.285.

11. Duchén K, Casas R, Fagerås-Böttcher M, et al. Human milk polyunsaturated long-chain fatty acids and secretory immunoglobulin A antibodies and early childhood allergy. Pediatr Allergy Immunol. 2000;11:29.

12. Firth MA, Shewen PE, Hodgins DC. Passive and active components of neonatal innate immune defenses. Anim Health Res Rev. 2005;6:143.

13. Labbok MH, Clark D, Goldman AS. Breastfeeding: maintaining an irreplaceable immunological resource. Nat Rev Immunol. 2004;4:565.

14. Armogida SA, Yannaras NM, Melton AL, Srivastava MD. Identification and quantification of innate immune system mediators in human breast milk. Allergy Asthma Proc. 2004;25:297.

15. LeBouder E, Rey-Nores JE, Rushmere NK, et al. Soluble forms of Toll-like receptor (TLR)2 capable of modulating TLR2 signaling are present in human plasma and breast milk. J Immunol. 2003;171:6680.

16. LeBouder E, Rey-Nores JE, Raby AC, et al. Modulation of neonatal microbial recognition: TLR-mediated innate immune responses are specifically and differentially modulated by human milk. J Immunol. 2006;176:3742.

17. Rigotti E, Piacentini GL, Ress M, et al. Transforming growth factor-beta and interleukin-10 in breast milk and development of atopic diseases in infants. Clin Exp Allergy. 2006;36:614.

18. Snijders BE, Damoiseaux JG, Penders J, et al. Cytokines and soluble CD14 in breast milk in relation with atopic manifestations in mother and infant (KOALA Study). Clin Exp Allergy. 2006;36:1609.

19. Kim BS. Atopic Dermatitis. In: James Wd (Ed). Medscape. Updated: Jul 27, 2022.https://emedicine.medscape.com/article/1049085-overview. Accessed online at December 3, 2022.

20. Spergel JM. From atopic dermatitis to asthma: the atopic march. Ann Allergy Asthma Immunol. 2010;105(2):99–106; quiz 107–9, 117.

21. Carlsten C, Dimich-Ward H, Ferguson A, Watson W, Rousseau R, Dybuncio A, et al. Atopic dermatitis in a high-risk cohort: natural history, associated allergic outcomes, and risk factors. Ann Allergy Asthma Immunol. 2013;110(1):24–8.

22. Eichenfield LF, Tom WL, Chamlin SL, Feldman SR, Hanifin JM, Simpson EL, et al. Guidelines of care for the management of atopic dermatitis: section 1. Diagnosis and assessment of atopic dermatitis. J Am Acad Dermatol. 2014;70(2):338–51. [Guideline]

23. D'Alessandro A, Scaloni A, Zolla L. Human milk proteins: an interactomics and updated functional overview. J Proteome Res. 2010;9:3339–73. https://doi.org/10.1021/pr100123f.

24. Davis MK. Breastfeeding and chronic disease in childhood and adolescence. Pediatr Clin N Am. 2001;48:125–41. https://doi.org/10.1016/S0031-3955(05)70289-3.

25. Giwercman C, Halkjaer LB, Jensen SM, Bønnelykke K, Lauritzen L, Bisgaard H. Increased risk of eczema but reduced risk of early wheezy disorder from exclusive breast-feeding in high-risk infants. J Allergy Clin Immunol. 2010;125:866–71. https://doi.org/10.1016/j.jaci.2010.01.026.

26. Munblit D, Treneva M, Peroni DG, Colicino S, Chow LY, Dissanayeke S, Pampura A, Boner AL, Geddes DT, Boyle RJ. Immune components in human milk are associated with early infant immunological health outcomes: a prospective three-country analysis. Nutrients. 2017;9:532. https://doi.org/10.3390/nu9060532.

27. Munblit D, Boyle R, Warner J. Factors affecting breast milk composition and potential consequences for development of the allergic phenotype. Clin Exp Allergy. 2015;45:583–601. https://doi.org/10.1111/cea.12381.
28. Guilbert TW, Stern DA, Morgan WJ, Martinez FD, Wright AL. Effect of breastfeeding on lung function in childhood and modulation by maternal asthma and atopy. Am J Respir Crit Care Med. 2007;176:843–8. https://doi.org/10.1164/rccm.200610-1507OC.
29. Nuzzi G, Di Cicco ME, Peroni DG. Breastfeeding and allergic diseases: what's new? Children (Basel). 2021;8(5):330. https://doi.org/10.3390/children8050330.
30. Björkstén B, Ait-Khaled N, Asher MI, Clayton T, Robertson C, Group I.P.T.S. Global analysis of breast feeding and risk of symptoms of asthma, rhinoconjunctivitis and eczema in 6–7 year old children: ISAAC Phase Three. Allergol Immunopathol. 2011;39:318–25. https://doi.org/10.1016/j.aller.2011.02.005.
31. Lodge CJ, Tan D, Lau M, Dai X, Tham R, Lowe AJ, Bowatte G, Allen K, Dharmage SC. Breastfeeding and asthma and allergies: a systematic review and meta-analysis. Acta Paediatr. 2015;104:38–53. https://doi.org/10.1111/apa.13132.
32. Kull I, Böhme M, Wahlgren CF, Nordvall L, Pershagen G, Wickman M. Breast-feeding reduces the risk for childhood eczema. J Allergy Clin Immunol. 2005;116:657–61.
33. Ehlayel MS, Bener A. Duration of breast-feeding and the risk of childhood allergic diseases in a developing country. Allergy Asthma Proc. 2008;29:386–91.
34. Flohr C, Nagel G, Weinmayr G, Kleiner A, Strachan DP, Williams HC, ISAAC Phase Two Study Group. Lack of evidence for a protective effect of prolonged breastfeeding on childhood eczema: lessons from the International Study of Asthma and Allergies in Childhood (ISAAC) Phase Two. Br J Dermatol. 2011;165:1280–9.
35. Chiu CY, Liao SL, Su KW, Tsai MH, Hua MC, Lai SH, et al. Exclusive or partial breastfeeding for 6 months is associated with reduced milk sensitization and risk of eczema in early childhood: the PATCH Birth Cohort Study. Medicine (Baltimore). 2016;95:e3391.
36. Gdalevich M, Mimouni D, David M, Mimouni M. Breast-feeding and the onset of atopic dermatitis in childhood: a systematic review and meta-analysis of prospective studies. J Am Acad Dermatol. 2001;45:520–7.
37. Schoetzau A, Filipiak-Pittroff B, Franke K, Koletzko S, Von Berg A, Gruebl A, et al. Effect of exclusive breast-feeding and early solid food avoidance on the incidence of atopic dermatitis in high-risk infants at 1 year of age. Pediatr Allergy Immunol. 2002;13:234–42.
38. Lee KS, Rha YH, Oh IH, Choi YS, Kim YE, Choi SH. Does breast-feeding relate to development of atopic dermatitis in young Korean children?: based on the Fourth and Fifth Korea National Health and Nutrition Examination Survey 2007–2012. Allergy Asthma Immunol Res. 2017;9:307–13.
39. Bergmann RL, Diepgen TL, Kuss O, Bergmann KE, Kujat J, Dudenhausen JW, et al. Breastfeeding duration is a risk factor for atopic eczema. Clin Exp Allergy. 2002;32:205–9.
40. Lin B, Dai R, Lu L, Fan X, Yu Y. Breastfeeding and atopic dermatitis risk: a systematic review and meta-analysis of prospective cohort studies. Dermatology. 2020;236:345–60. https://doi.org/10.1159/000503781.

Congenital Abnormalities of the Airway

Elad Azizli, Cemal Cingi, and Jeffrey C. Bedrosian

1 Introduction: Embryological Considerations

Already by weeks 4 and 5, the developing foetus is developing an airway, a structure which grows from the branchial arches. During the initial stages in pulmonary development, the dividing airways influence the layout of the expanding vasculature [1], a fact which helps to explain the common association between airway conditions and pulmonary or circulatory anomalies [2].

Furthermore, there are known to be multiple airway abnormalities linked to congenital syndromes or anomalous anatomy arising during embryological development. Abnormalities of the airway are currently likely to be diagnosed at an early stage, leading to surgical intervention and use of the neonatal intensive care unit. Therefore, neonatologists need knowledge of this important and growing area [2].

E. Azizli (✉)
Otorhinolaryngology Specialist, Private Practice, Istanbul, Türkiye

C. Cingi
Medical Faculty, Department of Otorhinolaryngology, Eskisehir Osmangazi University, Eskisehir, Türkiye
e-mail: cemal@ogu.edu.tr

J. C. Bedrosian
Rhinology and Skull Base Surgery, Specialty Physician Associates, St. Luke's Medical Center, Bethlehem, PA, USA

© The Author(s), under exclusive license to Springer Nature Switzerland AG 2023
Ö. N. Şahin et al. (eds.), *Breastfeeding and Metabolic Programming*,
https://doi.org/10.1007/978-3-031-33278-4_44

1.1   Development In Utero

Development of the foetus in utero can be separated into two distinct phases: embryogenesis (the first 8 weeks), during which all the major organ systems form (organogenesis), and the foetal phase, wherein these systems assume a more mature form [3].

1.2   Organogenesis

The cells that form the larynx originate from the endodermal layer of the foregut and contiguous mesenchymal tissue at a location between the fourth pharyngeal arch and the sixth. The first sign of the foregut appears on day 20, when the ventral laryngotracheal groove forms. Two days later, this structure has already given rise to the primordial laryngeal sulcus and the respiratory diverticula. By day 24, the lungs begin to bud bilaterally. The laryngotracheal groove deepens until the lateral edges fold over to create a tubular structure, which then begins its caudal descent. The tracheooesophageal septum then forms a boundary between the developing trachea and oesophagus. At first, there exists a linear opening between the developing respiratory system and the pharynx, but this slit fuses from the caudal pole towards the cranial pole. Failure of closure leads to an abnormal connection of the laryngotracheal and oesophageal regions. In normal development, however, the respiratory system and the gut from this stage onwards develop independently of each other [3].

By day 32, the earliest beginnings of the larynx are observable. Near to the cranial pole of the laryngotracheal tube, there appear mesenchymal arytenoid swellings arising from the paired sixth pharyngeal arches. As the swellings enlarge, they move towards the midline and towards each other. When they reach the caudal extent of the hypobranchial eminence, they form a T-shaped entrance into the laryngotracheal tube. These structures apply pressure on the laryngotracheal tube in the midline and this causes the tube to fuse shut, which means it no longer communicates at this stage with the pharynx. Continued expansion of the arytenoid swellings in a cranial direction eventually results in formation of the arytenoid and corniculate cartilages and the primordial aryepiglottic folds [3].

The structures above the level of the glottis, i.e. the epiglottic and cuneiform cartilages, develop from the hypobranchial eminence. The fourth pharyngeal arch supplies the thyroid cartilage, which grow from chondrification centres on each side, whilst the sixth pharyngeal arch supplies the cricoid and tracheal cartilages. By day 33, the superior laryngeal nerve can be seen, having arisen from the fourth pharyngeal arch, and on day 37, the recurrent laryngeal nerve has already arisen from the sixth pharyngeal arch [3].

Thus, by the 40th day of gestation, the larynx already possesses both its cartilaginous skeleton and intrinsic musculature. Four days later the cartilages have matured considerably and there is a complete ring of cricoid. On day 48, the concavity of the epiglottis is clearly perceptible. By day 51, the hyoid cartilage is in existence. Thus, as the embryonic period draws to a close, the larynx already possesses its own intrinsic muscles, nerve and vascular supply and cartilaginous framework. Furthermore, the tube now reopens, so that the tube is open as far as the trachea. Thereafter, there is ongoing stepwise maturation of the laryngeal structures for the rest of the pregnancy [3].

1.3 Maturation of Organ Systems

The vocal processes arise from the arytenoids and there is midline fusion of the thyroid cartilage during the third month of gestation. In the following month, mucous-secreting cells and glandular structures form in the submucosa. The cartilaginous framework of the epiglottis hardens into fibrocartilage at some point between months 5 and 7, which is also the time when the corniculate and cuneiform cartilages make their appearance. As the pregnancy draws to a close, the growth pattern of the cricoid cartilage alters from an interstitial to perichondrial type [3].

2 Laryngomalacia

2.1 Epidemiology

The most frequently occurring congenital laryngeal anomaly is laryngomalacia. This condition, where the cartilaginous framework is excessively soft, represents 60% of laryngeal structural anomalies. The male to female ratio in such cases is 2:1 [4].

2.2 Aetiology and Pathogenesis

A mechanism that accounts for every case of laryngomalacia has not yet been discovered. Possible hypotheses to explain the condition invoke immature growth or abnormal development of cartilage, gastrooesophageal reflux (GORD) or underdevelopment of neuromuscular control.

The epiglottis is formed by the third and fourth pharyngeal arches. In cases of laryngomalacia, the epiglottis is excessively elongated and extends too far laterally. This occurs due to overactive growth of the portion arising from the third arch. On histology, however, the cartilaginous appearances of the larynx taken from infants with laryngomalacia do not differ from the normal infant larynx.

It is possible that GORD is a cause of laryngomalacia. A recent histopathological study of surgical biopsies taken at aryepiglottoplasty found inflammatory exudates of varying degrees of severity in different regions of the epithelium. At a deeper level, oedema was observed in these specimens.

There is a significant association between GORD and greater symptomatic severity and higher risk of complications.

In cases of laryngomalacia, the arytenoid also prolapses, which indicates that dysfunction of neuromuscular control may be significant. However, it is noteworthy that in premature births hypotonicity is more common (indicative of immature neuromuscular control), but there is no increase in laryngomalacia [3].

2.3 Presenting Features

The usual presenting symptoms in cases of laryngomalacia are noisy breathing and stridor on inspiration. These symptoms are worsened by lying supine, whilst feeding and when distressed. The symptoms lessen if the child is placed on his or her front and the neck extended. The quality of the voice is generally normal. The onset is typically when the infant is a few weeks old, with progressive worsening lasting months followed by resolution at the age of 1½ to 2 years. It is unusual for symptoms to be already present at birth.

A less usual presentation is with difficulty feeding, but not to the extent of causing failure to thrive. Infants with laryngomalacia seldom experience respiratory distress or cyanosis [3].

When physically examined, infants with laryngomalacia are normally within the expected growth percentiles, have a healthy appearance and show no signs of distressed breathing, such as flared nostrils, rib retraction, use of accessory muscles or cyanosis. Their cry is powerful and has a normal quality. However, the following abnormal features may be observed on flexible endoscopy [3]:

- The epiglottis is both elongated and extends too far laterally, resembling the letter omega. When the child draws a breath, the epiglottis drops in a posteroinferior direction.
- The arytenoids have excessive bulkiness and prolapse in an anteromedial direction when breath is drawn.
- The aryepiglottic folds are shorter than usual and become tethered to the epiglottis.
- When the patient breathes in, the aryepiglottic folds (cuneiform cartilage) collapse inwards.
- When breath is expelled, however, these structures above the glottis are all lifted clear and air flows freely.
- The vocal folds have normal appearances and function in patients with laryngomalacia.

2.4 Diagnosis

The combination of suitable history and examination using the endoscope is generally adequate to allow laryngomalacia to be diagnosed. Imaging may support the diagnosis as well as allowing the assessment of other potential reasons for stridor, such as tracheomalacia, compression of the innominate artery or tracheal vascular rings. Plain X-ray obtained during inspiration may reveal inferomedial movement of the epiglottis and arytenoids. On fluoroscopic examination, it may be possible to see collapse of the structures above the glottis and widening of the hypopharynx. Where a paediatric patient shows signs of respiratory distress or where other abnormalities appear to be present in imaging studies, rigid bronchoscopy should be undertaken, for which the patient will require general anaesthesia [3].

2.5 Treatment

In the majority of patients, watchful waiting is appropriate. Attention should be paid to any breathing or feeding problems which may arise. If the child suffers from GORD, it is important to treat this condition actively since it may worsen laryngomalacia. The child may need to be put in particular positions to sleep and agents used in GORD may need to be utilised [3].

Somewhat rarely, where breathing becomes difficult in cases of laryngomalacia, surgery may be indicated [5]. If respiratory distress develops rapidly, a tracheotomy should be undertaken and the tube left in situ until the supraglottic structures have had time to develop normally. An alternative procedure to tracheotomy is epiglottoplasty. Epiglottoplasty consists of bilateral excision of a wedge-shaped portion of the aryepiglottic folds, reducing the size of the epiglottis, excision of the corniculate and cuneiform cartilages and removal of any excess mucosal tissue from the arytenoids. The result is a widened entrance into the larynx. The usual instrumentation employed is a laser. Extubation is normally arranged to occur one day after the operation. There is a review by Richter and Thompson dating from 2008 which examines indications for surgery, the methods available and perioperative management [6].

3 Vocal Cord Paralysis

3.1 Epidemiological Aspects

Paralysis of the vocal cords is responsible for between 15 and 20% of cases featuring congenital laryngeal abnormalities. It is thus the second most frequently occurring condition of this kind. Paralysis of the vocal cords affects both boys and girls equally [7].

3.2 Aetiology and Pathogenetic Mechanism

Most cases of paralysis of the cords occurring bilaterally are of unknown cause. In a proportion of patients, paralysis may be due to underdevelopment of central neuromuscular control. It can also occur secondary to central nervous system pathology, such as the Arnold-Chiari malformation, cerebral palsy, hydrocephalus, myelomeningocoele, spina bifida, hypoxia or a cerebral haemorrhage.

A temporary paralysis of the vocal cords lasting between half a year and 9 months may follow from traumatic injury to the cervical spine incurred at birth. Most cases of unilateral paralysis are of unknown cause, but some are a result of a peripheral nerve palsy. The recurrent laryngeal nerve is sometimes damaged at birth leading to paralysis of the vocal cords [3].

3.3 Clinical Presentation

The usual presentation is of an infant with stridor upon inspiration, even whilst resting, but worsening as a child becomes aroused. The vocal quality is almost normal and the airway becomes steadily less patent. Indeed, it may become obstructed to the degree that respiratory distress occurs and airway management is needed. Since patients with bilateral paralysis of the vocal cords frequently aspirate, the child may be prone to repeated lower respiratory tract infections.

When the child is physically examined, there may be signs of respiratory distress (flared nostrils, use of accessory muscles of respiration (e.g. supraclavicular), indrawing of the rib cage and cyanotic episodes) but some children will not show these signs. Examination of the head and neck may indicate abnormalities affecting the cranial nerves. The diagnosis can generally be confirmed by endoscopic examination, at which vocal cord paralysis is apparent. No other condition should be able to account for the symptoms.

Vocal cord paralysis affecting only one side may come to clinical attention shortly after birth or be subclinical. The most frequently occurring presentation is a dysphonic, breathy cry that becomes more evident with arousal. Infants in this situation may also have difficulty feeding and may aspirate [3].

3.4 Diagnosis

Unilateral paralysis of the vocal folds can be diagnosed endoscopically. If the patient has distressed breathing, rigid bronchoscopy should be employed to ensure there are no other obstructions to the passage of air. Radiological investigations are warranted to evaluate the possibility that the recurrent laryngeal nerve is affected by a lesion of the mediastinum or cervical region. The technique of laryngeal electromyography (EMG) is currently being used to assess mobility in conditions affecting the vocal cords and is useful to separate true paralysis from vocal fold fixation. This technique is also beneficial for estimating the outcome following the development of vocal fold paralysis [3].

3.5 Management

In cases where the vocal cords are paralysed bilaterally, urgent management of the airway may be required. This typically involves endotracheal intubation. To bypass the obstructed portion tracheotomy is required. The tubing should be left in situ for 2 years after placement, by which point the paralysis has completely resolved in above 50% of cases. Where the paralysis does not resolve, the patient may be able to be safely decannulated following surgical lateralisation of the vocal folds [3].

In the majority of cases where vocal cord paralysis affects a single side, watchful waiting is adequate, provided the patient does not develop problems with breathing and feeding. Aspiration can generally be prevented by ensuring the child is in an upright position. On rare occasions, a distressed patient may need to undergo intubation if a clear airway is to be provided [3].

4 Congenital Subglottic Stenosis

4.1 Epidemiology

The third most frequently occurring congenital laryngeal anomaly is congenital subglottic stenosis, which is responsible for some 15% of the total cases. It is also the laryngeal abnormality most likely to lead to tracheotomy in an infant patient. The male to female ratio is 2:1 [3].

4.2 Aetiology and Pathogenetic Mechanism

Congenital subglottic stenosis (CSS) occurs due to the laryngotracheal tube failing to reform a channel in foetal development. This should normally occur during the third month. Different degrees of severity are linked to how much recanalisation occurs. A total failure of recanalisation results in total atresia of the larynx [8].

There are two principal categories of CSS: membranous and cartilaginous. Membranous CSS results when the submucosal layer surrounding the lumen hypertrophies. Fibro-connective tissue overgrows, as does mucous glandular tissue. Membranous CSS is more common than the cartilaginous variant and is milder.

Cartilaginous CSS, by contrast, arises because the cricoid cartilage has an abnormal shape. Generally, the cartilage becomes narrower in a lateral direction, but it can become thickened overall or feature overgrowth of the anterior or posterior laminae [3].

4.3 Clinical Presentation

CSS typically first becomes evident at the age of a few months. Usually there is little indication that the stenosis exists until an infective episode occurs, which puts extra strain on the subglottic airway. In these situations, the child presents in the same way as a case of croup (infectious laryngotracheobronchitis). Thus, stridor exists during both phases of respiration, which may also be accompanied by respiratory distress. Some children develop a bark when they cough, but patients generally cry in the normal way. If such symptoms keep recurring or the length infection-related croup lasts exceeds expectations (i.e. beyond three days), clinicians have grounds to suspect an underlying diagnosis of CSS [3].

4.4 Diagnosis

CSS is usually suspected when the history reveals repeated episodes of croup. Rigid bronchoscopic examination is employed for diagnostic confirmation and to highlight any other abnormality in the airway. The stenotic portion needs to be measured – both its length and diameter. The latter can be conveniently estimated from the diameter of the largest scope able to pass through the stenosis. The criteria for diagnosing CSS are a lumen under 4 mm diameter in an infant or under 3 mm if the infant was born prematurely. Endoscopic examination of CSS usually reveals a less severe lesion than in cases where the subglottic stenosis is acquired later [3].

4.5 Management

In the majority of cases, CSS resolves without the need for intervention as the child matures. However, if the airway is compromised to a major extent, there may be a need to intubate the patient and perform a tracheotomy. In the latter case, the cannula can usually be removed when the child is 3 or 4 years old, by which point the subglottic space has enlarged.

The mortality rate following tracheostomy has been reported by Strang et al., based on a retrospective review of 132 procedures undertaken on infants. There were a number of indications for tracheostomy included in the sample namely subglottic stenosis, bronchopulmonary dysplasia, congenital cardiac disorders, craniofacial abnormalities or trisomies. The rate of death following tracheostomy regardless of indication was 14.4%, but this figure fell to 3.7% when only the indication for subglottic stenosis was considered [9].

Laser ablation is occasionally of value in managing CSS, but it is generally only employed for lesions that are composed of soft tissues and are no greater than 5 mm across. Surgical reconstruction of the laryngotracheal tube is generally not required, but is an option in cases where decannulation is otherwise impossible. Thus, laryngotracheoplasty is only appropriate where subglottic stenosis is of a high degree of severity [3].

5 Congenital Laryngeal Atresia

5.1 Epidemiological Features

Laryngeal atresia has the worst prognosis amongst congenital laryngeal abnormalities, but is fortunately the least frequently encountered. There are limited case studies indicating that patients with the condition have been able to survive [3].

5.2 Aetiology and Pathogenetic Mechanism

The condition arises when the laryngotracheal tube fails to recanalise during the third month of pregnancy. The larynx is therefore atretic [3].

5.3 Presenting Features

The condition presents as an acutely obstructed airway in a neonate. This is apparent as soon as the umbilical cord is clamped. The newborn child exhibits signs of severe respiratory distress with highly forceful attempts to breath but the inability to inspire or cry. Unless a tracheotomy is immediately performed, the child dies. Intubation is impossible in such cases. In a few cases, a child affected by laryngeal atresia also has further anomalous development which may paradoxically save his or her life. If the trachea and oesophagus are connected by a fistula of sufficient size to allow airflow into the lungs, the neonate may be able to breathe via the fistula [3].

5.4 Diagnosis

The presence of laryngeal atresia can be confirmed by diagnostic use of an endoscope, after the tracheotomy tube has been placed. In cases of polyhydramnios, the condition may be recognised prenatally, which then permits prior planning for tracheotomy. However, in those cases where there is fistulatory communication between the trachea and oesophagus, the condition will not be revealed prenatally, since there is no polyhydramnios in such cases [3].

5.5 *Management*

Treatment involves performing tracheotomy immediately after the child is born. In cases where prenatal diagnosis has occurred, the umbilical cord should not be clamped until after performing a tracheotomy. This ensures the neonate receives adequate oxygen throughout. In a neonate with a tracheoesophageal fistula, the child may be intubated via the oesophagus and a mask applied until a tracheotomy tube has been placed [3].

6 Laryngotracheoesophageal Clefts

Laryngotracheoesophageal clefts occur very infrequently. They are congenital lesions affecting the posterior wall of the laryngotracheal tune. Their presence means the oesophagus communicates with the larynx and trachea. Benjamin and Inglis divided clefts into four types (I–IV) on the basis of various features, in particular length and whether the lesion extended into the glottis, cricoid cartilage or trachea (cervical or thoracic portion) [10]. Types I and II are of minor importance. Repair may be undertaken endoscopically or transcervically, and rarely creates severe complications apart from a degree of dysphagia. Types III and IV, however, do result in more serious illness and may cause early death. If there are large of clefts, surgical repair often has to occur several times, and for this reason multidisciplinary working involving cardiothoracic, ENT and intensive care specialists is a must for good outcomes [2, 11, 12].

7 Congenital Tracheal Stenosis

Congenital stenosis of the trachea may be confined to one particular location or run some length along the airways. Uncommonly, it may affect the carina and a stretch of bronchus. Patients with this condition have been noted to have unusual morphology of the branching of the trachea and bronchi. The most frequently occurring atypical arborisation pattern is a tracheal right superior lobar bronchus and trifurcation pattern [13]. If congenital tracheal stenosis causes symptoms, surgical intervention is required. Symptoms generally depend on the severity of airway narrowing. If the stenotic region is short, the affected segment is frequently resected and the cut ends are rejoined. However, if the affected segment is lengthy, tracheal reconstruction may be required. Indeed, for lengthy sections of tracheal stenosis, surgery presents many challenges. Early attempts at surgical reconstruction of the trachea were associated with a raised risk of mortality [14, 15], which stimulated a search for a safer technique. Some of the techniques attempted included patch tracheoplasty and the use of external Hagl stents. At present, the most favoured option for cases of extensive tracheal stenosis is slide tracheoplasty. Using this method, the surgeon can enlarge the tracheal lumen by utilising sections of the patient's airway [16–18]. Although this method is known to shorten the trachea, the trachea subsequently lengthens spontaneously, particularly in the half-year following the procedure [19]. In cases where stenosis occurs in conjunction with an anomaly of the circulatory system (such as a pulmonary artery sling or reduplicated aorta, creating a vessel wrapping around the airway), the circulatory abnormality is addressed at the same operation, which calls for use of cardipulmonary bypass [11].

Tracheal repair should be evaluated bronchoscopically 1-week post-surgery, with additional balloon dilatation used for regions where the trachea remains narrowed. The objective is to extubate the patient at the earliest opportunity to avoid any complications which may arise due to instrumentation damaging the airway. The rate of complications is proven lower when the child is not kept on mechanical ventilation with the use of sedation and muscle relaxants [20]. There need to be regular checks on the airway shortly after surgery. For the initial weeks after the procedure, the airway should be checked multiple times using bronchography or bronchoscopy. This monitoring identifies any areas of granulation tissue which may potentially obstruct the airway, and identifies where any intervention is required [16].

7.1 Stents

If the airway has a tendency to re-stenose post-surgically even when balloon dilatation is employed, airway stenting may be called for. Stents for the airway first entered clinical use in the 1990s. Their insertion is straightforward and not especially risky and they are able to remain in situ for a considerable time, preventing a major airway becoming obstructed [21]. Furthermore, stents frequently prevent the need for artificial ventilation. Stents were originally of a fixed shape and calibre, but are now available in an expandable form of the type employed in angioplasty, so that they can be manipulated with a balloon catheter. The material used has also evolved from metal to silastic and is now even biodegradable [22–24]. Granulation tissue tends to form at the site of stents and where this occurs there may be a need to dilate the segment bronchoscopically and remove the stent earlier than anticipated. It is unusual for a stent to move out of place or erode into the adjacent tissues, however, if this does occur life is endangered. Stents which are custom-produced for each patient are now available. They are made from polydioxanone and they degrade naturally within the body, which means they are neither permanent nor require a procedure to remove them. This then means the patient's own airway can regenerate itself [24].

References

1. Hislop AA. Airway and blood vessel interaction during lung development. J Anat. 2002;201:325–34.
2. Mok Q. Airway problems in neonates-a review of the current investigation and management strategies. Front Pediatr. 2017;5:60. https://doi.org/10.3389/fped.2017.00060.
3. Tewfik TL. Congenital Malformations of the Larynx. In: Meyers AD (Ed). Medscape. Updated: Jan 13, 2021. https://emedicine.medscape.com/article/837630-overview#showall. Accessed online at July 3, 2022.
4. Klinginsmith M, Goldman J. Laryngomalacia. [Updated 2022 Feb 15]. In: StatPearls [Internet]. Treasure Island (FL): StatPearls Publishing; 2022 Jan. Available from: https://www.ncbi.nlm.nih.gov/books/NBK544266/
5. Del Do M, Song SA, Nesbitt NB, et al. Supraglottoplasty surgery types 1-3: a practical classification system for laryngomalacia surgery. Int J Pediatr Otorhinolaryngol. 2018;111:69–74.
6. Richter GT, Thompson DM. The surgical management of laryngomalacia. Otolaryngol Clin N Am. 2008;41(5):837–64.
7. Singh JM, Wang R, Kwartowitz G. Unilateral Vocal Fold Paralysis. [Updated 2021 Nov 22]. In: StatPearls [Internet]. Treasure Island (FL): StatPearls Publishing; 2022 Jan-. Available from: https://www.ncbi.nlm.nih.gov/books/NBK519060/
8. Groblewski JC, Shah RK, Zalzal GH. Microdebrider-assisted supraglottoplasty for laryngomalacia. Ann Otol Rhinol Laryngol. 2009;118(8):592–7.
9. Reinhard A, Gorostidi F, Leishman C, Monnier P, Sandu K. Laser supraglottoplasty for laryngomalacia; a 14 year experience of a tertiary referral center. Eur Arch Otorhinolaryngol. 2017 Jan.;274(1):367–74.
10. Benjamin B, Inglis A. Minor congenital laryngeal clefts: diagnosis and classification. Ann Otol Rhinol Laryngol. 1985;98:417–20.
11. Shehab ZP, Bailey CM. Type IV laryngotracheoesophageal clefts – recent 5 year experience at Great Ormond Street Hospital for Children. Int J Pediatr Otorhinolaryngol. 2001;60:1–9.
12. Mathur NN, Peek GJ, Bailey CM, Elliott MJ. Strategies for managing Type IV larybgotrachoesophageal clefts at Great Ormond Street Hospital for Children. Int J Pediatr Otorhinolaryngol. 2006;70:1901–10.
13. Speggiorin S, Torre M, Roebuck DJ, McLaren CA, Elliott MJ. A new morphologic classification of congenital tracheobronchial stenosis. Ann Thorac Surg. 2012;93:958–61.
14. Loeff DS, Filler RM, Vinograd I, Ein SH, Williams WG, Smith CR, et al. Congenital tracheal stenosis: a review of 22 patients from 1965 to 1987. J Pediatr Surg. 1988;23:744–8.
15. Filler RM. Current approaches in tracheal surgery. Pediatr Pulmonol Suppl. 1999;18:105–8.
16. Elliott M, Roebuck D, Noctor C, McLaren C, Hartley B, Mok Q, et al. The management of congenital tracheal stenosis. Int J Pediatr Otorhinolaryngol. 2003;67(Suppl 1):S183–92.
17. Beierlein W, Elliott MJ. Variations in the technique of slide tracheoplasty to repair complex forms of long-segment congenital tracheal stenosis. Ann Thorac Surg. 2006;82:1540–2.
18. Elliott M, Hartley BE, Wallis C, Roebuck D. Slide tracheoplasty. Curr Opin Otolaryngol Head Neck Surg. 2008;16:75–82.
19. Speggiorin S, Gilbert TW, Broadhead M, Roebuck DJ, McLaren CA, Elliott MJ. Do tracheas grow after slide tracheoplasty? Ann Thorac Surg. 2012;93:1083–6.
20. Jacobs BR, Salman BA, Cotton RT, Lyons K, Brilli RJ. Postoperative management of children after single-stage laryngotracheal reconstruction. Crit Care Med. 2001;29:164–8.
21. Filler RM, Forte V, Fraga JC, Matute J. The use of expandable metallic airway stents for tracheobronchial obstruction in children. J Pediatr Surg. 1995;30:1050–5. discussion 1055–6
22. Filler RM, Forte V, Chait P. Tracheobronchial stenting for the treatment of airway obstruction. J Pediatr Surg. 1998;33:304–11.
23. Wyatt ME, Hartley BE, Roebuck D, McLaren C, Elliott M, Pigott N, et al. Metallic tracheobronchial stenting in the paediatric airway. Otolaryngol Head Neck Surg. 2004;131:220.
24. Vondrys D, Elliott MJ, McLaren CA, Noctor C, Roebuck DJ. First experience with biodegradable airway stents in children. Ann Thorac Surg. 2011;92:1870–4.

Upper Airway Lesions in the Neonate

Mustafa Caner Kesimli

1 Introduction

There are a wide range of conditions which result from abnormalities in nasal development. This chapter addresses how the nose and nasal interior develops in utero, then discusses congenital nasal abnormalities, such as nasal dermoids, gliomas, encephalocoeles, nasal clefts, proboscis lateralis, arhinia, polyrrhinia, nasopharyngeal teratoma and epignathus [1]. There is a separate chapter dedicated to choanal atresia in this volume.

2 Nasal Embryological Development

There are three distinct stages in the development of the nose from an embryological perspective, namely the preskeletal, chondrocranial and ossification phases, which occur in that order. In the first stage, the mesenchyme around the external nasal placodes swells in size. The second stage involves the laying down of a cartilaginous framework to support the nasal structures. In the final stage, the different structures forming the framework of the nose fuse together and there is cellular infiltration of the nasal skeleton [2].

There is migration in a medial and caudal direction of proliferating cells from the ectoderm in week 3 of embryogenesis. These cells are destined to establish the notochord. At the same time, more specialised cells of ectodermal origin begin folding back on themselves within the primitive streak, also located medially and caudally within the embryo. The specialised cells find their way between the ectoderm and endoderm. During week 3, there are also key developments at the rostral pole.

M. C. Kesimli (✉)
Caner Kesimli Private ENT Clinic, Istanbul, Türkiye

Ö. N. Şahin et al. (eds.), *Breastfeeding and Metabolic Programming*,
https://doi.org/10.1007/978-3-031-33278-4_45

The ectodermal and endodermal layers stick to each other here and produce the buccopharyngeal membrane, a structure marking the anterior limit of the primitive foregut. As week 3 comes to an end, there is already a neural groove present dorsomedially. As this groove deepens and becomes thicker, the neural tube comes into existence. From the rostral pole of the neural tube, the primary brain vesicles subsequently form [1].

Around days 20–30 of embryological development, there is a bilateral thickening which appears in the midline, which will subsequently form the paraxial mesoderm cephalically. When this occurs, the buccopharyngeal membrane is no longer apparent, and a primordial nasal cavity can be seen [1].

There is medial migration of the nostrils, which meet with fusion of the soft tissue elements at the point where the orbits are also moving towards the midline. The anterior portion of the nasal septum, the medial portion of the superior lip and some of the anterior bony palate are all derived from the medial nasal processes. The posterior portion of the nasal septum and several bones – the ethmoid, nasal and premaxilla, are all derived from the nasofrontal process, which grows out of the floor of the anterior cranial fossa. Up to weeks 6 or 7 of embryogenesis, there is a division of the posterior nasal and oral cavities caused by presence of the oronasal membrane, a structure which subsequently undergoes resorption, allowing the primitive choanae to develop [3].

During embryological development, the prenasal space exists between the nasal and frontal bones. This space is bounded anteriorly by the skin of the nose and posteriorly by the foramen caecum. The dural membrane can potentially herniate in the area of the foramen caecum. The cribriform plate is produced when the fonticulus frontalis undergoes fusion with the foramen caecum [4].

3 Holoprosencephaly

The most frequently occurring abnormality of development affecting the forebrain is holoprosencephaly. In this condition, the forebrain fails partially or completely to separate into right and left hemispheres. In most patients, holoprosencephaly also causes abnormal development of the face in the midline [3].

The appearances in holoprosencephaly vary, with manifestations of abnormal midline development such as a single incisor in the upper jaw, cebocephaly (with the eyes less than one eye-width apart, microstomia and a fused nostril) or cyclopia. Although the brain may have developed normally, in many cases the right and left halves may remain fused (semilobar holoprosencephaly), the lateral ventricles may be conjoint or the corpus callosum may not be present (alobar holoprosencephaly). Typically, greater severity of facial abnormality correlates with more severely abnormal development of the central nervous system. There is a high likelihood of fatality occurring in infants with severe holoprosencephaly. In those who do not die from the condition, epilepsy and learning disability frequently occur. On the other hand, mental function may be normal and there may be no symptoms in some paediatric cases of semilobar holoprosencephaly.

It is probable that solitary median maxillary incisor syndrome is due to a degree of holoprosencephaly [5].

4 Frontonasal Dysplasia

The presentation in frontonasal dysplasia differs somewhat from holoprosencephaly. This condition may also be termed median cleft face syndrome. The clinical manifestations include wide-set eyes, a frontal hairline forming a V-shape in the midline, clefting of the calvarium (cranium bifidum occultum) and a midline cleft affecting the superior lip and palate [6]. The Tessier system used to classify cleft disorders of the face and cranium begins numbering in an anti-clockwise direction around the eye socket. In this system, frontonasal dysplasia is the 14th type.

The putative aetiology of frontonasal dysplasia is defective development of the nasofrontal process, which prevents cellular migration towards the midline. There is an association with mutated ALX homeobox family alleles, which render the gene product inactive [7]. Management potentially includes surgery to the face and cranium, for a better cosmetic outcome [8].

5 Nasal Dermoids

5.1 Embryological Aspects and Aetiology

Nasal dermoids are characterised by cysts or sinus tracts with a lining of epithelium, which may bear appendages typical of the skin, such as eccrine or exocrine glands or hair follicles. As a group they occur the most frequently of all congenital abnormalities affecting the nose. They may originate from islands of isolated epithelium formed within ectodermal tissues, or arise as remnants of ectoderm within the nasal septum after it has fused and ossified.

The majority of experts consider the most likely explanation for nasal dermoids to involve the prenasal space and fontanelle. This potential space opens up between the front wall of the nose and the frontal and nasal bones. As ossification occurs, skin may persist, joined to the fibrocartilaginous nasal capsule and occupying the prenasal space or fonticulus. Elements of the epidermis, including the appendages, may become isolated within the ossified tissues. A tract may develop. The island of epidermis may also be attached to the dura mater, and there is then a tract connecting the skin of the nose to the meninges via the prenasal space and foramen caecum or the fontanelle [1].

5.2   Clinical Presentation and Management

Between 3.7 and 12% of the dermoids affect the head and neck region, representing 1.1% of all dermoids in the body. Typically, nasal dermoids are in the midline and usually they are found on the dorsum of the nose. They appear as a mass or a pit in the nose and may be found along the entire length of the nose from the glabella down to the columella. They may occur singly or as a group. It is not unusual for the dermoid to contain hair and sebaceous secretion. A portion of these dermoids drain outwards. The characteristic time for a dermoid to present is up to the age of 1 month. By the age of 1 year, 73% of nasal dermoids have already been identified [1].

5.3   Operative Removal

A nasal dermoid that extends into the cranial cavity is a possible portal of entry for pathogens into the central nervous system and thus necessitates operative removal [9]. The traditional approach to surgical excision of nasal dermoids extending into the cranial cavity was craniotomy, usually as one part of a multi-stage procedure [10]. More recently, surgeons have favoured endoscopic surgery for lesions of the skull base or extending just into the cranial cavity, since these are far less invasive. An endoscopic approach may be combined with incision of the nose directly or with performance of open rhinoplasty. In the latter method, the nose may be degloved from the nasal tip to the dorsum [3, 11].

6   Glioma

6.1   Embryological Factors and Aetiogenesis

A glioma refers to collections of glial cells which lack a surrounding capsule and are found external to the central nervous system. Various hypotheses have been proposed to explain how gliomas form, such as [1]: (a) Part of the olfactory bulb remains separated by the fused halves of the cribriform plate or (b) nervous tissue develops in an ectopic location, or (c) they represent an encephalocoele which has been divided from the main lesion, or (d) the rostral neuropore closes abnormally, and mesodermal cells do not enter the region properly, leaving some areas deficient in osseous tissue growth [1].

6.2 Clinical Presentation and Management

Some 30% of paediatric gliomas are within the nose, 60% are outside the nose and 10% occur in combination with other cells. In contrast to dermoids, gliomas are not typically midline lesions, nor are they attached to the skin or sinuses. Gliomas cannot be easily compressed, they do not expand when the Valsalva manoeuvre is performed and they cannot be transilluminated. Gliomas occurring outside the nose are typically at the level of the glabella, although their location is often away from the midline [12].

Gliomas occurring in the nasal cavity are often attached to the middle turbinate or are superior. They may resemble a nasal polyp. Gliomas that are both within and outside the nose have a characteristic dumbbell appearance, being joined by a connecting band of tissue. In 15% of cases, the glioma is continuous with the dura mater, the connecting region passing through the foramen caecum or the fontanelle. Possible clinical presentations include one-sided nasal blockage, a mass on one side of the nose, nose bleeds or a nasal discharge of cerebrospinal fluid. Gliomas outside the cranial cavity more frequently cause telecanthus or wide spacing of the eyes. If both internal jugular veins are compressed by the examiner at the same time, the lesion does not grow in size, i.e. it is Furstenberg negative. Imaging with computed tomography (CT) is valuable for diagnostic purposes. CT can reveal osseous defects, whereas magnetic resonance imaging (MRI) is helpful for delineating the soft tissue elements. These lesions should not be biopsied. The treatment is to excise the lesion surgically.

Glioma removal for an extranasal lesion generally involves standard excision techniques. An intranasal glioma that does not enter the cranial cavity may call for lateral rhinotomy to achieve access. If the lesion extends into the cranial cavity, neurosurgical assistance will be required. To prevent the lesion recurring, the entire glioma must be removed [1].

Neither biopsy nor excision by surgery should occur unless the lesion has been imaged fully using CT and MRI [13]. The first-line management involves surgical excision [14]. If treatment is not undertaken in a timely manner, the lesion may cause an infection or damage the nasal septum +/− the nasal bone [3].

7 Encephalocoele

7.1 Embryological Factors and Aetiogenesis

In encephalocoeles, nervous tissue prolapses through a defective area of the cranium. Lesions consisting of meningeal tissues are termed meningocoeles, whereas if neural tissue is intermixed with meningeal elements, an encephalomeningocoele is formed. A lesion of this type that connects to a ventricle is termed an encephalomeningocystocoele. The aetiogenesis has some similarity with how gliomas form.

Despite the absence of a clear genetic basis for encephalocoeles, the fact that they occur in conjunction with some other disorders, notably Ehlers-Danlos syndrome or frontonasal dysplasia, does raise the suspicion that genetic factors are of significance, even if currently unknown [1].

7.2 Clinical Presentation and Management

Encephalocoeles which involve the cranial cavity represent 20% of such lesions. Amongst this 20%, 15% are within the nose. The encephalocoeles within the nose represent two types: sincipital (60%) and basal (40%).

Sincipital encephalocoeles may be further subdivided in the following way: (a) Nasofrontal type (two-fifths of lesions), where the lesion passes through a defect between the nasal bone and frontal bone. (b) Nasoethmoidal lesions (a further two-fifths of lesions), where the lesion passes between the nasal bone and the cartilages of the nose. (c) Nasoorbital type (the remaining fifth), where the lesion passes through a defective maxillary frontal process. The usual presentation of a sincipital encephalocoele is as a mass overlying the glabellar region that does not readily compress [1].

Basal encephalocoeles may also be further subdivided in the following way: (a) Transethmoidal lesions, which pass via the cribriform plate to enter the superior meatus. These lesions extend in a medial direction towards the middle turbinate. (b) Sphenoethmoidal type, which passes via the cribriform plate, then between the posterior ethmoid cells and sphenoid into the nasopharyngeal region. (c) Sphenoorbital type, which invades the eye socket through the superior orbital fissure. These lesions may present as exophthalmos. (d) Transsphenoidal type, in which the lesion prolapses into the nasopharyngeal region through defective bone behind the cribriform plate. All these types may fail to come to clinical attention for many years [1].

8 Nasopharyngeal and Oropharyngeal Teratoma (Epignathus)

Teratomas are rare tumours consisting of cellular elements derived from endodermal, mesodermal and ectodermal embryological tissues. Infrequently a teratoma shows features of a fully developed organ, such as a limb. This type of teratoma is referred to as an epignathus [1].

8.1   Embryological Factors and Aetiogenesis

Multiple hypotheses have been advanced to account for why teratomas occur. Amongst the better supported hypotheses are the following:

- The lesion is a result of abnormal development of germ cells. This may account for their occurrence in the ovary or testis, but not in the head and neck region.
- Certain totipotent cells may fail to differentiate and later begin differentiating, producing a teratoma.
- A teratoma is a separate embryo embedded within the body of the patient. It is, in effect, a conjoined twin [1].

8.2   Clinical Presentation and Management

The usual presentation is of acute respiratory distress in a neonate of sufficient severity to necessitate endotracheal intubation or a tracheotomy. If the teratoma is small, it may reveal itself due to problematic feeding. It is essential to exclude involvement of the cranial cavity by imaging studies. Both CT and MRI studies are utilised to delineate any osseous defect within the sphenoid and to ascertain how the lesion is related to the brain and meninges [1].

The majority of teratomas occurring within the nasopharynx do not extend into the cranial cavity and thus can be removed surgically by approaching through the mouth. It is generally straightforward to excise a nasopharyngeal teratoma if the palate is cleft, as is generally the case. For teratomas which extend into the cranial cavity, the approach must be craniofacial. The outcome following surgery is generally favourable and no teratomas have yet been reported to indicate features of developing malignancy [15].

Recently a new approach to the obstructed airway has been introduced. This approach, known as 'ex utero intrapartum treatment (EXIT)', involves opening the airway whilst the foetus is still attached to the uteroplacental circulation, thus ensuring a steady supply of oxygen [16].

9   Pyriform Aperture Stenosis

The pyriform aperture is the opening within the bones of the face that allows air to pass from the nasal cavity into the nasopharynx. This aperture may be stenotic at birth (a condition referred to as congenital pyriform aperture stenosis [CPAS]). CPAS may result in an obstructed airway in a neonate [17–20].

9.1 Presentation

The usual presentation of CPAS is an infant who breathes noisily and is in respiratory distress. This distress deepens when feeding is attempted, but lessens when the child cries [18, 20]. CPAS may be an isolated condition or form part of a set of abnormalities, such as in conjunction with a solitary upper central incisor, anomaly of the pituitary, craniosynostosis or holoprosencephaly [17, 21–25].

9.2 Treatment

If the degree of stenosis is relatively mild, stenting of the nose bilaterally using endotracheal tubes is sometimes sufficient. If, however, the stenosis is very marked, a tracheotomy may need to be undertaken, and the tube then remains in place up to the point when the child can tolerate surgical repair of the stenosis [21, 26]. Surgical intervention may still lead to a narrowed pyriform aperture, with the result that the patient is prone to recurrent respiratory infective episodes in early childhood. In some cases of severe CPAS, one alternative approach to consider is dilation of the nose without taking away any bone or use of stents [27].

References

1. Tewfik TL. Congenital Malformations of the Nose. In: Meyers AD (Ed). Medscape. Updated: Mar 25, 2021. https://emedicine.medscape.com/article/837236-overview. Accessed online at July 3rd, 2022.
2. Adil E, Huntley C, Choudhary A, Carr M. Congenital nasal obstruction: clinical and radiologic review. Eur J Pediatr. 2012;171(4):641–50.
3. Isaacson GC. Congenital anomalies of the nose. In: Messner AH, Wilkie L (Eds). UpToDate. Last updated: Jan 10, 2022.
4. Harley EH. Pediatric congenital nasal masses. Ear Nose Throat J. 1991;70:28.
5. Garcia Rodriguez R, Garcia Cruz L, Novoa Medina Y, et al. The solitary median maxillary central incisor (SMMCI) syndrome: associations, prenatal diagnosis, and outcomes. Prenat Diagn. 2019;39:415.
6. Chervenak FA, Tortora M, Mayden K, et al. Antenatal diagnosis of median cleft face syndrome: sonographic demonstration of cleft lip and hypertelorism. Am J Obstet Gynecol. 1984;149:94.
7. Bertola DR, Rodrigues MG, Quaio CR, et al. Vertical transmission of a frontonasal phenotype caused by a novel ALX4 mutation. Am J Med Genet A. 2013;161A:600.
8. Laure B, Batut C, Benouhagrem A, et al. Addressing hypertelorism: indications and techniques. Neurochirurgie. 2019;65:286.
9. Paller AS, Pensler JM, Tomita T. Nasal midline masses in infants and children. Dermoids, encephaloceles, and gliomas. Arch Dermatol. 1991;127:362.
10. Denoyelle F, Ducroz V, Roger G, Garabedian EN. Nasal dermoid sinus cysts in children. Laryngoscope. 1997;107:795.
11. Livingstone DM, Brookes J, Yunker WK. Endoscope-assisted nasal dermoid excision with an open rhinoplasty approach. Int J Pediatr Otorhinolaryngol. 2018;109:101.

12. Okumura M, Francisco RP, Lucato LT, Zerbini MC, Zugaib M. Prenatal detection and postnatal management of an intranasal glioma. J Pediatr Surg. 2012;47(10):1951–4.
13. Myer CM 3rd, Cotton RT. Nasal obstruction in the pediatric patient. Pediatrics. 1983;72:766.
14. Rahbar R, Resto VA, Robson CD, et al. Nasal glioma and encephalocele: diagnosis and management. Laryngoscope. 2003;113:2069.
15. Diakite C, Benateau H, Dakpe S, Guerreschi P, Galinier P, Veyssiere A. Management of nasopharyngeal teratomas associated with cleft palate. Int J Oral Maxillofac Surg. 2019;48(3):291–7.
16. Chiu HH, Hsu WC, Shih JC, et al. The EXIT (Ex Utero Intrapartum Treatment) Procedure. J Formos Med Assoc. 2008;107(9):745–8.
17. Szeremeta W, Parikh TD, Widelitz JS. Congenital nasal malformations. Otolaryngol Clin N Am. 2007;40:97.
18. Brown OE, Myer CM 3rd, Manning SC. Congenital nasal pyriform aperture stenosis. Laryngoscope. 1989;99:86.
19. Rombaux P, Hamoir M, Francois G, et al. Congenital nasal pyriform aperture stenosis in newborn: report on three cases. Rhinology. 2000;38:39.
20. Ramadan H, Ortiz O. Congenital nasal pyriform aperture (bony inlet) stenosis. Otolaryngol Head Neck Surg. 1995;113:286.
21. Van Den Abbeele T, Triglia JM, François M, Narcy P. Congenital nasal pyriform aperture stenosis: diagnosis and management of 20 cases. Ann Otol Rhinol Laryngol. 2001;110:70.
22. Godil MA, Galvin-Parton P, Monte D, et al. Congenital nasal pyriform aperture stenosis associated with central diabetes insipidus. J Pediatr. 2000;137:260.
23. Lo FS, Lee YJ, Lin SP, et al. Solitary maxillary central incisor and congenital nasal pyriform aperture stenosis. Eur J Pediatr. 1998;157:39.
24. Beregszàszi M, Léger J, Garel C, et al. Nasal pyriform aperture stenosis and absence of the anterior pituitary gland: report of two cases. J Pediatr. 1996;128:858.
25. Guilmin-Crépon S, Garel C, Baumann C, et al. High proportion of pituitary abnormalities and other congenital defects in children with congenital nasal pyriform aperture stenosis. Pediatr Res. 2006;60:478.
26. Pérez CG, Gabaldon Masse P, Cocciaglia A, Rodríguez H. Congenital pyriform aperture stenosis: ten years experience. Acta Otorrinolaringol Esp. 2021;72:252.
27. Wine TM, Dedhia K, Chi DH. Congenital nasal pyriform aperture stenosis: is there a role for nasal dilation? JAMA Otolaryngol Head Neck Surg. 2014;140:352.

Newborn Hearing Screening

Taylan Bilici, Nuray Bayar Muluk, and Yusuf Dundar

1 Introduction

The first recommendation for the development and nationwide implementation of "universally applied procedures for early identification and evaluation of hearing impairment" came in 1965 from the Babbidge Report, a report of the Advisory Committee on Education of the Deaf. Efforts have continued since this time to further reduce the age at which a child is identified as having hearing loss, with the ultimate goal that "all infants with hearing loss be identified before 3 months of age and receive intervention services initiated by 6 months of age." The Joint Committee on Infant Hearing (JCIH) issued a statement in 2000 recommending universal screening for hearing loss before hospital discharge in addition to principles and guidelines for hospital and state programs [1]. Identification of newborn hearing loss is addressed in the Healthy People 2010 goals (Goal 28–11) stated as "increasing the proportion of newborns who are screened for hearing loss by age 1 month, have audiologic evaluation by age 3 months, and are enrolled in appropriate intervention services by age 6 months." [2, 3].

T. Bilici (✉)
Department of Otorhinolaryngology, Adana Seyhan State Hospital, Adana, Türkiye

N. B. Muluk
Faculty of Medicine, Department of Otorhinolaryngology, Kırıkkale University, Kırıkkale, Türkiye

Y. Dundar
Department of Otolaryngology-Head and Neck Surgery, Texas Tech University, Health Sciences Center, Lubbock, TX, USA

© The Author(s), under exclusive license to Springer Nature Switzerland AG 2023
Ö. N. Şahin et al. (eds.), *Breastfeeding and Metabolic Programming*,
https://doi.org/10.1007/978-3-031-33278-4_46

561

Significant permanent hearing loss is a common disorder at birth and can lead to delayed language development, difficulties with behavior and psychosocial interactions, and poor academic achievement. Detection of hearing loss during infancy can initiate intervention resulting in improved language, cognitive, behavioral, and academic outcomes [4]

2 Epidemiology

2.1 General Newborn Population

Clinically significant bilateral hearing loss occurs in 1 to 3 per 1000 live births [5–7]. In the United States, data from the Centers for Disease Control and Prevention (CDC) reported a rate of permanent hearing loss of 1.7 per 1000 infants screened for hearing loss, with an overall screening rate of 98.4% for all newborns, excluding infant deaths and parental refusal [7]. There was no documented diagnosis reported in 38.0% of infants who failed the newborn hearing screening.

The prevalence of moderate, severe, and profound bilateral permanent hearing loss is estimated at 1 in 900 to 2500 newborns [6, 8]. The prevalence of unilateral hearing impairment above 30 decibels (dB) has been reported as 6 out of 1000 newborns [9].

Congenital hearing loss may be due to genetic/hereditary disorders or acquired conditions due to perinatal problems (e.g., congenital infections) [5]. Permanent hearing loss is often associated with other congenital abnormalities, and there are >400 syndromes reported to be associated with permanent hearing loss. In approximately one-quarter to one-half of infants and children with permanent hearing loss, the cause is not identified [9, 10].

2.2 NICU Setting

Infants cared for in a neonatal intensive care unit (NICU), which includes neonatal level II, III, and IV care units, are at greater risk of hearing loss compared with healthy term infants [11–13]. In particular, sensorineural hearing loss (SNHL) and auditory neuropathy (AN) are much more common with reported rates of 16.7 and 5.6 per 1000 infants, respectively, among infants cared for in a NICU compared with an estimated incidence of 0.06 per 1000 infants among a healthy newborn population [11, 12]. If infants with hyperbilirubinemia are included in the healthy newborn population, the incidence of SNHL rises to 0.3 per 1000 infants, still one-tenth of the rate seen in infants cared for in the NICU [4].

Risk factors associated with acquired SNHL and AN include very low birth weight (<1500 g), congenital infections, severe hyperbilirubinemia, perinatal asphyxia, and exposure to ototoxic medications (e.g., aminoglycosides, diuretics) [8].

3   Risk Factors for Hearing Loss

Major risk factors for neonatal hearing loss include the following [4, 6, 14]:

- Neonatal intensive care unit (NICU) admission for at least 5 days.
- Syndromes associated with hearing loss.
- Family history of permanent childhood hearing loss.
- Craniofacial anomalies (e.g., anomalies of the pinna or ear canal, cleft lip, and palate).
- Congenital or neonatal infection (e.g., cytomegalovirus, toxoplasmosis, rubella, syphilis, herpes, Zika) or bacterial meningitis.
- Severe hyperbilirubinemia (defined as serum bilirubin >35 mg/dL (599 micro/L) or requiring exchange transfusion) [15].
- Perinatal complications (e.g., perinatal asphyxia, neonatal encephalopathy, low five-minute Apgar score).
- Ototoxic mediation (e.g., aminoglycosides, diuretics).

4   Prevention of Deafness with Early Hearing Loss Detection and Intervention Programs

Before the establishment of universal newborn hearing screening (UNHS), the typical age at which a kid in the United States was diagnosed as profoundly deaf was 2 years. Children with mild-to-severe hearing loss were seldom diagnosed until they started school [1, 16].

The early detection of hearing loss in neonates has been revolutionized by universal newborn hearing screening (UNHS) programs [3].

There are three essential features that define early hearing detection and intervention programs (EHDI):

- "Screening (the initial test for hearing loss), conducted through universal newborn hearing screening (UNHS)"
- "Audiologic evaluation to confirm for hearing loss"
- "Early intervention to enhance communication, thinking, and behavioral skills needed to achieve academic and social success" [16].

Even the most attentive parents may miss the signs of hearing loss in their infants and toddlers before the first birthday [16].

The early worries of parents concerning hearing difficulties are often dismissed by doctors and other health experts, even when they turn out to be right. In most cases, parents don't become concerned that their kid has a hearing problem until he or she misses developmental milestones in speech and language around the age of 1 or 2 [3, 17].

After a baby is diagnosed with hearing loss, an audiologist may equip them with an amplification device as early as 4 weeks of age. Cochlear implants may be placed in children as young as 12 months if necessary. Infants born deaf may be expected to catch up to their hearing counterparts in linguistic, cognitive, and social development with the help of early intervention [18].

Spread the word to expectant and new parents as well as the general public about the value of a routine hearing test for their child. A hearing test should be given to infants who were delivered at home or in other nontraditional birth settings between 2 and 3 months of age. Please check with your state's program for eligibility criteria. The screening process must be transparent to parents, and the findings must be communicated to them without undue delay. Provide parents the facts and point them in the direction of facilities that can do the hearing tests quickly [3].

5 Rationale for Screening

Screening newborns for hearing loss leads to earlier detection and intervention in patients with congenital hearing impairment. Early intervention can significantly improve language acquisition and educational achievement in affected patients [19–25].

5.1 Earlier Detection

The available evidence demonstrates that screening newborns detects hearing loss at an earlier age than relying solely on identifying clinical signs of hearing loss [17, 26–30]. This is because caregivers and clinicians are often not able to detect hearing loss in infants until there are signs of delayed speech and language development.

This point was best illustrated by a clinical trial carried out in the 1990s at four hospitals in England [26, 30]. Over a 3-year period, the hospitals alternated between 6-month periods of screening all newborns and periods of no screening. Among the 25,609 infants born during screening periods, 27 were found to have bilateral permanent hearing loss (incidence 105 per 100,000 live born infants) and among the 28,172 infants born during periods without screening, 26 were found to have bilateral permanent hearing loss (incidence 92 per 100,000 live born infants). Compared with infants with hearing loss who were born during periods without screening, those born during screening periods were more likely to have the hearing loss confirmed before age 10 months (59 versus 38%) and to start intervention before age 10 months (56 versus 27%; odds ratio 2.4, 95% confidence interval [CI]: 1.0–6.0) [4].

5.2 Language and Developmental Outcomes

Earlier diagnosis and intervention for permanent hearing loss in infants appear to improve language and developmental outcomes [19, 21–25, 31]. Earlier diagnosis allows for earlier introduction of hearing aids.

In a study of 120 children with bilateral permanent hearing loss identified from a large birth cohort in England, children whose hearing loss was confirmed by 9 months of age had better receptive and general language abilities compared with those confirmed after 9 months of age [21, 22, 26, 30]. In subsequent follow-up reports, patients from this cohort who were identified before 9 months had better reading and communication skills than those diagnosed after 9 months of age through adolescence [4, 21, 23].

6 Types of Hearing Loss

The pinna and ear canal make up the outer ear, while the tympanic membrane, ossicles, and middle ear cavity make up the middle ear, and the cochlea and vestibular system make up the inner ear (the cochlea). Hearing loss is classified according to the site of the anatomic or physiological dysfunction that leads to it [32].

If there is a problem with the system that transfers external sounds to the inner ear, the person will suffer from conductive hearing loss. There is damage to either the external or middle ear, or both, in this case. Loss of loudness or sensitivity to inaudible noises is common symptoms of conductive hearing loss. Foreign bodies, impacted ear wax, fluid in the ear from things like colds, allergies, or ear infections, and a malfunctioning eustachian tube are common causes of conductive losses. If a kid has conductive hearing loss, it can typically be treated medically or surgically, and if not, a hearing aid helps tremendously [3].

Damage to the cochlea (inner ear) or auditory nerve causes sensorineural hearing loss. Deficits in speech comprehension or amplification are only two of the symptoms of sensorineural hearing loss. Diseases, injuries, ototoxic medicines, and genetic disorders are only few of the many potential root causes of sensorineural hearing loss. Exposure to loud noise, infections, traumatic brain injury, old age, and tumors are additional potential causes. Twenty) The likelihood of this kind of hearing loss is particularly significant for NICU grads. Hypoxia, intraventricular hemorrhage, hyperbilirubinemia, exposure to ototoxic medications, infection, and convulsions all increase the risk of hearing loss in premature infants with a birth weight of less than 1500 g [33] Sensorineural hearing loss is currently treated with no medicinal options. Educational and communicative therapy, as well as a hearing aid or cochlear implant, may help a kid who has trouble hearing [3].

Occasionally, a sensorineural loss may occur with conductive hearing loss. Such a condition is known as "mixed hearing loss," and it may affect both ears. The degree of deafness may be further broken down into two categories: unilateral and bilateral. Most cases of congenital hearing loss in a Colorado infant study were of the sensorineural type, affecting both ears (68%). Unilateral conductive (7%), unilateral sensorineural (20%), and bilateral conductive (5%) losses also occurred [34].

The degree to which someone has lost their hearing is also measured. Dependent on the decibel (dB) level or loudness of a sound, it may range from barely audible to completely deafening for a young kid. Deafness is a term used to identify children with severe (71–90 dB) and profound (91+ dB) hearing losses, while hard of hearing is used to describe those with mild (26–40 dB) to moderately severe (70 dB) losses. Hearing impairment varies from person to person and from the lowest to the highest sound frequencies [32].

There are four primary consequences for children with hearing loss [3]:

One of its effects is a halt in the development of both receptive and expressive language (speech and language).

Second, because of difficulties in learning and retention, academic performance suffers because of the language barrier.

[3] Isolation from others and a low opinion of oneself are common results of having trouble communicating

This factor could influence the career paths people choose [3, 18].

The first screening test may not pick up on certain moderate hearing impairments that only impact certain pitches. It's also possible for some newborns to have normal hearing but later acquire a kind of hearing loss. There are genetic, drug, and medical factors that may contribute to this. Assist parents in understanding typical speech and language development patterns. Parents should be on the lookout for signs of hearing loss and should contact their doctor immediately if they have concerns [3].

7   Severity of Hearing Loss

The extent of hearing loss is defined by measuring the hearing threshold in decibels (dB) at various frequencies. Normal hearing has a threshold of -10 to 15 dB [4].

Hearing loss ranges from slight to profound. In individuals with bilateral hearing loss, the severity of loss is based on the better-functioning ear.

Severity of hearing loss defined by the American Speech-Language Hearing Association as follows [9, 19, 35]:

- No hearing loss—-10 to 15 dB.
- Slight—16 to 25 dB.
- Mild—26 to 40 dB.
- Moderate—41 to 55 dB.
- Moderately severe—56 to 70 dB.
- Severe—71 to 90 dB, or 61 to 80 dB based on the World Health Organization (WHO) definition [9].
- Profound—>91 dB, or >80 dB based on WHO definition.

8   Tests Used in UNHS Programs

A loss of hearing of more than 30 dB may have a negative impact on a child's ability to learn language. Hearing evaluation methods for babies aged 3 months and younger should be sensitive enough to pick up on this level of damage. Automated auditory brainstem response (AABR) and otoacoustic emissions (OAE) are two physiological measurements that have shown potential for this purpose [3].

Oscillatory auditory emissions (OAE) are noises produced by the cochlea that are not perceptible to the human ear when stimulated by audible sounds. The middle ear receives an inaudible signal from the cochlea's outer hair cells, which vibrate and generate an echo. A tiny probe placed within the ear canal can accurately quantify this sound. Emissions are made by people with typical hearing. Individuals with a hearing loss of more than 25–30 dB do not. Outer-ear-canal obstruction, middle-ear fluid, and outer-hair-cell injury in the cochlea may all be detected by OAEs. OAE requires fewer throwaway components, so it's cheaper overall, and it works quickly. Transient evoked otoacoustic emissions (TEOAE) and distortion product otoacoustic emissions (DPOAE) are two types of OAE (DPOAE). When the middle ear has not been properly ventilated after delivery or when there is still dirt in the ear canal, the test may provide false results [34]. It cannot identify problems with the auditory or nervous systems either. When an infant has auditory neuropathy or a brain conduction issue in addition to sensory (i.e., outer hair cell) malfunction, OAEs will not be able to identify the condition [1].

The auditory evoked potential (AABR) is a signal that is generated in the auditory nerve. Infants often utilize it. Electrodes are attached to the scalp in order to capture the brain's electrical activity while it processes sound. Cochlear, auditory nerve, and auditory pathways in the brainstem may all be damaged, but AABR can identify this. In the context of early hospital discharge, the AABR is recommended since it is unaffected by middle ear fluid or ear canal debris, both of which are common in the first 12–24 h of birth. Because to the increased risk of auditory neuropathy in NICU grads, this screening is recommended [33, 34]. Babies must be napping or otherwise calm during AABR testing [3, 36].

Both exams are trustworthy and may be finished in about ten minutes [34]. Both of these testing procedures may be employed alone or together. When used together, the OAE and AABR may evaluate more of the auditory system and lower the amount of false positives. Several hospitals use OAEs as a first step in baby screening, with the AABR being used on those who don't pass [3].

A research was conducted to examine the referral rates and costs of the three universal newborn hearing screening (UNHS) protocols (TEOAE alone, AABR alone, and the 2-step TEOAE/AABR). Three screening techniques were compared, with AABR attaining the lowest referral rate at discharge (3.21%), followed by the 2-step approach (4.67%), and the TEOAE methodology (6.49%) (P 0.01). Costs per identified kid were comparable amongst programs using any of the three approaches (AABR, $32.81; 2-step, $33.05; TEOAE, $28.69) [37].

8.1 Screening Tests for Hearing

A credible newborn hearing screening test is one that can identify a better-ear hearing loss of 35 dB or less in babies less than 3 months of age [38].

Based on these four requirements, two electrophysiological methods exist:

Otoacoustic emissions (OAEs) Automatic auditory brainstem responses (AABRs) (OAE).

Low-cost, easily transportable, and repeatable, OAE and AABR methods may be fully automated. They can test for issues with the ear's periphery and the cochlea, but not with the most core parts of the ear. Every youngster who does not pass one of these tests has to be evaluated further by an audiologist to determine whether they have a hearing loss. Furthermore, slight hearing loss will be missed by both approaches [4].

8.2 Automated Auditory Brainstem Response

AABR is a test that analyzes how many times a click stimulus causes an increase in electrical activity in the inferior colliculus of the midbrain, which is part of the eighth cranial nerve (the cochlear nerve). Sensorineural hearing loss (SNHL) and auditory neuropathy are two forms of impairment that may be identified (AN). The screening auditory brainstem response (SABR) or screening brainstem auditory evoked response are other names for this evaluation (BAER). Around 4% of newborns screened with AABR are sent on for a more in-depth audiologic examination, which often involves a diagnostic ABR and an assessment by an audiologist with experience working with young children [38].

Methodology: The AABR makes use of 35 dB of click or chirp stimulation. The waveform recordings produced by the ABR in response to the stimuli are recorded using three surface electrodes placed on the forehead, neck, and mastoid or shoulder. The screening AABR compares the waveforms' morphology and latency to typical newborn templates, producing a pass or fail reading without the requirement for examiner interpretation if the waveforms are in plain sight. Most AABR screenings take between 4 and 15 min to complete, yet with the most up-to-date technology, a newborn baby may have their screening finished in as little as 8 min [4].

Automatic acoustic brainstem response (AABR) is not the same as an acoustic brainstem response (ABR) used for diagnosis. AABR is a machine that can instantly tell you whether or not you passed a screening. Diagnostic ABR, on the other hand, gives quantifiable data (e.g., waveforms) that, when assessed by a qualified audiologist, may pinpoint the precise kind and extent of a hearing loss. Delays or complete lack of waves, for instance, may indicate a problem with the brain or the inner ear. It is common practice for NICUs to do the diagnostic ABR on newborns who failed the screening AABR before discharging them. More explanations of ABR are found elsewhere [4].

8.3 Otoacoustic Emissions

What the test is measuring: Otoacoustic emissions (OAEs) are sound waves produced by the inner ear's cochlear outer hair cells in response to acoustic stimulation. These weak OAEs may be picked up by placing a microphone in the external auditory canal. OAE is utilized for screening for SNHL but cannot identify AN since it analyzes hearing only from the middle ear to the outer hair cells of the inner ear [4].

    Methodology: A tiny microphone is inserted into the external auditory canal of a newborn to perform the OAE screening. A stimulus (clicks or tones) is generated by the microphone, and the resulting sound waves are detected as they leave the cochlea. It also checks the signal-to-noise ratio to make sure the results are reliable. OAE screening typically takes no more than two minutes per ear under optimum circumstances.

    Types of OAEs may be broken down into subcategories based on the stimulus that was utilized to trigger the vibrations of the cochlear basal membrane. Transient Otoacoustic Emissions (TOAEs) and Distortion Product Otoacoustic Emissions (DPOAEs) are the most often utilized tests in clinical practice [4].

8.4 Comparison of AABR and OAE

Automatic auditory brainstem response (AABR) and otoacoustic emissions (OAE) are two different kinds of hearing tests, however they are both used for screening.

    Time: OAE tests often take less time overall and less time for patient preparation than AABR tests [39]. Time restrictions may also be an issue with AABR due to the fact that newborns must either be sleeping or quietly awake throughout testing. OAE, on the other hand, may be done when the baby is awake, whether it be for feeding or pacifier use [40]. Yet, OAE response time is much improved whether the newborn is asleep or quietly awake.

    Interference: OAE is very susceptible to environmental noise and the infant's own physiological noise [41]. Physiological noise, myogenic noise, and poor acoustics may all make it challenging to get OAE responses at low frequencies. When the recorded frequency is less than 1500 Hz, this noise interference becomes more noticeable (Hz). As a result, modifying protocol parameters to include select high frequencies, which are more critical for interpreting speech, may enhance screening with OAE [41–43]. A pediatric audiologist is the ideal candidate to execute these protocol adjustments. Muscle artifacts do not affect OAE the way they do AABR [40, 44]. Moreover, electrical artifacts may muddy the waters of AABR [40].

9 Protocols

Single- and two-stage universal screening methods are the two most common forms of screening procedures [4].

OAE or AABR are used in a single-stage NHS to identify 80–95% of hearing-impaired ears, making this kind of NHS the most efficient. The total cost of universal NHS would rise because of the high false-positive rate associated with each individual test; this would cause many newborns with normal hearing to be sent for audiologic screening. Just 4% of newborns tested with AABR [45, 46] and between 5% and 21% of infants screened with OAE [45, 46] need to be referred for audiologic assessment [17, 47]. One in 900–2500 newborns is born with severe-to-profound hearing loss, according to some studies. As a result, anywhere between 40 and 500 newborns with normal hearing would be referred for audiologic examination after a single-stage screen for a single incidence of substantial hearing loss. Thus, most U.S. maternity wards use two-stage procedures [4].

Patients who do not pass the first test are given a second opportunity to do so before being sent for an audiological evaluation [48]. The two-step procedure is preferable since it cuts down on both the number of false-positive results and the number of patients sent for audiologic evaluation [49, 50].

Researchers found that between 900 and 1400 newborns would need to be tested in a two-stage NHS in order to detect a single occurrence of bilateral hearing loss [26, 51]. A two-tiered NHS predicts that 1 in 45 babies in the newborn nursery will have moderate to severe bilateral irreversible hearing loss [6].

Yet, because of an unfounded assumption that all newborns who fail the first test but pass the second have normal hearing, the two-stage screening may overlook infants with hearing loss [48, 52, 53]. Moreover, the existing screening instruments have thresholds of roughly 35 dB, missing minor hearing loss and delaying diagnosis. This discovery has led the JCIH and the AAP to propose routine monitoring of children's language and hearing abilities in accordance with the AAP's periodicity plan [4].

10 Significance of Hearing Screen Results

Despite its growing popularity, universal newborn hearing screening (UNHS) is not endorsed by all experts due to concerns about its high false-positive rate [54]. There are a variety of potential drawbacks associated with false-positive findings for universal newborn hearing screening (UNHS). They include emotional distress, incorrect disease labeling, iatrogenic illness due to unneeded testing, and higher financial and time expenditures. The number of false positives is drastically decreased when a two-stage testing methodology is used (OAE followed by AABR or AABR performed twice) [3, 54].

Two-stage testing (AABR followed by ABR administered by an audiologist for neonates who failed the first stage) was compared to AABR testing alone in one study of infants not in the NICU. After doing the test again, the percentage of false positives dropped from 3.9% to 0.8%, a decrease of 80%. A comprehensive retrospective assessment of 148,240 newborns assessed with one of three procedures (AABR, OAE, or OAE/AABR) confirmed differences in referral rates [26]. Referral rates to OAE testing were 11% compared to 1.5% to AABR screening. There was an 8.4% referral rate after completing the two-step procedure (OAE and AABR)). It is evident that AABR testing seems to provide the lowest false-positive rate, with OAE and AABR testing giving the next best alternative [3].

11 Conclusion

Early diagnosis is very important for the children with HL, and it plays an essential role in reducing its destructive results. Lingual development of babies during the initial period is rather fast. It is important for the babies to have a normal hearing capability from the points of social, emotional, and mental progress along with speech development. In case the infant's hearing loss is not detected at an early stage, this leads to a disability which will have a lifelong influence in the person such as impediment in speech, intellectual performance weakness, social inadaptability, and emotional disorders [2].

References

1. Joint Committee on Infant Hearing. Year 2000 position statement: principles and guidelines for early hearing detection and intervention programs. Pediatrics. 2000;106:798–817.
2. Ulusoy S, Ugras H, Cingi C, Yilmaz HB, Muluk NB. The results of national newborn hearing screening (NNHS) data of 11,575 newborns from west part of Turkey. Eur Rev Med Pharmacol Sci. 2014;18(20):2995–3003.
3. Gracey K. Current concepts in universal newborn hearing screening and early hearing detection and intervention programs. Adv Neonatal Care. 2003;3(6). https://www.medscape.com/viewarticle/466531_2. Accessed online at February 22, 2023.
4. Vohr BR. Screening the newborn for hearing loss. Abrams SA, Duryea TK, Wilkie L (Eds). UpToDate. Last updated: Aug 10, 2022.
5. Anastasio ART, Yamamoto AY, Massuda ET, et al. Comprehensive evaluation of risk factors for neonatal hearing loss in a large Brazilian cohort. J Perinatol. 2021;41:315.
6. Thompson DC, McPhillips H, Davis RL, et al. Universal newborn hearing screening: summary of evidence. JAMA. 2001;286:2000.
7. 2019 Summary of National CDC EHDI Data. Available at: https://www.cdc.gov/ncbddd/hearingloss/2019-data/01-data-summary.html. Accessed 25 July 2022.
8. Vos B, Senterre C, Lagasse R, et al. Newborn hearing screening programme in Belgium: a consensus recommendation on risk factors. BMC Pediatr. 2015;15:160.
9. Lang-Roth R. Hearing impairment and language delay in infants: Diagnostics and genetics. GMS Curr Top Otorhinolaryngol Head Neck Surg. 2014;13:Doc05.

10. Declau F, Boudewyns A, Van den Ende J, et al. Etiologic and audiologic evaluations after universal neonatal hearing screening: analysis of 170 referred neonates. Pediatrics. 2008;121:1119.

11. Xoinis K, Weirather Y, Mavoori H, et al. Extremely low birth weight infants are at high risk for auditory neuropathy. J Perinatol. 2007;27:718.

12. Korver AM, van Zanten GA, Meuwese-Jongejeugd A, et al. Auditory neuropathy in a low-risk population: a review of the literature. Int J Pediatr Otorhinolaryngol. 2012;76:1708.

13. Nair V, Janakiraman S, Whittaker S, et al. Permanent childhood hearing impairment in infants admitted to the neonatal intensive care unit: nested case-control study. Eur J Pediatr. 2021;180:2083.

14. Bielecki I, Horbulewicz A, Wolan T. Risk factors associated with hearing loss in infants: an analysis of 5282 referred neonates. Int J Pediatr Otorhinolaryngol. 2011;75:925.

15. Wickremasinghe AC, Risley RJ, Kuzniewicz MW, et al. Risk of Sensorineural Hearing Loss and Bilirubin Exchange Transfusion Thresholds. Pediatrics. 2015;136:505.

16. Centers for Disease Control. Commission on Education of the Deaf. Available at www.cdc.gov/ncbddd/ehdi. Accessed 30 Apr 2003.

17. Yoshinaga-Itano C, Sedey AL, Coulter DK, Mehl AL. Language of early- and later-identified children with hearing loss. Pediatrics. 1998;102:1161–71.

18. American Speech-Language-Hearing Association. Hearing facts on newborn hearing loss and screening, 2003. Available at: www.asha.org. Accessed 30 Apr 2003.

19. Korver AM, Konings S, Dekker FW, et al. Newborn hearing screening vs later hearing screening and developmental outcomes in children with permanent childhood hearing impairment. JAMA. 2010;304:1701.

20. Preventive US. Services Task Force. Universal screening for hearing loss in newborns: US Preventive Services Task Force recommendation statement. Pediatrics. 2008;122:143.

21. Pimperton H, Blythe H, Kreppner J, et al. The impact of universal newborn hearing screening on long-term literacy outcomes: a prospective cohort study. Arch Dis Child. 2016;101:9.

22. Kennedy CR, McCann DC, Campbell MJ, et al. Language ability after early detection of permanent childhood hearing impairment. N Engl J Med. 2006;354:2131.

23. McCann DC, Worsfold S, Law CM, et al. Reading and communication skills after universal newborn screening for permanent childhood hearing impairment. Arch Dis Child. 2009;94:293.

24. Vohr B, Jodoin-Krauzyk J, Tucker R, et al. Early language outcomes of early-identified infants with permanent hearing loss at 12 to 16 months of age. Pediatrics. 2008;122:535.

25. Pimperton H, Kreppner J, Mahon M, et al. Language Outcomes in Deaf or Hard of Hearing Teenagers Who Are Spoken Language Users: Effects of Universal Newborn Hearing Screening and Early Confirmation. Ear Hear. 2017;38:598.

26. Wessex Universal Neonatal Hearing Screening Trial Group. Controlled trial of universal neonatal screening for early identification of permanent childhood hearing impairment. Lancet. 1998;352:1957.

27. Russ SA, Rickards F, Poulakis Z, et al. Six year effectiveness of a population based two tier infant hearing screening programme. Arch Dis Child. 2002;86:245.

28. Ghogomu N, Umansky A, Lieu JE. Epidemiology of unilateral sensorineural hearing loss with universal newborn hearing screening. Laryngoscope. 2014;124:295.

29. Moeller MP. Early intervention and language development in children who are deaf and hard of hearing. Pediatrics. 2000;106:E43.

30. Kennedy C, McCann D, Campbell MJ, et al. Universal newborn screening for permanent childhood hearing impairment: an 8-year follow-up of a controlled trial. Lancet. 2005;366:660.

31. Meinzen-Derr J, Wiley S, Grove W, Altaye M, Gaffney M, Satterfield-Nash A, Folger AT, Peacock G, Boyle C. Kindergarten Readiness in Children Who Are Deaf or Hard of Hearing Who Received Early Intervention. Pediatrics. 2020;146(4):1–9.

32. Knott C. Universal newborn hearing screening coming soon: "Hear's why". Neonatal Netw. 2001;20:25–33.

33. Stolz JW. Hearing loss in neonatal intensive care graduates. In: Cloherty JP, Stark AR, editors. Manual of neonatal care. Philadelphia, PA: Lippincott-Raven; 1998. p. 648–50.

34. Mehl AL, Thomson V. The Colorado Newborn Hearing Screening Project, 1992–1999: on the threshold of effective population-based universal newborn hearing screening. Pediatrics 2002;109. Available at www.pediatrics.org/cgi/content/full/109/1/e7. Accessed 30 Jan 2023.
35. www.asha.org/public/hearing/degree-of-hearing-loss/. Accessed on 28 Nov 2022.
36. Mehl AL, Thomson V. Newborn hearing screening: the great omission. Pediatrics 1998;101. Available at www.pediatrics.org/cgi/content/full/101/1/e4. Accessed 30 Apr 2003.
37. Vohr BR, Oh W, Stewart EJ, Bentkover JD, Gabbard S, et al. Comparison of costs and referral rates of 3 universal newborn hearing screening protocols. J Pediatr. 2001;139:238–44.
38. www.jcih.org/JCIH_2019_Executive_Summary.pdf. Accessed on 28 Nov 2021.
39. Hahn M, Lamprecht-Dinnesen A, Heinecke A, et al. Hearing screening in healthy newborns: feasibility of different methods with regard to test time. Int J Pediatr Otorhinolaryngol. 1999;51:83.
40. Choo D, Meinzen-Derr J. Universal newborn hearing screening in 2010. Curr Opin Otolaryngol Head Neck Surg. 2010;18:399.
41. Hall JW 3rd. Screening for and assessment of infant hearing impairment. J Perinatol. 2000;20:S113.
42. Headley GM, Campbell DE, Gravel JS. Effect of neonatal test environment on recording transient-evoked otoacoustic emissions. Pediatrics. 2000;105:1279.
43. Akinpelu OV, Peleva E, Funnell WR, Daniel SJ. Otoacoustic emissions in newborn hearing screening: a systematic review of the effects of different protocols on test outcomes. Int J Pediatr Otorhinolaryngol. 2014;78:711.
44. Callison DM. Audiologic evaluation of hearing-impaired infants and children. Otolaryngol Clin N Am. 1999;32:1009.
45. Pickett BP, Ahlstrom K. Clinical evaluation of the hearing-impaired infant. Otolaryngol Clin N Am. 1999;32:1019.
46. van Straaten HL. Automated auditory brainstem response in neonatal hearing screening. Acta Paediatr Suppl. 1999;88:76.
47. Finitzo T, Albright K, O'Neal J. The newborn with hearing loss: detection in the nursery. Pediatrics. 1998;102:1452.
48. Johnson JL, White KR, Widen JE, et al. A multicenter evaluation of how many infants with permanent hearing loss pass a two-stage otoacoustic emissions/automated auditory brainstem response newborn hearing screening protocol. Pediatrics. 2005;116:663.
49. Lin HC, Shu MT, Lee KS, et al. Comparison of hearing screening programs between one step with transient evoked otoacoustic emissions (TEOAE) and two steps with TEOAE and automated auditory brainstem response. Laryngoscope. 2005;115:1957.
50. Holster IL, Hoeve LJ, Wieringa MH, et al. Evaluation of hearing loss after failed neonatal hearing screening. J Pediatr. 2009;155:646.
51. Prieve BA, Stevens F. The New York State universal newborn hearing screening demonstration project: introduction and overview. Ear Hear. 2000;21:85.
52. Norton SJ, Gorga MP, Widen JE, et al. Identification of neonatal hearing impairment: evaluation of transient evoked otoacoustic emission, distortion product otoacoustic emission, and auditory brain stem response test performance. Ear Hear. 2000;21:508.
53. Levit Y, Himmelfarb M, Dollberg S. Sensitivity of the Automated Auditory Brainstem Response in Neonatal Hearing Screening. Pediatrics. 2015;136:e641.
54. Clemens CJ, Davis SA. Minimizing false-positives in universal newborn hearing screening: a simple solution. Pediatrics 2001;107. Available at www.pediatrics.org/cgi/content/full/107/3/e29. Accessed 30 Apr 2003.

Hearing Loss in Neonates and Infants

Bilal Sizer, Nuray Bayar Muluk, and Nitin R. Ankle

1 Introduction

A high societal and economic cost is incurred due to infant and child hearing loss due to the subsequent delay in speech and language development. By early diagnosis and therapy, children with hearing loss may improve their language and communication skills to the point that they can fully participate in and contribute to a hearing society [1, 2]. The public is becoming more aware of hearing loss, which has spurred the development of medical infrastructure and associated medical advancements to assist those with hearing loss. The diagnosis and treatment of hearing loss in newborns and babies have undergone a sea change with the implementation of a screening approach for congenital hearing loss [3, 4].

2 Epidemiology

According to global data, two to three out of every 1000 newborns are born with profound bilateral hearing loss, and another two to four are born with moderate or unilateral hearing loss [5]. Premature babies and those hospitalized in the neonatal

B. Sizer (✉)
Faculty of Medicine, Department of Otorhinolaryngology, İstanbul Arel University, İstanbul, Türkiye

N. B. Muluk
Faculty of Medicine, Department of Otorhinolaryngology, Kırıkkale University, Kırıkkale, Türkiye

N. R. Ankle
J. N. Medical College, Department of ENT & Head-Neck Surgery, KLE Academy of Higher Education & Research (KAHER), Belagavi, Karnataka, India

Ö. N. Şahin et al. (eds.), *Breastfeeding and Metabolic Programming*, https://doi.org/10.1007/978-3-031-33278-4_47

intensive care unit are more likely to develop hearing loss (NICU). Previous studies found that between 1.2 and 11% of premature newborns were diagnosed with a hearing loss depending on their gestational age [6]. There is an elevated incidence of hearing loss among infants admitted to the NICU, ranging from 1.6 to 13.7%. [7]. Research out of Korea found that while 4.6% of healthy infants were projected to have hearing loss, the rate increased to 28.8% of newborns hospitalized for more than 4.5 days in the NICU [8, 9].

In the United States, the rate of congenital hearing loss varies by race and method of diagnosis, making it difficult to compile reliable data. Several industrialized nations were able to quantify the prevalence of congenital hearing loss once they instituted national newborn hearing loss screening programs [10].

About 1.07–2.7 per 1000 preschoolers and 2.05–3.5 per 1000 teenagers are affected by hearing loss, respectively [11]. Cochlear implantation, which is used for auditory rehabilitation on patients with severe-to-profound hearing loss, was performed significantly later in the "refer" group compared to the "suspect" and "delay" groups in the Korean study involving infants with suspected acquired or delayed hearing loss after they passed the NHS [8, 9, 11] Since the permanent hearing loss at this age, which grows over that time, imposes severe language development delays, communication challenges, and societal expenses, early and precise identification of hearing loss in newborns and toddlers is critical. Pure tone audiometry should be routinely done around five or throughout puberty to prevent a delay in identifying hearing loss, particularly the late-onset or progressive variety [4, 11].

In order to effectively treat congenital or perinatal hearing loss, it is crucial to diagnose the condition and initiate early intervention before the child's sixth month of life [3, 4]. The normal hearing has a significant role in the development of speech and language, as well as intellectual and emotional growth, throughout the first year of life, making prompt treatment essential [12, 13].

3 Importance of Hearing Loss in Neonates and Infants

Children with hearing loss are at risk for delays in several cognitive skills, including working memory and executive abilities, despite the dramatic advances in speech and language [14, 15]. The effects of these issues in the classroom and on the job are far-reaching. In a population survey of Danish young men who were called to appear before a draft board, 51% of those with normal hearing continued their education above the age of 16; this number dropped to 42% for those with mild-to-moderate hearing loss and 34% for those with more severe hearing loss [16]. Norwegian cohort research revealed similar results, showing that those with hearing loss were 50% less likely to complete college [17].

A child's quality of life may be negatively impacted by hearing loss, research shows, especially in school and social life, as well as in terms of conduct and behavioral problems. Internalizing behaviors, conduct and hyperactivity issues, and other emotional difficulties were all linked to hearing loss in an unquantified but elevated way, according to one systematic study [18]. For youngsters who are deaf or hard of hearing, one research indicated that as many as half suffered from mental health issues [19]. As a result, typical childhood activities may be more challenging for 17–48% of children with unilateral hearing loss and the 50% with a cochlear implant who also have vestibular dysfunction. Studies that follow the same group of people over time show a correlation between women's early hearing loss and later anxiety, sadness, and worse well-being [20].

4 Etiology

Congenital hearing loss has several causes, but genes and the environment are the most important. Over half of all instances of congenital hearing loss have been thought to have a genetic component; another 25% were considered idiopathic, and the other 10% were unknown. Ongoing genetic research has led to findings that suggest that up to 80% of instances of congenital hearing loss in wealthy countries are caused by hereditary factors, with the other 20% caused by environmental or acquired causes [21, 22] such as toxoplasmosis, syphilis, rubella, cytomegalovirus, and herpes (TORCH) infections during pregnancy; postnatal bacterial meningitis [23]. It is becoming more apparent that congenital cytomegalovirus (CMV) infection is the leading environmental cause of congenital hearing loss, especially in affluent nations. [4, 21].

Branchiootorenal syndrome and CHARGE syndrome are only two examples of the many anatomical anomalies with known genetic roots. Those affected with branchiootorenal syndrome often have problems with their external ears, hearing, and kidneys. Coloboma, cardiac problems, atresia of choanae, growth retardation, genital abnormalities, and atypical olfactory development are all features of CHARGE syndrome. Ear abnormalities include exterior, middle, and internal ear malformations.

The risk of hearing impairment is most remarkable among infants born at less than 24 weeks of gestation. It decreases with increasing gestational age, birth weight, and the absence of other medical complications (1.2–7.5% among infants born at 24–31 weeks and 1.4–4.8% among those who weighed 750–1500 g at birth). Babies in NICUs have a 1.2–7.5% incidence rate of hearing loss (NICUs). Hyperbilirubinemia, sepsis, newborn bacterial meningitis, necrotizing enterocolitis, extended breathing, ototoxic drug exposure, and extracorporeal membrane oxygenation all enhance the risk of hearing loss in the neonatal intensive care unit [10, 24].

Because of congenital CMV's prevalence, various genetic or structural temporal bone etiologies can coexist with it. Due to the widespread immunization of pregnant women, congenital sensorineural hearing loss caused by the rubella virus is uncommon. While being very rare, the prevalence of congenital syphilis increased to 23.3% per 100,000 live births in 2017; this was particularly true in metropolitan areas and demographics [24, 25].

The most common syndromic and non-syndromic causes of hearing loss are listed in Table 1. [26]. Mutations in the GJB2 gene (encoding for gap junction protein beta 2) are the leading cause of congenital deafness in industrialized countries. DFNB1 was the first identified locus for non-syndromic deafness with autosomal recessive inheritance [27]. Connexin 26 is encoded by this gene (gap junction beta 2). Connexin 26 is expressed in the cochlea between the supporting cells and stria vascularis, spiral ligament, and spiral limbus. An action potential is generated in hair cells in response to sound waves, and this protein plays a role in the recycling of potassium used in this process [27]. Because of this, it is generally agreed that mutations in the GJB2 gene result in sensorineural hearing loss. Mutations in the SLC26A4 (solute carrier family 26 members 4) gene on chromosome 7, which encodes the pendrin protein, cause Pendred syndrome, the most common syndromic hearing loss [28]. Due to the recessive nature of Pendred syndrome, a child must inherit two mutant SLC26A4 genes, one from each parent. A predisposition characterizes Pendred syndrome to hearing loss, which is often but not always present at birth, often increases with time, and is linked to repeated mild head trauma. This condition is characterized by enlarged vestibular aqueducts, which increase the susceptibility of the inner ear to trauma. Also possible is vertigo. Goiter is a hallmark of this condition, seen in 75% of patients [28].

5 Screening for Congenital Hearing Loss

In 1957, Larry Fisch proposed the idea of a newborn hearing screening (UNHS) [29]. It became widespread in wealthy nations in the late twentieth century, however. In the beginning, NHS was only done to those at a high risk for hearing loss. Nevertheless, only around half of newborns with hearing loss had a risk factor for hearing loss; the other half of instances occurred in infants without risk factors [30]. Babies in most industrialized nations now have a hearing test soon after birth. For the first 28 days of life, the UNHS screens infants using an automated auditory brainstem response (AABR) and an automated otoacoustic emission (AOAE). Premature children that undergo UNHS have their accurate ages determined by their estimated birth dates. The stated ranges for AOAE's sensitivity and specificity are 50–100% and 13–91%, whereas those for AABR are 96% and 98%. [4]. Table 2 displays the 2019 recommendations of the American Joint Committee on Infant Hearing on causes of hearing loss [4]. Regardless of the newborn hearing screening findings, infants with these risk factors should be sent to the otolaryngology department for a thorough hearing examination and frequent checks. While audiometric tests are not commonly done, after a newborn has passed the NHS, the hearing state is monitored periodically using questionnaires designed for infant medical checks till 71 months of age. The NHS may not pick up on specific causes of hearing loss since they manifest in the early stages only as moderate hearing loss. As a result, several industrialized nations now provide pure-tone audiometry hearing exams to children as young as 5 years old [4]. For instance, a missed diagnosis is possible even after UNHS in cases of auditory neuropathy spectrum disorder (characterized by signal processing dysfunction along the auditory nerve or compromised signal transmission to the auditory nerve by presynaptic inner hair cells with fully functional outer hair cells). Since its creation, the UNHS has been applied well in affluent countries, yet inequities still exist worldwide. Even though certain nations, like Ireland and the Netherlands, have a screening percentage above 99%, many others have not [31]. Around a third of nations (representing about 38% of the world's population) provided no or very little screening, while another third had UNHS programs that were either virtually or entirely implemented. The average living level in nations where screening is wholly or almost universal is 10 times greater than in countries with less than 10% coverage. [31]. Moreover, with the fast development of sequencing technology, molecular genetic testing may compensate for the shortcomings of UNHS. Unfortunately, this is impossible due to the high uncertainty accompanying such testing.

Infants at increased risk of delayed-onset or progressive hearing loss.
**Infants with toxic levels or a known genetic susceptibility remain at risk.*
***Syndromes* [32].
****Parental/caregiver concerns should always prompt further evaluation.*

6 Hearing Rehabilitation for Bilateral Sensorineural Hearing Loss

Binaural listening is crucial for the development of spoken language, for effective communication in everyday listening and learning environments, and ultimately for academic success, and there is physiological and behavioral evidence to support the idea that bilateral input to the auditory system, as opposed to unilateral input, facilitates these abilities [17]. For children with bilateral sensorineural hearing loss, two ears equipped with a device are preferable to one in one ear since this maximizes hearing in both ears, which is crucial for developing spoken language. Children with both ears affected by sensorineural hearing loss may choose to use two hearing aids, two cochlear implants, or one cochlear implant in one ear and one hearing aid in the other (referred to as bimodal devices). Patients' audiometric hearing thresholds are considered while making these recommendations. An ideal listening environment would include hearing levels within the average range for both ears. It is common practice to prescribe bilateral hearing devices for children with bilateral sensorineural hearing loss who have significant quantities of residual hearing. Since hearing aids alone may not help children with severe-to-profound hearing loss, cochlear implant technology should be investigated. Bimodal devices may be an option for kids whose residual hearing is somewhere in the middle or who have noticeably different hearing in each ear [17].

Cochlear implants, unlike hearing aids, do not magnify acoustic information but instead provide an electrical signal straight to the auditory nerve. A cochlear implant consists of a receiver-stimulator and an electrode array surgically implanted into the inner ear, stimulating the cochlea to produce auditory signals. A microphone, magnetic transmission coil, and processor comprise a cochlear implant's exterior components.

7 Children with Hearing Aids

Two recent studies indicated that children with moderate-to-severe hearing loss who used hearing aids performed worse on average on some spoken language outcomes than their usually hearing peers. Compared to their usually hearing counterparts, their scores on receptive language, expressive language, speech production, and vocabulary tests fell within a range of 0.5–2 standard deviations (SDs) [33]. Children's disadvantages relative to their usually hearing classmates were mitigated by the severity of their remaining hearing loss. In addition to superior language results, we found higher mother education and nonverbal cognitive abilities, earlier hearing aid receipt, more consistent device usage, and stronger audibility [33].

8 Children with Cochlear Implants

Before the clinical availability of cochlear implants, children with bilateral severe-to-profound hearing loss using traditional hearing aids learned to talk at about half the rate of similar-aged children with normal hearing. By the time they attend primary school, many children with bilateral severe-to-profound hearing loss have acquired age-appropriate speech perception, speech production, and expressive and receptive language abilities due to cochlear implant development. Despite favorable language-learning conditions, 30–50% of kids still need to catch up in this area [34]. Age-appropriate spoken language outcomes for children with cochlear implants have been associated with higher preimplant residual hearing, earlier cochlear implant and early intervention service receipt, an emphasis on auditory and oral instruction, and the use of updated cochlear implant processor technology. It has been shown that children with cochlear implants have superior academic outcomes and a higher overall quality of life [35]. Cochlear implant patients' educational, vocational, and occupational achievement rates have continuously fallen below those of the normative population over the long run [17].

It is widely held in the medical community that children with profound hearing loss have a far better chance of acquiring language with the help of bilateral cochlear implants [36]. Some kids will get both cochlear implants at once, while others may get them in phases, with each step requiring a variable length (e.g., a few months to several years). The available research supports increased binaural processing capacities. Since there is not much time between the first and second implant, the implications of timing for the second implant need to be discussed [37]. Notably, as the threshold for cochlear implant eligibility in the United States rises to include children with greater levels of residual hearing in at least one ear, many children may present with bimodal device settings (cochlear implant combined with a hearing aids at the nonimplanted ear). Doctors assessing these children must choose whether continuing bimodal use or proceed with bilateral implants [36, 37].

Before the clinical availability of cochlear implants, children with bilateral severe-to-profound hearing loss who used traditional hearing aids acquired spoken language skills at about half the rate of similarly aged children with normal hearing. Cochlear implants have allowed many children with bilateral severe-to-profound hearing loss to reach their full linguistic potential in elementary school. 30–50% of children still do not acquire age-appropriate spoken language abilities, even when exposed to environmental and pedagogical elements that favor optimal language development [34]. Age-appropriate spoken language outcomes for pediatric recipients of cochlear implants have been linked to higher levels of nonverbal intelligence and maternal education, higher levels of preimplant residual hearing, earlier receipt of cochlear implant and early intervention services, a focus on auditory and oral instruction, and the use of updated cochlear implant processor technology. It has been demonstrated that children with cochlear implants do better in school and have a higher quality of life [35]. Cochlear implant recipients' long-term educational, vocational, and occupational attainment rates continue to lag well below the general population's [17].

Medical professionals agree that children with profound hearing loss have a far better chance of acquiring language if they get dual cochlear implants [36]. Cochlear implantation might co-occur for some children or at various periods for others (e.g., a few months to several years). Despite evidence suggesting superior binaural processing, Because the interval between implants is short, it is crucial to analyze how scheduling affects the outcome of the procedure [37]. As the standards for cochlear implant candidacy in the United States continue to expand, more and more children may be accepted with some degree of residual hearing in at least one ear, increasing the likelihood that many children may come with bimodal device setups (cochlear implant combined with a hearing aid at the nonimplanted ear). While evaluating these children, clinicians must choose between recommending continued bimodal use or progressing to bilateral implants [36, 37] to treat single-sided sensorineural hearing loss.

There is mounting evidence that unintended loss of hearing may negatively impact a child's development in several areas, including language, speech, and learning, as well as their conduct [38]. As a result, there has been a rise in the use of conventional hearing aids, frequency-modulating systems, devices for contralateral routing of signals, bone-conduction hearing aids, and cochlear implants for children with unilateral hearing loss. Transmitting sounds from the transmitter to the receiver, frequency-modulating devices lessen the effects of environmental noise, ear fatigue, and physical separation between the speaker and the listener. Hearing aids with contralateral signal routing gather sound from the damaged ear and transmit it to the healthy ear. Hearing aids that transmit sound through the skull's skeleton may help those with trouble hearing by avoiding the middle ear and activating the auditory nerve in either the affected or the normal ear on the same side. A cochlear implant is a device that uses an electrode implanted in the cochlea to stimulate the auditory nerve. Bone-conduction hearing aids have been demonstrated to help children with severe-to-profound unilateral sensorineural hearing loss hear better, particularly in noisy situations and at lower sound levels (the speech recognition threshold) [39]. Children aged over 5 years with substantial unilateral hearing loss (often called single-sided deafness) may undergo cochlear implant treatment. Speech outcome metrics in calm and loud settings, bimodal speech reception thresholds in noise, and sound localization have all been found to improve via research [40, 41]. Reports of success with hearing aids that route signals contralaterally are inconsistent. Frequency-modulating systems and traditional hearing aids may be helpful even in cases with milder unilateral loss. Children'sHomeInventory for ListeningDifficulties (CHILD) scores demonstrate that with traditional hearing aids, kids report feeling better at home and in the classroom after using them to help with speech recognition in noise, word recognition in both quiet and loud environments, and sound localization [42]. Objective hearing tests, such as the Bamford-Kowal-Bench sentence list and word recognition scores in loud and quiet settings, have also been proven to improve using frequency-modulating devices. Studies are needed to determine whether or not auditory rehabilitation can mitigate the adverse effects of unilateral hearing loss on speech and language, communication, academic performance, and social functioning; the evidence thus far is consistent only in showing improvement in audiological measures.

9 The Financial Burden of Newborn Hearing Impairment

The cost of hearing aids used in the rehabilitation process might vary widely. A cochlear implant device may cost around $20,000, whereas a set of hearing aids may only cost $6000. These estimates do not include ongoing expenses like speech therapy, cochlear implant programming, and medical and surgical bills. On the other hand, uncorrected hearing loss may result in significant financial burdens; for example, one research revealed that special education and lost productivity cost families of children with prelingual severe-to-profound hearing loss more than $1 million throughout their lifetimes [17].

10 Conclusion

Many advancements have been made in detecting and treating hearing loss in neonates and babies. The prognosis and counseling of families affected by hearing loss may be improved by early detection and knowledge of the condition's causes.

Furthermore, knowing about the many types of hearing aids, cochlear implants, and other assistive devices may help guide patient care and improve results.

References

1. Yoshinaga-Itano C, Sedey AL, Coulter DK, Mehl AL. Language of early-and later-identified children with hearing loss. Pediatrics. 1998;102(5):1161–71.
2. Mohr PE, Feldman JJ, Dunbar JL, McConkey-Robbins A, Niparko JK, Rittenhouse RK, Skinner MW. The societal costs of severe to profound hearing loss in the United States. Int J Technol Assess Health Care. 2000;16(04):1120–35.
3. Joint Committee on Infant Hearing. Year 2007 position statement: principles and guidelines for early hearing detection and intervention programs. Pediatrics. 2007;120(4):898–921.
4. Choe, G., Park, S. K., & Kim, B. J. (2023). Hearing loss in neonates and infants. Clinical and Experimental Pediatrics.
5. Cox C, Hack M, Metz D. Brainstem-evoked response audiometry: normative data from the preterm infant. Audiology. 1981;20(1):53–64.
6. Frezza S, Catenazzi P, Gallus R, Gallini F, Fioretti M, Anzivino R, Corsello M, Cota F, Vento G, Conti G. Hearing loss in very preterm infants: should we wait or treat? Acta Otorhinolaryngol Ital. 2019;39(4):257.
7. Di Stadio A, Molini E, Gambacorta V, Giommetti G, Della Volpe A, Ralli M, Lapenna R, Trabalzini F, Ricci G. Sensorineural hearing loss in newborns hospitalized in neonatal intensive care unit: an observational study. Int Tinnitus J. 2019;23(1):31–6.
8. Li PC, Chen WI, Huang CM, Liu CJ, Chang HW, Lin HC. Comparison of newborn hearing screening in well-baby nursery and NICU: a study applied to reduce referral rate in NICU. PLoS One. 2016;11(3):e0152028.
9. Chang J, Oh SH, Park SK. Comparison of newborn hearing screening results between well babies and neonates admitted to the neonatal intensive care unit for more than 5 days: analysis based on the national database in Korea for 9 years. PLoS One. 2020;15(6):e0235019.
10. Korver AM, Smith RJ, Van Camp G, Schleiss MR, Bitner-Glindzicz MA, Lustig LR, Usami SI, Boudewyns AN. Congenital hearing loss. Nat Rev Dis Primers. 2017;3(1):1–17.
11. Fortnum HM, Summerfield AQ, Marshall DH, Davis AC, Bamford JM. Prevalence of permanent childhood hearing impairment in the United Kingdom and implications for universal neonatal hearing screening: questionnaire based ascertainment studyCommentary: universal newborn hearing screening: implications for coordinating and developing services for deaf and hearing impaired children. BMJ. 2001;323(7312):536.
12. Ruben RJ, Umano H, Silver M. Assessment of efficacy of intervention in hearing impaired children with speech and language deficits. Laryngoscope. 1984;94(1):10–5.
13. Bielecki I, Horbulewicz A, Wolan T. Risk factors associated with hearing loss in infants: an analysis of 5282 referred neonates. Int J Pediatr Otorhinolaryngol. 2011;75(7):925–30.
14. Beer J, Kronenberger WG, Pisoni DB. Executive function in everyday life: implications for young cochlear implant users. Cochlear Implants Int. 2011;12(sup1):S89–91.
15. Kronenberger WG, Pisoni DB, Harris MS, Hoen HM, Xu H, Miyamoto RT. Profiles of verbal working memory growth predict speech and language development in children with cochlear implants. J Speech Lang Hear Res. 2013;56(3):805–25.
16. Teasdale TW, Sorensen MH. Hearing loss in relation to educational attainment and cognitive abilities: a population study: Hipoacusia en relación con los logros educativos y las habilidades cognitivas: Estudio en una población. Int J Audiol. 2007;46(4):172–5.
17. Kileny PR. Evoked potentials in the management of patients with cochlear implants: research and clinical applications. Ear Hear. 2007;28(2):124S–7S.

18. Bigler D, Burke K, Laureano N, Alfonso K, Jacobs J, Bush ML. Assessment and treatment of behavioral disorders in children with hearing loss: a systematic review. Otolaryngol Head Neck Surg. 2019;160(1):36–48.

19. Hindley PA, Hill PD, McGuigan S, Kitson N. Psychiatric disorder in deaf and hearing impaired children and young people: a prevalence study. J Child Psychol Psychiatry. 1994;35(5):917–34.

20. Idstad M, Tambs K, Aarhus L, Engdahl BL. Childhood sensorineural hearing loss and adult mental health up to 43 years later: results from the HUNT study. BMC Public Health. 2019;19(1):1–9.

21. Shearer AE, Hildebrand MS, Smith RJ. Hereditary hearing loss and deafness overview. GeneReviews®[Internet]; 2017.

22. Shave S, Botti C, Kwong K. Congenital sensorineural hearing loss. Pediatr Clin. 2022;69(2):221–34.

23. Ko H, Dehority W, Maxwell JR. The impact of maternal infection on the neonate. Congenital anomalies in newborn infants: clinical and etiopathological perspectives; 2021. p. 41.

24. Lieu JE, Kenna M, Anne S, Davidson L. Hearing loss in children: a review. JAMA. 2020;324(21):2195–205.

25. Cuffe KM, Torrone EA, Hong J, Leichliter JS, Gift TL, Thorpe PG, Bernstein KT. Identification of United States counties at elevated risk for congenital syphilis using predictive modeling and a risk scoring system, 2018. Sex Transm Dis. 2022;49(3):184–9.

26. Chang KW. Genetics of hearing loss—non-syndromic. Otolaryngol Clin N Am. 2015;48(6):1063–72.

27. Kelsell DP, Dunlop J, Stevens HP, Lench NJ, Liang JN, Parry G, Mueller RF, Leigh IM. Connexin 26 mutations in hereditary non-syndromic sensorineural deafness. Nature. 1997;387(6628):80–3.

28. Coyle B, Coffey R, Armour JA, Gausden E, Hochberg ZE, Grossman A, Britton K, Pembrey M, Reardon W, Trembath R. Pendred syndrome (goitre and sensorineural hearing loss) maps to chromosome 7 in the region containing the non-syndromic deafness gene DFNB4. Nat Genet. 1996;12(4):421–3.

29. Fisch L. The importance of auditory communication. Arch Dis Child. 1957;32:230–5.

30. Ptok M. Early detection of hearing impairment in newborns and infants. Dtsch Arztebl Int. 2011;108(25):426.

31. Neumann K, Euler HA, Chadha S, White KR. A survey on the global status of newborn and infant hearing screening. J Early Hear Detect Interv. 2020;5(2):63–84.

32. Van Camp G, Smith RJH. Hereditary hearing loss homepage. 2005; 2007. URL: http://www. uia.ac.be/dnalab/hhh.

33. Cupples L, Ching TY, Button L, Leigh G, Marnane V, Whitfield J, Gunnourie M, Martin L. Language and speech outcomes of children with hearing loss and additional disabilities: identifying the variables that influence performance at five years of age. Int J Audiol. 2018;57(sup2):S93–S104.

34. Geers AE, Nicholas J, Tobey E, Davidson L. Persistent language delay versus late language emergence in children with early cochlear implantation. J Speech Lang Hear Res. 2016;59(1):155–70.

35. Ballard KJ, Wambaugh JL, Duffy JR, Layfield C, Maas E, Mauszycki S, McNeil MR. Treatment for acquired apraxia of speech: a systematic review of intervention research between 2004 and 2012. Am J Speech Lang Pathol. 2015;24(2):316–37.

36. Peters BR, Wyss J, Manrique M. Worldwide trends in bilateral cochlear implantation. Laryngoscope. 2010;120(S2):S17–44.

37. Burrows PE, Mason KP. Percutaneous treatment of low flow vascular malformations. J Vasc Interv Radiol. 2004;15(5):431–45.

38. Anne S, Lieu JE, Cohen MS. Speech and language consequences of unilateral hearing loss: a systematic review. Otolaryngol Head Neck Surg. 2017;157(4):572–9.

39. Christensen L, Richter GT, Dornhoffer JL. Update on bone-anchored hearing aids in pediatric patients with profound unilateral sensorineural hearing loss. Arch Otolaryngol Head Neck Surg. 2010;136(2):175–7.
40. Urík M, Hošnová D, Šlapák I, Jančíková J, Odstrčilík J, Jarkovský J, Baumgartner WD. First experiences with a new adhesive bone conduction hearing device in children. Int J Pediatr Otorhinolaryngol. 2019;126:109614.
41. Zeitler DM, Sladen DP, DeJong MD, Torres JH, Dorman MF, Carlson ML. Cochlear implantation for single-sided deafness in children and adolescents. Int J Pediatr Otorhinolaryngol. 2019;118:128–33.
42. Priwin C, Jönsson R, Hultcrantz M, Granström G. BAHA in children and adolescents with unilateral or bilateral conductive hearing loss: a study of outcome. Int J Pediatr Otorhinolaryngol. 2007;71(1):135–45.

Programming the Auricle

Ergun Sevil, Cemal Cingi, and Mario Milkov

1 Introduction

The incidence rate of ear abnormalities in neonates is between 15 and 50%. [1]. Mental anguish might result from an odd auricular appearance [2]. Evidence suggests that children born with ear abnormalities are more likely to struggle with anxiety, low self-esteem, and relationship issues [3]. As a result, correcting ear abnormalities is crucial for the emotional well-being of kids [3, 4].

Malformations and deformations are the two most common types of congenital auricle abnormalities. The partial lack of skin and/or cartilage characterizes auricle abnormalities, which arise from a failure in embryologic development. As a consequence, the pinna becomes undeveloped, necessitating auricular restoration. Deformities of the auricle manifest as a completely formed pinna with no missing skin or cartilage [5].

After the ear has finished 85–90% of its development, usually just before school age, surgical correction is the primary therapy for these auricular abnormalities. Many studies have indicated that beginning the process of shaping a malformed ear as early as possible after birth (ideally within the first 3 days) may provide desirable outcomes and avoid the need for surgical surgery. Peak levels of maternal estrogen and tissue hyaluronic acid, which promote pliability in the infant auricle, occur

E. Sevil (✉)
Alanya Training and Research Hospital, Department of Otorhinolaryngology, Alaaddin Keykubat University, Alanya, Antalya, Türkiye

C. Cingi
Medical Faculty, Department of Otorhinolaryngology, Eskisehir Osmangazi University, Eskisehir, Türkiye
e-mail: cemal@ogu.edu.tr

M. Milkov
Faculty of Medicine, Department of Otorhinolaryngology, Varna University, Varna, Bulgaria

Ö. N. Şahin et al. (eds.), *Breastfeeding and Metabolic Programming*, https://doi.org/10.1007/978-3-031-33278-4_48

"

during the first 72 hours after delivery and return to baseline by 6 weeks of age, when the auricle becomes more elastic and solid [6].

A shorter molding treatment and less frequent need for surgical correction may result from establishing criteria for early detection of congenital auricular abnormalities so that molding therapy may begin within 3 days of birth [6, 7]. Use of foam, adhesives, wires, and putty were among the novelties. Maternal estrogen circulates through the body, keeping hyaluronic acid levels in cartilage high and enhancing the cartilage in the ear's capacity to be flexible. It has been shown that estrogen receptors are present in human auricular chondrocytes, and animal models have shown that estrogen injection into the auricle causes the ear to become soft and malleable [6–10].

2 Epidemiology

Auricular abnormalities are quite common in newborns, with a reported prevalence of 55.2–57%. [6]. Delays in treatment have occurred in the past due to the common belief that infants born with earlobe abnormalities would grow out of them naturally.

3 Etiology

Congenital auricle abnormalities may be traced back to a combination of hereditary (25%) and environmental (10%) causes, with genetic interaction accounting for the remaining 65% of cases. In the fifth to ninth week of pregnancy, if the embryo is inadequately formed, the baby may be born without key ear anatomical features. Auricular morphologic abnormalities including prominent ear, cup ear, and lop ear may occur as a consequence of aberrant auricle cartilage formation in the latter stages of embryogenesis. Single or numerous hillock loss and division may be at the root of these abnormalities [11]. Auricle morphological malformations may also be caused by antenatal intrauterine and external pressures, as well as by labor canal resistance, with the kind of deformity correlating with the direction of the pressure. The typical form of the auricle relies heavily on the work of the internal and exterior auricle muscles [12].

4 Evaluation of Auricular Anomaly

Auricular malformation (Table 1) should have been identified on the first visit. Photographs of the patient's clinical condition before, during, and after therapy are required. Whether or not the ear could be molded, the parents should have been informed of the potential outcomes, dangers, and alternatives [12].

Table 1 Auricle anomalies (Adopted from Reference 6)

Ear anomalies	Characteristics
Prominent ear	Auricle inclines forward, cranial ear angle increases, and the auricle is large and flat. The normal anatomic morphology of the auricle and anti-auricle is unknown
Cryptotia ear	The upper pole of the auricle is buried under the temporal subcutaneous tissues
Stahl's ear	The superior auricle is flat and has an abnormal bulge
Cup ear	The auricle length becomes shorter, the triangular fossa become narrower but do not disappear, and the shape of the supine position is like a cup
Lop ear	The upper part of the auricle is pendulous
Conchal crus	The auricular foot is abnormally raised in the auricular cavity
Helical rim	The ear rim does not curl, and the ear wheel is flat or not present
Grade I microtia	The auricle is slightly smaller but its shape is not significantly altered

Auricle abnormalities are best treated non-surgically between days 5 and 7 following delivery. The levels of residual maternal estrogen after delivery are highest during the first 72 h after birth and decline to their initial levels after 6 weeks. Auricular cartilage's adaptability is enhanced by estrogen, which may raise its hyaluronic acid levels. Around 6 weeks, the auricle loses a lot of its pliability since the estrogen and hyaluronic acid levels in the baby's blood have dropped [9, 13]. Patients have a 30% probability of self-healing if they are born within a week. Certain auricular malformations, including lobed ears with mild and severe deformities and Stahl's ears, may enhance their self-healing rate if the patient's parents massage and manipulate them appropriately within 14 days after birth [5, 8]. According to Tan et al., the effectiveness of noninvasive correction was maximized if it occurred during the first 3 months after birth, and the timeliness of therapy was strongly correlated with the durability of its therapeutic benefits [9]. Byrd et al. found that kids older than 3 weeks of age required a longer treatment course, and that the therapy's effectiveness was reduced by 50%. [5].

Auricular abnormalities may be treated in a variety of manner. Stahl's ear and lop ears had the quickest recovery times. When the helix of one ear folds over onto the upper leg of the helix of the other ear, a condition known as a lop ear is manifested. This causes the top half of the auricle to droop down and cover the upper helix of the opposite ear, resulting in a shorter auricle. The ear morphology of a child with a lop is drastically different from that of a child with normal ears, and this difference is usually readily apparent to parents from an early age. Thus, lop ears are detected at an earlier age and treated for a shorter period of time than other forms of abnormalities. When the posterior cerebral sulcus is insufficiently deep or nonexistent and there is also no discernible posterior auricular sulcus, this condition is known as cryptotia. A full look may be restored by pulling the top auricle outward, but the deformity will return as the pull is removed. Individuals with extreme cryptotia have a significant lack of auricular skin and upper auricular chondrodysplasia. A cryptotia ear is a malformation of the upper auricle that is often missed by parents and, as a result, requires more time spent on treatment if detected at a later age [6]. After approximately 2 weeks of care, the initial step of therapy is pulling out the auricle's top edge from beneath the scalp [14]. In the second phase, a lower frame is used to mold the auricle, a process that takes a considerable amount of time. Byrd felt that the diagnosis could only be established when the distance between the middle helium and the lateral cranial wall was >1 cm [5], making early identification of the prominent ear the most difficult and often disregarded. Patients older than 14 days after birth were included in this research, and all three of them had prominent ears that needed therapy lasting longer than 4 weeks. Overgrowth of auricular cartilage [15] causes cranio-auricular angle enlargement, which is difficult to cure and often results in a rebound. An increase in awareness regarding large ears is crucial, since this might lead to earlier diagnosis and treatment.

Molding methods may be used to non-surgically treat Stahl's ears, cup ears, and prominent ears, three common congenital auricular malformations [6].

5   Techniques

Non-surgical methods for fixing congenital ear abnormalities have been documented on several occasions [6, 16]. Metal wire, surgical tape, foam, and silicone tape are the traditional molding materials for ears [16, 17].

5.1   Traditional Ear-Shaping

First Step: Before to ear molding, the patient's hair was cut around the ear (to protect the skin) and the patient's skin oil was washed away with isopropyl alcohol to provide a good bond between the cradle and the skin.

Second Step: The splint was chosen, bent, and put on the auricle's anterolateral surface such that its form mimicked that of a helix.

Third Step: We used surgical tape to secure the helix to the antihelix groove on the auricle's anterolateral surface. The auricle was brought closer to the scalp with the use of surgical tape.

Fourth Step: Foam was used to shield the ear from the mold's contents.

Taping was employed during the first week of therapy to offset the considerable resistive forces to expansion caused by tissue shortage. The splint was then bent into the correct helix form and adhered to the ear's anterolateral surface. All day, every day, the babies wore the splint.

Don't stop therapy only because skin problems manifested themselves; foam-covered molding materials absorb exudate and improve skin lesions. As pressure ulcers developed, the splinting was discontinued. Patients were instructed to return to the clinic 3 days following ear-molding to be evaluated for any adverse reactions. Infants were routinely scheduled for weekly follow-up after it was established that none of the initial five patients had any complications 3 days after treatment. This allowed for the monitoring of complications and auricle changes, as well as the adjustment of devices to achieve better correcting conditions. It was standard practice to continue splinting until 1 week after the auricular anatomy had returned to normal, and in cases where no correction had taken place, splinting was discontinued after a maximum of 6 weeks of therapy [17].

5.2 EarWell Is an Infant Hearing Correction System (Becon Medical Ltd., Naperville, Ill.)

Four basic parts make up the EarWell system: The posterior cradle, the retractors, the conchal former, and the anterior shell. Positioned in the antihelix and the suggested upper limb of the triangular fossa, the posterior conformer completes the posterior cradle. The helical rim is held in place by the retractors. The sticky inner surface of the posterior cradle secures these retractors in place. After that, a conchal former made of a soft, compressible material is inserted into the conchal space. Finally, the anterior shell is fastened to the posterior cradle, causing the conchal former and retractor system to experience direct anterior forces [5].

The average time each gadget was used was 2 weeks. When the first problem was fixed, additional EarWell molding occurred for another 2 weeks. Weekly patient assessments looked for problems and treatment halts due to things like equipment movement [5, 18].

5.3 Non-Surgical Ear Molding for Infants with InfantEar (TalexMedical LLC, Malvern, Pa.)

The InfantEar set consists of the base plate, conformer, rim piece, silicone gel, and the protective cap, which has since been discontinued. Following the manufacturer's instructions, a normal ear molding kit was used [19].

5.3.1 Earlimn (Cihui Ltd., Hunan, China) (Cihui Ltd., Hunan, China)

For both deformations and malformations, the Earlimn system (Cihui Ltd., Hunan, China) was implemented. A cradle, retractors of varying sizes, a conchal mold, and a cover are all part of the system. The cradle was sewn into place on the abnormal ear's skin. The helical rim's form was fashioned with the aid of the retractors. The concha was given a helping hand when a mold was inserted inside of it. The cradle was covered by a lid that also served to secure the retractors and conchal mold [20].

6 Conclusion

A majority of babies are born with ear abnormalities, and only around 30% of them fix themselves. Appropriate shaping begun in the first week of life may fix these defects. Compared to the alternative, surgical correction, the outcomes of neonatal molding are generally superior.

Ear molding is cheap, simple, and requires no surgery. It is a vital technique for correcting auricular abnormalities in newborns, and it has to be extensively disseminated in clinical practice. Treatment is more likely to be successful if it is started right away once the problem is discovered.

References

1. Daniali LN, Rezzadeh K, Shell C, Trovato M, Ha R, Byrd HS. Classification of newborn ear malformations and their treatment with the EarWell infant ear correction system. Plast Reconstr Surg. 2017;139(3):681–91. https://doi.org/10.1097/PRS.0000000000003150.
2. Jiamei D, Jiake C, Hongxing Z, Wanhou G, Yan W, Gaifen L. An investigation of psychological profiles and risk factors in congenital microtia patients. J Plastic Reconstr Aesthet Surg. 2008;61 Suppl 1:S37–43. https://doi.org/10.1016/j.bjps.2007.09.002.
3. Li D, Chin W, Wu J, Zhang Q, Xu F, Xu Z, Zhang R. Psychosocial outcomes among microtia patients of different ages and genders before ear reconstruction. Aesthet Plast Surg. 2010;34(5):570–6. https://doi.org/10.1007/s00266-010-9502-1.
4. Horlock N, Vögelin E, Bradbury ET, Grobbelaar AO, Gault DT. Psychosocial outcome of patients after ear reconstruction: a retrospective study of 62 patients. Ann Plast Surg. 2005;54(5):517–24. https://doi.org/10.1097/01.sap.0000155284.96308.32.
5. Byrd HS, Langevin CJ, Ghidoni LA. Ear molding in newborn infants with auricular deformities. Plast Reconstr Surg. 2010;126(4):1191–200. https://doi.org/10.1097/PRS.0b013e3181e617bb.
6. Matsuo K, Hayashi R, Kiyono M, Hirose T, Netsu Y. Nonsurgical correction of congenital auricular deformities. Clin Plast Surg. 1990;17(2):383–95.
7. Petersson RS, Recker CA, Martin JR, Driscoll CL, Friedman O. Identification of congenital auricular deformities during newborn hearing screening allows for non-surgical correction: a Mayo Clinic pilot study. Int J Pediatr Otorhinolaryngol. 2012;76(10):1406–12. https://doi.org/10.1016/j.ijporl.2012.06.011.
8. Kurozumi N, Ono S, Ishida H. Non-surgical correction of a congenital lop ear deformity by splinting with Reston foam. Br J Plast Surg. 1982;35(2):181–2. https://doi.org/10.1016/0007-1226(82)90160-6.
9. Tan ST, Shibu M, Gault DT. A splint for correction of congenital ear deformities. Br J Plast Surg. 1994;47(8):575–8. https://doi.org/10.1016/0007-1226(94)90144-9.
10. Ullmann Y, Blazer S, Ramon Y, Blumenfeld I, Peled IJ. Early nonsurgical correction of congenital auricular deformities. Plast Reconstr Surg. 2002;109(3):907–15. https://doi.org/10.1097/00006534-200203000-00013.
11. Porter CJ, Tan ST. Congenital auricular anomalies: topographic anatomy, embryology, classification, and treatment strategies. Plast Reconstr Surg. 2005;115(6):1701–12. https://doi.org/10.1097/01.prs.0000161454.08384.0a.
12. Chen Y, Wang W, Wang Y, Mao X. Using ear molding to treat congenital auricular deformities. Front Pediatr. 2021;9:752981. https://doi.org/10.3389/fped.2021.752981.
13. Kenny FM, Angsusingha K, Stinson D, Hotchkiss J. Unconjugated estrogens in the perinatal period. Pediatr Res. 1973;7(10):826–31. https://doi.org/10.1203/00006450-197310000-00006.

14. Marsh D, Sabbagh W, Gault D. Cryptotia correction--the post-auricular transposition flap. J Plast Reconstr Aesthet Surg. 2011;64(11):1444–7. https://doi.org/10.1016/j.bjps.2011.06.037.
15. Schultz K, Guillen D, Maricevich RS. Newborn ear deformities: early recognition and novel nonoperative techniques. Semin Plast Surg. 2017;31:141–5. https://doi.org/10.1055/s-0037-1603958.
16. van Wijk MP, Breugem CC, Kon M. Non-surgical correction of congenital deformities of the auricle: a systematic review of the literature. J Plast Reconstr Aesthet Surg. 2009;62(6):727–36. https://doi.org/10.1016/j.bjps.2009.01.020.
17. Kim J, Jo T, Choi J, Kim J, Jeong W. Efficacy of classic ear molding for neonatal ear deformity: case series and literature review. J Clin Med. 2022;11(19):5751. https://doi.org/10.3390/jcm11195751.
18. Chan SLS, Lim GJS, Por YC, Chiang MF, Ho S, Saffari SE, Chia HL. Efficacy of ear molding in infants using the EarWell infant correction system and factors affecting outcome. Plastic Reconstr Surg. 2019;144(4):648e–58e. https://doi.org/10.1097/PRS.0000000000006057.
19. Patel V, Mazzaferro DM, Swanson JW, Taylor JA, Bartlett SP. Public perception of helical rim deformities and their correction with ear molding. J Craniofac Surg. 2020;31(3):741–5. https://doi.org/10.1097/SCS.0000000000006400.
20. Zhuang Q, Wei N, Zhou Q, Wang H, Wu Y, Chen Z, Yu D, Wang P, Shi H. Efficacy and timing of neonatal ear correction molding. Aesthet Plast Surg. 2020;44(3):872–8. https://doi.org/10.1007/s00266-019-01596-y.

The Effect of Breastfeeding on Childhood Otitis Media

Muhammet Pamukcu, Nuray Bayar Muluk, and Peter Catalano

1 Introduction

Throughout history, breastfeeding has been the obvious and natural way for mothers to feed their infants. Despite the widespread availability of alternatives to mothers breastfeeding their own offspring, in every culture and country the option to breastfeed remains a significant method for the nutrition of neonates. Breastfeeding, however, like other cultural practices, has waxed and waned over the years. Three hundred years ago, the infants born to mothers of high social class tended to be breastfed by wet nurses, and this trend then spread towards members of lower socioeconomic groups over the next 200 years [1, 2]. The trend in the twentieth century was towards fewer mothers breastfeeding infants, from a peak of around 90% to the current rate of 42%. Unlike many determinants of health, where less healthy practices are more common amongst lower income groups, breastfeeding is actually more prevalent in societies which are poorer overall. The decline in breastfeeding comes despite the accumulating evidence that breast milk has numerous advantages over artificial baby milk, such as providing immunity against frequently occurring pathogens encountered in infancy [3, 4].

M. Pamukcu (✉)
Medical Faculty, Department of Otorhinolaryngology, Istanbul Altinbas University, İstanbul, Türkiye

N. B. Muluk
Faculty of Medicine, Department of Otorhinolaryngology, Kırıkkale University, Kırıkkale, Türkiye

P. Catalano
School of Medicine, St. Elizabeth's Medical Center, Department of Otolaryngology, Tufts University, Boston, MA, USA

© The Author(s), under exclusive license to Springer Nature Switzerland AG 2023
Ö. N. Şahin et al. (eds.), *Breastfeeding and Metabolic Programming*,
https://doi.org/10.1007/978-3-031-33278-4_49

"><

2 The Burden of Otitis Media

The pathogens responsible for acute otitis media (AOM) are generally viral or bacterial. In the latter case, antibiotic treatment is frequently prescribed. The risk in early childhood increases due to the narrowness of the middle ear cavity and the fact that the Eustachian tubes drain the cavity inefficiently due to their twisting course. Frequent presenting features of AOM are significant otalgia, abrupt onset deafness, pyrexia and malaise. There are several complications associated with AOM. Patients who are predisposed towards AOM commonly experience recurrent bouts of the infection as infants and young children. After the acute infection resolves, it is common for an effusion to develop in the middle ear, causing the condition known as otitis media with effusion (OME). This then results in auditory loss. OME may become chronic, which then causes more long-lasting deafness and problems with linguistic development, academic performance and some behavioural issues. The tympanic membrane may be perforated following AOM and a chronic discharge may occur (known as chronic suppurative otitis media). Although less frequently encountered, other more grave complications are also possible, including mastoiditis, cerebral abscess formation or meningitis [1, 2].

The annual number of cases of AOM worldwide is thought to be 709 million, which equates to an incidence of 10.85% [5]. The age range most affected is between 1 and 4 years, where the incidence is 60.99%. There is considerable variation in incidence according to geographical location, with an incidence of 3.64% in Central Europe, but a much higher rate of 43.36% in Africa south of the Sahara [5]. There is a major health burden arising from AOM, both in developed and developing countries. For developed countries, AOM is the number one reason for antibiotics to be employed and the condition affects at least 60% of infants (up to the age of 1 year), whilst 80% of children have had at least one episode of AOM by the age of 3 years [6–8]. The complications of AOM also create considerable morbidity. The prevalence worldwide of chronic suppurative otitis media is calculated to be close to 31 million cases and irreversible auditory loss following AOM occurs at a frequency of 30.82 per 10,000 cases [1]. Moreover, AOM results in 21,000 deaths each year. The risk of mortality is most elevated in children up to the age of 5 years [5].

Despite the fact that the latest official guidance on treating AOM of mild severity, short duration and without complications advises against routine antibiotic use [9], AOM remains the most frequent indication for prescribing antibiotics in many different countries [10]. Not only does this result in an unwarranted strain on healthcare budgets, it also makes the development of antibiotic-resistant organisms in the community more probable [11, 12].

3 How Does Breastfeeding Potentially Protect Against AOM?

At one time the dominant theory to explain how breastfeeding protects against AOM posited the idea that the effect largely relied on the increased drainage of the eustachian tubes brought about when infants suckle at the breast. This theory suggests that the negative pressure created and the position of the infant when nursing are the key factors. A rival theory explains the reduced frequency of AOM in infants who receive breastfeeding as due to immunity conferred by constituents in breast milk which exert an active immune function. Interest in the second theory has increased recently following the greater research focus on the microbial flora of the gut, especially that established during infancy. It is increasingly evident that a healthy gastrointestinal microbiome develops at this stage in life, conferring several advantages to the infant, including protection against a number of pathogenic organisms [13–15].

The development of a healthy microbial flora in the infant is contributed to by particular constituents of breast milk, namely specific beneficial microbes themselves and several kinds of human milk oligosaccharides (HMOs). HMOs are carbohydrates secreted in milk and are especially abundant in colostrum. Primates secrete milk oligosaccharides with several features unique to this sub-grouping within the mammals, namely a high level of diversity and a significant degree of fucosylation [16]. More than 200 distinct HMOs have been identified in breast milk [17]. Fucosylation occurs in some 50–80% of these. Maternal genetics determines which HMOs are present [18]. HMOs are highly abundant in colostrum, with a concentration of 20–25 g/L, with a somewhat lower concentration in mature milk, namely 5–20 g/L [19]. It appears that infants cannot metabolise these carbohydrates to generate energy, but instead they act as nutrition for several different species of bacterial organisms that are beneficial to the health of the neonatal and infant gastrointestinal tract.

There has been extensive research interest in the composition of the gastrointestinal microbiome in infants and in how the microbial flora both offers a protective effect against gastrointestinal infections and helps to train the developing immune system to distinguish between pathogens and beneficial commensals. The evidence base for the nasopharyngeal microbiome is more slender and less has been learnt about how the bacterial flora may prevent AOM. A recent study undertaken by Biesbroek et al. [20] compared the microbial flora of the nasopharynx in 202 infants, half of whom received exclusive breastfeeding whilst the other half consumed artificial baby milk only. This study concluded that the floral composition correlated with the type of feeding. The breastfed infants had a flora at age 6 weeks with higher numbers of organisms from the genera *Dolosigranulum* and *Corynebacterium* than in the flora of formula-fed infants. Furthermore, the levels of Staphylococci, *Prevotella* and *Veillonella* spp. were lower in the breastfed infants [20].

Breast milk constituents act directly to regulate bacterial numbers, but the live microbes present within breast milk also cause modulate the numbers of pathogenic species known to cause middle ear infections. Milk has lactobacilli within it, and these organisms take up residence in the nasopharynx within the initial months of breastfeeding. This colonisation helps to lower the rate of middle ear infections [21, 22]. According to some studies, the presence of commensal bacterial species in the nose in breastfed infants also leads to lower number of *Staphylococcus aureus* and may result in fewer middle ear infections, although this has not yet been definitively established to occur [23, 24]. Breast milk also reduces inflammation in epithelia, which likely alters any epigenetic effects (reflected in histone activation or DNA methylation). The effect of these epigenetic alterations is a less severe reaction to the presence of pathogens within the middle ear. However, at present the epigenetic changes and how they affect middle ear infections is not well understood and more research is needed [25, 26].

4 The Duration of Breastfeeding

There are differences between studies in terms of the length of time for which breastfeeding continued. Generally, it has been concluded that breastfeeding which continues for longer than 3 months offers a greater degree of protection against otitis media than shorter periods [2, 27–29]. Furthermore, a minimum of 6 months duration of breastfeeding was also more beneficial than a briefer duration in terms of preventing middle ear infections [30, 31]. Studies rarely examine the situation where breastfeeding continues beyond 6 months, with studies where the duration of breastfeeding was up to 9 months or 1 year a minority. Nonetheless, one study which did examine these lengthier durations of breastfeeding concluded that 9 months of breastfeeding was superior to 3 months in the degree of protection it conferred [32].

5 The Effect of Duration and Method of Feeding

Overall, the evidence shows that breastfed infants have a lower risk of middle ear infections up to the age of 1 year. Multiple studies have concluded that breastfed infants benefit from a lower risk of otitis media at the ages of 6 months or 1 year [31–33]. In one study, a risk reduction was detectable for 3 years after breastfeeding, but undetectable after a further 3 years [31–33]. In a different study, it was concluded that being exclusively breastfed when younger still conferred a protective effect in children at the age of 6 years [34]. When exclusive breastfeeding is compared to mixed feeding, the former appears to offer a greater reduction in risk. Moreover, if formula milk is introduced at an early stage, this reduces the protective advantage of breastfeeding and makes middle ear infections more likely.

6 Conclusion

There seems to be a general consensus that breastfeeding confers a reduced risk of infectious diseases in infants generally, not just AOM. Infants who are exclusively breastfed for 6 months are more protected than those breastfed for shorter durations; however, there is no apparent additional protection if breastfeeding extends beyond

1 year in duration, despite the fact that breastfeeding for 18 months still lowers the incidence of middle ear infections. The incidence of middle ear infections is raised in children who are offered artificial baby milk from a very young age. The reduction in the incidence of middle ear infections is more apparent in data relying on parental reporting of episodes of otitis media or AOM than for recurrent middle ear infections, those involving a serous effusion or where the child required hospital admission.

The promotion of breastfeeding is justified not just by its protective effects in AOM but because of other advantages it offers, both for maternal and infant health and for the economic health of families. For this reason, there is a need for worldwide governmental endorsement and encouragement of the WHO breastfeeding guidelines.

References

1. Kørvel-Hanquist A, Djurhuus BD, Homøe P. The effect of breastfeeding on childhood otitis media. Curr Allergy Asthma Rep. 2017;17(7):45. https://doi.org/10.1007/s11882-017-0712-3.
2. Lodge CJ, Bowatte G, Matheson MC, Dharmage SC. The role of breastfeeding in childhood otitis media. Curr Allergy Asthma Rep. 2016;16(9):68. https://doi.org/10.1007/s11882-016-0647-0.
3. Stevens EE, Patrick TE, Pickler R. A history of infant feeding. J Perinat Educ. 2009;18:32–9.
4. Victora CG, Bahl R, Barros AJ, França GV, Horton S, Krasevec J, Murch S, Sankar MJ, Walker N, Rollins NC, et al. Breastfeeding in the 21st century: epidemiology, mechanisms, and lifelong effect. Lancet. 2016;387:475–90. A comprehensive review of the effect of breastfeeding on mother and child health status and a general description of the breastfeeding rates worldwide
5. Monasta L, Ronfani L, Marchetti F, Montico M, Vecchi Brumatti L, Bavcar A, et al. Burden of disease caused by otitis media: systematic review and global estimates. PLoS One. 2012;7(4):e36226.
6. Gonzales R, Malone DC, Maselli JH, Sande MA. Excessive antibiotic use for acute respiratory infections in the United States. Clin Infect Dis. 2001;33(6):757–62.
7. Teele DW, Klein JO, Rosner B. Epidemiology of otitis media during the first seven years of life in children in greater Boston: a prospective, cohort study. J Infect Dis. 1989;160(1):83–94.
8. Vergison A, Dagan R, Arguedas A, Bonhoeffer J, Cohen R, Dhooge I, et al. Otitis media and its consequences: beyond the earache. Lancet Infect Dis. 2010;10(3):195–203.
9. Le Saux N, Robinson JL, Canadian Paediatric Society. Management of acute otitis media in children six months of age and older. Paediatr Child Health. 2016;21(1):1–8.
10. Kørvel-Hanquist A, Koch A, Niclasen J, Dammeye J, Lous J, Olsen SF, Homøe P. Risk factors of early otitis Media in the Danish National Birth Cohort. PLoS One. 2016;11:e0166465.
11. Palmeira P, Carneiro-Sampaio M. Immunology of breast milk. Rev Assoc Méd Bras. 2016;62:584–93. A general description of the immunological roll of breast milk on the immune system of the newborn child
12. Brandtzaeg P. The mucosal immune system and its integration with the mammary glands. J Pediatr. 2010;156:S8–S15.
13. Stenfors LE. Non-specific and specific immunity to bacterial invasion of the middle ear cavity. Int J Pediatr Otorhinolaryngol. 1999;49(Suppl 1):S223–6.

14. Björck L, Rosén C, Marshall V, Reiter B. Antibacterial activity of the lactoperoxidase system in milk against pseudomonads and other gram-negative bacteria. Appl Microbiol. 1975;30:199–204.

15. de Steenhuijsen Piters WA, Sanders EA, Bogaert D. The role of the local microbial ecosystem in respiratory health and disease. Philos Trans R Soc Lond Ser B Biol Sci. 2015;370(1675):20140294.

16. Goto K, Fukuda K, Senda A, Saito T, Kimura K, Glander KE, et al. Chemical characterization of oligosaccharides in the milk of six species of New and Old World monkeys. Glycoconj J. 2010;27(7–9):703–15.

17. Bode L. Recent advances on structure, metabolism, and function of human milk oligosaccharides. J Nutr. 2006;136(8):2127–30. A very good introduction to human milk oligosaccharides and an insight into how they may relate to health and disease authored by international expert in HMOs

18. Oliveira D, Wilbey R, Grandison A, Roseiro L. Milk oligosaccharides: a review. Int J Dairy Technol. 2015;68(3):305–21.

19. Coppa GV, Pierani P, Zampini L, Carloni I, Carlucci A, Gabrielli O. Oligosaccharides in human milk during different phases of lactation. Acta Paediatr Suppl. 1999;88(430):89–94.

20. Biesbroek G, Bosch AA, Wang X, Keijser BJ, Veenhoven RH, Sanders EA, et al. The impact of breastfeeding on nasopharyngeal microbial communities in infants. Am J Respir Crit Care Med. 2014;190(3):298–308.

21. Biesbroek G, Bosch AATM, Wang X, Keijser BJF, Veenhoven RH, Sanders EA, Bogaert D. The impact of breastfeeding on nasopharyngeal microbial communities in infants. Am J Respir Crit Care Med. 2014;140612135546007.

22. Hilty M, Qi W, Brugger SD, Frei L, Agyeman P, Frey PM, Aebi S, Mühlemann K. Nasopharyngeal microbiota in infants with acute otitis media. J Infect Dis. 2012;205:1048–55.

23. Maldonado J, Cañabate F, Sempere L, Vela F, Sánchez AR, Narbona E, López-Huertas E, Geerlings A, Valero AD, Olivares M, et al. Human milk probiotic lactobacillus fermentum CECT5716 reduces the incidence of gastrointestinal and upper respiratory tract infections in infants. J Pediatr Gastroenterol Nutr. 2012;54:55–61.

24. Patel JA, Alvarez-Fernandez P, Jennings K, Loeffelholz M, McCormick D, Chonmaitree T. Factors affecting *Staphylococcus aureus* colonization of the nasopharynx in the first 6 months of life. Pediatr Infect Dis J. 2015;34:826–30.

25. Claycombe KJ, Brissette CA, Ghribi O. Epigenetics of inflammation, maternal infection, and nutrition. J Nutr. 2015;145:1109S–15S.

26. Wiertsema SP, Veenhoven RH, Sanders EA, Rijkers GT. Immunologic screening of children with recurrent otitis media. Curr Allergy Asthma Rep. 2005;5:302–7.

27. Sale MM, Chen W-M, Weeks DE, et al. Evaluation of 15 functional candidate genes for association with chronic otitis media with effusion and/or recurrent otitis media (COME/ROM). PLoS One. 2011;6:e22297.

28. Hörnell A, Lagström H, Lande B, Thorsdottir I. Breastfeeding, introduction of other foods and effects on health: a systematic literature review for the 5th Nordic nutrition recommendations. Food Nutr Res. 2013;57:20823.

29. Bowatte G, Tham R, Allen K, Tan D, Lau M, Dai X, Lodge C. Breastfeeding and childhood acute otitis media: a systematic review and meta-analysis. Acta Paediatr. 2015;104:85–95.

30. Salone LR, Vann WF, Dee DL. Breastfeeding: an overview of oral and general health benefits. J Am Dent Assoc. 2013;144:143–51.

31. Martines F, Salvago P, Ferrara S, Messina G, Mucia M, Plescia F, Sireci F. Factors influencing the development of otitis media among Sicilian children affected by upper respiratory tract infections. Braz J Otorhinolaryngol. 2016;82:215–22.

32. Jensen RG, Koch A, Homøe P, Bjerregaard P. Tobacco smoke increases the risk of otitis media among Greenlandic Inuit children while exposure to organochlorines remain insignificant. Environ Int. 2013;54:112–8.

33. Salah M, Abdel-Aziz M, Al-Farok A, Jebrini A. Recurrent acute otitis media in infants: analysis of risk factors. Int J Pediatr Otorhinolaryngol. 2013;77:1665–9.
34. Fisk CM, Crozier SR, Inskip HM, Godfrey KM, Cooper C, Roberts GC, Robinson SM, the Southampton Women's Survey Study Group. Breastfeeding and reported morbidity during infancy: findings from the Southampton Women's survey: breastfeeding and reported morbidity during infancy. Matern Child Nutr. 2011;7:61–70.

Candidiasis During Breastfeeding

Mehtap Koparal, Nuray Bayar Muluk, and Gabriela Kopacheva Barsova

1 Introduction

The earliest published description of oral infection with *Candida albicans* dates from 1838. François Valleix, a paediatric specialist in France noted the infection within the buccal cavity. Candidiasis (thrush) generally occurs in newborn children or those under the age of 1 year, or in older patients who are on antibiotic or corticosteroid pharmacotherapy, have multiple endocrine abnormalities or are immunodeficient. Candidiasis is a potential initial presentation of underlying HIV (human immunodeficiency virus) infection. When observed at a late stage in HIV, it is an ominous sign. Children using corticosteroid inhalers are also at a raised risk of thrush [1].

2 Pathophysiological Aspects

Candidiasis occurs where the host becomes immunodeficient or there is a disturbance in the normal oral flora. When Candidal organisms multiply on the mucosal surfaces of the mouth, epithelial cells are sloughed off and accumulate with bacterial debris, keratin and dead cells, appearing as a pseudomembrane. The

M. Koparal (✉)
Adıyaman Training and Research Hospital, Department of Otorhinolaryngology, Health Sciences University, Adıyaman, Türkiye

N. B. Muluk
Medical Faculty, Department of Otorhinolaryngology, Kirikkale University, Kirikkale, Türkiye

G. K. Barsova
Faculty of Medicine, Cyril and Methodius University of Skopje,
Skopje, Republic of Macedonia

Ö. N. Şahin et al. (eds.), *Breastfeeding and Metabolic Programming*,
https://doi.org/10.1007/978-3-031-33278-4_50

pseudomembrane may be stuck tightly to the mucosal tissues. Whilst its extent is usually limited, from time to time there may be large areas of swelling, ulcers and necrotic destruction of the mucosal tissues underlying the plaque [1].

In most cases occurring neonatally, *C. albicans* is transferred from the maternal vagina during birth. Accordingly, the infants of mothers who have active candidiasis of the vagina are more in danger. It has also been established that yeast may be transferred by breastfeeding if the breast is colonised by *C. albicans*, through hands and via teats that have been insufficiently sterilised. Kissing the child may also transfer the microorganisms.

In a large number of both adults and paediatric patients, the gut is colonised by *C. albicans* without symptoms occurring. This is likely to be the source of Candida found on the perineum. It is not uncommon to observe that a child with oral candidiasis also has a candidal nappy rash [1].

3   History

Typically, the parents notice that there is a white coating in the oral cavity of their offspring. If it is very marked, the child may not be able to feed adequately. Patients frequently disclose recent treatment with antibiotics or corticosteroids, which are known to predispose to oral candidiasis [1].

A study which addressed negative outcomes associated with prescribing antibiotics noted that use of amoxicillin or co-amoxiclav was commonly associated with oral thrush, but this was rarely actually reported. The authors concluded that better knowledge of the advantages and disadvantages of antibiotic use is needed by doctors [2, 3].

If candidiasis occurs in conjunction with diarrhoeal illness, exanthemata, failure to thrive, pathological enlargement of the liver and spleen or recurrent infections, an underlying immunodeficiency should be investigated [4].

The mother should be specifically questioned about the following:

- Vaginal thrush at the time of birth, which may explain transfer of yeasts.
- If the mother is HIV positive, this is likely to explain the infection.

4   Physical Examination

Thrush frequently initially presents as white dots that grow and become white-coloured plaques on the mucosal tissues of the mouth [1].

If the clinician scrapes a plaque with the spatula, the lesion may be strongly adherent to the tissues and when removed, the base may be noted to be painful, inflamed and liable to bleed [1].

Oral candidiasis may occur in conjunction with a nappy rash. A baby with a nappy rash should be checked for thrush in the mouth [5].

It is essential to avoid confusing candidal plaques with a tongue coating.

It is vital to perform a careful physical examination, particularly where candidiasis recurs or the child is no longer an infant. Note the growth overall, where any exanthem occurs, painful swollen lymph nodes, enlargement of the liver and spleen and any further infected mucocutaneous areas [6–8].

5 Laboratory Investigations

The most straightforward method for identifying candidal plaques is by scraping the lesions with a spatula. Candidal plaques have inflammation around the base and tend to bleed [1].

It is possible to send a plaque for microbiological culture; however, this is seldom necessary. Microscopy reveals gram-positive yeasts that are large and ovoid in shape [1].

Tooyama *et al.* studied methods by which oral thrush could be reliably confirmed in the laboratory [9] and concluded that concentrated rinse sampling was effective for this purpose.

6 Treatment

Candida spp. are susceptible to a considerable number of antimycotic agents. The most frequently prescribed antimicrobials for thrush are nystatin or an imidazole. However, it is vital to be aware of any local variation in antimicrobial susceptibility. Some strains of *C. albicans* are no longer sensitive to fluconazole. There are some newer agents which have received US FDA approval for paediatric use, such as the echinocandins (caspofungin, micafungin). Anidulafungin, another agent in the echinocandin group, does also have FDA approval, but not for paediatric use. All the echinocandins work by disrupting the integrity of the fungal cell wall via inhibition of 1,3 beta-D-glucan synthase. There are now multiple agents of this type in licensed clinical use [10].

The use of antimicrobials typically leads to quicker recovery from oral candidiasis [11]. The first-line therapy involves fluconazole or an oral suspension of nystatin. Several other antimicrobials also have proven efficacy. It is unusual for *C. albicans* to be resistant to nystatin. However, this agent achieves its microbicidal action by coming into direct contact with the organisms. Thus, it needs to be swirled over all the mucosae where plaques are present, in contrast to systemic agents, such as fluconazole. Treatment failure occurs more often with nystatin than fluconazole [12].

If the patient is an older child or an adult, the antimicrobial solutions need to be swirled around in the mouth before being ingested. If this does not occur, posterior pharyngeal and oesophageal lesions may remain untreated. In a young child, the carers should smear 1 or 2 mL of the suspension over the buccal mucosa each time. Nystatin can be painted on the plaques using a swab (not the absorbent type) or an applicator. Ideally, the treatment should be provided in the interval between feeding, so that the suspension remains in more prolonged contact with the yeasts [1].

7 Candidiasis Affecting the Nipple and Breast in Lactating Women

It is challenging to confirm the existence of candidal organisms in breast milk since lactoferrin, a normal component of breast milk, interferes with mycological culture [13–18]. Culture is more sensitive if iron is added to the sample first [15]. Iron-containing culture medium, although selective for *C. albicans*, is difficult to obtain. In clinical practice, standard laboratory mycological culture is not helpful given the inhibitory effect of breast milk lactoferrin. In cases where a bacterial pathogen may be responsible, and antibiotic pharmacotherapy has not resolved the problem, breast milk should be cultured and antibiotic susceptibility testing undertaken [13].

7.1 History and Physical Examination

Alongside clinical physical examination, a lactating patient should be referred to a clinician with a special interest in breastfeeding or another professional with special training on lactation to ensure that breastfeeding occurs in the most suitable way to prevent problems [13].

The history needs to thoroughly cover any pain, how delivery occurred and details of any breastfeeding. The mother should be asked about use of antibiotics during labour or thereafter, any previous problems with cracked nipples and whether her child has a dummy or uses a bottle [19–21]. From a number of studies, it has emerged that vaginal candidiasis peripartum, antibiotics at that time or subsequently and utilisation of dummies, bottle feeders and breast pumps are all risks for a yeast infection of the breast. These associations were all found based on clinical diagnosis or self-reported breast infection [20, 22, 23]. A different study where diagnosis was confirmed microbiologically found, however, that the sole significant association with breast infection was with bottle feeding in the initial fortnight following delivery (odds ratio [OR]: 6.4; confidence interval [CI]: 2.8–71.4; $P < 0.001$) [14].

The history should also cover factors suggesting papillary or areolar dermatitis or Raynaud's syndrome. The clinical observation that the breast exhibits cyanosis is sufficient to diagnose Raynaud's syndrome. It is a common mistake to diagnose and treat apparent mammary candidiasis in cases of papillary pain, where in fact this is due to Raynaud's syndrome [24].

7.2 Therapy for Papillary Candidasis

Pharmacotherapy for papillary or ductal candidiasis is complicated by insufficient evidence from trials. Although a number of agents are employed for treating papillary or mamillary candidiasis, there is no trial evidence to confirm benefit. The agent most frequently utilised for papillary candidiasis is topical nystatin (mycostatin), an antimicrobial with activity against *C. albicans* [14, 19, 21]. Nonetheless, resistance to nystatin is present in above 40% of strains of *C. albicans* and thus maternal treatment with concomitant miconazole or clotrimazole as topically applied creams is advisable. Pharmacological management generally also includes a topical antibiotic to be applied to papillary fissures, which are frequently seen in cases of papillary candidiasis and may harbour *S. aureus*. For this purpose, suitable choices include mupirocin (Bactroban) or a combination product, such as neosporin [25, 26]. If papillary candidiasis results in severe oedema or erythema, corticosteroid ointment may be used, either of low or mid-potency, as this aids healing [18]. Whatever the management approach taken, both the mother and infant must be treated at the same time. For infants, the most frequently preferred approach is to use a suspension of nystatin in conjunction with fluconazole (Diflucan) by mouth [21, 27].

7.3 Management of Ductal Candidiasis

It is common to treat persistent papillary or presumed ductal candidiasis with fluconazole by mouth [19, 21]. Nonetheless, given that no trial has yet established that fluconazole is both safe and efficacious in managing candidal infections of the breast, treatment should only be undertaken where the diagnosis appears very clear. Indeed, the US FDA has so far not licensed fluconazole in this application. The dosages used in treating breast infections are the same as those used in candidal infections of other internal organs, namely the bladder, liver or oesophagus, which occur in patients whose immune systems are severely compromised. Thus, the initial loading dose of between 200 and 400 mg is followed by a daily course of 100–200 mg lasting 2–3 weeks [28–30]. According to the data from randomised controlled trials, the side effect burden at these doses is slight [29]. It is common for clinicians to prolong the fluconazole course for between 1 and 2 weeks following symptomatic resolution to guarantee the infection has been eradicated and recurrence will not occur [13].

The recommendation is for breastfeeding not to stop while mothers are prescribed fluconazole. Nonetheless, breastfeeding women should be advised prior to commencing the course that there is a lack of trial data about fluconazole and they should weigh up the advantages and disadvantages when deciding about breastfeeding and weaning. In pregnant women fluconazole is a category C agent (i.e. it has teratogenic potential according to animal models where high does were employed.

It is therefore contraindicated. Fluconazole also interacts with other medications, resulting in raised concentrations of phenytoin, warfarin, cisapride and certain sulfonylureas [31]. It is advisable to discuss potential drug interactions with patients prior to prescription. There is excretion of fluconazole into breast milk, but this is only equivalent to around 1% of the dose provided to the mother and is under 5% of the dosage licensed in children. Overall, fluconazole is rated as safe for the infant when prescribed to breastfeeding mothers [32].

References

1. Kumar M. Thrush. In: Steele RW (Ed). Medscape. Updated: Jan 17, 2019. https://emedicine.medscape.com/article/969147-overview#a5. Accessed online at 2 July 2022.
2. Gillies M, Ranakusuma A, Hoffmann T, Thorning S, McGuire T, Glasziou P, et al. Common harms from amoxicillin: a systematic review and meta-analysis of randomized placebo-controlled trials for any indication. CMAJ. 2015 Jan 6;187(1):E21–31.
3. Pullen LC. Amoxicillin Adverse Effects Underreported, Underrecognized. Medscape Medical News. Available at http://www.medscape.com/viewarticle/835143. November 19, 2014; Accessed: June 16, 2015.
4. Pappas PG, Kauffman CA, Andes D, et al. Clinical practice guidelines for the management of candidiasis: 2009 update by the Infectious Diseases Society of America. Clin Infect Dis. 2009;48(5):503–35. (Guideline)
5. Hoppe JE. Treatment of oropharyngeal candidiasis and candidal diaper dermatitis in neonates and infants: review and reappraisal. Pediatr Infect Dis J. 1997;16(9):885–94.
6. Kalfa VC, Roberts RL, Stiehm ER. The syndrome of chronic mucocutaneous candidiasis with selective antibody deficiency. Ann Allergy Asthma Immunol. 2003 Feb.;90(2):259–64.
7. Liu X, Hua H. Oral manifestation of chronic mucocutaneous candidiasis: seven case reports. J Oral Pathol Med. 2007;36(9):528–32.
8. Rowen JL. Mucocutaneous candidiasis. Semin Perinatol. 2003;27(5):406–13.
9. Tooyama H, Matsumoto T, Hayashi K, Kurashina K, Kurita H, Uchida M, et al. Candida concentrations determined following concentrated oral rinse culture reflect clinical oral signs. BMC Oral Health. 2015;15:150.
10. Tsekoura M, Ioannidou M, Pana ZD, Haidich AB, Antachopoulos C, Iosifidis E, et al. Efficacy and safety of echinocandins for the treatment of invasive candidiasis in children: a meta-analysis. Pediatr Infect Dis J. 2019;38(1):42–9.
11. Lewis MAO, Williams DW. Diagnosis and management of oral candidosis. Br Dent J. 2017;223(9):675–81.
12. Lyu X, Zhao C, Yan ZM, Hua H. Efficacy of nystatin for the treatment of oral candidiasis: a systematic review and meta-analysis. Drug Des Devel Ther. 2016;10:1161–71.
13. Wiener S. Diagnosis and Management of Candida of the Nipple and Breast. J Midwifery Womens Health. 2006;51(2):125–128. https://www.medscape.com/viewarticle/527409_3. Accessed online at 2 July 2022.
14. Morrill JF, Heinig MJ, Pappagianis D, Dewey KG. Risk factors for mammary candidosis among lactating women. J Obstet Gynecol Neonatal Nurs. 2005;34:37–45.
15. Morrill JF, Pappagianis D, Heinig MJ, Lonnerdal B, Dewey KG. Detecting Candida albicans in human milk. J Clin Microbiol. 2003;41:475–8.
16. Andersson Y, Lindquisit S, Lagerqvist C, Hernell O. Lactoferrin is responsible for the fungistatic effect of human milk. Early Hum Dev. 2000;59:95–105.
17. Soukka T, Tenovuo J, Lenander-Lumikari M. Fungicidal effect of human lactoferrin against Candida albicans. Microbiol Lett. 1992;90:223–8.

18. Okutomi T, Abe S, Tansho S, Wakabayashi H, Kawase K, Yamaguchi H. Augmented inhibition of growth of Candida albicans by neutrophils in the presence of lactoferrin. Immunol Med Microbiol. 1997;18:105–12.
19. Porter J. Treating sore, possibly infected nipples. J Hum Lact. 2004;20:221–2.
20. Dinsmoor MJ, Viloria R, Lief L, Elder S. Use of intrapartum antibiotics and the incidence of postnatal maternal and neonatal yeast infections. Obstet Gynecol. 2005;106:19–22.
21. Brent NB. Thrush in the breastfeeding dyad: results of a survey on diagnosis and treatment. Clin Pediatr. 2001;40:503–6.
22. Thomassen P, Johansson VA, Wassberg C, Petrini B. Breastfeeding, pain and infection. Gynecol Obstet Investig. 1998;46:73–4.
23. Tanguay K, McBeab M, Jain E. Nipple candidosis among breastfeeding mothers. Can Fam Physician. 1994;40:1407–13.
24. Anderson JE, Held N, Wright K. Raynaud's phenomenon of the nipple: a treatable cause of painful breastfeeding. Pediatrics. 2004;113:360–4.
25. Amir L, Garland S, Debberstein L, Farish S. Candida albican: Is it associated with nipple pain in lactating women? Gynecol Obsetet Invest. 1996;41:30–4.
26. Graves S, Wright W, Harman R, Bailet S. Painful nipples in nursing mothers: fungal or staphylococcal? A preliminary study. Aust Fam Physician. 2003;32:570–1.
27. Goins A, Ascher D, Waecker N, Arnold J, Moorefield E. Comparison of fluconazole and nyststin oral suspensions for treatment of oral candidiasis in infants. Pediatr Infect Dis J. 2002;21:1165–7.
28. Hale T. Medications and mothers' milk. Amarillo (TX): Pharmasoft; 2004. p. 326–30.
29. Sobel J, Kauffman C, McKinsey D, et al. Candiduria: A randomized double-blind study of treatment with fluconazole and placebo-controlled trial. Clin Infect Dis. 2000;30:19–24.
30. Wainer S, Cooper PA, Gouws H, Akierman A. Prospective study of fluconazole therapy in systemic neonatal fungal infection. Pediatr Infect Dis J. 1997;16:763–7.
31. Bennett JE. Antimicrobial agents, antifungal agents. In: Hardman JJ, Limbird LE, editors. Gooodman & Gilmans: The pharmacological basis of therapeutics. 9th ed. New York: McGraw-Hill; 1996.
32. Force RW. Fluconazole concentrations in breast milk. Pediatr Infect Dis. 1995;14:235–6.

Frenotomy for Tongue-Tie in Neonates

Selis Gülseven Güven and Ahmet Köder

1 Introduction

Tongue-tie, or ankyloglossia, refers to a condition in which the frenulum of the tongue is so shortened that it prevents the tongue executing its normal range of movement. There is uncertainty about the exact frequency with which ankyloglossia occurs, with estimates ranging from below one in a hundred to one in ten infants. This unclarity about prevalence is likely to result from there being no universally-agreed criteria for diagnosing ankyloglossia [1–5].

In certain cases, ankyloglossia has been linked to mutation of the TBX22 gene. In these patients, ankyloglossia occurs are part of an X-linked cleft palate syndrome.

2 Anatomical Considerations

It is common to describe the lingual frenulum as consisting of connective tissue in the form of a cord or band underlying the mucosa. This description fails to do justice to the dynamic function of the frenulum. There is a fascial layer attached to the medial border of the mandible, somewhat in the manner of a diaphragm. The midline fold in this layer forms the frenulum. The fascial layer lies submucosally within the mouth. It is fused in the midline with the ventral connective tissue of the tongue. The fascia envelops the sublingual salivary glands and the duct of the submandibular gland. Deep to the fascia lies the anterior genioglossus muscle [5]. The frenulum is a dynamic structure insofar as it changes in position and thus overlies different parts of the mouth as the tongue moves. When the frenulum is in a tense state, the appearance varies significantly from patient to patient. The point of insertion may

S. G. Güven (✉) · A. Köder
Medical Faculty, Department of Otorhinolaryngology, Trakya University, Edirne, Türkiye

© The Author(s), under exclusive license to Springer Nature
Switzerland AG 2023
Ö. N. Şahin et al. (eds.), *Breastfeeding and Metabolic Programming*,
https://doi.org/10.1007/978-3-031-33278-4_51

be at the furthest anterior aspect of the tongue or some way further back. Indeed, for some infants who appear fully healthy, there is no identifiable frenulum attaching the oral floor to the tongue. When these infants raise their tongue, the muscular fibres of the genioglossus bunch up to form a fold resembling the frenulum, but connected more posteriorly than is usually the case [6].

The lingual nerve ramifies over the lingual ventral surface. These nerves lie just under the fascial layer and are at risk of being damaged when a frenotomy is performed [7].

3   Epidemiology

It appears that ankyloglossia is more common in boys than girls, the ratio of male to female lying somewhere between 1.1:1 and 3:1. The majority of cases of ankyloglossia are thought not to be genetic in origin and typically there are no other associated abnormalities. In a certain number of cases, there are reports which link ankyloglossia to specific genetic syndromes [1].

The frequency of tongue-tie is between less than 1 in 100 and 1 in 10 infants, with estimates affected by which population is sampled and the criteria applied in diagnosis [8–14]. There is no universally accepted clinical definition for ankyloglossia, nor has an entirely objective grading system so far been accepted by all practitioners. Certain methods of grading, e.g. the Coryllos scheme, are ways to identify the nature of the frenulum rather than grade the severity of any dysfunction, whilst other methods of grading, namely the Hazelbaker Assessment Tool for Lingual Frenulum Function and the Bristol Tongue Assessment Tool, involve evaluation of both the type and function of any tongue-tie [15].

In the majority of studies, male infants are more commonly affected by ankyloglossia than females, the condition being between 1.5 and 2.6 times more common in boys [8]. Although tongue-tie is typically not clearly genetic, in heritable X-linked ankyloglossia, mutated alleles for the T box transcription factor, TBX22, lead to ankyloglossia which may be associated with cleft lip or palate or hypodontia [16].

4   Pathophysiological Mechanism

Standardised diagnostic criteria for tongue-tie do not exist, nor is there a standard scheme for classifying cases. In a neonate, normally there should be at least 16 mm of 'free tongue' movement. If this figure is below 11 mm, the infant has moderately severe tongue-tie, whilst a free tongue length of under 7 mm is considered severe. For children older than this, the utility of this classification is in doubt. If the point of frenal attachments is located in the midline and posteriorly on the ventral lingual aspect, this situation is termed 'posterior ankyloglossia'. There are numerous methods that may be helpful for distinguishing between cases, either on anatomical or functional grounds [1].

One such method is the Hazelbaker Assessment for Lingual Frenulum Function, which takes into account both anatomical and functional characteristics of the lesion [1].

- Anatomical characteristics which are scored include appearance when the tongue is raised, how elastic the frenulum is and how long and where it is attached to the tongue and the inferior alveolar ridge [1].
- Functional characteristics to consider include ability to move from side-to-side, raise tongue, protrude tongue, spread the tongue, perform a cupping movement, propel food back towards the throat and whether snap-back occurs [1].

5   Clinical Presentation

The following are all features that may present in cases of ankyloglossia [8, 11, 14, 17]:

- The frenulum is shorter than normal and its point of insertion is on the lingual tip or close to it.
- The child cannot place the tongue on the superior teeth and jaw.
- The tongue cannot be extended beyond 1 or 2 mm beyond the inferior mesial incisors.
- The tongue cannot be fully lateralised.
- The tongue develops a notch or becomes heart-shaped when extended.
- In children who lack the ability to follow a request to stick the tongue out, if the examiner is unable to insert a finger between the inferior lingual surface and the lower jaw, this counts as evidence of tongue-tie.

It is unknown exactly how ankyloglossia develops if no intervention is undertaken [17]. It is hypothesised that the frenulum may naturally elongate as a result of the constant pressure exerted by tongue movements, but whether this actually occurs awaits validation using a prospective study design [17].

5.1   Posterior Ankyloglossia

This condition lacks a standard definition. In some writing, the term 'posterior ankyloglossia' refers to frenular attachment on the posterior lingual underside, but elsewhere this term refers to the tongue being tethered submucosally. Indeed, certain authors argue that posterior ankyloglossia is not a distinct abnormality and deprecate the use of this concept [15].

5.2 *Superior Labial Frenulum*

There is little consensus about when an upper lip tie can be identified, how it should be classified and what the implications are. The current schemes proposed for classification lack reliability, even amongst specialists with an interest in the condition [18]. A labial frenulum of some sort is invariably present in neonates, the majority with attachment to the gums [19, 20]. On rare occasions, a baby may not be able to latch on during breastfeeding because the superior lip cannot be adequately everted. In these infants, it has been suggested that the upper lip tie should be divided surgically. However, there are no data to prove how effective this procedure is, nor when it should be undertaken.

6 Differential Diagnosis

- Glossoschissis.
- Congenital fissured tongue.
- Lingual thyroid.
- Lymphatic vessel anomalies.
- Intraoral ranula.
- Macroglossia [1].

7 Possible Complications

The most frequently occurring complications in cases of ankyloglossia are as follows [17, 21]:

- Neonates or infants may have problems feeding from the breast.
- Young children, including toddlers, may have difficulty saying words clearly.
- In older children or teenagers, there may be specific problems caused by the tongue's limited range of movement, such as being unable to lick their lips or kiss properly.

There is little agreement amongst experts on how far ankyloglossia can cause problems of an extent to come to clinical attention [17]. The evidence base is poor, with most studies in ankyloglossia comprising either case series or studies of observational design [8, 22]. In spite of this situation, the frequency with which tongue-tie is diagnosed and surgical remediation sought has increased almost twofold since a decade ago, and this frequency varies widely across centres [23].

7.1   Difficulties Related to Breastfeeding

Most infants are still able to feed from the breast, in spite of ankyloglossia [10]. Nonetheless, difficulties related to breastfeeding more commonly arise in tongue-tied infants than in those with a normal lingual frenulum. According to a published case series, difficulty latching on or the mother experiencing papillary pain occurs in 25% of cases with tongue-tie, but in only 3% in those without [10, 14]. If a child is solely breastfeeding and cannot fully latch on, the amount of milk transferred may be so low as to cause failure to thrive [14, 24]. Researchers have not highlighted any issues related to bottle feeding in tongue-tied infants. This is likely to be because the movements needed are so different between bottle and breastfeeding [6].

If a child has begun to breastfeed but then experiences difficulties, clinicians should be suspicious of tongue-tie and examine the child accordingly [8]. It is beneficial to seek the advice of a breastfeeding specialist to ensure no other problem is present that may explain the difficulty [17]. In certain patients, frenotomy is required before the infant is able to continue breastfeeding adequately [12, 13, 25–27].

- **Speech articulatory issues**. It remains unclear exactly how tongue-tie affects the development of speech [17, 28]. In some paediatric patients, tongue-tie is linked to articulatory difficulties, although the child is still able to vocalise and speech begins at a normal age [17, 29]. A lingual frenulum attached to the lingual tip and of a length that does not permit the tongue to articulate with the alveolar ridge is potentially the most likely to explain the problem. The phonemes likely to be misarticulated are /t/, /d/, /z/, /s/, /ð/, /θ/, /n/ and /l/, i.e. dental and alveolar consonants plus fricatives. Ankyloglossia does not cause speech delay. The rate of language acquisition in affected children does not differ from their peers.
- Difficulties related to clear articulation may pass unnoticed or unremarked on by the parents [9]. A speech and language therapy referral should be made for any child with tongue-tie who cannot accurately produce the phonemes listed above [17].

7.2   Mechanical or Social Difficulties

A number of mechanical or social issues may arise from the limited range of movement in individuals with ankyloglossia, namely [17]:

- Periodontal disorders may arise from the child being unable to sweep food away from the teeth with the tongue or lick his or her lips.
- Poor dental hygiene may be noted.
- There may be localised discomfort.
- The patient may be unable to lick or kiss, which may make older children feel socially discomfited.

There may be a diastema in the inferior mesial incisors.

8 Management

Surgical intervention (i.e. frenotomy) consists in raising the tongue to tension the frenulum prior to making an incision through the mucosa and fascia in a direction parallel to the tongue and near to the point of attachment. This incision can be done in a single movement and is very swift. The child can be held by being swaddled or attached to a papoose board. If an assistant can hold the infant's head still, the procedure is easier to accomplish. This procedure is usually performed when the child is between 6 day and 18 days old. A study which enrolled 200 infant subjects where frenotomy was performed without analgesia found that 18% of subjects cried whilst frenotomy was being undertaken, and 60% did so afterward. Griffiths, in an article titled 'Do tongue ties affect breastfeeding?' states that infants who undergo frenotomy only cry for 15 seconds on average. Some clinicians administer sucrose prior to incision, which may reduce pain. On rare occasions, the frenulum re-grows in a similar abnormal fashion [1].

Prior to a decision for frenotomy, it is important that other diagnostic possibilities to account for difficulty breastfeeding and low weight gain be considered. A nurse with expertise in breastfeeding advice should undertake an evaluation of the infant-mother dyad and ensure the mother is well-informed about the best technique to use when feeding the infant [1].

Although it is rare for frenotomy to result in complications or additional risks, there are reports indicating these do sometimes occur. The most frequent complication is bleeding, which usually resolves with applied pressure. The relatives should be questioned about bleeding disorders in family members, or in the child him or herself if older than a few weeks, prior to performing frenotomy [1].

Laser surgery is increasingly replacing various conventional surgical instruments due to a number of associated benefits, in particular shorter operation times, the ability to cauterise and sterilise the tissues, rapid restoration of haemostasis, lower levels of associated pain and less frequent post-surgical complications, such as pain, oedema or infection [30, 31]. Laser surgery additionally permits improved access and better visualisation of the operative field, since no instruments block the view and bleeding is minimised. Furthermore, wounds frequently do not require suturing and any incisions can be at a definite depth, thereby preventing inadvertent injury to the underlying lingual musculature [31–33].

The most frequently undertaken treatment for ankyloglossia is frenotomy, which has the advantage of being a straightforward, rapid and largely non-destructive procedure that can be undertaken even in an outpatient first appointment [34, 35]. The level of pain experienced by the patient is low and breastfeeding can occur even straight afterwards. The lingual frenulum is easily pierced and is not a highly vascular structure. However, frenotomy has the disadvantage that the tongue-tie may recur and it may be necessary to undertake further interventions before the tongue gains a normal range of movement [34–36].

Frenectomy is a more invasive operation and less easily undertaken in infants, albeit the outcome is more guaranteed and recurrent tongue-tie seldom occurs. It involves excising the frenulum in its entirety [36, 37]. The evidence base is inadequate to answer the question of when the optimal timing is for frenectomy to be undertaken [11, 36]. It is clear, nonetheless, that frenectomy should occur before any abnormality in speech or swallowing has begun to be apparent. If frenectomy is delayed, the involvement of a speech and language therapy specialist is essential to ensure that the child goes on to develop the normal tongue movements needed for eating and speech [36].

Frenotomy (or frenulotomy) is a procedure whereby the tension in the frenulum is released by clipping the structure [17]. It is often indicated for infants unable to breastfeed adequately and generally does not require local anaesthetic injections to be performed first [14, 17, 38].

In undertaking frenotomy, the frenulum should be directly visualised, since this ensures the incision is adequate and helps prevent inadvertent damage to adjacent oral structures. The patient should first be immobilised by being swaddled or placed in a papoose board, and the baby's head should be kept in position by a suitable assistant. A headlight or operating microscope are suitable for illumination. A pair of surgical forceps may be used to grasp and lift the tongue. Alternatively, a grooved retractor or simply two gloved fingers may be sufficient to place the tongue in the desired position. When the frenulum is divided, bleeding is usually only minor [6].

Where bleeding occurs, applied pressure using a gauze sponge generally stops any oozing from the capillaries. In some centres, there is a preference for dividing the tongue-tie by means of a laser (carbon dioxide or diode type). This then prevents bleeding. The use of laser has the disadvantage of making the intervention more costly without any corresponding improvement in surgical outcome [39]. As soon as frenotomy has been completed, the infant may be permitted to feed at the breast [17].

Lingual frenotomy may be complicated by bleeding, the airway becoming obstructed, damage to the salivary ducts or glands, aversion to feeding, cicatrisation and the possibility the lesion may recur. Although the frequency of complications is low, the risks must be explained to parents whilst obtaining written, informed consent. The majority of studies indicate that patients experience little pain and adverse consequences are rare [12, 25, 35, 40–42]. Frenotomy in an infant is relatively contraindicated in the following conditions (not an exhaustive list): retrognathia, micrognathia, neuromuscular disease, hypotonia and clotting disorders [15].

Some experts favour getting patients to undertake tongue strengthening exercises after frenotomy. These exercises may include lingual massage or stretching the tongue and muscles of the oral cavity floor. There is, however, no clinical trial evidence to show benefit from these interventions [43].

Frenuloplasty involves cutting the tongue-tie and performing plastic reconstruction. This procedure is only used for cases of tongue-tie where basic frenotomy fails, there is posterior insertion of the frenulum or revision surgery is required [6].

Frenuloplasty is undertaken under general anaesthesia with ventilation occasionally secured by a mask, or more usually intubation via the nose or mouth. For this operation, the surgeon grasps the tongue with forceps and raises it to expose the frenulum, which is then incised in the midline, as in frenotomy. The surgeon then dissects submucosally as far as the genioglossal fibres medially. This then completely releases any tongue-tie. The dissection may be carried out with bipolar electrosurgical scissors or monopolar cautery, this instrumentation being preferred due to the ability to establish haemostasis, an important consideration given the rich lingual blood supply. Provided the operative field is well-illuminated and the loupe or operative microscope are employed, the frenulum can usually be divided with minimal risks to the adjacent ducts of the submandibular gland. By dissection in the midline, there is less likelihood of damaging the lingual nerve on each side [6].

Following the dissection portion of frenuloplasty, an ellipse of tissue remains missing in the area of the oral cavity floor. Unless this area is replaced, cicatrisation may occur and the tongue become tethered again. Generally wound closure is achieved by placing several absorbable sutures in a coronal plane. This produces a V-Y advancement flap on each side. To stop fibrotic contraction of the area, it is recommended to create several converging triangular flaps. There is currently no trial evidence to substantiate the claim that multiple z-plasties are superior to a single z-plasty [44]. Patients may begin eating normally again after surgery as soon as they feel able to do so. If the patient is an older child and the indication for frenuloplasty is faulty articulation, provision is usually made for continuing speech therapy accompanied by particular tongue-strengthening exercises following surgery [45].

References

1. Becker S, Mendez MD. Ankyloglossia. [Updated 2022 Mar 15]. In: StatPearls [Internet]. Treasure Island (FL): StatPearls Publishing; 2022 Jan-. Available from: https://www.ncbi.nlm. nih.gov/books/NBK482295/. Accessed online at 2 July 2022.
2. Campanha SMA, Martinelli RLC, Palhares DB. Association between ankyloglossia and breastfeeding. Codas. 2019;31(1):e20170264.
3. Hill R. Implications of Ankyloglossia on Breastfeeding. MCN Am J Matern Child Nurs. 2019;44(2):73–9.
4. Wood NK. Home-based interventions in a case of first latch at 27 days. Nurs Womens Health. 2019 Apr;23(2):135–40.
5. Mills N, Pransky SM, Geddes DT, Mirjalili SA. What is a tongue tie? Defining the anatomy of the in-situ lingual frenulum. Clin Anat. 2019;32(6):749–61.
6. Isaacson GC. Ankyloglossia (tongue-tie) in infants and children. In: Messner AH, Wilkie L (Eds). UpToDate. Last updated: Mar 12, 2021.
7. Mills N, Keough N, Geddes DT, et al. Defining the anatomy of the neonatal lingual frenulum. Clin Anat. 2019;32:824.
8. Hall DM, Renfrew MJ. Tongue tie. Arch Dis Child. 2005;90:1211.
9. Cinar F, Onat N. Prevalence and consequences of a forgotten entity: ankyloglossia. Plast Reconstr Surg. 2005;115:355.
10. Messner AH, Lalakea ML, Aby J, et al. Ankyloglossia: incidence and associated feeding difficulties. Arch Otolaryngol Head Neck Surg. 2000;126:36.
11. Segal LM, Stephenson R, Dawes M, Feldman P. Prevalence, diagnosis, and treatment of ankyloglossia: methodologic review. Can Fam Physician. 2007;53:1027.
12. Hogan M, Westcott C, Griffiths M. Randomized, controlled trial of division of tongue-tie in infants with feeding problems. J Paediatr Child Health. 2005;41:246.

13. Ricke LA, Baker NJ, Madlon-Kay DJ, DeFor TA. Newborn tongue-tie: prevalence and effect on breast-feeding. J Am Board Fam Pract. 2005;18:1.
14. Ballard JL, Auer CE, Khoury JC. Ankyloglossia: assessment, incidence, and effect of frenuloplasty on the breastfeeding dyad. Pediatrics. 2002;110:e63.
15. Messner AH, Walsh J, Rosenfeld RM, et al. Clinical Consensus Statement: Ankyloglossia in Children. Otolaryngol Head Neck Surg. 2020;162:597.
16. Kantaputra PN, Paramee M, Kaewkhampa A, et al. Cleft lip with cleft palate, ankyloglossia, and hypodontia are associated with TBX22 mutations. J Dent Res. 2011;90:450.
17. Lalakea ML, Messner AH. Ankyloglossia: does it matter? Pediatr Clin N Am. 2003;50:381.
18. Santa Maria C, Aby J, Truong MT, et al. The superior labial frenulum in newborns: what is normal? Glob Pediatr Health. 2017;4:2333794X17718896.
19. Ray S, Golden WC, Walsh J. Anatomic distribution of the morphologic variation of the upper lip frenulum among healthy newborns. JAMA Otolaryngol Head Neck Surg. 2019;145:931.
20. Kotlow LA. Diagnosing and understanding the maxillary lip-tie (superior labial, the maxillary labial frenum) as it relates to breastfeeding. J Hum Lact. 2013;29:458.
21. Lalakea ML, Messner AH. Ankyloglossia: the adolescent and adult perspective. Otolaryngol Head Neck Surg. 2003;128:746.
22. National Institute for Health and Clinical Excellence (NICE) interventional procedure guidance [IPG149]. Division of ankyloglossia (tongue-tie) for breastfeeding. Available at: https://www.nice.org.uk/guidance/ipg149/chapter/1-Guidance. Accessed on 09 June 2016.
23. Joseph KS, Kinniburgh B, Metcalfe A, et al. Temporal trends in ankyloglossia and frenotomy in British Columbia, Canada, 2004-2013: a population-based study. CMAJ Open. 2016;4:E33.
24. Forlenza GP, Paradise Black NM, McNamara EG, Sullivan SE. Ankyloglossia, exclusive breastfeeding, and failure to thrive. Pediatrics. 2010;125:e1500.
25. Dollberg S, Botzer E, Grunis E, Mimouni FB. Immediate nipple pain relief after frenotomy in breast-fed infants with ankyloglossia: a randomized, prospective study. J Pediatr Surg. 2006;41:1598.
26. Geddes DT, Langton DB, Gollow I, et al. Frenulotomy for breastfeeding infants with ankyloglossia: effect on milk removal and sucking mechanism as imaged by ultrasound. Pediatrics. 2008;122:e188.
27. Power RF, Murphy JF. Tongue-tie and frenotomy in infants with breastfeeding difficulties: achieving a balance. Arch Dis Child. 2015;100:489.
28. Messner AH, Lalakea ML. Ankyloglossia: controversies in management. Int J Pediatr Otorhinolaryngol. 2000;54:123.
29. Messner AH, Lalakea ML. The effect of ankyloglossia on speech in children. Otolaryngol Head Neck Surg. 2002;127:539.
30. Junqueira MA, Cunha NN, Costa e Silva LL, Araújo LB, Moretti AB, Couto Filho CE, Sakai VT. Surgical techniques for the treatment of ankyloglossia in children: a case series. J Appl Oral Sci. 2014 Jun;22(3):241–8.
31. Kara C. Evaluation of patient perceptions of frenectomy: a comparison of Nd:YAG laser and conventional techniques. Photomed Laser Surg. 2008;26(2):147–52.
32. Aras MH, Göregen M, Güngörmüs M, Akgül HM. Comparison of diode laser and Er: YAG lasers in the treatment of ankyloglossia. Photomed Laser Surg. 2010;28(2):173–7.
33. Puthussery FJ, Shekar K, Gulati A, Downie IP. Use of carbon dioxide laser in lingual frenectomy. Br J Oral Maxillofac Surg. 2011;49(7):580–1.
34. Hong P, Lago D, Seargeant J, Pellman L, Magit AE, Pransky SM. Defining ankyloglossia: a case series of anterior and posterior tongue ties. Int J Pediatr Otorhinolaryngol. 2010;74(9):1003–6.
35. Masaitis NS, Kaempf JW. Developing a frenotomy policy at one medical center: a case study approach. J Hum Lact. 1996;12(3):229–32.
36. Manfro AR, Manfro R, Bortoluzzi MC. Surgical treatment of ankyloglossia in babies: case report. Int J Oral Maxillofac Surg. 2010;39(11):1130–2.
37. Kupietzky A, Botzer E. Ankyloglossia in the infant and young child: clinical suggestions for diagnosis and management. Pediatr Dent. 2005;27(1):40–6.

38. Froom SR, Stewart J. Novel local anaesthetic analgesic technique for tongue-tie. Anaesthesia. 2007;62:97.
39. Ghaheri BA, Cole M, Fausel SC, et al. Breastfeeding improvement following tongue-tie and lip-tie release: a prospective cohort study. Laryngoscope. 2017;127:1217.
40. Griffiths DM. Do tongue ties affect breastfeeding? J Hum Lact. 2004;20:409.
41. Interventional procedures overview - division of anklyloglossia (tongue-tie) for breastfeeding. www.nice.org.uk/ip279overview. Accessed on 25 June 2008.
42. Amir LH, James JP, Beatty J. Review of tongue-tie release at a tertiary maternity hospital. J Paediatr Child Health. 2005;41:243.
43. Pransky SM, Lago D, Hong P. Breastfeeding difficulties and oral cavity anomalies: The influence of posterior ankyloglossia and upper-lip ties. Int J Pediatr Otorhinolaryngol. 2015;79:1714.
44. Ottawa (ON): Canadian Agency for Drugs and Technologies in Health. Frenectomy for the Correction of Ankyloglossia: A Review of Clinical Effectiveness and Guidelines, CADTH Rapid Response Reports; 2016.
45. Tecco S, Baldini A, Mummolo S, et al. Frenulectomy of the tongue and the influence of rehabilitation exercises on the sEMG activity of masticatory muscles. J Electromyogr Kinesiol. 2015;25:619.

Dietary Modifications and Supplementation in Breastfeeding Mothers

İlke Özer Aslan and Keziban Doğan

1 Introduction

Breastfeeding mothers usually feel torn between the need to diet in order to lose excess weight gained during pregnancy and the need to maintain an adequate dietary intake to ensure milk is available for the infant. Different cultures approach this matter in different ways. Older people frequently offer contradictory advice about the best thing to do, leaving mothers bemused by how to behave.

Lactation involves a complex interaction of different factors, including nutrition, endocrine effects and the mother's behaviour. Recently there have accumulated important insights into how the nutritional status of the mother influences breastfeeding and the infant's healthy development. Nonetheless, much is still unknown regarding the necessary dietary intake of trace elements in breastfeeding women. Some studies have examined how dietary supplementation with zinc, copper or iodine affects the level of these ions in human milk [1–3]. One trial, carried out in the Italian city of Ferrara, administered a particular dietary supplement tailored for breastfeeding to healthy lactating mothers. These women were socio-economically above average and their infants in good health. Of 32 women who completed enrolment, 22 continued until the end of the trial. All the infants were delivered at term, not part of a multiple pregnancy and were initially breastfed within the first 12 h after being born. Each of the 22 women who completed the trial filled out a diary of their diet over a 3-day period. Analysis of the diet showed that their average intake for the trace elements under study was as follows: Zn = 12 mg, Cu = 1.4 mg and

İ. Özer Aslan (✉)
Department of Obstetrics and Gynecology, Faculty of Medicine, Tekirdag Namık Kemal University, Tekirdag, Türkiye

K. Doğan
Department of Obstetrics and Gynecology, University of Health Sciences, Bakırköy Dr. Sadi Konuk Training and Research Hospital, İstanbul, Türkiye

Ö. N. Şahin et al. (eds.), *Breastfeeding and Metabolic Programming*,
https://doi.org/10.1007/978-3-031-33278-4_52

I = 145 µg. The level of intake for zinc and copper ions fell within the recommended limits for breastfeeding mothers in Italy, but the iodine intake was deficient, since the recommended daily allowance is 200 µg. For the purposes of the trial, the groups were split into two. Each subgroup contained seven women with their first child, and four women who had already given birth before. The dietary intake between the two groups differed. One group ate a normal diet for the region and had no supplementation with vitamins or minerals. The other group received a PerMamma dietary supplement manufactured by Abbott, which supplied 20 mg $ZnSO_4$, 2 mg $CuSO_4$ and 116 µg KI (equating to approximately 60–90% of the daily requirements whilst breastfeeding). All the women were actively breastfeeding. Breast milk was analysed at 3 days, 30 days and 90 days after delivery. The sample volume was 10 mL. The results indicated a significant fall in the level of zinc in milk, with no differences between the two study groups. There was no alteration in copper level between day 3 and day 30, but the final sample in both groups showed a lower level and the groups were statistically identical in this regard. Iodine levels fells rapidly in both groups at an early stage, regardless of whether additional iodine had been supplied. The iodine concentration in breast milk remained steady in both groups after the first month of breastfeeding. This study found that the groups did not differ at the level of statistical significance in terms of breast milk concentrations of the elements under investigation. Earlier studies reporting iodine concentrations in human milk are not, however, in accord with the findings from this Italian study. However, the Ferrara study does appear to show that if mothers are in good health and receiving a satisfactory diet, supplements, at least in the short term, do not affect the breast milk availability of zinc, copper or iodine. For these elements, breast milk concentrations are as expected, regardless of whether any supplement is used. There is now a need for a study of longitudinal design to establish exactly how maternal dietary iodine relates to breast milk concentration. The homeostatic mechanisms operative in breast milk production call for more intensive investigation in the future [3].

2   Obesity

The numbers of women suffering from obesity is increasing globally, in high-, middle- and low-income countries [4, 5]. There are several stages at which women are more prone to obesity, such as after giving birth and in middle age. The reasons for this propensity include physiological, endocrine, psychological and dietary alterations at these stages in life [6, 7]. There are also a number of incorrect beliefs held by particular cultures that can increase obesity, such as feeling that pregnant women should eat to excess or specific food items high in lipids and sugar that are said to increase breast milk production after birth [2]. Unfortunately, becoming overweight or obese may lead to cardiovascular and metabolic disorders, notably type 2 diabetes mellitus, dyslipidaemia, elevated blood pressure, cerebrovascular accidents and even specific malignancies, e.g. those of the breast or ovary [8, 9]. Because of these complications, it is a key clinical responsibility to pay close attention to managing weight gain in women.

3 Objectives in Losing Weight and Calorie Counting

Women whose body mass index (BMI) indicates they are overweight or obese should be encouraged to lose excess weight. It is worth advising weight loss even in women whose BMI indicates a normal weight but whose waist measurement exceeds 80 cm, or whose body fat comprises above 30–38% of the total body mass. Likewise, if they have retained 4.5 kg or more compared to their weight prior to conception [10]. When setting targets for a patient to lose weight, they should be achievable, based on the patient's wishes, and result in a more healthy ratio of lean to fat mass whilst not harming the overall nutritional status [11, 12]. If a patient is able to lose between 5 and 10% of her body weight, this is of clinical significance as it results in reduced adipose intra-abdominally as well as intra-hepatically [12]. This then has beneficial effects on the glycaemic level, arterial tension and lipids in the circulation, regardless of BMI [13]. This degree of weight loss is usually achievable by dietary means, which allows a loss of between half and one kilo each week for around half a year. Clinicians should, however, ensure the diet still fulfils the patient's energy requirements [11]. There is also a need to make allowance for the lengthier time taken to go from a very high BMI (i.e. one exceeding 30 kg/m^2, termed obesity II) to a more healthy one than from a less severe degree of overweight (obesity I, where BMI is between 25 and 29.9 kg/m^2). To achieve the necessary diet, account should be taken, in calculating the calories to supply, of BMI, basal metabolic rate (BMR) and the extent to which the patient is physically active. This figure is also affected by the woman's life stage, in particular whether she has recently given birth or is in middle age.

4 Principles Behind Dietary Prescriptions

There are a number of principles to bear in mind when prescribing a diet, to ensure patients can stick to it. Dietary prescriptions should be individualised, achievable and written in terms the patient can understand. This then facilitates patient concordance and greater success. A number of key considerations in improving the sustainability of a prescribed diet are outlined in the following sections [4].

4.1 Achievable Objectives

Women should aim to return either to the body mass they had prior to conception or the ideal weight. Likewise, women in middle age who are overweight or suffer from obesity should aim to achieve the ideal weight through following realistic, attainable objectives within a time-limited period [11, 12]. An example of a suitable objective is to eat between four and five portions of fruit and vegetables daily, consume a maximum of two teaspoons of sucrose in 24 h and aim to lose around half to one kilo weekly.

4.2 Mixture of Macro- and Micro-Nutrients

When prescribing a sustainable diet, the clinician should construct it in such a way as to provide a perfectly balanced, healthy mixture of macro- and micro-nutrients as well as allowing weight loss. There have been several dieting methods advocated that alter the usual macro-nutrient balance, e.g. balanced nutrient reduction, in which carbohydrates are plentiful, alongside moderate levels of lipids and protein, protein-rich diets with moderate lipids and depleted carbohydrates (Zone or South Beach diets), high lipids, moderate protein and low carbohydrates (Atkin's) or carbohydrate-rich, moderate protein and depleted lipids (Dr Dean Ornish) [13, 14]. Nonetheless, a diet based on the usual balance of macro-nutrients is also suitable for achieving sustained weight loss. In such a balanced diet, between 50 and 60% of calories are supplied by carbohydrates, between 15 and 25% come from protein sources and no more than 30% from lipids [15, 16].

4.3 Tailoring Advice on Diet According to the Patient

To ensure a higher degree of patient concordance with a prescribed diet, the patient's choices and usual habits should be borne in mind [17]. A vegetarian patient, for example, should be offered a diet offering appropriate protein-rich items, namely dairy products, pulses and cereals and soya. A diet involving egg albumen, chicken meat and fish would not be acceptable to the majority of vegetarians.

4.4 Meals Should be Frequent, Not Too Large, and Contain Balanced Nutrition

The total daily calorific intake should be spread out over the day in the form of three main meals of moderate size and two or three snacks in-between. This type of eating pattern allows appetite to be controlled, stops the urge to binge, lessens food cravings and stops patients eating massive, calorie-intense meals [17, 18].

4.5 *Low-Calorie Meals Rich in Nutrients*

Low-calorie diets aim to achieve weight loss by reducing the habitual caloric intake by between 500 and 750 kcal, which puts the patient in negative energy balance [17]. For women of middle age seeking to lose excess weight, the usual recommended daily calorie allowance is 1200–1500 kcal [6]. Women carrying excess weight after giving birth require a negative energy balance of 500 kcal, which can be achieved by providing between 1200 and 1800 kcal daily. For lactating women, this allowance should be increased by 300 kcal [2, 7]. The daily calorie allowance is made up of the main meals and snacks consumed during the day, with the bulk of the calories coming from main meals. A good practice is to ensure the plate consists of 50% vegetables high in dietary fibre and 25% of the plate should be a protein-rich item [19]. This will then ensure the patient feels full after eating, which prevents appetite surges and bingeing, and, inevitably, excessive consumption of calories. For a small meal or snack with less than 200 kcal, vegetable or fruit salads or thick vegetable soups are an excellent choice, as they are not highly calorific, but contain a rich mixture of nutrients [11, 20, 21].

5 Adjusting the Diet in the Light of Frequent Co-Morbidities

Dyslipidaemia, diabetes mellitus and high blood pressure are frequent co-morbid conditions in obese patients [8, 9]. Any recommended diet needs to be suitable for women who may have such co-morbidities. It is especially important to consider women who have suffered from diabetes of pregnancy or pregnancy-related hypertension, to reduce the incidence of complications. The following sections outline some of the factors to consider when treating patients in this situation.

5.1 *Diabetes Mellitus*

If a diabetic woman can lose at least 2% of her body weight, an improvement in diabetic control becomes evident through the blood glucose level and glycosylated haemoglobin. Glycaemia becomes increasingly normal as weight is lost [13]. Realistic weight loss is possible if the patient follows a low-calorie balanced diet tailored to achieve a negative energy balance of 500 kcal. There should be complex carbohydrates included and these may be made available at different meals, matched to the insulin-dosing regimen for diabetic individuals. Complex carbohydrates give a sense of satiety and do not raise blood glucose too high, hence they are of value in a diet focused on weight loss [7, 21]. Breakfast cereals and foods high in added sucrose need to be eliminated from the diet as far as possible. The patient may be advised to eat high-quality sources of protein that are low in fat (both cholesterol and saturated lipids), so that any calories consumed have maximal nutritional value [21]. Dairy products with full fat should be swapped for those made with skimmed or semi-skimmed milk. Red meat can be replaced by egg albumen, fish, lean cuts or poultry. Some culinary spices have beneficial effects on glycaemic levels. The seeds of fenugreek are rich in soluble fibre and trigonelline, and are potentially helpful in lowering circulating sugar levels, as well as cholesterol and triacylglycerides. Despite these purported benefits, fenugreek may interact with specific drugs, including anticoagulants, and thus it should only be advised by fully trained nutritionists. Cinnamon also potentially lowers glycaemic levels, since it contains procyanidin type-A polymer, which possesses bioactivity. Caution is required in patients with known hepatic disorders, as high doses of cinnamon, or prolonged use, may be toxic to the liver. Patients should be advised against the extremes of prolonged fasting and high levels of consumption at a single meal [7, 21].

5.2   Dyslipidaemia

The levels of triacylglycerides and cholesterol partially normalise in obese patients who achieve a loss of between 5 and 10% of body mass [19]. There are several different types of diets that may be used with benefit in patients with dyslipidaemia, in particular the DASH – dietary approach to stop hypertension – diet, which emphasises replacement of milk products with low-fat options, plentiful fruits and vegetables, nuts and seeds, but restricted consumption of red meat and food items high in sugar or fat, Mediterranean-style diets, involving plentiful fruit and vegetables, olive oil but lower amounts of protein and lipids, and vegetarian diets, which have low levels of saturated fat and large amounts of dietary fibre from whole grains, fruit and vegetables. The patient should be advised to consume complex carbohydrates plus protein-containing food items that have reduced levels of cholesterol and saturated fats, since this allows for loss of weight and a more healthy lipid profile. To counter the raised levels of triacylglycerides, patients are recommended to consume items rich in omega-3 fatty acids and to eliminate food items that are high in fat, salt and sugar (termed HFSS). Furthermore, lifestyle changes should be advocated, in particular the need to get exercise and avoid tobacco and alcohol [19–24].

5.3   Hypertension

Hypertension can be both prevented and managed in obese subjects by the patient losing 5–10% of his/her bodyweight. There are significant reductions in the systolic blood pressure in subjects with both normal and elevated blood pressure who are on the DASH diet, in which fruit and vegetables, minimal fat-content dairy products, whole grain cereals, lean cuts of meat and nuts are major constituents. It is recommended that dietary sodium not exceed the range 1500–2000 mg daily. Fruit and vegetables may contain varying amounts of sodium. Bananas, apples, peaches, most green and leafy vegetables and beans contain low levels of sodium. Cabbage, cauliflower, spinach and beetroot, on the other hand, are rich in sodium and therefore consumption of them needs to be limited.

Patients should be advised to severely restrict consumption of food items with an unexpectedly high sodium level, e.g. tinned fruit or vegetables, or highly processed items like gravy powders, dressings or crisps. Better still, these items may be omitted completely. Some sources of sodium may be overlooked if a drug history is not obtained from the patient. Enquiry should be specifically made about antacids, amongst other medications. The other essential ions in the diet, namely calcium, potassium and magnesium, need to exist in the diet for proper management of hypertension to occur. These minerals can be provided in the form of nuts, vegetables (locally sourced and seasonal, ideally) or some grains (such as millet) [19, 24].

5.4 Polycystic Ovary Syndrome (PCOS)

Female patients with polycystic ovary syndrome should receive advice to lose 2–5% of body weight initially, then 5–10% in the longer term, if they want to improve ovarian function through lifestyle modification [13]. These patients should increase dietary fibre whilst reducing their intake of high-sugar foods. Sources of protein that are not high in fat are preferable, thus red meat, if consumed, should be a lean cut. Some dietary items have an anti-inflammatory effect, in particular, tomatoes, spinach, nuts and sources of omega-3 fatty acids (including walnuts or flax seeds) or turmeric, whereas others tend to stimulate inflammation, in particular fried food, red meat and processed items [20]. Consumption of the former should be favoured over the latter. In any case, omitting or severely restricting highly processed food items and other types of food that have high lipid, sodium and sucrose levels is a vital step in dietary management.

6 Conclusion

Management of diet should proceed stepwise. The important factors to consider in recommending a suitable diet are the individual's basal metabolic requirements, the balance of macro- and micro-nutrients needed and the objectives aimed for. If dietary management is approached from a realistic, personalised perspective, and any prescribed diet is provided in a patient-friendly format, weight loss can be achieved in women following pregnancy and in middle age. Whatever diet is followed, however, one constant feature is that all breastfeeding mothers will require additional fluid intake and a varied diet to ensure milk production is sufficient and of high quality.

References

1. Ares Segura S, Arena Ansótegui J, Díaz-Gómez NM. en representación del Comité de Lactancia Materna de la Asociación Española de Pediatría. La importancia de la nutrición materna durante la lactancia, ¿necesitan las madres lactantes suplementos nutricionales? [The importance of maternal nutrition during breastfeeding: Do breastfeeding mothers need nutritional supplements?]. An Pediatr (Barc). 2016;84(6):347.e1–7. https://doi.org/10.1016/j.anpedi.2015.07.024. Spanish. Epub 2015 Sep 14

2. Kajale N, Khadilkar A, Chiponkar S, Unni J, Mansukhani N. Effect of traditional food supplements on nutritional status of lactating mothers and growth of their infants. Nutrition. 2014;30(11–12):1360–5. https://doi.org/10.1016/j.nut.2014.04.005. Epub 2014 Apr 19

3. Chierici R, Saccomandi D, Vigi V. Dietary supplements for the lactating mother: influence on the trace element content of milk. Acta Paediatr Suppl. 1999 Aug;88(430):7–13. https://doi.org/10.1111/j.1651-2227.1999.tb01294.x.

4. Malhotra A, Verma A, Kaur D, Ranjan P, Kumari A, Madan J. A stepwise approach to prescribe dietary advice for weight management in postpartum and midlife women. J Obstet Gynaecol India. 2022;72(2):114–24. https://doi.org/10.1007/s13224-022-01643-w. Epub 2022 Mar 29

5. Bhurosy T, Jeewon R. Overweight and obesity epidemic in developing countries: a problem with diet, physical activity, or socioeconomic status? Sci World J. 2014;2014:964236. https://doi.org/10.1155/2014/964236.

6. Chopra S, Sharma KA, Ranjan P, Malhotra A, Vikram NK, Kumari A. Weight management module for perimenopausal women: a practical guide for gynecologists. J Midlife Health. 2019;10(4):165–72. https://doi.org/10.4103/jmh.JMH_155_19.

7. Kaur D, Malhotra A, Ranjan P, Chopra S, Kumari A, Vikram NK. Weight management in postpartum women—an Indian per- spective. Diabetes Metab Syndr. 2021;15(6):102291. https://doi.org/10.1016/j.dsx.2021.102291.

8. Hruby A, Hu FB. The epidemiology of obesity: a big picture. PharmacoEconomics. 2015;33(7):673–89. https://doi.org/10.1007/s40273-014-0243-x.

9. Vesco KK, Leo MC, Karanja N, Gillman MW, McEvoy CT, King JC, Eckhardt CL, Smith KS, Perrin N, Stevens VJ. One-year post- partum outcomes following a weight management intervention in pregnant women with obesity. Obesity. 2016;24(10):2042–9. https://doi.org/10.1002/oby.21597.

10. Bennion KA, Tate D, Muñoz-Christian K, Phelan S. Impact of an internet-based lifestyle intervention on behavioral and psychosocial factors during postpartum weight loss. Obesity. 2020;28(10):1860–7. https://doi.org/10.1002/oby.22921.

11. Willoughby D, Hewlings S, Kalman D. Body composition changes in weight loss: strategies and supplementation for maintaining lean body mass, a brief review. Nutrients. 2018;10(12):1876. https://doi.org/10.3390/nu10121876.

12. Yumuk V, Tsigos C, Fried M, Schindler K, Busetto L, Micic D, Toplak H. Obesity management task force of the european association for the study of obesity. european guidelines for obesity management in adults. Obes Facts. 2015;8(6):402–24. https://doi.org/10.1159/000442721. Epub 2015 Dec 5. Erra- tum in: Obes Facts. 2016;9(1):64.

13. Ryan DH, Yockey SR. Weight loss and improvement in comorbidity: differences at 5%, 10%, 15%, and over. Curr Obes Rep. 2017;6(2):187–94. https://doi.org/10.1007/s13679-017-0262-y.

14. Van Horn L, Carson JA, Appel LJ, Burke LE, Economos C, Karmally W, Lancaster K, Lichtenstein AH, Johnson RK, Thomas RJ, Vos M. Recommended dietary pattern to achieve adherence to the American Heart Association/American College of Cardiology (AHA/ACC) guidelines: a scientific statement from the American Heart Association. Circulation. 2016;134(22):e505–29.

15. Rebello CJ, O'Neil CE, Greenway FL. Dietary fiber and satiety: the effects of oats on satiety. Nutr Rev. 2016;74(2):131–47. https://doi.org/10.1093/nutrit/nuv063.

16. Schreiber DR, Dautovich ND. Depressive symptoms and weight in midlife women: the role of stress eating and menopause status. Menopause. 2017;24(10):1190–9. https://doi.org/10.1097/GME.0000000000000897.
17. Steenhuis I, Poelman M. Portion size: latest developments and interventions. Curr Obes Rep. 2017;6(1):10–7. https://doi.org/10.1007/s13679-017-0239-x.
18. Viola GC, Bianchi F, Croce E, Ceretti E. Are food labels effec- tive as a means of health pre- vention? J Public Health Res. 2016;5(3):768. https://doi.org/10.4081/jphr.2016.768.
19. Soeliman FA, Azadbakht L. Weight loss maintenance: a review on dietary related strategies. J Res Med Sci. 2014;19(3):268–75.
20. Casazza K, Brown A, Astrup A, Bertz F, Baum C, Brown MB, Dawson J, Durant N, Dutton G, Fields DA, Fontaine KR, Heymsfield S, Levitsky D, Mehta T, Menachemi N, Newby PK, Pate R, Raynor H, Rolls BJ, Sen B, Smith DL Jr, Thomas D, Wansink B, Allison DB. Weighing the evidence of common beliefs in obesity research. Crit Rev Food Sci Nutr. 2015;55(14):2014–53.
21. Gray A, Threlkeld RJ. Nutritional recommendations for individuals with diabetes. 2019 Oct 13. In: Feingold KR, Anawalt B, Boyce A, Chrousos G, de Herder WW, Dhatariya K, Dungan K, Hershman JM, Hofland J, Kalra S, Kaltsas G, Koch C, Kopp P, Korbonits M, Kovacs CS, Kuohung W, Laferrère B, Levy M, McGee EA, McLachlan R, Morley JE, New M, Purnell J, Sahay R, Singer F, Sperling MA, Stratakis CA, Trence DL, Wilson DP, editors. Endotext [Internet]. South Dartmouth (MA): MDText. com, Inc.; 2000. PMID: 25905243.
22. Salehi B, Ata A, Anil Kumar VN, Sharopov F, Ramírez-Alarcón K, Ruiz-Ortega A, Abdulmajid Ayatollahi S, Tsouh Fokou PV, Kobarfard F, Amiruddin Zakaria Z, Iriti M, Taheri Y, Martorell M, Sureda A, Setzer WN, Durazzo A, Lucarini M, Santini A, Capasso R, Ostrander EA, Atta-ur-Rahman CMI, Cho WC, Sharifi-Rad J. Antidiabetic potential of medicinal plants and their active components. Biomolecules. 2019;9(10):551. https://doi.org/10.3390/biom9100551.
23. Locke A, Schneiderhan J, Zick SM. Diets for, health: goals and guidelines. Am Fam Physician. 2018;97(11):721–8.
24. Lee TS, Kim JS, Hwang YJ, Park YC. Habit of eating breakfast is associated with a lower risk of hypertension. J Lifestyle Med. 2016;6(2):64–7. https://doi.org/10.15280/jlm.2016.6.2.64.

Human Milk Banking: A Brief Overview

Güniz Yaşöz, Esra Polat, and Despina D. Briana

1 Introduction

Human breast milk is the most nutrient-rich and ideal nutrition for all infants. Breast milk is convenient, hygienic, safe, affordable, and contains antibodies that contribute to preventing many common pediatric diseases. Additionally, infants who are exclusively breastfed for six months have significantly lower rates of gastrointestinal and respiratory tract infections. Breastfeeding is beneficial for brain development and lowers the incidence of sudden infant death [1]. Human milk constitutes bioactive and nutritional factors; microorganisms, stem cells, and oligosaccharides are also present, contributing to brain development and the maturation of the immune system and gut [2]. Children fed with human breast milk also demonstrated better white and gray matter development, resulting in higher language scores and a higher neurodevelopment level, such as better intelligence quotient (IQ), memory, and academic success in the subsequent years [3, 4]. Consequently, breast milk microbiota contributes to the colonization of an infant's gut, possibly contributing to a child's health [5].

G. Yaşöz (✉)
Department of Pediatrics, University of Kyrenia, Kyrenia, Cyprus
e-mail: guniz.yasoz@kyrenia.edu.tr

E. Polat
Umraniye Education and Research Hospital, Department of Pediatrics, Division of Pediatric Gastroenterology, Health Sciences University, Istanbul, Türkiye

D. D. Briana
NICU, Third Department of Pediatrics, National and Kapodistrian University of Athens, University General Hospital "ATTIKON", Athens, Greece

© The Author(s), under exclusive license to Springer Nature Switzerland AG 2023
Ö. N. Şahin et al. (eds.), *Breastfeeding and Metabolic Programming*,
https://doi.org/10.1007/978-3-031-33278-4_53

2   Breastfeeding

The World Health Organization (WHO), the American Academy of Pediatrics (AAP), and the European Society for Pediatric Gastroenterology, Hepatology, and Nutrition Committee on Nutrition (ESPGHAN) recommend breastfeeding as the primary source of nutrition for the first six months [6–8]. The AAP has recently updated its policy statement and technical report on "Breastfeeding and the Use of Human Milk" and included recommendations and evidence of significant health advantages of breastfeeding till two years of age or older to both mothers and infants [9]. Donor human milk (DHM) should be considered the first alternative whenever a mother is unable to breastfeed, has insufficient milk production, or suffers any other circumstance that may prevent her from nursing her child [10]. It is universally acknowledged that no commercial formula can be compared to breast milk. According to the WHO and the United Nations International Children's Emergency Fund (UNICEF) if the newborn cannot be fed by the mother's own milk, or if supplementation is necessary, especially for those of low birth weight and other vulnerable infants, DHM should be given [6]. The World Health Organization recommends that low birth weight newborns, who are susceptible to infection, necrotizing enterocolitis, bronchopulmonary dysplasia, and feeding intolerance, should be fed DHM when the maternal milk is not accessible [11]. In 2018, a systematic review and meta-analysis showed that donor human milk, as compared to formula feeding, significantly decreases the risk of necrotizing enterocolitis among low birth weight and preterm infants [12]. Another study found that very low birth weight infants with a higher breastfeeding rate, including DHM during hospital stay and reduced exposure to formula, did not develop bronchopulmonary dysplasia or sepsis [13]. According to the findings of a recent study, in addition to being recommended for preterm infants, donor human milk should also be used in healthy and at-risk term infants [14].

3   Milk Banking

Several national and global policy groups such as AAP and ESPGHAN have declared DHM the preferred feeding method if the mother's own milk is insufficient, missing, inaccessible, or contraindicated. When there is no breast milk, the World Health Organization recommends DHM for its nutritional properties and proven guidance for nursing and lactation. Furthermore, findings of the literature concluded that DHM not only contributes to infant development and health but also may benefit mothers' well-being and parents' mental health [15]. There is also evidence that newborns fed donor human milk rather than formula accept full feeds more quickly and leave the hospital sooner. Thus, donor human milk possibly contributes to lowering costs of hospitalization [16]. In a recent study, preterm neonates born at less than 37 weeks of gestation who received donor human milk or formula showed lower rates of necrotizing enterocolitis, intracranial hemorrhage, and sepsis [17]. Therefore, human milk banks (HMBs) were established so that mothers could provide their babies with human milk if their own milk was insufficient, unavailable, or not recommended. The purpose of a human milk bank is to serve as a bridge between donors and recipients by collecting, storing, screening, processing, and distributing donor milk in a safe and ethical manner [18].

Although the issue and importance of donor human milk banks have recently come to the fore, its history is quite old, dating back to the 1900s. The first breast milk bank was established in Vienna, Austria, in 1909 [19]. During the 1980s, many human milk banks closed due to different conditions and increased disease risks [20]. Today efforts to achieve standardization in most human milk banks are being made by applying strict rules and criteria for milk donors. However, a global coordinating committee has not been established to issue minimum standards for quality, safety, and ethics in the storage and distribution of human milk by donors [21].

Current knowledge indicates that breast milk is a complex biological liquid but not sterile since many pathogenic, commensal, and probiotic microbes including bacteria and viruses have been isolated, such as *Streptococci*, *Staphylococci*, *Lactobacilli*, *Micrococci*, *Enterococci* species, hepatitis B, C viruses, herpes simplex virus, cytomegalovirus, human immunodeficiency virus, and human T-lymphotrophic virus. Although many microbes are potentially pathogenic, some are also found in fresh breast milk of women, which means some of them are part of the natural microbiome of human milk [22–24]. Donor human milk is pasteurized for its microbial safety by the human milk banks to eliminate pathogens. Currently, the Holder technique is the one that is most frequently advised for pasteurizing human donor milk. In addition to pasteurization, donor selection includes stringent rules and serological testing for the safety of human milk prepared by HMB. Generally, donors do not receive any payment; they give their milk altruistically. However, there are some for-profit milk banks that compensate donors [25]. Paying donors for breast milk remains an ethical dilemma.

After donor human milk reaches the HMB, it is frozen and stored in the laboratory. The milk from two to four donors is pooled, carefully mixed, and poured into bottles. The bottles are pasteurized by using Holder pasteurization, in which DHM is heated to 62.5°C for 30 min and then rapidly cooled down [26–28]. Using Holder pasteurization, most pathogens can be removed from donor milk, but some of their biological properties are also significantly reduced. Some nutrients, anti-infective components, enzymes, growth factors, as well as stem cells may be affected by the pasteurization process. Nevertheless, some essential compounds, such as oligosaccharides and some vitamins, are relatively heat resistant [27, 29]. Thus, for the time being, there is no ideal method for pasteurization. Therefore, there is growing interest in developing new techniques that can inactivate hazardous pathogens and retain the functional and essential components of human donor milk.

The best nutrition for an infant is typically regarded as breast milk from the mother. The composition of every mother's milk differs individually. It is also important to note that breast milk content changes as the baby grows. When there is no mother's own milk available, the use of donor human milk is also advised. On the other hand, the donor milk banks are known to provide mature or pooled milk from breastfeeding mothers at various phases of the lactation process. The nutritional content of different donor human milk samples might vary considerably due to changes in maternal characteristics, lactational phase, donor milk bank procedures, and environmental conditions [30]. As a result, donor mothers at various phases of breastfeeding contribute milk to the pool in the HMB. If donor human milk is used, the ideal stage of breastfeeding and gestation should be identical [31]. A recent study about the nutritional content of human donor milk reveals that its fat, calorie, and protein compositions can fluctuate by twice or more, and that the mineral and vitamin composition is missing. There is currently a limited amount of information available regarding the constituents of donor human milk. Targeting donor human milk fortification, protein and energy assessments are reasonable strategies [32]. Future research should focus on the development of individualized methods of preparing human donor milk (Table 1).

Human milk banks are expanding around the globe providing human donor milk to improve infant health. In 2020, there were approximately over 65 countries with more than 750 human milk banks. A growing number of milk banks are being founded in low- and middle-income nations. A 2020 Global Milk Banking Leaders Network report estimated that at least 800,000 newborns get human donor milk worldwide each year [34]. The 19th of May has been celebrated internationally as World Day of Human Milk Donation for over a decade.

Since there is a growing interest in spreading and investing in HMBs worldwide, efforts are being made to standardize procedures and regulations to establish HMBs. An international expert meeting on human milk banks was organized by the WHO and the University of Zurich in 2019 to emphasize that the use of donor human milk should be regulated wherever necessary in the setting of encouraging, protecting, and enhancing the use of mother's own milk. Furthermore, the WHO recently called for the development of guidelines for human milk banking, which are expected to be released in 2022–2023 [21].

Various factors contribute to differences in human milk banking organization worldwide, including economics and funding, as well as religious and cultural

Table 1 Flowchart of the human milk process

Selection of donor mother
Health check of donor mother
Donor mother expresses breastmilk
Milk stored in home freezer or refrigerator
Milk is transported to milk bank
Milk is stored in bank freezer
Milk is thawed and pooled
Milk is aliquoted
Milk is pasteurized (usually Holder 62.5°C for 30 min)
Milk is cultured (at random)
Milk is delivered to the recipient (baby)

Adapted from Haiden N, Ziegler EE. Human Milk Banking. Ann Nutr Metab. 2016;69 Suppl 2:8–15. doi: 10.1159/000452821. Epub 2017 Jan 20. PMID: 28103607 [33]

factors. Accordingly, legislation should be developed according to the needs of each country. Various countries around the world have systematically developed HMB networks. For example, by implementing a nationalized, integrated human milk banking program in Brazil, significant progress has been made in promoting breast-feeding, providing lactation support, and providing donor milk to families in need. Brazil's HMB program is an excellent example for low- and middle-income countries. On the other hand, Kenya, which is located in a continent with a high neonatal mortality rate, started an integrated program with the UK in 2016. The program includes a learning exchange to support and train staff and to establish standard operating procedures for HMB. On the other hand, Vietnam has created standards for establishing human milk banks that align with government standards for hospitals [21]. Muslim countries face a slightly different situation. As a result of the traditional practice of milk kinship, establishing human milk banks in Muslim countries is challenging. The concept of milk kinship in the Muslim faith is based on the belief that breastfeeding creates a kinship between women and their nonbiological nursing infants and the biological infants they are nursing, preventing future marriages for "milk brothers and sisters." As a result, many Muslim families are reluctant to use human donor milk as a source of breast milk due to the anonymity of human donor milk and the fact that a large number of donors have contributed to such banks [35]. The first HMB was launched in the Al-Zahra Hospital of Tabriz, Iran, in 2016. In 2021, a retrospective study from Iran was published on the short-term outcomes of this hospital's donor human milk bank, and as a result of launching the HMB, premature infant outcomes significantly improved [36].

Several organizations such as the European Milk Bank Association (EMBA) have also been established worldwide. There have been already 281 human milk banks in 30 countries, according to EMBA. EMBA is a nonprofit organization dedicated to promoting milk banking in Europe and encouraging international cooperation among European milk banks, which was founded in 2008 [37].

Several studies showed similarities in the microbiome between the mother's own milk and donor human milk, which differs from the microbiome of formula. Thus, it is possible that the microbiome of infants who get donor milk functions similarly to the microbiome of those who receive their mothers' own milk [38, 39].

In late 2019, the severe acute respiratory syndrome coronavirus 2 (SARS-CoV-2) emerged among humans, resulting in the coronavirus disease-2019 (COVID-19) pandemic throughout the world. There has been a rise in uncertainty regarding breast milk and feeding in light of the global COVID-19 pandemic. During the early phases of the COVID-19 pandemic, most clinical practices involved anti-breastfeeding strategies, such as separating mothers from their babies [40]. As the pandemic progressed, new evidence has emerged confirming the benefit and importance of human milk and the significance of protecting and supporting breastfeeding. Moreover, it is been repeatedly confirmed that infected mother's milk supplies anti-SARS-CoV-2 IgG and IgA, which neutralize SARS-CoV-2 activity in babies. In light of the recent results, it is suggested that mothers keep feeding with their own milk throughout mild or moderate maternal COVID-19 illness as milk likely provides newborns with immunological benefits [41]. Therefore, breast milk was once again found to be the best option for nutrition, regardless of the pandemic conditions.

4 Conclusion

It is well known that human breast milk is the ideal source of nutrition for an infant. It has been suggested that DHM would be the best option for babies who do not get adequate milk supply from their mothers for several reasons. Human milk banks were established so mothers could feed their babies with human milk if their milk was insufficient, unavailable, or not recommended. Human milk banks serve as a bridge between donors and recipients, collecting, storing, screening, processing, and distributing donor milk, ensuring its quality and safety.

Developing an integrated approach to human milk banking worldwide is crucial to enhancing newborn care. Therefore, it is necessary to develop and implement global standards for operating human milk banks among all countries around the world.

References

1. Rouw E, von Gartzen A, Weißenborn A. [The importance of breastfeeding for the infant]. Bundesgesundheitsblatt Gesundheitsforschung Gesundheitsschutz. 2018;61(8):945–951.
2. Selma-Royo M, et al. Human milk microbiome: From actual knowledge to future perspective. Semin Perinatol. 2021;45(6):151450.
3. Belfort MB, et al. Breast milk feeding, brain development, and neurocognitive outcomes: a 7-year longitudinal study in infants born at less than 30 weeks' gestation. J Pediatr. 2016;177:133–139.e1.
4. Deoni SC, et al. Breastfeeding and early white matter development: a cross-sectional study. NeuroImage. 2013;82:77–86.
5. García-Ricobaraza M, et al. Short- and long-term implications of human milk microbiota on maternal and child health. Int J Mol Sci. 2021;22(21):11866.
6. Bass JL, Gartley T, Kleinman R. World Health Organization baby-friendly hospital initiative guideline and 2018 implementation guidance. JAMA Pediatr. 2019;173(1):93–4.
7. Agostoni C, et al. Breast-feeding: a commentary by the ESPGHAN Committee on Nutrition. J Pediatr Gastroenterol Nutr. 2009;49(1):112–25.
8. WHO Guidelines Approved by the Guidelines Review Committee, in Baby-Friendly Hospital Initiative: Revised, Updated and Expanded for Integrated Care. 2009, World Health Organization, Copyright © 2009, World Health Organization and UNICEF.: Geneva.
9. Meek JY, Noble L, S.o. Breastfeeding. Policy statement: breastfeeding and the use of human milk. Pediatrics. 2022;150(1):e2022057988.
10. Velmurugan S, et al. Perceptions on human milk donation and banking: maternal optimism. J Family Med Prim Care. 2020;9(11):5820–1.
11. WHO Guidelines Approved by the Guidelines Review Committee, in Guidelines on Optimal Feeding of Low Birth-Weight Infants in Low- and Middle-Income Countries. 2011, World Health Organization, Copyright © 2011, World Health Organization.: Geneva.

12. Quigley M, McGuire W. Formula versus donor breast milk for feeding preterm or low birth weight infants. Cochrane Database Syst Rev. 2014(4):Cd002971.
13. Oliveira MG, Valle Volkmer DF. Factors associated with breastfeeding very low birth weight infants at neonatal intensive care unit discharge: a single-center brazilian experience. J Hum Lact. 2021;37(4):775–83.
14. McCune S, Perrin MT. donor human milk use in populations other than the preterm infant: a systematic scoping review. Breastfeed Med. 2021;16(1):8–20.
15. Brown A, Shenker N. Receiving screened donor human milk for their infant supports parental wellbeing: a mixed-methods study. BMC Pregnancy Childbirth. 2022;22(1):455.
16. Wight NE. Donor human milk for preterm infants. J Perinatol. 2001;21(4):249–54.
17. Torres-Muñoz J, et al. Clinical results of the implementation of a breast milk bank in premature infants (under 37 weeks) at the Hospital Universitario del Valle 2018-2020. Nutrients. 2021;13(7):2187.
18. Public health round-up. Bull World Health Organ. 2021;99(6):408–9.
19. Cassidy TM. Historical research: more than milk: the origins of human milk banking social relations. J Hum Lact. 2022;38(2):344–50.
20. Kim J, Unger S. Human milk banking. Paediatr Child Health. 2010;15(9):595–602.
21. Tyebally Fang M, et al. Developing global guidance on human milk banking. Bull World Health Organ. 2021;99(12):892–900.
22. Strom K, et al. Microbiological quality of milk donated to the regional human milk bank in warsaw in the first four years of activity. Healthcare (Basel). 2022;10(3):144.
23. Urbaniak C, Burton JP, Reid G. Breast, milk and microbes: a complex relationship that does not end with lactation. Womens Health (Lond). 2012;8(4):385–98.
24. Clarke NM, May JT. Effect of antimicrobial factors in human milk on rhinoviruses and milk-borne cytomegalovirus in vitro. J Med Microbiol. 2000;49(8):719–23.
25. Thibeau S, Ginsberg HG. Bioethics in practice: the ethics surrounding the use of donor milk. Ochsner J. 2018;18(1):17–9.
26. Moro GE, et al. Processing of donor human milk: update and recommendations from the european milk bank association (EMBA). Front Pediatr. 2019;7:49.
27. Kontopodi E, et al. Testing the effects of processing on donor human milk: analytical methods. Food Chem. 2022;373(Pt A):131413.
28. Arslanoglu S, et al. Guidelines for the establishment and operation of a donor human milk bank. J Mater Fetal Neonatal Med. 2010;23(sup2):1–20.
29. Bertino E, et al. Effects of Holder pasteurization on human milk oligosaccharides. Int J Immunopathol Pharmacol. 2008;21(2):381–5.
30. Ballard O, Morrow AL. Human milk composition: nutrients and bioactive factors. Pediatr Clin N Am. 2013;60(1):49–74.
31. Sánchez Luna M, Martin SC, Gómez-de-Orgaz CS. Human milk bank and personalized nutrition in the NICU: a narrative review. Eur J Pediatr. 2021;180(5):1327–33.
32. Perrin MT, et al. The nutritional composition and energy content of donor human milk: a systematic review. Adv Nutr. 2020;11(4):960–70.
33. Haiden N, Ziegler EE. Human milk banking. Ann Nutr Metab. 2016;69(Suppl 2):8–15.
34. Shenker N. Maintaining safety and service provision in human milk banking: a call to action in response to the COVID-19 pandemic. Lancet Child Adolesc Health. 2020;4(7):484–5.
35. Subudhi S, Sriraman N. Islamic beliefs about milk kinship and donor human milk in the United States. Pediatrics. 2021;147(2):e20200441.
36. Hosseini M, et al. Short-term outcomes of launching mother's milk bank in neonatal intensive care unit: a retrospective study. Arch Iran Med. 2021;24(5):397–404.
37. Weaver G, et al. Recommendations for the establishment and operation of human milk banks in europe: a consensus statement from the european milk bank association (EMBA). Front Pediatr. 2019;7:53.
38. Cacho NT, et al. Personalization of the microbiota of donor human milk with mother's own milk. Front Microbiol. 2017;8:1470.

39. Dessì A, et al. Metabolomics of breast milk: the importance of phenotypes. Metabolites. 2018;8(4):79.
40. Hu YJ, Wake M, Saffery R. Clarifying the sweeping consequences of COVID-19 in pregnant women, newborns, and children with existing cohorts. JAMA Pediatr. 2021;175(2):117–8.
41. Pace RM, et al. Characterization of SARS-CoV-2 RNA, antibodies, and neutralizing capacity in milk produced by women with COVID-19. mBio. 2021;12(1):e03192–20.

Emotional Communication During Breastfeeding

Can Cemal Cingi and Dilek Eroğlu

1 Introduction

The ability to lactate is unique to mammals. Lactation arose due to evolutionary pressures favouring high efficiency in delivering nutrients to offspring, both in quality and quantity. There is complete consensus that breastfeeding is the optimal way for neonates and infants to feed for the initial part of their lives. The recommendation from both the World Health Organisation and the American Academy of Pediatrics is for infants to be breastfed for a minimum of six months, without additional sources of nutrition. Besides the immediate benefits of supplying the infant's nutritional requirements, it has been demonstrated that breastfeeding creates major and long-lasting effects on children's cognitive and behavioural development, as well as their mental health. Furthermore, the act of breastfeeding an infant results in a durable and significant communicative exchange between mother and child [1–3].

C. C. Cingi (✉)
Faculty of Communication Sciences, Department of Communication Design and Management, Anadolu University, Eskişehir, Türkiye
e-mail: ccc@anadolu.edu.tr

D. Eroğlu
School of Foreign Languages, Department of Foreign Languages, Anadolu University, Eskişehir, Türkiye
e-mail: dteroglu@anadolu.edu.tr

© The Author(s), under exclusive license to Springer Nature Switzerland AG 2023
Ö. N. Şahin et al. (eds.), *Breastfeeding and Metabolic Programming*,
https://doi.org/10.1007/978-3-031-33278-4_54

2 How Breastfeeding Influences Affective State and Stress in the Mother

Evidence suggests that breastfeeding affects mothers' affective state and their response to stress [4]. A comparison of breastfeeding *vs* bottle-feeding mothers indicated that breastfeeding mothers were less anxious, had a more positive affect and felt less stressed than those feeding their infants formula milk [5]. This research was based on mothers' self-reported emotions, but there is also objective evidence confirming that breastfeeding fosters good emotional health, such as studies indicating that breastfeeding was associated with increased activity of the tenth cranial nerve on the heart, lower blood pressure and a decrease in the tendency for cardiac rate to speed up, compared to women feeding their infants formula. These physiological effects suggest the breastfeeding mothers are calmer and less anxious [6, 7]. It has also been shown that lactating mothers secrete lower levels of cortisol in reaction to social stress [4]. Furthermore, mothers of breastfed infants sleep longer and more deeply than mothers using formula for feeding, with one study demonstrating a 45-minute lengthening in sleep duration and fewer arousals from sleep [8]. Breastfeeding mothers also respond in different ways to displays of emotion in other people, an effect that has the potential to raise the quality of social relationships and interactions. In particular, research published recently has found an association between breastfeeding infants as the sole method for lengthy periods and responding more readily to emotionally warmer-looking faces. If a mother breastfed more than usual on a particular day, she also tended to react less to faces exhibiting hostile emotions [9].

Thus, to summarise the evidence on the effects of breastfeeding on maternal affect, mood and responsiveness to stress, it has been demonstrated that there is a protective effect on emotional health and an increased tendency to perceive emotional warmth in other people. The emotional effects of breastfeeding resemble those seen when oxytocin was supplied via the nose, using a placebo comparator, which may indicate that the effects in lactating mothers occur secondary to a rise in endogenous oxytocin [10, 11]. Oxytocin has an established role in lactation and is known to increase during breastfeeding [12]. A genetic study, moreover, established an association between polymorphism of the CD38 rs3796863 single nucleotide polymorphism (SNP) and how rapidly cortisol levels fall when the mother breastfeeds her child. In particular, in those subjects who had the genotype associated with higher levels of oxytocin, cortisol levels fell more sharply. This more rapid fall in cortisol was, surprisingly, also observed in the infants [13]. We may therefore conclude that the physiological mechanism that accounts for the emotional and other beneficial effects described earlier operates through an increase in endogenous oxytocin in women who are breastfeeding.

3 Breastfeeding and Attachment Between Mother and Infant

It is believed that breastfeeding plays a key role in ensuring attachment of the mother and infant and ensuring the mother understands the child's needs [14, 15]. Studies indicate that, compared to mothers whose infants are formula-fed, breastfeeding mothers are more tactile with their children, show greater responsiveness and the mother and infant gaze at each other to a greater extent during feeding [16–18]. A study consisting of 675 pairs of mother and infant followed up longitudinally found that mothers who breastfed for longer responded more sensitively to the infant's needs, the attachment was more secure and the disoriented attachment style was rarer when the child reached the age of 14 months [19]. Evidence from neuroimaging studies also indicates that breastfeeding reinforces the bond between mother and infant. In one such study, where functional magnetic resonance was the imaging modality, a difference was noted in the region of the central nervous system activated when mothers heard their infant crying. The mothers who breastfed exclusively showed higher levels of limbic activation, consistent with emotional involvement, than the mothers who fed their infants formula [20, 21].

Despite this evidence, it is noteworthy that not all researchers have found a direct connection between breastfeeding and the type of attachment that develops. Britton et al. [23] found that there was no relationship between breastfeeding and attachment formation at the age of 12 months. There was, however, a significant correlation between how sensitive the mother was to the infant's needs at the age of three months and the likelihood of continuing to breastfeed up to one year. Mothers with greater sensitivity have been shown to bond more effectively with their infants [22–24]. These results may be interpreted as hinting that breastfeeding and attachment are linked through the increased maternal sensitivity seen in breastfeeding mothers. The way mothers act towards their infants is also likely impacted by the emotional benefits that breastfeeding confers on mothers, namely greater emotional positivity, lower stress and improved emotional responsiveness towards other people [8, 9].

4 How Being Breastfed Affects Psychological Development

Evidence from studies in many different countries has now accumulated to support the idea that breastfeeding leads to better cognitive outcomes as the child develops, such as greater ability to remember things, higher linguistic abilities and improved intelligence quotient (IQ) [25–29].

Studies of longitudinal type undertaken prospectively have the advantage that they do not rely on mothers' reporting on breastfeeding retrospectively, which may be a source of inaccuracy. The authors of a longitudinal study of this type ascertained that being breastfed more frequently or for a longer period had a positive association with higher scores on the Bayley Scales of Infant Development. In particular, memory improved, as did linguistic performance and motor development, assessed at ages 14 and 18 months. It is also noteworthy that this beneficial effect on cognitive development in breastfed infants persists right into adolescence [30–32]. A study undertaken by Bernard et al. [33] evaluated the cognitive abilities and motor skills of children at the ages of two and three years, noting that cognitive development was greater in those children who had been breastfed. This study used the Communicative Development Inventory [34] and Ages and Stages Questionnaire [35] to assess cognitive development.

The results from this study indicated that children exclusively breastfed for lengthy periods were better at solving problems than other children. A different study, involving a large cohort taken from the general population, assessed executive function (i.e. sequencing, etc.) at the age of four years. Those children who had received exclusive breastfeeding for more than half a year outperformed those who never received breastfeeding, or in whom breastfeeding continued for under six months [36]. A cohort study that assessed children from the first to sixth years of life concluded that the length of time children were breastfed correlated in a dose-dependent manner with verbal intelligence, assessed by means of the Revised Peabody Picture Vocabulary Test (PPVT-R) [37]. The results demonstrated that, for children aged five years, the highest performance on the test was seen in those children who had received breastfeeding for half a year or more, whereas the lowest scores occurred in those who were always bottle-fed. A different study, also of longitudinal type, evaluated cognitive ability in children aged between one and seven years. The measurements were made using the Wechsler Intelligence Scale for Children [38]. Longer exclusive breastfeeding correlated consistently with higher performance on the scale [39]. Moreover, a comparison between those children who received only breast milk and those who got both breast and artificial milk showed that the former kept on raising their scores higher for the age range studied. Although one explanation for the difference between the groups is that maternal intelligence is a confounder, a study involving large numbers and also of longitudinal design did in fact control for this and still established that breastfeeding was beneficial in terms of cognitive development [40].

The claim has also been asserted that starting breastfeeding straight after birth is protective against the development of cognitive impairments in children. One clinic-based study compared children aged between 4 and 11 years with a specific language impairment with their neurotypical peers. The researchers asked about breastfeeding and concluded that specific language impairment was significantly more likely if children had not been breastfed from birth onwards [41]. Although the data support the fact that early breastfeeding and specific cognitive impairments are negatively correlated, they cannot be used to prove a definite causal link between breastfeeding and a reduction in risk.

There is even more persuasive evidence to suggest that breastfeeding affects cognitive development. One randomised controlled study enrolled 13,000 pairs of mothers and infants [28]. The intervention consisted of a programme advocating breastfeeding, following which seven times as many mothers were still breastfeeding when the infant was three months old. The study had a longitudinal design. At follow-up, when the children were 6.5 years old, they were assessed for intelligence level and their teachers asked to rate their academic ability [28]. In terms of both outcome measures the children who were exclusively breastfed did better than the non-intervention group. When this same cohort was followed up ten years later, the breastfed individuals continued to have an advantage in terms of linguistic competence, but this difference did not persist for other measures of neurocognition [42]. The researchers involved speculated that the benefits of breastfeeding may become weaker over time, as other factors, for example intellectual stimulation by the parents, or association with other children, play a more determining role in cognitive development.

Nonetheless, the idea that breastfed children continue to have an advantage in cognitive abilities, even as adults, does seem to be justified. Mortensen et al. [25] assessed cognitive abilities in different groups via a variety of psychometric instruments. Their results reveal that being breastfed for a lengthier period as an infant increased cognitive abilities as an adult, an effect that was demonstrable in different groups and regardless of the psychometric technique employed [43]. Yet another study, where the subjects were aged 30 years, revealed that a longer time being exclusively breastfed correlated with higher IQ, better academic performance and higher earnings [44]. Indeed, one study went as far as to argue that the length of time an individual was breastfed as an infant influenced reading ability even in middle age (i.e. at the age of 53 years). The test applied in this case was the National Adult Reading Test [43].

It is important to observe that the studies we have been discussing so far attempted to control for many of the potential confounders, such as the mother's educational attainment, employment status, income level, age, how the child was delivered, smoking whilst pregnant and weight at birth. One study that enrolled many subjects controlled for a large number of commonly considered potential confounders, including the mother's IQ, socioeconomic status and educational attainment, but also less obvious confounders, e.g. mother's mental health, attachment style and risk of environmental toxins. Despite factoring all these into the analysis, there was still a powerful effect linking a long duration of being exclusively breastfed with improved neuropsychological development [45]. There have been studies, however, where the relationship between breastfeeding and psychological benefit was much less clear after confounders were taken into consideration. One such study was that of Jacobsen et al., which discovered an apparent association between breastfeeding and children's IQ scores at the ages of 4 and 11 years. Once the mother's IQ and the level of parenting skill were factored in (the latter having been evaluated via the Home Observation Measurement of the Environment [HOME] instrument), the association appeared less definite [45]. Likewise, in a study undertaken by von Stumm and Plomin [46], once socioeconomic status and gestational age were factored in, only a small effect of breastfeeding was noted on children's IQ. Moreover, this effect was only observable at the age of two years and only in female children. At age 16 years no effect was observable. Thus, in general terms, since there are so many potential confounders and it is so complex to factor them into any analysis, any results that appear to show that breastfeeding has an unequivocal impact on cognition need to be interpreted cautiously [47, 48]. This issue of confounders in studies investigating the benefits of breastfeeding has been discussed in depth in a review article [49]. Despite the caution needed in interpreting results from individual studies, it is clear that, overall, the evidence supports the notion that exclusively breastfeeding for a lengthy period does indeed benefit the child in neuropsychological terms.

If breastfeeding does influence neuropsychological development, it is reasonable to ask how this effect may be mediated. It has been hypothesised that certain components of breast milk, notably the long-chain polyunsaturated fatty acids (LC-PUFAs), found in breast milk but not typically in artificial substitutes, may play a role [50]. Two principal fatty acids of this type are docosahexaenoic acid (DHA) and arachidonic acid (ARA). These molecules have a neurodevelopmental role since they are needed for normal growth of neurones, repair processes and myelin sheath formation [51]. It is probably significant that the myelin sheaths mainly develop up to the age of 18 months. Neonates are able to synthesise a limited amount of DHA up to the age of 14 days, but synthesis then ceases until the child is 6 months old [52]. Because endogenous production halts during this period, the provision of exogenous LC-PUFAs may be significant for neural development, which explains why breast milk has an advantage.

5 Conclusion

Besides the nutritional benefits of breastfeeding, the action of breastfeeding is important in establishing communication between the mother and infant. It is a part of bonding. Beyond its nutritional role, breastfeeding helps to form loving bonds between the child and mother that grow over time. Mothers who understand the value of breastfeeding know that an aspect of this act is communication. Just as knowledge of metabolic programming is growing, so is our appreciation of the importance of early communication between mother and child.

References

1. Krol KM, Grossmann T. Psychological effects of breastfeeding on children and mothers. Bundesgesundheitsblatt Gesundheitsforschung Gesundheitsschutz. 2018;61(8):977–85. https://doi.org/10.1007/s00103-018-2769-0.
2. Alarcon J. The Impact of Interpersonal Communication on Breastfeeding; 2013. Open Access Theses & Dissertations. 1775. https://digitalcommons.utep.edu/open_etd/1775
3. Raju TN. Breastfeeding is a dynamic biological process—not simply a meal at the breast. Breastfeed Med. 2011;6:257–9. https://doi.org/10.1089/bfm.2011.0081.
4. Heinrichs M, Neumann ID, Ehlert U. Lactation and stress: protective effects of breast-feeding in humans. Stress. 2002;5:165–203. https://doi.org/10.1080/1025389021000010530.

5. Groër MW. Differences between exclusive breastfeeders, formula-feeders, and controls: a study of stress, mood, and endocrine variables. Biol Res Nurs. 2005;7:106–17. https://doi.org/10.1177/1099800405280936.

6. Mezzacappa ES, Kelsey RM, Katkin ES. Breast feeding, bottle feeding, and maternal autonomic responses to stress. J Psychosom Res. 2005;58:351–65. https://doi.org/10.1016/j.jpsychores.2004.11.004.

7. Hahn-Holbrook J, Holt-Lunstad J, Holbrook C, Coyne SM, Lawson ET. Maternal defense: breast feeding increases aggression by reducing stress. Psychol Sci. 2011;22:1288–95. https://doi.org/10.1177/0956797611420729.

8. Doan T, Gardiner A, Gay CL, Lee KA. Breast-feeding increases sleep duration of new parents. J Perinat Neonatal Nurs. 2007;21:200–6. https://doi.org/10.1097/01.JPN.0000285809.36398.1b.

9. Krol KM, Kamboj SK, Curran HV, Grossmann T. Breastfeeding experience differentially impacts recognition of happiness and anger in mothers. Sci Rep. 2014;4:7006. https://doi.org/10.1038/srep07006.

10. de Oliveira DC, Zuardi AW, Graeff FG, Queiroz RH, Crippa JA. Anxiolytic-like effect of oxytocin in the simulated public speaking test. J Psychopharmacol. 2012;26:497–504. https://doi.org/10.1177/0269881111400642.

11. Marsh AA, Yu HH, Pine DS, Blair RJ. Oxytocin improves specific recognition of positive facial expressions. Psychopharmacology. 2010;209:225–32. https://doi.org/10.1007/s00213-010-1780-4.

12. Dawood MY, Khandawood FS, Wahi RS, Fuchs F. Oxytocin release and plasma anterior-pituitary and gonadal-hormones in women during lactation. J Clin Endocrinol Metab. 1981;52:678–83. https://doi.org/10.1210/jcem-52-4-678.

13. Krol KM, Monakhov M, Lai PS, Ebstein RP, Heinrichs M, Grossmann T. Genetic variation in the maternal oxytocin system affects cortisol responsiveness to breastfeeding in infants and mothers. Adapt Human Behav Physiol. 2018; https://doi.org/10.1007/s40750-018-0090-7.

14. Zetterström R. Breastfeeding and infant-mother interaction. Acta Paediatr. 1999;88:1–6. https://doi.org/10.1111/j.1651-2227.1999.tb01293.x.

15. Brandt KA, Andrews CM, Kvale J. Mother-infant interaction and breastfeeding outcome 6 weeks after birth. J Obstet Gynecol Neonatal Nurs. 1998;27:169–74. https://doi.org/10.1111/j.1552-6909.1998.tb02607.x.

16. Kennell J, McGrath S. Starting the process of mother-infant bonding. Acta Paediatr. 2005;94:775–7. https://doi.org/10.1080/08035250510035634.

17. Bernal J, Richards MP. Effects of bottle and breast feeding on infant development. J Psychosom Res. 1970;14:247. https://doi.org/10.1016/0022-3999(70)90050-4.

18. Wiesenfeld AR, Malatesta CZ, Whitman PB, Granrose C, Uili R. Psychophysiological response of breast-feeding and bottle-feeding mothers to their infants signals. Psychophysiology. 1985;22:79–86. https://doi.org/10.1111/j.1469-8986.1985.tb01563.x.

19. Lavelli M, Poli M. Early mother-infant interaction during breast- and bottle-feeding. Infant Behav Dev. 1998;21:667–83. https://doi.org/10.1016/S0163-6383(98)90037-6.

20. Tharner A, Luijk MPCM, Raat H, et al. Breastfeeding and its relation to maternal sensitivity and infant attachment. J Dev Behav Pediatr. 2012;33:396–404. https://doi.org/10.1097/DBP.0b013e318257fac3.

21. Kim P, Feldman R, Mayes LC, et al. Breastfeeding, brain activation to own infant cry, and maternal sensitivity. J Child Psychol Psychiatry. 2011;52:907–15. https://doi.org/10.1111/j.1469-7610.2011.02406.x.

22. Jansen J, de Weerth C, Riksen-Walraven JM. Breastfeeding and the mother-infant relationship—a review. Dev Rev. 2008;28:503–21. https://doi.org/10.1016/j.dr.2008.07.001.

23. Britton JR, Britton HL, Gronwaldt V. Breastfeeding, sensitivity, and attachment. Pediatrics. 2006;118:E1436–43. https://doi.org/10.1542/peds.2005-2916.

24. Belsky J, Fearon RM. Early attachment security, subsequent maternal sensitivity, and later child development: does continuity in development depend upon continuity of caregiving? Attach Hum Dev. 2002;4:361–87.

25. Mortensen EL, Michaelsen KF, Sanders SA, Reinisch JM. The association between duration of breastfeeding and adult intelligence. JAMA. 2002;287:2365–71. https://doi.org/10.1001/jama.287.18.2365.

26. Oddy WH. Long-term health outcomes and mechanisms associated with breastfeeding. Expert Rev Pharmacoecon Outcomes Res. 2002;2:161–77. https://doi.org/10.1586/14737167.2.2.161.

27. Oddy WH, Kendall GE, Blair E, de Klerk NH, Silburn S, Zubrick S. Breastfeeding and cognitive development in children. Adv Exp Med Biol. 2004;554:365–9. https://doi.org/10.1007/978-1-4757-4242-8_42.

28. Kramer MS, Aboud F, Mironova E, et al. Breastfeeding and child cognitive development—new evidence from a large randomized trial. Arch Gen Psychiatry. 2008;65:578–84. https://doi.org/10.1001/archpsyc.65.5.578.

29. Daniels MC, Adair LS. Breast-feeding influences cognitive development in Filipino children. J Nutr. 2005;135:2589–95. https://doi.org/10.1093/jn/135.11.2589.

30. Ludington SM, Hadeed A, Anderson G. Cardiorespiratory, thermal and state effects of Kangaroo Care for preterm infants—randomized control trial. Pediatr Res. 1991;29:A223.

31. Bayley N. Mental growth during the first three years. A developmental study of sixty-one children by repeated tests. Genet. Psychol Monogr. 1933;14:1–92. [Google Scholar]

32. Guxens M, Mendez MA, Molto-Puigmarti C, et al. Breastfeeding, long-chain polyunsaturated fatty acids in colostrum, and infant mental development. Pediatrics. 2011;128:E880–9. https://doi.org/10.1542/peds.2010-1633.

33. Bernard JY, De Agostini M, Forhan A, et al. Breastfeeding duration and cognitive development at 2 and 3 years of age in the EDEN Mother-Child Cohort. J Pediatr. 2013;163:36–U414. https://doi.org/10.1016/j.jpeds.2012.11.090.

34. Fenson L, Marchman VA, Thal DJ, Dale PS, Reznick JS, Bates E. The MacArthur-Bates communicative development inventories user's guide and technical manual. 2nd ed. Baltimore: Paul H. Brookes Publishing Co Inc; 2006. [Google Scholar]

35. Squires J, Potter L, Bricker D. The ASQ user's guide for the ages and stages questionnaires: a parent-completed child-monitoring system. 2nd ed. Baltimore: Paul H. Brookes Publishing Co Inc; 1999. [Google Scholar]

36. Julvez J, Guxens M, Carsin AE, et al. A cohort study on full breastfeeding and child neuropsychological development: the role of maternal social, psychological, and nutritional factors. Dev Med Child Neurol. 2014;56:148–56. https://doi.org/10.1111/dmcn.12282.

37. Dunn LM, Dunn LM. Peabody picture vocabulary test-revised. Circle Pines: American Guidance Service; 1981. [Google Scholar]

38. Wechsler D. Manual of the Wechsler Intelligence Scale for children-revised. New York: Psychological Corporation; 1974. [Google Scholar]

39. Jedrychowski W, Perera F, Jankowski J, et al. Effect of exclusive breastfeeding on the development of children's cognitive function in the Krakow prospective birth cohort study. Eur J Pediatr. 2012;171:151–8. https://doi.org/10.1007/s00431-011-1507-5.

40. Kanazawa S. Breastfeeding is positively associated with child intelligence even net of parental IQ. Dev Psychol. 2015;51(12):1683–9. https://doi.org/10.1037/dev0000060.

41. Diepeveen FB, van Dommelen P, Oudesluys-Murphy AM, Verkerk PH. Specific language impairment is associated with maternal and family factors. Child Care Health Dev. 2017;43:401–5. https://doi.org/10.1111/cch.12451.

42. Yang S, Martin RM, Oken E, et al. Breastfeeding during infancy and neurocognitive function in adolescence: 16-year follow-up of the PROBIT cluster-randomized trial. PLoS Med. 2018;15:e1002554. https://doi.org/10.1371/journal.pmed.1002554.

43. Richards M, Hardy R, Wadsworth ME. Long-term effects of breast-feeding in a national birth cohort: educational attainment and midlife cognitive function. Public Health Nutr. 2002;5:631–5. https://doi.org/10.1079/PHN2002338.

44. Victora CG, Horta BL, de Mola CL, et al. Association between breastfeeding and intelligence, educational attainment, and income at 30 years of age: a prospective birth cohort

study from Brazil. Lancet Glob Health. 2015;3:E199–205. https://doi.org/10.1016/S2214-109X(15)70002-1.

45. Jacobson SW, Chiodo LM, Jacobson JL. Breastfeeding effects on intelligence quotient in 4- and 11-year-old children. Pediatrics. 1999;103:e71. https://doi.org/10.1542/peds.103.5.e71.

46. von Stumm S, Plomin R. Breastfeeding and IQ growth from toddlerhood through adolescence. PLoS One. 2015;10:e0138676. https://doi.org/10.1371/journal.pone.0138676.

47. Jain A, Concato J, Leventhal JM. How good is the evidence linking breastfeeding and intelligence? Pediatrics. 2002;109:1044–53. https://doi.org/10.1542/peds.109.6.1044.

48. Der G, Batty GD, Deary IJ. Effect of breast feeding on intelligence in children: prospective study, sibling pairs analysis, and meta-analysis. BMJ. 2006;333:945–948a. https://doi.org/10.1136/bmj.38978.699583.55.

49. Walfisch A, Sermer C, Cressman A, Koren G. Breast milk and cognitive development—the role of confounders: a systematic review. BMJ Open. 2013;3:e003259. https://doi.org/10.1136/bmjopen-2013-003259.

50. Drover J, Hoffman DR, Castaneda YS, Morale SE, Birch EE. Three randomized controlled trials of early long-chain polyunsaturated fatty acid supplementation on means-end problem solving in 9-month-olds. Child Dev. 2009;80:1376–84. https://doi.org/10.1111/j.1467-8624.2009.01339.x.

51. Guesnet P, Alessandri JM. Docosahexaenoic acid (DHA) and the developing central nervous system (CNS)—Implications for dietary recommendations. Biochimie. 2011;93:7–12. https://doi.org/10.1016/j.biochi.2010.05.005.

52. Deoni SC, Dean DC 3rd, Piryatinksy I, O'Muircheartaigh J, Waskiewicz N, Lehman K, et al. Breastfeeding and early white matter development: a cross-sectional study. NeuroImage. 2013;82:77–86. https://doi.org/10.1016/j.neuroimage.2013.05.090.

Tobacco Use in Breastfeeding Mothers

Ali Timucin Atayoglu and Ayten Guner Atayoglu

1 Introduction

Smoking is a major health hazard that remains very common worldwide. Nicotine is a highly addictive substance. There are in excess of 250 million female smokers globally. When expectant mothers continue to smoke, they not only harm themselves, but also damage the health of their foetus [1]. Postpartum smoking mothers continue to damage infant health as the child is exposed to passive smoking and the nicotine and other harmful constituents of tobacco smoke linger in the air and are passed on through breastfeeding [1–3].

Nicotine and the other toxic constituents of tobacco are present in all types of tobacco products, namely cigarettes, cigars, pipe tobacco and chewing tobacco. Whether the infant is breastfed or given artificial formula milk, if the mother smokes, there is a raised risk of sudden infant death syndrome (SIDS), infections of the ear and lower respiratory tract (especially bronchitis and pneumonia) and less effective pulmonary function in infancy and later childhood [4].

All infants whose mothers smoke are exposed to the hazards of passive smoking and therefore inhale the toxic compounds released by burning tobacco, including nicotine. Furthermore, these same toxic compounds may be passed on during breastfeeding. The nicotine in tobacco is probably also the reason why smoking mothers produce less breast milk, since it suppresses the circulating maternal prolactin concentration [4].

A. T. Atayoglu (✉)
Department of Family Medicine, Istanbul Medipol University, International School of
Medicine, Istanbul, Türkiye
e-mail: atatayoglu@medipol.edu.tr

A. G. Atayoglu
Department of Family Medicine, Beylikdüzü State Hospital, Istanbul, Türkiye
e-mail: ayten.atayoglu@saglik.gov.tr

© The Author(s), under exclusive license to Springer Nature
Switzerland AG 2023
Ö. N. Şahin et al. (eds.), *Breastfeeding and Metabolic Programming*,
https://doi.org/10.1007/978-3-031-33278-4_55

Consumption of electronic cigarettes and vaping generally involves inhaling nebulised nicotine, flavour molecules and other ingredients produced by a small electrical vaping device. The potential harms that vaping presents to infant health have not yet been fully elucidated, however it is clear that the vapour produced by these devices still contains toxic and harmful molecules, including nicotine, flavour molecules and solvents [4].

Clinicians should provide support to smoking or vaping mothers to enable them to give up smoking altogether. In mothers who continue their tobacco use breast-feeding is still the best option for infant nutrition, as it remains superior in terms of both balanced nutrition and its clear advantages for health [4].

The following advice should be provided to smoking mothers, to enable them to reduce some of the harm to the infant [4]:

- Smoking should not occur in the vicinity of the infant.
- Smoking inside or in confined areas should stop.
- In vehicles and at home, a no smoking rule should be made.
- After smoking, mothers should wash their hands thoroughly and change their clothes.

2 Breastfeeding

Breast milk is generally accepted to be the optimal way for infants to feed, since it has the ideal nutritional balance for the child and assists with healthy growth and development. There are above 200 individual constituents in breast milk. It contains the essential nutrition for the infant, supplying water, carbohydrates, protein, fat, electrolytes and vitamins. In addition, milk contains various immunoactive elements, both cellular (i.e. macrophages, lymphocytes, neutrophils and epithelio-cytes) and humoral (immunoglobulins from classes M, A, D, G and E, complement proteins, interleukin-6, -8 and -10, cytokines, bifid factor, resistance factor, lactofer-rin and antioxidants). Finally, it also contains numerous endocrine signals, including (but not limited to) insulin, erythropoietin, bombesin and thyroxine [5, 6].

Breastfeeding offers benefits in various ways, such as improving infant and maternal health, as well as aiding family cohesion and social function. In terms of infant health, there are several domains in which breastfeeding offers benefits. It lowers the infant death rate, particularly deaths resulting from diarrhoeal illness and infections of the respiratory tract. Breastfed infants are less prone to atopy. It results in better neurological, motor and psychological development. It is linked to reductions in the rates of various chronic disorders, including systemic hypertension, diabetes mellitus, Crohn's disease, ulcerative colitis, coeliac disease, disorders involving autoimmunity and lymphoma. Furthermore, breastfeeding also protects against malocclusion syndromes, mouth breathing and speech and language disorders involving faulty articulation [7].

Besides benefits to the infant's health, breastfeeding also provides benefits for maternal health. Nursing an infant causes more rapid involution of the uterus, since it causes increased oxytocin levels. It leads to a reduction in postpartum haemorrhage and hence lower levels of maternal anaemia. There are associated reductions in the risk of developing diabetes mellitus, malignant neoplasia of the breast, ovary or uterus and bony fractures secondary to osteoporosis. Nursing also improves bonding between the infant and mother. Breastfeeding also acts like a contraceptive and helps to space out pregnancies. In mothers whose infants are exclusively breastfed for at least six months, it aids weight loss after delivery. Furthermore, breastfeeding is also good for the family budget as it avoids the cost of purchasing artificial formula milk and the related equipment, and means lower costs for prescribed medicines, since breastfed infants enjoy better health in general [5–7].

3 Breastfeeding in Smoking Mothers

Despite acknowledging that breast milk entails numerous benefits, many clinicians have concerns that toxic compounds from cigarette smoke, including nicotine, may be transferred to the infant in milk, in addition to the damage caused by passive smoking. There is plentiful published evidence about the negative effects of passive smoking in childhood, such as triggering or exacerbating allergic disorders (including allergic rhinitis and asthma [8]), provoking chronic disorders of the respiratory system [9], lengthier and more frequently occurring infections of the respiratory tract (upper and lower) [10] and higher rates of admission to hospital [11].

Cigarette smoke contains a number of compounds with established toxicity, including cyanide, aluminium, dichlorodiphenyltrichloroethane (DDT), arsenic, ammonia, formaldehyde, benzene, lead, carbon monoxide and nicotine [12]. The toxic effects of these compounds on breastfed infants are not yet understood, and the evidence base so far is inconclusive about the harms these compounds may produce [6].

The concentration of nicotine in breast milk is at least twice that found in the mother's peripheral circulation [13]. Nonetheless, it seems clear that breastfeeding still protects infants against various disorders. Acute respiratory conditions occurred more frequently in the infants of smoking mothers if they were fed artificial baby milk than if they were breastfed [14]. The balance of risk still favours breastfeeding over formula feeding and thus nicotine consumption is no longer recognised as a reason to advise mothers not to breastfeed [15]. Whilst every mother who smokes should receive smoking cessation advice, even if the woman continues to smoke, breastfeeding should still be recommended since it is the ideal nutrition for the infant and there is a lack of definite evidence showing harm linked to consumption of breast milk. There is, however, reason for concern that smoking mothers produce milk that is depleted in iodine [16]. One reason that there appears limited evidence for harm may be because the subject is inadequately researched. Furthermore, studies that examined how infants of smoking mothers develop suffered from the absence of key data, such as for how long breastfeeding occurred, whether the mother continued smoking after delivery, and what level of exposure to tobacco through breast milk actually occurred [3].

Although the guidelines do advise smoking mothers still to breastfeed their offspring, the rate of breastfeeding amongst smokers is lower than in non-smokers and the duration for which breastfeeding occurs is shorter [17]. There have been various theories advanced as to why this is so. One theory is that smoking at least ten cigarettes each day interferes with lactation, causing the breast to secrete less milk than usual and changing the constituents in the milk [18]. The endocrine processes by which these changes in lactation occur are not understood yet, nor what the effects of lower tobacco consumption are. A second theory hypothesises that smoker mothers are more inclined to judge the amount of breast milk secreted to be insufficient [19] and to have lower than usual motivation to continue [20]. Finally, the behaviour of the infants of smoking mothers with tobacco use equivalent to at least five cigarettes a day might encourage the mothers to attempt weaning. Such behaviours may include showing signs of colic and crying more than usual [21].

After their mothers had been smoking cigarettes, infants had alterations in their sleeping pattern. The duration of active and quiet sleep was significantly diminished and early waking from naps also occurred. There appears to be a dose–response relationship between the nicotine in breast milk and the degree of sleep disturbance in the infant [3].

It is unclear from the data available so far if shorter infant naps connected to smoke exposure are compensated by longer sleeps at other times. The effects of nicotine withdrawal in infants also require investigation. It has been observed that adults who quit smoking do enjoy better sleep, albeit they suffer from withdrawal symptoms during the initial period of quitting [22]. In a study examining the effects of alcohol exposure on breastfed infants, the infants were noted to recover any temporary sleep debt induced by this exposure [23]. Mothers typically want their infants to sleep for longer [24] and not to exhibit signs of colic and lengthy crying, and this generally occurs when infants are weaned. This may be the explanation for why smoking mothers cease breastfeeding earlier than their non-smoking peers.

There are a number of different factors affecting infants' sleep patterns, both physiological and related to the surrounding environment. One study attempted to link alterations in the sleep patterns of infants to breast milk consumption by eliminating other possible confounding variables. The observation of sleep was scheduled for the same time each day and in a private room. The mothers who smoked did so in a separate place from the child to avoid passive inhalation of cigarette smoke by the infant. The infants were fitted with an actigraph and lay in a supine position on a carpet or crib, so that any movements were not artefacts of the mother's movement [25]. The volume of breast milk consumed by infants of smoking mothers and that of infants of non-smoking mothers were compared and found to match, showing that infants did not show any aversion for the tobacco flavours in breast milk [2]. All in all it seems, therefore, that any change in sleep pattern of infants breastfed by smoking mothers is due to the actual breast milk itself, not some other factor [3].

The precise way in which breast milk containing tobacco causes alterations in infant sleep architecture has not been established, but the fact that sleep is altered in this way is consistent with the known pharmacodynamic profile of nicotine, the most potent pharmacological agent in cigarette smoke [26]. Consumption of nicotine has a direct effect on spike activity in the pontogeniculo-occipital region, and this spiking is known to be of importance in sleep beginning and continuing [27]. Furthermore, the neurones of the ventrolateral preoptic region, which encourage sleep, are also indirectly inhibited by nicotine [28]. Exposure to tobacco smoke is the factor that most increases the risk of SIDS (sudden infant death syndrome) [29]. There are several potential mechanisms for this risk: one is via changed sleep and arousal reactions; another is that agents in tobacco are neurotoxic and can cause death in infants with pre-existing susceptibility, as may occur with alcohol [30, 31]. At present it is not known which of the two possibilities (if either) is the correct explanation.

Nicotine has complex effects upon neurotransmission in numerous different neural pathways and affects functionality in the long term of synapses [32]. It therefore follows that the injurious effects of being exposed to nicotine as an infant may not appear until later, following apparently normal development. Neonates exposed to nicotine via breastfeeding have increased expression of nicotinic receptors, as occurs both in utero [32] and in adults with prolonged tobacco use [33]. There may be long-term harmful consequences on behaviour and cognitive development if neonates are exposed to nicotine [1]. Sleep is a key factor in how infants learn and it is known that nicotine disrupts sleep, hence nicotine may disturb cognitive development in this way [34]. From studies in experimental animals, it has been established that hindering active sleep prevents effective learning and interferes with the ability to remember [35].

The likelihood that an adolescent will begin smoking is increased if the mother was a smoker when the adolescent was a young child [36]. Animals exposed to nicotine in utero via amniotic fluid or through milk express nicotinic receptors in the central nervous system at the same level as in adult smokers [33]. Where the mother smokes, both breast milk and amniotic fluid contain taste molecules from tobacco. It therefore appears probable, since it has been shown for other tastes that exposure via milk increases liking for specific flavours [37, 38], that taste-bearing molecules from tobacco also increase liking for smoking. This effect operates alongside the neurodevelopmental alterations induced by nicotine. Children who grow up in a smoking environment come to attach particular emotions to tobacco, linked to the way tobacco was used by the parents [39].

4   Nicotine in Breast Milk

There are a number of significant toxic effects of nicotine exposure through breast milk on neonates [21]. The degree of toxicity depends on the mother's daily tobacco use and the time elapsed between smoking and commencing breastfeeding [40].

Nicotine has a half-life of around 2 h in human milk [41]. Nicotine undergoes rapid absorption from the infant gut and there is the potential for accumulation to occur in particular tissues, leading to apnoea, agitation and vomiting [42]. The age at which infants become competent to fully metabolise nicotine has not yet been established. Nicotine is water-soluble and undergoes extensive hepatic metabolism before entering the systemic circulation [40]. Further research focus on how infants metabolise nicotine is warranted [43, 44].

A study that examined the level of cotinine (a metabolite of nicotine) in the urine of mothers who smoke, concentrating on the effect of breastfeeding on urinary excretion, ascertained that metabolites of tobacco are concentrated in breast milk, particularly nicotine. The authors suggested that the focus on harmful passive smoking by children was only one part of the total exposure, and that breastfeeding actually considerably increases tobacco exposure [6, 40].

Researchers have now discovered that the nicotine concentration in breast milk of mothers who smoke is nearly three-fold (actually 2.9) times the level in the peripheral circulation. Indeed, when the urine of breastfed infants was analysed, the concentration of cotinine was found to be ten-fold that of children whose mothers also smoked but were fed artificial formula milk. The concentration of cotinine in breastfed offspring of smoking mothers is similar to that measured in adult smokers [40].

There are alterations in the length of time infants sleep and remain awake if they breastfeed straight after the mother has smoked. The average sleeping time if the mother did not smoke was 84.5 min, whereas it was 53.4 min if the mother smoked [3]. This reduction in the time spent actively and quietly asleep by infants has been definitely linked to maternal tobacco consumption just before infant feeding. Furthermore, smoking also has a broader effect on the pattern of sleeping and waking in breastfed infants of smoking mothers. A different study also noted that the infants of mothers who smoked had disordered sleep [19]. When nicotine is inhaled, it also causes discomfort to infants, resulting in infants becoming more irritable, crying excessively, displaying lack of energy, exhibiting symptoms of colic and appearing paler than usual [10, 12, 13, 19, 21].

It has also been reported that smoking reduces the iodine content of breast milk. In the breast milk of non-smoking mothers the concentration is 53.8 g/L, but this is reduced to 26.9 g/L in smoking mothers [43]. The infant also excretes a lower concentration of iodine in the urine, with the average being 33.3 g/dL, compared to 50.4 g/dL in children of non-smokers. There is an inverse correlation between the cotinine concentration in maternal urine and the concentration of iodine in breast milk. Cotinine is the biomarker for smoking that has the highest reliability and has a $t_{1/2}$ of around 20 h. It has been speculated that the lowered breast milk concentration of iodine in the breast milk of smoking mothers may lead to iodine deficiency in infants. This may then cause endocrine problems since thyroid hormones are synthesised by infants using iodine from the breast milk. Thiocyanate levels in the maternal peripheral circulation were also found to be significantly raised in smokers, which may provide the mechanism by which the transport of iodide ions into the breast milk is inhibited, since thiocyanate acts as a competitive inhibitor of the sodium-iodide transporter protein. The transporter protein moves two substances in the same direction, i.e. it is a secondary active transport mechanism [6].

Using an animal model (rats), researchers have also ascertained that exposing the animal mother to nicotine causes the thyroid in the newborn rat to dysfunction and may result in secondary hypothyroidism in adult rats. The hepatic deiodinase I (also known as iodine peroxidase) level of the rat young was measured 15 and 180 days after birth. Hepatic deiodinase I is a biomarker for thyroid dysfunction, since its level falls in hypothyroid animals but rises in hyperthyroidism. Whilst maternal nicotine exposure did not affect the body mass of the young, either positively or negatively, at the period of lactation, following weaning the rats of mothers exposed to nicotine had a higher body mass than those of non-nicotine-exposed mothers. Nicotine exposure in the mother increased the serum leptin concentration at days 15, 21, 90 and 180 of life. At 180 days the rat is considered adult and the increase at that point was statistically significant. Both whilst lactation was still underway (at day 15) and at day 180 (adult stage) the rats with maternal exposure to nicotine had a higher level of body fat than controls. At day 15 the proportion of body fat was 27%, and at day 180, it was 33%. Furthermore, compared to rats without the maternal nicotine exposure, the exposed rats had a higher concentration of body protein and adipose surrounding the viscera. The lipid profiles in the exposure group adults were, however, normal [45].

References

1. DiFranza JR, Aligne CA, Weitzman M. Prenatal and postnatal environmental tobacco smoke exposure and children's health. Pediatrics. 2004;113:1007–15.
2. Mennella JA, Beauchamp GK. Smoking and the flavor of breast milk. N Engl J Med. 1998;339:1559–60.
3. Mennella JA, Yourshaw LM, Morgan LK. Breastfeeding and smoking: short-term effects on infant feeding and sleep. Pediatrics. 2007;120(3):497–502. https://doi.org/10.1542/peds.2007-0488.
4. Tobacco and E-Cigarettes. Centers for Disease Control and Prevention (CDC). https://www.cdc.gov/breastfeeding/breastfeeding-special-circumstances/vaccinations-medications-drugs/tobacco-and-e-cigarettes.html. Accessed online at 3 Nov 2022.
5. Brasil - Ministério da Saúde. *Secretaria de atenção à saúde - departamento de atenção básica. Saúde da criança: nutrição infantil - Aleitamento materno e alimentação complementar.* Brasília: Ministério da Saúde; 2009.
6. Primo CC, Ruela PB, Brotto LD, Garcia TR, Lima EF. Effects of maternal nicotine on breastfeeding infants. Rev Paul Pediatr. 2013;31(3):392–7. https://doi.org/10.1590/S0103-05822013000300018.
7. Carvalho MR, Tamez RN. Amamentação: bases científicas para a prática profissional. Rio de Janeiro: Guanabara Koogan; 2002.
8. Weitzman M, Gortmaker S, Walker DK, Sobol A. Maternal smoking and childhood asthma. Pediatrics. 1990;85:505–11.

9. Mannino DM, Siegel M, Husten C, Rose D, Etzel R. Environmental tobacco smoke exposure and health effects in children: results from the 1991 National Health Interview Survey. Tob Control. 1996;5:13–8.

10. Stoddard JJ, Miller T. Impact of parental smoking on the prevalence of wheezing respiratory illness in children. Am J Epidemiol. 1995;141:96–102.

11. Jin C, Rossignol AM. Effects of passive smoking on respiratory illness from birth to age eighteen months, in Shanghai, People's Republic of China. J Pediatr. 1993;123:553–8.

12. Einarson A, Riordan S. Smoking in pregnancy and lactation: a review of risks and cessation strategies. Eur J Clin Pharmacol. 2009;65:325–30.

13. Ferguson BB, Wilson DJ, Schaffner W. Determination of nicotine concentrations in human milk. Am J Dis Child. 1976;130:837–9.

14. Woodward A, Douglas RM, Graham NM, Miles H. Acute respiratory illness in Adelaide children: breast feeding modifies the effect of passive smoking. J Epidemiol Community Health. 1990;44:224–30.

15. American Academy of Pediatrics, Committee on Drugs. Transfer of drugs and other chemicals into human milk. Pediatrics. 2001;108:776–89.

16. Laurberg P, Nohr SB, Pedersen KM, Fuglsang E. Iodine nutrition in breast-fed infants is impaired by maternal smoking. J Clin Endocrinol Metab. 2004;89:181–7.

17. Liu J, Rosenberg KD, Sandoval AP. Breastfeeding duration and perinatal cigarette smoking in a population-based cohort. Am J Public Health. 2006;96:309–14.

18. Hopkinson JM, Schanler RJ, Fraley JK, Garza C. Milk production by mothers of premature infants: influence of cigarette smoking. Pediatrics. 1992;90:934–8.

19. Hill PD, Aldag JC. Smoking and breastfeeding status. Res Nurs Health. 1996;19:125–32.

20. Donath SM, Amir LH. The relationship between maternal smoking and breastfeeding duration after adjustment for maternal infant feeding intention. Acta Paediatr. 2004;93:1514–8.

21. Matheson I, Rivrud GN. The effect of smoking on lactation and infantile colic. JAMA. 1989;261:42–3.

22. Soldatos CR, Kales JD, Scharf MB, Bixler EO, Kales A. Cigarette smoking associated with sleep difficulty. Science. 1980;207:551–3.

23. Mennella JA, Garcia-Gomez PL. Sleep disturbances after acute exposure to alcohol in mothers' milk. Alcohol. 2001;25:153–8.

24. Weissbluth M, Liu K. Sleep patterns, attention span, and infant temperament. J Dev Behav Pediatr. 1983;4:34–6.

25. Kahn A, Groswasser J, Sottiaux M, Rebuffat E, Franco P, Dramaix M. Prone or supine body position and sleep characteristics in infants. Pediatrics. 1993;91:1112–5.

26. Zhang L, Samet J, Caffo B, Punjabi NM. Cigarette smoking and nocturnal sleep architecture. Am J Epidemiol. 2006;164:529–37.

27. Vazquez J, Guzman-Marin R, Salin-Pascual RJ, Drucker-Colin R. Transdermal nicotine on sleep and PGO spikes. Brain Res. 1996;737:317–20.

28. Saint-Mleux B, Eggermann E, Bisetti A, et al. Nicotinic enhancement of the noradrenergic inhibition of sleep-promoting neurons in the ventrolateral preoptic area. J Neurosci. 2004;24:63–7.

29. Anderson ME, Johnson DC, Batal HA. Sudden infant death syndrome and prenatal maternal smoking: rising attributed risk in the Back to Sleep era. BMC Med. 2005;3:4.

30. Hayes MJ. Methodological issues in the study of arousal and awakening in infants. In: Salzarulo P, Ficca G, editors. Awakening and sleep-wake cycle across development. Amsterdam: John Benjamins Publishing; 2002. p. 23–45.

31. Chang AB, Wilson SJ, Masters IB, et al. Altered arousal response in infants exposed to cigarette smoke. Arch Dis Child. 2003;88:30–3.

32. Slotkin TA. Fetal nicotine or cocaine exposure: which one is worse? J Pharmacol Exp Ther. 1998;285:931–45.

33. Narayanan U, Birru S, Vaglenova J, Breese CR. Nicotinic receptor expression following nicotine exposure via maternal milk. Neuroreport. 2002;13:961–3.

34. Gomez RL, Bootzin RR, Nadel L. Naps promote abstraction in language-learning infants. Psychol Sci. 2006;17:670–4.
35. McDermott CM, LaHoste GJ, Chen C, Musto A, Bazan NG, Magee JC. Sleep deprivation causes behavioral, synaptic, and membrane excitability alterations in hippocampal neurons. J Neurosci. 2003;23:9687–95.
36. Osler M, Clausen J, Ibsen KK, Jensen G. Maternal smoking during childhood and increased risk of smoking in young adulthood. Int J Epidemiol. 1995;24:710–4.
37. Mennella JA, Jagnow CP, Beauchamp GK. Prenatal and post-natal flavor learning by human infants. Pediatrics. 2001;107(6) Available at: www.pediatrics.org/cgi/content/full/107/6/e88
38. Mennella JA, Beauchamp GK. Flavor experiences during formula feeding are related to preferences during childhood. Early Hum Dev. 2002;68:71–82.
39. Forestell CA, Mennella JA. Children's hedonic judgments of cigarette smoke odor: effects of parental smoking and maternal mood. Psychol Addict Behav. 2005;19:423–32.
40. Mascola MA, Van Vunakis H, Tager IB, Speizer FE, Hanrahan JP. Exposure of young infants to environmental tobacco smoke: breast-feeding among smoking mothers. Am J Public Health. 1998;88:893–6.
41. Schulte-Hobein B, Schwartz-Bickenbach D, Abt S, Plum C, Nau H. Cigarette smoke exposure and development of infants throughout the first year of life: influence of passive smoking and nursing on cotinine levels in breast milk and infant's urine. Acta Paediatr. 1992;81:550–7.
42. Luck W, Nau H. Nicotine and cotinine concentrations in serum and milk of nursing smokers. Br J Clin Pharmacol. 1984;18:9–15.
43. Laurberg P, Nøhr SB, Pedersen KM, Fuglsang E. Iodine nutrition in breast-fed infants is impaired by maternal smoking. J Clin Endocrinol Metab. 2004;89:181–7.
44. Bruin JE, Kellenberger LD, Gerstein HC, Morrison KM, Holloway AC. Fetal and neonatal nicotine exposure and postnatal glucose homeostasis: identifying critical windows of exposure. J Endocrinol. 2007;194:171–8.
45. Oliveira E, Moura EG, Santos-Silva AP, Fagundes AT, Rios AS, Abreu-Villaça Y, et al. Short- and long-term effects of maternal nicotine exposure during lactation on body adiposity, lipid profile, and thyroid function of rat offspring. J Endocrinol. 2009;202:397–405.